Essentials of Spinal Stabilization

Langston T. Holly • Paul A. Anderson
Editors

Essentials of Spinal Stabilization

Springer

Editors
Langston T. Holly
Department of Neurosurgery
and Orthopaedics
David Geffen UCLA School
of Medicine
Los Angeles, CA, USA

Paul A. Anderson
Department of Orthopedics and
Rehabilitation
University of Wisconsin UWMF
Madison, WI, USA

ISBN 978-3-319-59712-6   ISBN 978-3-319-59713-3 (eBook)
DOI 10.1007/978-3-319-59713-3

Library of Congress Control Number: 2017951102

Printed on acid-free paper

This Springer imprint is published by Springer Nature
The registered company is Springer International Publishing AG
The registered company address is: Gewerbestrasse 11, 6330 Cham, Switzerland

Contents

Contributors

Vincent J. Alentado, MD Indiana University, Department of Neurological Surgery, Indianapolis, IN, USA

R. Todd Allen, MD UCSD Department of Orthopaedics, San Diego, CA, USA

Paul A. Anderson, MD University of Wisconsin, Department of Orthopedic Surgery and Rehabilitation, Madison, WI, USA

Farbod Asgarzadie, MD Department of Neurosurgery, Kaiser Permanente Hospital, Fontana, CA, USA

Tyler Atkins Carolina NeuroSurgery and Spine, Charlotte, NC, USA

Rahul Basho, MD Department of Orthopaedic Surgery, Hannibal Regional Hospital, Hannibal, MO, USA

Carolina Gesteira Benjamin, MD Department of Neurosurgery, NYU Langone Medical Center, New York, NY, USA

Emily Bennett, MD Department of Neurosurgery, Cleveland Clinic, Neurological Institute, Cleveland, OH, USA

Edward C. Benzel, MD Department of Neurosurgery, Cleveland Clinic, Neurological Institute, Cleveland, OH, USA

Sigurd H. Berven, MD Department of Orthopaedic Surgery, University of California, San Francisco, CA, USA

Charles L. Branch Jr. Department of Neurosurgery, Wake Forest Baptist Medical Center, Winston Salem, NC, USA

J. Kenneth Burkus, MD Attending Physician, Spine Service, The Hughston Clinic, Columbus, GA, USA

Zorica Buser, PhD Department of Orthopaedic Surgery, Keck School of Medicine, University of Southern California, Los Angeles, CA, USA

Alvin Y. Chan, BS Department of Neurosurgery, Froedtert Hospital and the Medical College of Wisconsin, Milwaukee, WI, USA

Victor Chang, MD Department of Neurosurgery, Henry Ford Hospital, Detroit, MI, USA

Ken Hsuan-kan Chang, MD Department of Neurological Surgery and Rehabilitation Medicine, University of Miami Miller School of Medicine, Lois Pope Life Center, Miami, FL, USA

Kevin S. Chen Department of Neurosurgery, University of Michigan, Ann Arbor, MI, USA

Domagoj Coric Carolina NeuroSurgery and Spine, Charlotte, NC, USA

John Dimar, MD Norton Leatherman Spine Center, Department of Orthopaedic Surgery, University of Louisville, Louisville, KY, USA

Mladen Djurasovic, MD Norton Leatherman Spine Center, Department of Orthopaedic Surgery, University of Louisville, Louisville, KY, USA

Richard G. Fessler, MD, PhD Department of Neurological Surgery, Rush University Medical Center, Chicago, IL, USA

Jeffrey S. Fischgrund, MD Department of Orthopaedic Surgery, William Beaumont Hospital, Royal Oak, MI, USA

Anthony Frempong-Boadu, MD Department of Neurosurgery, NYU Langone Medical Center, New York, NY, USA

Mark Benjamin Frenkel, MD, MA Department of Neurosurgery, Wake Forest Baptist Medical Center, Winston Salem, NC, USA

Tristan B. Fried, BS Thomas Jefferson University Hospital, Department of Orthopedics, Philadelphia, PA, USA

Benjamin J. Geddes Department of Orthopedic Surgery, Yale University, New Haven, CT, USA

Zoher Ghogawala Department of Neurosurgery, Alan and Jacqueline Stuart Spine Research Center, Lahey Hospital and Medical Center, Burlington, MA, USA

Department of Neurosurgery, Tufts University School of Medicine, Boston, MA, USA

Jeffrey Gum, MD Norton Leatherman Spine Center, Department of Orthopaedic Surgery, University of Louisville, Louisville, KY, USA

James S. Harrop, MD, FACS Department of Neurological and Orthopedic Surgery, Division of Spine and Peripheral Nerve Surgery, Neurosurgery Director of Delaware Valley SCI Center, Thomas Jefferson University, Philadelphia, PA, USA

David J. Hart, MD Department of Neurosurgery, Wake Forest Baptist Medical Center, Winston Salem, NC, USA

Robert F. Heary, MD Department of Neurological Surgery, New Jersey Medical School, Rutgers, The State University of New Jersey, Newark, NJ, USA

Randall J. Hlubek, MD Department of Neurosurgery, Barrow Neurological Institute, St. Joseph's Hospital and Medical Center, Phoenix, AZ, USA

Douglas A. Hollern, MD Thomas Jefferson University Hospital, Department of Orthopedics, Philadelphia, PA, USA

Wellington K. Hsu, MD Department of Orthopaedic Surgery, Northwestern University Feinberg School of Medicine, Chicago, IL, USA

Andre Jakoi, MD Department of Orthopaedic Surgery, Keck School of Medicine, University of Southern California, Los Angeles, CA, USA

Jacob Januszewski Department of Neurosurgery, Barrow Neurological Institute, Phoenix, AZ, USA

Kevin L. Ju, MD Texas Back Institute, Rockwall, TX, USA

Adam S. Kanter, MD, FAANS Department of Neurological Surgery, University of Pittsburgh Medical Center, Pittsburgh, PA, USA

Dean G. Karahalios, MD Advocate Medical Group, Advocate Health Care, Downers Grove, IL, USA

Osama N. Kashlan Department of Neurosurgery, University of Michigan, Ann Arbor, MI, USA

Bhavesh Katbamna, BS Medical College of Wisconsin, Milwaukee, WI, USA

Mena Kerolus, MD Department of Neurosurgery, Rush University Medical Center, Chicago, IL, USA

Saad A. Khairi, MD Indiana University Health Neuroscience Center, Indianapolis, IN, USA

Jad G. Khalil, MD Department of Orthopaedic Surgery, William Beaumont Hospital, Royal Oak, MI, USA

Frank La Marca, MD Department of Neurosurgery, University of Michigan, Ann Arbor, MI, USA

Darren R. Lebl, MD, MBA Hospital for Special Surgery, New York, NY, USA

Gohar Majeed, DO, MSc Neurosurgery Resident, Riverside University Health System Medical Center, Moreno Valley, CA, USA

Melvin C. Makhni, MD, MBA The Spine Hospital, Columbia University Medical Center, New York, NY, USA

Michael Markowitz, DO Rowan Medical College, Philadelphia, PA, USA

David McCarthy, BS Department of Neurological Surgery and Rehabilitation Medicine, University of Miami Miller School of Medicine, Lois Pope Life Center, Miami, FL, USA

Michael M. McDowell, MD Department of Neurological Surgery, University of Pittsburgh Medical Center, Pittsburgh, PA, USA

Stephen K. Mendenhall, MD Indiana University Health Neuroscience Center, Indianapolis, IN, USA

Andrew Z. Mo, MD Lenox Hill Hospital, New York, NY, USA

Jean-Pierre Mobasser, MD Goodman Campbell Brain and Spine, Department of Neurological Surgery, Indiana University School of Medicine, Indianapolis, IN, USA

Thomas E. Mroz, MD Departments of Orthopaedic and Neurological Surgery, Cleveland Clinic, Cleveland, Ohio, USA

Jeffrey P. Mullin, MD Department of Neurosurgery, Cleveland Clinic, Neurological Institute, Cleveland, OH, USA

Praveen V. Mummaneni, MD Department of Neurological Surgery, University of California, San Francisco, CA, USA

Michael J. Musacchio Jr, MD NorthShore University HealthSystem, Neurosurgery and Spine Center, Evanston, IL, USA

Naveed Nabizadeh, MD UCSD Department of Orthopaedics, San Diego, CA, USA

Ryan Nazar, MD Department of Neurological Surgery, University of Louisville, Louisville, KY, USA

Eric W. Nottmeier, MD Department of Neurosurgery, St. Vincent's Spine and Brain Institute, Jacksonville, FL, USA

Marc R. Nuwer, MD, PhD Department of Neurology, David Geffen School of Medicine at UCLA, Los Angeles, CA, USA

Clinical Neurophysiology, Ronald Reagan UCLA Medical Center, Los Angeles, CA, USA

Josiah N. Orina, MD Department of Orthopaedic Surgery, University of California, San Francisco, CA, USA

David W. Polly Jr, MD Department of Orthopaedic Surgery, University of Minnesota, Minneapolis, MN, USA

Eric Potts, MD Goodman Campbell Brain and Spine, Department of Neurological Surgery, Indiana University School of Medicine, Indianapolis, IN, USA

John C. Quinn, MD Department of Neurological Surgery, New Jersey Medical School, Rutgers, The State University of New Jersey, Newark, NJ, USA

Vijay M. Ravindra Department of Neurosurgery, Clinical Neurosciences Center, University of Utah, Salt Lake City, UT, USA

Department of Neurosurgery, Alan and Jacqueline Stuart Spine Research Center, Lahey Hospital and Medical Center, Burlington, MA, USA

J.J. Renfrow Department of Neurosurgery, Wake Forest Baptist Medical Center, Winston Salem, NC, USA

John M. Rhee, MD Emory University, Orthopaedic Surgery, Atlanta, GA, USA

K. Daniel Riew, MD The Spine Hospital, Columbia University Medical Center, New York, NY, USA

Richard V. Roberts, MD Department of Orthopaedic Surgery, William Beaumont Hospital, Royal Oak, MI, USA

Gregory D. Schroeder, MD Thomas Jefferson University Hospital, Department of Orthopedics, Philadelphia, PA, USA

Jonathan N. Sembrano, MD Department of Orthopaedic Surgery, University of Minnesota, Minneapolis, MN, USA

Karin Swartz, MD Department of Neurosurgery, Froedtert Hospital and the Medical College of Wisconsin, Milwaukee, WI, USA

Oliver Tannous, MD Georgetown University Department of Orthopaedics, Washington, DC, USA

Nicholas Theodore, MD Barrow Neurological Institute, St. Joseph's Hospital and Medical Center, Phoenix, AZ, USA

Jason Toy Department of Orthopedic Surgery, Yale University, New Haven, CT, USA

Vincent Traynelis, MD Department of Neurosurgery, Rush University Medical Center, Chicago, IL, USA

Luis M. Tumialán, MD Department of Neurosurgery, Barrow Neurological Institute, St. Joseph's Hospital and Medical Center, Phoenix, AZ, USA

Juan S. Uribe Department of Neurosurgery, Barrow Neurological Institute, Phoenix, AZ, USA

Alexander R. Vaccaro, MD, PhD, MBA Thomas Jefferson University Hospital, Department of Orthopedics, Philadelphia, PA, USA

Payman Vahedi, MD Department of Neurosurgery at Tehran Medical Sciences Branch, Islamic Azad University, Tehran, Iran

Department of Neurosurgery, Thomas Jefferson University Hospitals, Philadelphia, PA, USA

Michael S. Virk, MD, PhD Department of Neurological Surgery, University of California, San Francisco, CA, USA

Michael Y. Wang, MD, FACS Department of Neurological Surgery and Rehabilitation Medicine, University of Miami Miller School of Medicine, Lois Pope Life Center, Miami, FL, USA

Jeffrey C. Wang, MD Department of Orthopaedic Surgery, Keck School of Medicine, University of Southern California, Los Angeles, CA, USA

Joseph A. Weiner, MD Department of Orthopaedic Surgery, Northwestern University Feinberg School of Medicine, Chicago, IL, USA

Ian K. White, MD Goodman Campbell Brain and Spine, Department of Neurological Surgery, Indiana University School of Medicine, Indianapolis, IN, USA

Robert G. Whitmore Department of Neurosurgery, Alan and Jacqueline Stuart Spine Research Center, Lahey Hospital and Medical Center, Burlington, MA, USA

Department of Neurosurgery, Tufts University School of Medicine, Boston, MA, USA

Jeff Wilson, MD PhD FRCSC St. Michael's Hospital, University of Toronto, Li Ka Shing Knowledge Institute, Toronto, ON, Canada

Christopher D. Witiw, MD Department of Neurological Surgery, Rush University Medical Center, Chicago, IL, USA

Division of Neurosurgery, Department of Surgery, University of Toronto, Toronto, ON, Canada

Jau-Ching Wu, MD, PhD Department of Neurosurgery, Taipei Veterans' General Hospital, Taipei, Taiwan

School of Medicine, National Yang-Ming University, Taipei, Taiwan

Jang W. Yoon, MD, MS Department of Neurosurgery, Mayo Clinic, Jacksonville, FL, USA

Sharon C. Yson, MD Department of Orthopaedic Surgery, University of Minnesota, Minneapolis, MN, USA

James J. Yue Department of Orthopedic Surgery, Yale University, New Haven, CT, USA

Hesham Mostafa Zakaria, MD Department of Neurosurgery, Henry Ford Hospital, Detroit, MI, USA

FeiFei Zhou, MD Peking University Third Hospital, Orthopaedics, Beijing, China

Cervical Traction and Reduction Techniques

1

Tristan B. Fried, Douglas A. Hollern, Michael Markowitz, Gregory D. Schroeder, and Alexander R. Vaccaro

Introduction

The current role of nonoperative techniques for the cervical spine is controversial, but it is critical that all spine surgeons have the ability to perform a closed reduction in their repertoire [1]. Closed reduction may be followed by treatment in a halo orthosis or a cervical collar as the definitive method of treatment, or it may be used in the initial phase as an adjunct to eventual surgical stabilization [1]. A closed reduction is almost exclusively performed for injuries in the cervical spine, but there are a variety of fractures and dislocations of the cervical vertebrae that can be corrected using closed reduction techniques.

Indications and Patient Selection

The primary indication for a closed reduction of a spinal injury is a displaced cervical fracture or dislocation that is either compressing the neural elements or a cervical injury that is unstable and has the possibility of compressing the neural elements [2]. Specifically, cervical traction can be used to treat cervical facet subluxations/dislocations, AOSpine C type (Translation) injuries, burst fractures, displaced odontoid fractures, and displaced hangman's fractures (with the exception of IIa fractures) [1, 3]. If a patient has an incomplete neurologic injury with continued spinal cord compression, urgent spinal cord decompression is recommended [4]. Surgeons should know the capabilities of their institution, and if a surgical decompression cannot be done expeditiously, a closed reduction should be performed [2].

Pre-procedure Considerations

Before inserting the Gardner-Wells tongs, the patient must be checked for coexisting injuries. If fractures of the skull are discovered, then other options should be explored; however not all skull fractures are a contraindication to traction (such as base of the skull fractures), and so traction may still be used if the fracture and its distribution are thoroughly understood. The use of

T.B. Fried, BS (✉) • D.A. Hollern, MD
G.D. Schroeder, MD • A.R. Vaccaro, MD, PhD, MBA
Thomas Jefferson University Hospital, Department of Orthopedics, Philadelphia, PA, USA
e-mail: tristanbfried@gmail.com; doughollern@gmail.com; gregdschroeder@gmail.com; alex.vaccaro@rothmaninstitute.com

M. Markowitz, DO
Rowan Medical College, Philadelphia, PA, USA
e-mail: mmarkowitz22@gmail.com

L.T. Holly, P.A. Anderson (eds.), *Essentials of Spinal Stabilization*,
DOI 10.1007/978-3-319-59713-3_1

Gardner-Wells tongs is contraindicated if there are soft tissue injuries near the traction site [1]. Another consideration is the choice of traction tong to be used during the reduction. Although there are tongs that are compatible with MRI, these tongs are not able to bear as much weight. Therefore when using traction for injuries in which a significant amount of weight may be needed, such as a C7/T1 facet dislocations, stainless steel tongs should be used as opposed to MRI compatible tongs [2].

Before any intervention begins, it must be assured that the facilities used have the proper equipment to handle a reduction, as well as the possible complications. This must include access to an MRI which is necessary if there is any rapid deterioration of neurological signs. Before beginning the procedure, a neurological examination should be taken to serve as a baseline for repeat neurological exams during the procedure [5].

Technique

Gardner-Wells Traction

The first step is clear identification of the injury using CT or radiographs of the cervical spine. After identification, the patient is prepared in a RotoRest bed (KCI, San Antonio, Texas) or Stryker bed (Stryker, Kalamazoo, Michigan), and the skin is prepped with an iodine solution [5]. Most commonly Gardner-Wells tongs are applied approximately 5–10 mm above the pinna of the ear in line with the external auditory meatus. It is critical that the pins are located below the equator of the skull to prevent the pins from pulling out after weight is applied. The pins should be tightened until the force indicator is approximately 1 mm above the surface, which is 31 lbs of force [1]. Importantly, while the risk of overtightening the spring-loaded pins exists, penetration of the inner table of the skull leading to abscess or hemorrhage is a rare complication. Cadaveric studies demonstrated nearly 162 pounds of force were necessary to penetrate the inner table of the skull, whereas only 30 pounds were needed to secure the pins appropriately [6]. A folded towel may be used under the patient's neck in order to get an improved angle for the reduction. Intravenous narcotics for pain control and muscle relaxation can be administered, but it is critical the patient be awake and alert and able to participate in a reliable neurologic exam [1]. The placement of the tongs more anteriorly or posteriorly depends on the direction in which the vector of force must be applied. Anterior application of the tongs will lead to extension of the neck, while posterior placement will lead to flexion of the cervical spine. Posterior placement of the pins can be beneficial in cervical facet dislocations, as often a significant flexion moment is needed in the reduction. If an anterior application of the tongs is used, they must avoid the temporalis muscle and superficial temporal artery and vein [5].

Patient positioning is crucial when administering tong traction. While supine positioning is preferred, the use of reverse Trendelenburg or the application of arm/leg weights should be utilized to counteract the traction weight as it is added to the skull throughout treatment. When using beds designed for traction, often shoulder rests are present to prevent translation of the entire body when traction is applied [2]. Prior to placing any weight on the tongs, a thorough neurologic exam should be performed and documented. Similarly, every time any weight is added, a thorough neurologic exam should be performed and documented. If at any time the patient begins to have new neurologic symptoms, the closed reduction should be aborted, and the patient should undergo urgent MR scanning prior to surgical intervention. Traction should begin at 5–10 pounds and steadily increased with 5–10-pound increments every 10–20 min in concurrence with serial neurologic and radiographic studies [7]. The patient must remain alert and oriented and able to participate in the exam after the addition of increased weight [2]. This method helps prevent over distraction of an already unstable injury as well as avoidance of muscle spasms derived from the traction itself. It is important to note that physical manipulation to recreate some of the deforming forces (i.e., increased cervical flexion in a flexion distraction injury) may be needed to help unlock the injury, but this should be done with caution, as excessive manipulation may result in further compression on the spinal cord. Additionally, in a unilaterally dislocated cervical facet, an axial load applied directly to the located facet while the head is rotated 30–40° past midline toward the injured facet may aid in the reduction [8].

Once reduction has been accomplished, the cervical pathology will then dictate the next step. In a cervical facet dislocation, once the facets are relocated, all but 10–20 pounds of weight can be removed, and the patient can remain in the RotoRest bed until surgical stabilization is performed. Alternatively the patient may be placed in slight cervical extension in a halo vest. If traction is being used in the setting of a burst fracture with retropulsion, the weight needed to decompress the spine through ligamentotaxis may remain on the tongs (10–20 lbs) until surgical decompression occurs.

Halo Traction

The initial evaluation and the actual reduction technique are almost identical when performing a reduction with halo traction compared to Gardner-Wells tongs; however attachment of the halo to the patient is significantly different. Initially the ring should be appropriately sized to fit with at least 1 cm of clearance between all points of the head and attached via the four pin sites [7]. With halo traction the optimal pin sites anteriorly are the anterolateral areas of the skull, about 1 cm superior to the orbital rim, superior to the lateral two thirds of the orbit, and inferior to the greatest circumference of the skull bilaterally [9]. While lateral placement is more ideal, attention to the temporal fossa is also critical as this bone is thin and in close proximity to the muscles of mastication and the zygomaticotemporal nerve [10]. The exact pin placement posteriorly is not as crucial, as the skull is more uniform and thicker, and neither neuromuscular nor vascular structures are not in harm's way. Initial data suggested that pins only be inserted with a torque of 5–6 inches/pound, but that changed when cadaveric studies determined up to 10 inches/pound of torque can be used to secure pins in place safely. Recently, it has been determined that a torque of 8 inches/pound was preferred during traction-reduction with minimal incidence of pin loosening and infection [9]. While the authors routinely use Gardner-Wells tongs for traction if the patient is going to require surgery, if the injury is to be treated definitely in a halo orthosis, the authors will use a halo for traction, and once the reduction is achieved, the reduction can be locked into place with the halo vest orthosis.

Head-Halter Traction

A third, however rarely used way to perform cervical traction is through a head-halter apparatus. This apparatus is preferred by some because it is entirely noninvasive; however it is not the author's choice because it is unable to handle the same amount of weight as tongs. Head-halter traction is also associated with the complication of temporomandibular joint pain. As a result of these factors, this device is not commonly used outside of pediatric atlantoaxial subluxation/fixation [8].

Illustrative Case

This is a 45-year-old man who slipped and fell down the steps in his house. He was brought to the emergency room with severe neck pain, but neurologically intact. A cervical spine computed tomography (CT) scan demonstrated a Type III odontoid fracture that was anteriorly displaced by 7.5 mm (Fig. 1.1). The decision was made to perform a closed reduction and treatment in a halo vest. The patient was placed prone on a RotorRest bed, and the aforementioned technique for halo traction was performed. Initial radiographs demonstrated continued anterior displacement of the odontoid fracture (Fig. 1.2a), and 10 pounds of weight was added in a posterior vector, and 10 pounds of weight was added in superior (distraction) vector (bivector traction). A neurologic exam showed no changes, but radiographic alignment also did not change (Fig. 1.2b). Another 10 pounds was added in both the

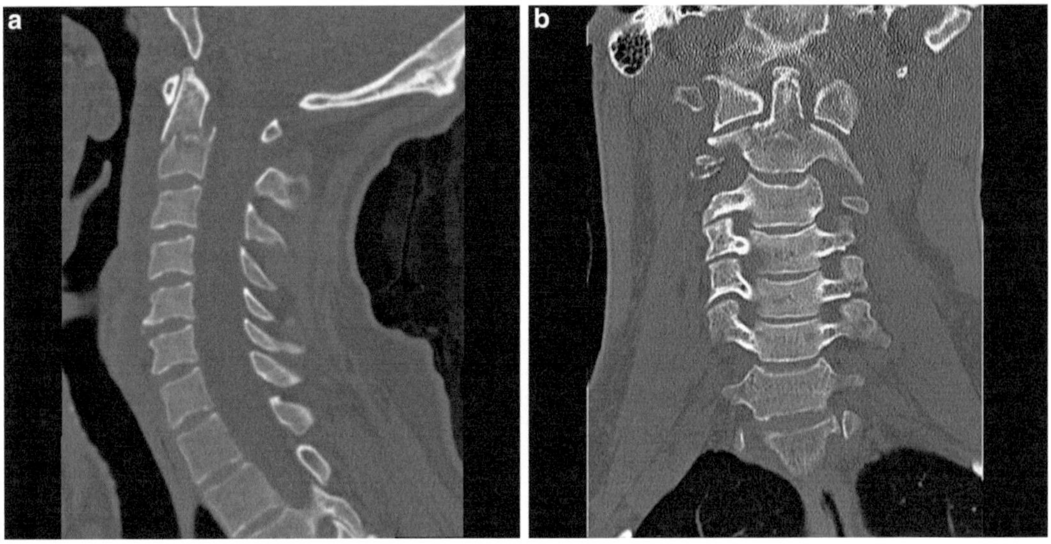

Fig. 1.1 Sagittal (**a**) and coronal (**b**) CT scan demonstrating a type III odontoid fracture with 7.5 mm of anterior translation

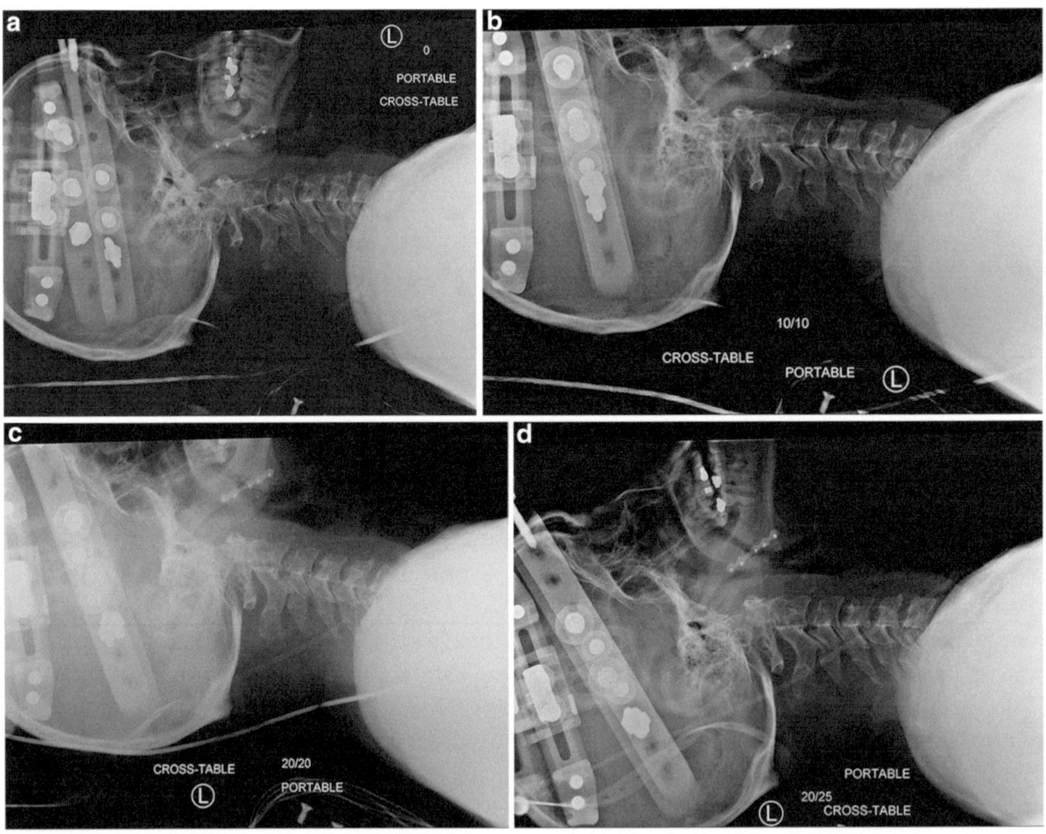

Fig. 1.2 Initial radiographs demonstrated continued anterior displacement of the odontoid fracture (**a**); 10 pounds of weight was added in a posterior vector, and 10 pounds of weight was added in superior (distraction) vector (**b**). Another 10 pounds was added in both the posterior and superior vectors (**c**), followed by an additional five pounds to the superior vector (**d**). The patient had no neurologic changes, but also had no significant change in radiographic alignment

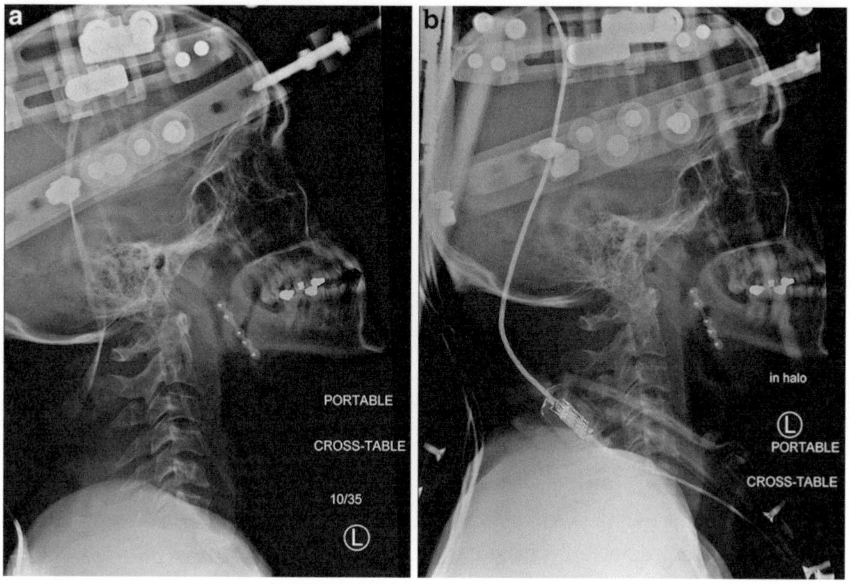

Fig. 1.3 After gentle manipulation of the fracture, a significant reduction was achieved (**a**), and final upright radiographs in the halo orthosis demonstrated 2.7 mm of anterior translation (down from 7.5 mm)

posterior and superior vectors, followed by an additional five pounds to the superior vector. The patient experienced no neurologic changes, but there was significant change in radiographic alignment (Fig. 1.2c, d). The decision was made to gently manipulate the fracture. The weight was taken off of the posterior vector, and a small flexion moment was placed by the surgeon on the halo. This recreation of the deformity "unlocked the fracture," and then 35 lbs of weight was placed in a superior vector, and 10 lbs was placed in a posterior vector. No neurologic changes were noted after manipulation, and a significant reduction was achieved (Fig. 1.3a). The halo ring was connected to the halo vest, and the weight was removed. Final upright radiographs demonstrated 2.7 mm of anterior fracture displacement, and so the patient was treated definitively in a halo orthosis (Fig. 1.3b).

Technical Pearls

- All patients should be awake, alert, and able to cooperate with a neurologic exam prior to the closed reduction of a cervical spine injury. After every incremental increase in weight, a repeat neurologic exam must be performed.
- The use of a bed designed for a closed reduction is critical. These beds will often allow for multivector traction that allows for both a distraction and a flexion moment. Additionally, it is often possible to remove the headpiece to create an extension moment. These complex vectors may be needed for different fracture patterns (such as the one in the case illustration), and achieving them on a bed not designed for cervical traction can be challenging.
- Tong pin placement is critical [1]. When flexion is required a more posterior pin placement relative to the tragus of the ear is beneficial, and when extension is desired, pins should be placed more anteriorly. Additionally, if the pins are placed asymmetric, there may be an unwanted rotational vector on the cervical spine [8].
- If possible have a digital X-Ray machine in the room, so time is not wasted as the technician is running to develop the film.
- Similar to fractures elsewhere, slight manipulation to "recreate the deformity" may be needed

to allow for fracture site disengagement in order to achieve an adequate reduction. Any manipulation should be done with extreme caution, particularly in patients with spinal cord compression.

- If the patient is going to be treated definitively in a halo vest orthosis, consider using the halo ring for traction rather than Gardner-Wells tongs.

Complications and Strategies for Avoidance

Since Fehlings et al. demonstrated superior long-term neurologic improvement in patients who underwent early decompression of the cervical spinal cord after injury, it is clear that expeditiously decompressing the neurologic elements is paramount [4]. However, cases of neurologic worsening during a closed reduction leading to displacement of a large disk herniation into the spinal cord have made the exact treatment algorithm of cervical facet dislocations controversial [11]. Often the diagnosis of a facet dislocation can be made on a cross table radiograph in the trauma bay, and the quickest way to decompress the spinal cord would be to perform a closed reduction at that time; however at many institutions, surgeons prefer to initially obtain an MRI to evaluate for the presence of a herniated disk or hematoma. The need for this delay was questioned by Vaccaro et al. when they reported on nine patients who had dislocated cervical facets. All nine patients had a prereduction MRI, and two of the nine had disk herniation identified on the MRI. A closed reduction was then performed on all patients, and none had worsening of their neurologic status. Additionally, all patients underwent a postreduction MRI, and five patients had a herniated disk after closed reduction. Based on these results, the authors stated that it was likely safe to perform a closed reduction in an awake, alert, and cooperative patient [12].

In patients with a cervical facet dislocation, the authors propose the following algorithm. If the patient has dislocated cervical facets, but is neurologically intact or has an incomplete spinal cord injury, an initial closed skeletal reduction may be safely performed prior to obtaining an MRI in an awake, alert, and examinable patient. Alternatively, an MRI may be obtained prior to an open or closed reduction. The urgency of a decompression is significantly less in a neurologically intact patient, and the delay in obtaining an MRI is negligible. Conversely, if the patient has a complete spinal cord injury, they should undergo a closed reduction as soon as the injury is identified, as there is little risk of worsening the neurologic outcome. Any patients who are not awake, alert, and cooperative should undergo an MRI prior to reduction. Lastly, the closed reduction should be stopped immediately if the patient begins to have worsening neurologic symptoms.

While halo and Gardner-Wells traction are effective methods of cervical traction, the pin placements for each may be problematic if placed improperly. Halo pin placement should take place with the patient's eyes closed. This is to reduce tethering of the skin and to avoid the inability to close the eyes. Incorrect anterior pin placement has been noted to cause injury to the supraorbital and supratrochlear nerve, while penetration directly into the frontal sinus or orbit is possible with excessive pin tightening [7]. To avoid complication, areas where pin placement can be safely applied have been defined at approximately 1 cm above the orbital rim, remaining below the equator of the skull, and above the lateral two thirds of the orbit [9]. It is also of importance to avoid too lateral pin placement as there is risk of compromising the temporalis muscle and the zygomaticotemporal nerve. Complications include impedance of mandibular motion and increased risk of skull penetration in this area. Posterior pin sites, while less dangerous to the immediate anatomic structures, should be placed inferior to the widest portion of the skull but superior enough to minimize potential cephalad pin migration and to avoid ring impingement on the upper helix of the ear [7].

Garner-Wells tongs unlike halo devices only require the placement of two pins. Appropriate pin site insertion is most effective at 1 cm above the pinna, lined up with external auditory meatus, and inferior to the equator of the skull [2]. With pin site insertion, care must be taken as there is risk of puncturing the superficial temporal artery or penetration to the temporalis muscle. Similar to complications of halo pin placement, effects of this complication include impedance of mandibular motion and increased risk of skull penetration [7]. Pins should also be angled upward with simultaneous tightening on insertion until the spring-loaded indicator protrudes 1 mm above the flat surface of the pin head. Avoid overtightening as it may result in penetration of the skull leading to potential abscess or hemorrhage [2, 13].

Other issues common to both treatment modalities include loosening and infection at pin sites. This is much more of an issue when patients are treated definitively in a halo orthosis; however this also can happen if patients undergo a closed reduction to temporarily stabilize the cervical spine, and surgical management is delayed. It has been reported that the pins loosen in up to 36–60% of patients treated with a halo orthosis. Pin site infection has been seen to occur in 20% of patient cases [14]. When suspicious of infection exists, measures must be taken immediately to prevent long-term complications. First, it is appropriate to obtain bacterial cultures, begin antibiotic therapy, and determine appropriate alternative pin location. Rarely the pin can penetrate the skull; failure to resolve an infected pin within the skull has been seen to cause abscess formation and severe neurologic sequelae. Alarming symptoms include generalized signs of infection, headaches, seizures, disorientation, and psychosis. While skull penetration is often a cause of pin overtightening, care must be taken to appropriately fixate the pins with the right amount of pressure. Typical pressures to achieve skull penetration are much lower than necessary to secure the pins appropriately, making this error rare. Application with routine pin tightening at 1 day and 1 week after halo fixation and every 24 h for Garner-Wells tongs has been proven safe to secure and minimize pin penetration into the skull [14].

Conclusion

Devices designed to provide cervical traction deliver the necessary support for correction of the pathologic process while simultaneously risking the development of dangerous complications. These complications surrounding cervical traction vary in severity but should always be addressed and corrected immediately upon discovery. Cervical traction is indicated for numerous cervical spine pathologies with the goal of spinal reduction and prevention or recovery of neurologic damage. While the ideal protocol for handling cervical spine pathologies remains controversial, the use of traction-reduction can be beneficial for many injuries.

References

1. Vaccaro AR, Betz RR, Zeidman SM. Principles and practice of spine surgery, vol. xxi. St. Louis: Mosby; 2003. p. 864.
2. Vaccaro AR, Albert TJ. Spine surgery: tricks of the trade. 3rd ed. New York: Thieme; 2016.
3. Vaccaro AR, Koerner JD, Radcliff KE, Oner FC, Reinhold M, Schnake KJ, et al. AOSpine subaxial cervical spine injury classification system. Eur Spine J. 2015;25(7):2173–2184.
4. Fehlings MG, Vaccaro A, Wilson JR, Singh A, David WC, Harrop JS, et al. Early versus delayed decompression for traumatic cervical spinal cord injury: results of the surgical timing in acute spinal cord injury study (STASCIS). PLoS One. 2012;7(2):e32037.
5. Vaccaro AR, Baron EM. Spine surgery, vol. xviii. Philadelphia: Saunders/Elsevier; 2008. p. 481.
6. Lerman JA, Dickman CA, Haynes RJ. Penetration of cranial inner table with Gardner-Wells tongs. J Spinal Disord. 2001;14(3):211–3.
7. Wang JH, Daniels AH, Palumbo MA, Eberson CP. Cervical traction for the treatment of spinal injury and deformity. JBJS Rev. 2014;2(5):1.
8. Vaccaro AR. Fractures of the cervical, thoracic, and lumbar spine, vol. xvii. New York: M. Dekker; 2003. p. 751.
9. Botte MJ, Byrne TP, Abrams RA, Garfin SR. Halo skeletal fixation: techniques of application and prevention of complications. J Am Acad Orthop Surg. 1996;4(1):44–53.
10. Lauweryns P. Role of conservative treatment of cervical spine injuries. Eur Spine J. 2010;19(Suppl 1):S23–6.

11. Eismont FJ, Arena MJ, Green BA. Extrusion of an intervertebral disc associated with traumatic subluxation or dislocation of cervical facets. Case report. J Bone Joint Surg Am. 1991;73(10):1555–60.
12. Vaccaro AR, Falatyn SP, Flanders AE, Balderston RA, Northrup BE, Cotler JM. Magnetic resonance evaluation of the intervertebral disc, spinal ligaments, and spinal cord before and after closed traction reduction of cervical spine dislocations. Spine (Phila Pa 1976). 1999;24(12):1210–7.
13. Saeed MU, Dacuycuy MA, Kennedy DJ. Halo pin insertion-associated brain abscess: case report and review of literature. Spine (Phila Pa 1976). 2007;32(8):E271–4.
14. Gelalis ID, Christoforou G, Motsis E, Arnaoutoglou C, Xenakis T. Brain abscess and generalized seizure caused by halo pin intracranial penetration: case report and review of the literature. Eur Spine J. 2009;18(Suppl 2):172–5.

Halo Vest Immobilization

2

Randall J. Hlubek and Nicholas Theodore

Abbreviations

CT Computed tomography
MR Magnetic resonance

Introduction

Cervical orthoses are used to restrict movement and maintain proper spinal alignment in patients with a wide range of spinal pathology, including trauma, deformity, and tumor. Halo vest immobilization with pin fixation to the skull has been considered the gold standard for external immobilization of the cervical spine since it was first introduced by Perry and Nickel in 1959 [1]. A number of biomechanical studies have quantified the degree of cervical immobilization provided by the halo vest [2–5]. Schneider et al. [6] performed a biomechanical evaluation of intervertebral motion for seven cervical orthoses in 45 healthy adult volunteers. The halo vest was the most effective orthosis for limiting axial rotation and lateral bending. Although the halo vest is most effective in restricting motion below the C2 level compared to more cranial levels [4], Richter et al. [7] demonstrated that it is still the most effective brace for restricting motion in the upper cervical spine (C1-2,C2-3). The halo may provide superior immobilization compared to other braces; however, the device is less effective in restricting motion at levels with instability and at the occipitocervical junction and in cervicothoracic regions [5]. Thus, careful clinical and radiographic follow-up of each patient should be conducted in all cases of spinal instability to ensure that the halo is adequately restricting motion and that alternative treatment (i.e., surgical fixation and fusion) is not warranted.

External immobilization with the halo device has several advantages to surgical fixation and fusion. First, the halo device may be motion-sparing when treating pathology such as hangman's fractures and odontoid fractures. After the injured portion of the spine has healed, the patient will most likely regain range of motion, which would not be the case with most surgical techniques that require fixation and fusion. Another advantage is that the halo device eliminates the risks of surgery, which may be substantial in some patients, such as those that have suffered trauma with multisystem injuries. Finally, halo vest immobilization can be used as a temporizing

R.J. Hlubek, MD
Department of Neurosurgery, Barrow Neurological Institute, St. Joseph's Hospital and Medical Center, Phoenix, AZ, USA

N. Theodore, MD (✉)
Barrow Neurological Institute, St. Joseph's Hospital and Medical Center, Phoenix, AZ 85013, USA
e-mail: Neuropub@dignityhealth.org

L.T. Holly, P.A. Anderson (eds.), *Essentials of Spinal Stabilization*,
DOI 10.1007/978-3-319-59713-3_2

measure to treat highly unstable spinal injuries while preparing patients for surgery, and it can be used in the operating room for positioning because the halo can be attached directly to the Mayfield head holder.

Although the halo device may be the most effective device for external immobilization of the cervical spine, it is not completely benign. The halo device has been shown to impair vital functions such as swallowing [8], respiratory function [9], and mobilization [10] because of the vest's significant weight and constriction. Complications associated with the halo device include infection at the pin site, pin loosening, decubitus ulcers, cerebral abscess, nonunion, and death [11–14]. The elderly are particularly vulnerable to serious complications with the halo device. Horn et al. [14] performed a retrospective review of patients 70 years of age or older who were treated with halo vest immobilization. Of the 53 patients identified, four patients developed respiratory distress, six developed dysphagia, and ten developed pin-related complications. Eight deaths occurred, of which six were secondary to respiratory distress and cardiovascular collapse. Thus, it is imperative to consider whether the patient is healthy enough to tolerate halo vest placement.

Indications and Patient Selection

The indications for halo vest application remain a topic of considerable debate. Pathological entities that may be treated with halo vest immobilization include fractures of the cervical spine that do not significantly compress the spinal cord or spinal nerves. Examples of fractures of the upper cervical spine that may be treated with the halo vest include: Jefferson fractures, type II and type III odontoid fractures, hangman's fractures, and various combinations of C1 and C2 fractures [15]. Other indications for the use of halo devices include preoperative traction for spinal deformity. Halo-gravity traction has been shown to achieve partial correction of cervical deformity and may decrease the extent of the osteotomy needed to achieve correction of spinal alignment in some cases [16].

Absolute contraindications for halo vest placement include skull fractures and scalp lacerations at the pin sites. Relative contraindications include elderly patients, impairment of pulmonary function, and barrel-shaped chest.

Preoperative Considerations

Several factors must be considered before nonoperative management with a halo vest is attempted. One of the most important considerations is whether the patient will tolerate halo vest immobilization. Elderly patients and patients with poor pulmonary function may not tolerate the significant weight and constriction of the halo vest. Instead, these patients may require nonoperative management with a rigid cervical collar or operative intervention if more rigid fixation is required to treat the instability.

Before application of the halo vest, the computed tomography (CT) of the patient's head (if available) should be carefully analyzed. It is important to note the location and extent of the frontal sinus in order to prevent perforation of the sinus. In additional, the patient should be evaluated for any skull fractures that may preclude placement of halo pins.

The preoperative alignment of the cervical spine must be evaluated to determine which maneuvers are necessary to achieve immobilization in the ideal alignment. For example, if the patient has a fracture with subsequent cervical kyphosis, the patient's spine may need to be immobilized in extension to achieve a more lordotic alignment.

During halo placement, appropriate placement of the pins is key to avoid complications. Careful preoperative planning should include evaluation of CT of the head to determine the location and extent of the frontal sinus. Perforation of an enlarged frontal sinus with a pin can result in intracranial infection, cerebrospinal fluid leak, or pneumocephaly [17, 18]. Options for safe zones for the anterior pins include the supraorbital location and the frontolateral location. The supraorbital location is 1 cm above the lateral two-thirds of the orbital rim (Fig. 2.1).

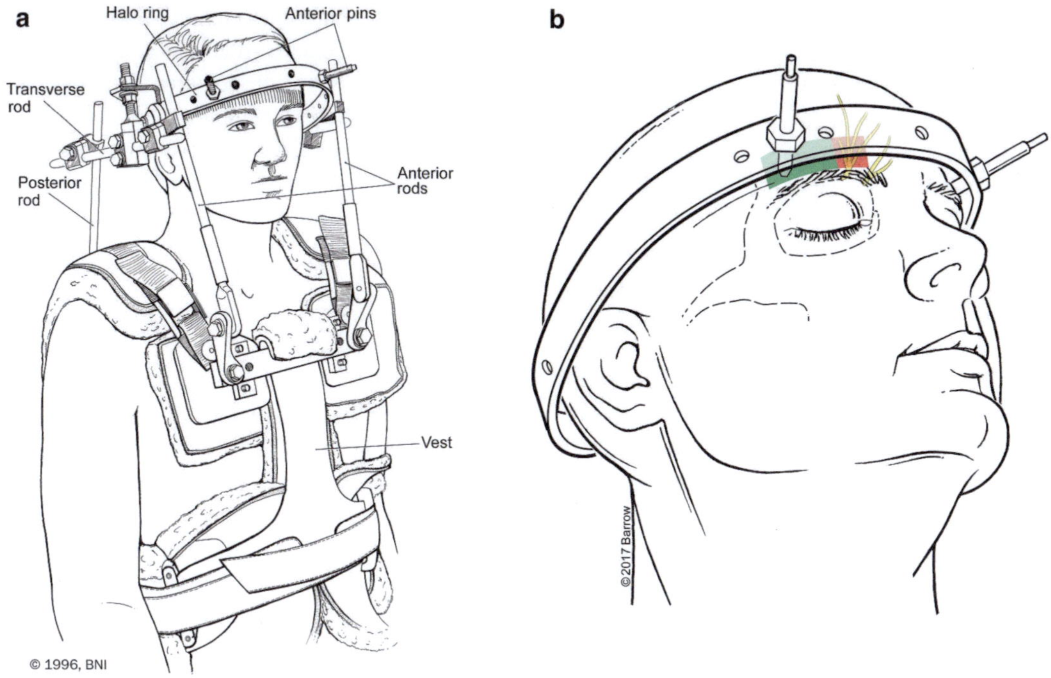

Fig. 2.1 (**a**) Illustration of the halo vest components. (**b**) Locations of the safe zone for the anterior pin (*green*) and the danger zone (*red*) where the supraorbital nerve resides (Used with permission from Barrow Neurological Institute, Phoenix, Arizona)

This area avoids the supratrochlear nerve, the supraorbital nerve, and the frontal sinus [13, 19]. The frontolateral location is just anterior to the triangular portion of the temporal hairline and thus may produce a more cosmetically acceptable result [20]. For either the supraorbital or frontolateral location, another key structure to avoid is the temporalis muscle, because pin penetration of the temporalis muscle, given its role as a muscle of mastication, is painful. The typical posterior pin placement is posterior and cranial to the ear in the temporo-occipital region, with the pins placed diagonal to the contralateral anterior pins [13, 19].

Surgical Technique

Before the halo vest is applied, intravenous muscle relaxants may be administered to provide mild sedative and musculoskeletal relaxant effects, as well as analgesic effects. However, it is important that the patient be alert enough to cooperate with the placement of the halo vest. The patient is placed supine on a flat bed, with the patient's cervical spine in a neutral position with the cranial-most portion of the head partially overhanging the bed. Strict cervical spine precautions should be maintained throughout the procedure. The circumference of the patient's head is measured across the greatest circumference of the skull, which is approximately one-half inch above the ears, to determine the appropriate ring size. The ring size should allow for 1 to 2 cm between the ring and the skull for patient comfort and for cleaning purposes. The chest circumference should then be measured at the level of the xiphoid process to determine the size of the vest. The sternal length is then measured and is used to determine the vest size.

One of the most important steps in applying the halo vest is ensuring that the spine is in an ideal alignment. A rolled-up towel may be placed under the neck/interscapular region to modify the alignment as desired. If the roll is placed closer to the interscapular region, then the cervical spine will achieve a more lordotic position. If it is placed in a more cranial position along the neck, then the cervical spine will be in a more kyphotic position.

A cotton stockinette liner is then rolled up from the patient's waist to just below the patient's axillae.

With the help of an assistant to ensure that strict cervical spine precautions are maintained, the patient is logrolled to one side, and the posterior vest is placed before the patient is rolled back to the supine position. The anterior vest is then applied, and care is taken to ensure that the sternal notch and clavicles are not compressed.

The appropriate pin sites are then chosen (see Technical Pearls), and the hair is then clipped at the desired sites. The pin sites are prepared using sterile technique with chlorhexidine swabs and then anesthetized with 1% lidocaine with epinephrine. The patient's head and neck are stabilized manually by the assistant during placement of the ring. The ring should be placed as low as possible without allowing it to touch the ears or eyebrows. The pins are then placed at their desired locations. The pins should be finger tightened in opposing pairs. The pins are then tightened with a torque driver to 8 in-lb in adults and 4 in-lb in small children. Typically, 4–6 pins are used in adult patients, and 8 pins are used in pediatric patients. Studies have shown that 8 in-lb of force is safe and optimal for anterior and posterior pin placement [21, 22]. Again, the pins should be tightened in an opposing fashion so that the ring is equidistant to the skull circumferentially. The jam nuts are tightened against the halo ring to prevent inadvertent protrusion of the pins. The pins are tightened again after 24 h to the same torque initially used.

Once the ring is secured, the head position is maintained as the bilateral posterior, and anterior rods are attached and secured to the ring via the superstructure composed of ring attachment disk, distraction assembly, and a transverse rod (Fig. 2.1).

All bolts and straps are then rechecked to ensure that they are adequately secured. Cervical radiographs are obtained in supine and upright positions to ensure preservation of optimal alignment. If alignment is not adequate, then the upright rods and halo ring may be adjusted accordingly to find the optimal position for healing.

Finally, daily hygiene is important for the prevention of pin-site infections. Pin sites should be cleaned daily with either hydrogen peroxide or normal saline.

Illustrative Case

History and Examination

A 40-year-old man presented to the trauma bay after a motor vehicle accident. Physical examination revealed tenderness to palpation in his cervical spine but no neurological deficits. The patient reported no significant past medical history.

Imaging

CT imaging of the cervical spine demonstrated a C2 hangman's fracture (Fig. 2.2). CT angiography revealed a traumatic dissection of the right vertebral artery along the distal V2 and V3 segment. The patient administered a 325 mg dose of aspirin for treatment of the dissection and to prevent thromboembolic stroke.

Treatment

The patient was considered for surgical fixation and fusion to treat the hangman's fracture. However, several factors persuaded us to attempt treatment with external immobilization with a halo vest. First, the patient had no injury to the C2-3 disk space and no compression of the spinal cord on magnetic resonance (MR) imaging. Second, the risk of injury to the left vertebral artery during surgical fixation and fusion was concerning given the traumatic dissection of the right vertebral artery. Third, the patient was young and healthy without any contraindications for halo placement.

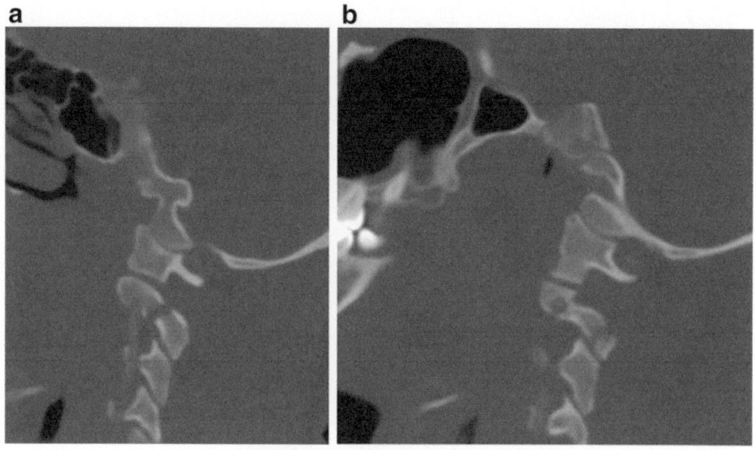

Fig. 2.2 Sagittal computed tomography (CT) images of the cervical spine showing a C2 hangman's fracture in a patient who suffered a neck injury in a motor vehicle accident. CT images showing fractures of the (**a**) right and (**b**) left C2 pars (Used with permission from Barrow Neurological Institute, Phoenix, Arizona)

Outcome

After placement of the halo, upright lateral radiography of the cervical spine was obtained to ensure ideal alignment (Fig. 2.3). At the patient's 2-month follow-up, CT imaging revealed evidence of a healing fracture, with bone beginning to bridge the fracture (Fig. 2.4). The halo vest was continued for another month, after which flexion/extension radiography of the cervical spine was obtained. The radiographs revealed complete fusion of the fracture and no instability (Fig. 2.5). The halo vest was removed at this time, and the patient was placed in a rigid cervical collar. The purpose of the cervical collar was to wean the patient from immobilization of the neck muscles and allow him to gradually build up his paraspinal muscle strength. This collar was continued for 2 weeks, at which time he was instructed to wean himself from it as tolerated.

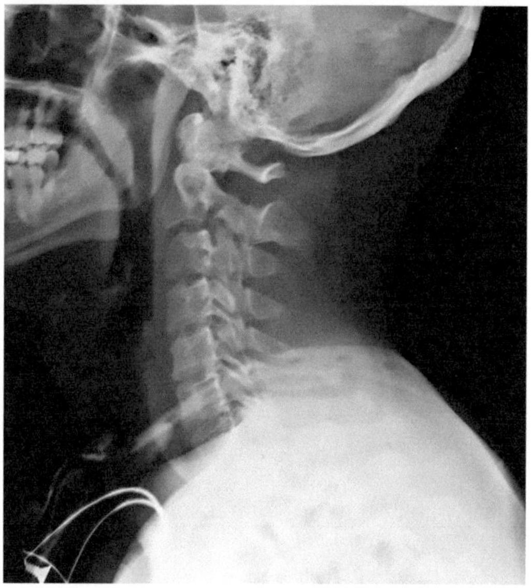

Fig. 2.3 After halo placement, proper alignment of the spine is verified by upright lateral radiography of the cervical spine (Used with permission from Barrow Neurological Institute, Phoenix, Arizona)

Technical Pearls

- Appropriate placement of the pins is key to avoiding complications. Careful preoperative planning should include evaluation of CT of the head to determine the location and extent of the frontal sinus.
- Safe zones for the anterior pins include a supraorbital location or a frontolateral location. The supraorbital location is 1 cm above the lateral two-thirds of the orbital rim. The frontolateral location is located just anterior to the triangular portion of the temporal hairline and may produce a more cosmetically acceptable result [20].
- During insertion of the anterior skull pins, it is imperative for the patient to close his or her eyes to prevent skin bunching.
- Avoid pin penetration of the temporalis muscle.
- Posterior pin placement is posterior and cranial to the ear in the temporo-occipital region

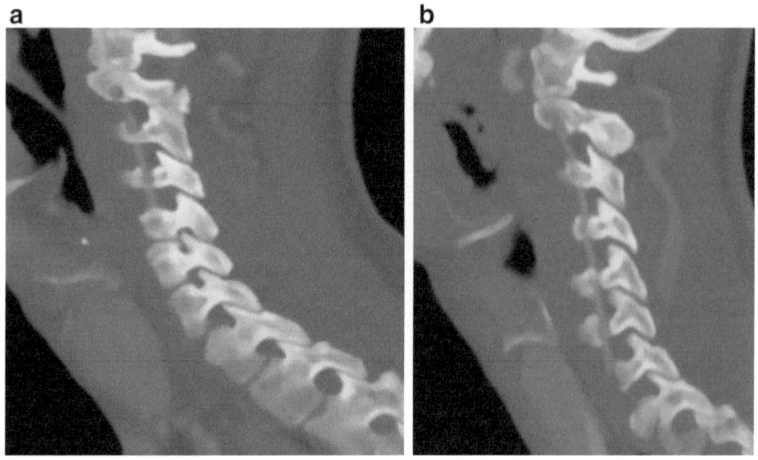

Fig. 2.4 Computed tomography (CT) images at the patient's 2-month follow-up revealed evidence of a healing fracture with bone beginning to bridge the fracture. CT images showing fractures of the (**a**) left and (**b**) right C2 pars (Used with permission from Barrow Neurological Institute, Phoenix, Arizona)

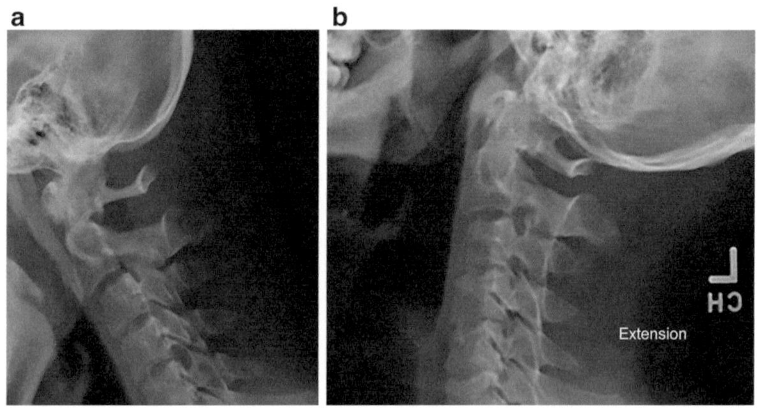

Fig. 2.5 One month later, (**a**) flexion and (**b**) extension radiographs of the cervical spine revealed no instability and complete fusion of the fracture (Used with permission from Barrow Neurological Institute, Phoenix, Arizona)

and diagonal to the contralateral anterior pins [13, 19].

- Care should be taken to place pins completely perpendicular to the skull in order to achieve the most rigid fixation and prevent slippage and subsequent scalp laceration.
- The vest should be carefully inspected after placement to ensure that all bony prominences are adequately padded in order to prevent skin ulcerations.

Complications and Strategies for Avoidance

Pin loosening is the most common complication of halo fixation, and compressive forces decrease an average of 83% during the halo treatment period, thereby compromising immobilization [12]. It is important that the pins be torqued to 8 in-lb, because doing so may help prevent loosening compared to lower torque pressures. Additionally, the torque should be rechecked 24–36 h after application and retightened if necessary. Periodic follow-up should be established, and pin torque should be assessed during the clinical visits.

Another potential complication is infection at the pin sites. Botte et al. retrospectively reviewed 179 patients and found the incidence of pin-site infections to be 20% [13]. The best protection against pin-site infection is sterile technique during application of the pins and optimal pin care. When applying the halo ring, a 1–2 cm gap must be present between the ring and the skull. This gap allows for daily cleaning with soap and water.

Injury to the supraorbital and supratrochlear nerve is a potential complication of halo vest application. This complication can occur if the pins are not placed in the appropriate supraorbital or frontolateral location. The nerves at risk reside in the medial third of the supraorbital rim; therefore, no pins should be placed in this area.

Perforation of an enlarged frontal sinus with a pin can result in intracranial infection, cerebrospinal fluid leak, or pneumocephaly [17, 18]. CT of the head should be analyzed before pin placement to evaluate the relevant cranial anatomy, and care should be taken to avoid the frontal sinus. The frontolateral location of the anterior pin is typically farther from the frontal sinus and may be a more appropriate location in patients with enlarged or aberrant frontal sinuses [20].

Follow-up is critical in patients who are immobilized with the halo vest to ensure that excessive motion is not occurring [23]. Supine and upright radiographs should be evaluated immediately after placement of the halo and at regular clinical follow-up examinations. If excessive motion is apparent on radiographs, then alternative management strategies (e.g., surgical fixation) may be warranted.

Conclusion

Halo vest immobilization can be an effective treatment strategy for the management of cervical fractures and instability. It is imperative to consider the patient's ability to tolerate the weight and constriction of the vest prior to its application. After the halo has been applied, close clinical follow-up is necessary to ensure that the patient is tolerating the vest and that it is effectively immobilizing the cervical spine.

References

1. Perry J, Nickel VL. Total cervical spine fusion for neck paralysis. J Bone Joint Surg Am. 1959;41:37–60.
2. Benzel EC, Hadden TA, Saulsbery CM. A comparison of the Minerva and halo jackets for stabilization of the cervical spine. J Neurosurg. 1989;70(3):411–4. doi:10.3171/jns.1989.70.3.0411.
3. Tomonaga T, Krag MH, Novotny JE. Clinical, radiographic, and kinematic results from an adjustable four-pad halovest. Spine (Phila Pa 1976). 1997;22(11):1199–208.
4. Lind B, Sihlbom H, Nordwall A. Forces and motions across the neck in patients treated with halo-vest. Spine (Phila Pa 1976). 1988;13(2):162–7.
5. Koch RA, Nickel VL. The halo vest: an evaluation of motion and forces across the neck. Spine (Phila Pa 1976). 1978;3(2):103–7.
6. Schneider AM, Hipp JA, Nguyen L, Reitman CA. Reduction in head and intervertebral motion provided by 7 contemporary cervical orthoses in 45 individuals. Spine (Phila Pa 1976). 2007;32(1):E1–6. doi:10.1097/01.brs.0000251019.24917.44.
7. Richter D, Latta LL, Milne EL, Varkarakis GM, Biedermann L, Ekkernkamp A, et al. The stabilizing effects of different orthoses in the intact and unstable upper cervical spine: a cadaver study. J Trauma. 2001;50(5):848–54.
8. Morishima N, Ohota K, Miura Y. The influences of halo-vest fixation and cervical hyperextension on swallowing in healthy volunteers. Spine (Phila Pa 1976). 2005;30(7):E179–82.
9. Lind B, Bake B, Lundqvist C, Nordwall A. Influence of halo vest treatment on vital capacity. Spine (Phila Pa 1976). 1987;12(5):449–52.
10. Ohnishi K, Miyamoto K, Kato T, Shimizu K. Effects of wearing halo vest on gait: three-dimensional analysis in healthy subjects. Spine (Phila Pa 1976). 2005;30(7):750–5.
11. Gelalis ID, Christoforou G, Motsis E, Arnaoutoglou C, Xenakis T. Brain abscess and generalized seizure caused by halo pin intracranial penetration: case report and review of the literature. Eur Spine J. 2009;18(Suppl 2):172–5. doi:10.1007/s00586-008-0759-x.
12. Fleming BC, Krag MH, Huston DR, Sugihara S. Pin loosening in a halo-vest orthosis: a biomechanical study. Spine (Phila Pa 1976). 2000;25(11):1325–31.
13. Botte MJ, Byrne TP, Abrams RA, Garfin SR. Halo skeletal fixation: techniques of application and prevention of complications. J Am Acad Orthop Surg. 1996;4(1):44–53.
14. Horn EM, Theodore N, Feiz-Erfan I, Lekovic GP, Dickman CA, Sonntag VK. Complications of halo fixation in the elderly. J Neurosurg Spine. 2006;5(1):46–9. doi:10.3171/spi.2006.5.1.46.
15. Vieweg U, Schultheiss R. A review of halo vest treatment of upper cervical spine injuries. Arch Orthop Trauma Surg. 2001;121(1–2):50–5.
16. Yang C, Wang H, Zheng Z, Zhang Z, Wang J, Liu H, et al. Halo-gravity traction in the treatment of severe spinal deformity: a systematic review and meta-analysis. Eur Spine J. 2016; doi:10.1007/s00586-016-4848-y.
17. Garfin SR, Botte MJ, Waters RL, Nickel VL. Complications in the use of the halo fixation device. J Bone Joint Surg Am. 1986;68(3):320–5.
18. Cheong ML, Chan CY, Saw LB, Kwan MK. Pneumocranium secondary to halo vest pin penetration through an enlarged frontal sinus. Eur

Spine J. 2009;18(Suppl 2):269–71. doi:10.1007/s00586-009-1004-y.
19. Kang M, Vives MJ, Vaccaro AR. The halo vest: principles of application and management of complications. J Spinal Cord Med. 2003;26(3):186–92.
20. Stone JL, Gulabani A, Gorelick G, Vannemreddy SN, Vannemreddy PS. Frontolateral pins for halo ring placement: reassessment of a common neurosurgical procedure with CT measurements of skull thickness. J Neurosurg Spine. 2013;19(6):744–9. doi:10.3171/2013.8.SPINE121020.
21. Ebraheim NA, Liu J, Patil V, Sanford CG Jr, Crotty MJ, Haman SP, et al. Evaluation of skull thickness and insertion torque at the halo pin insertion areas in the elderly: a cadaveric study. Spine J. 2007;7(6):689–93. doi:10.1016/j.spinee.2006.09.007.
22. Rizzolo SJ, Piazza MR, Cotler JM, Hume EL, Cautilli G, O'Neill DK. The effect of torque pressure on halo pin complication rates. A randomized prospective study. Spine (Phila Pa 1976). 1993;18(15):2163–6.
23. Anderson PA, Budorick TE, Easton KB, Henley MB, Salciccioli GG. Failure of halo vest to prevent in vivo motion in patients with injured cervical spines. Spine (Phila Pa 1976). 1991;16(10 Suppl):S501–5.

3 Occipitocervical Fusion

Vijay M. Ravindra, Robert G. Whitmore, and Zoher Ghogawala

Introduction

Cranial-cervical instability can be caused by systemic illnesses or traumatic injuries and often requires urgent attention and surgical stabilization. The cranial-cervical junction is a complex region of the spine with challenging anatomical and biomechanical considerations. The occipital-C1 joint is responsible for 15° of flexion and extension of the cervical spine; C1-C2 provides 45% of the axial rotation [1–3]. Surgical techniques and fusion constructs have evolved over time, mostly because of the historical difficulty of dealing with surgical stabilization and the associated high failure rates [4]. In spite of early failures, however, the evolution of rigid fixation and the adoption of short-segment fixation have resulted in fusion rates nearing 100% [5, 6]. In this chapter, we discuss the causes, both traumatic and systemic, of cranial-cervical instability and describe its surgical management.

V.M. Ravindra, MD, MSPH
Department of Neurosurgery, Clinical Neurosciences Center, University of Utah, 175 N. Medical Drive East, Salt Lake City, UT 84132, USA

Department of Neurosurgery, Alan and Jacqueline Stuart Spine Research Center, Lahey Hospital and Medical Center, 41 Mall Road, Burlington, MA 01805, USA
e-mail: Vijay.ravindra@hsc.utah.edu

R.G. Whitmore, MD • Z. Ghogawala, MD (✉)
Department of Neurosurgery, Tufts University School of Medicine, Boston, MA, USA

Department of Neurosurgery, Alan and Jacqueline Stuart Spine Research Center, Lahey Hospital and Medical Center, 41 Mall Road, Burlington, MA 01805, USA
e-mail: zoher.ghogawala@lahey.org

Indications and Patient Selection

Causes of Cranial-Cervical Instability

Cranial-cervical instability results from laxity or disruption of the occipital condyle-C1-C2 relationship; it is also described as and encompasses the terms occipitocervical instability (O-C1) or atlantoaxial instability (C1-2). We will focus on occipitocervical instability as it relates to cranial-cervical instability. Many conditions can lead to occipitocervical instability, including congenital cranial settling, trauma, rheumatoid arthritis, inflammatory arthropathies, tumor burden, and infection, and it can also develop after surgical decompression (Table 3.1) [5, 7, 8].

L.T. Holly, P.A. Anderson (eds.), *Essentials of Spinal Stabilization*,
DOI 10.1007/978-3-319-59713-3_3

Table 3.1 Common causes for cranial-cervical instability requiring surgical stabilization

Systemic	
Inflammatory	Rheumatoid arthritis Reiter syndrome Psoriatic arthritis Inflammatory bowel disease-related arthritis Calcium pyrophosphate deposition disease
Infection	Bacterial (osteomyelitis) Fungal
Neoplasm	Osteolytic Osteoblastic
Traumatic/surgical	
Trauma	Atlanto-occipital dislocation (AOD) Atlantoaxial dislocation Occipital condyle avulsion fracture
Postsurgical	After Chiari decompression or foramen magnum surgery After upper cervical laminectomy

Traumatic Cranial-Cervical Instability

Traumatic occipitocervical dislocation, which is defined as the traumatic dislocation of the occipital condyle and C1 lateral mass (O-C1 joint), is the most common presentation of traumatic cranial-cervical instability [8]. Patients often present with neurological dysfunction consistent with acute spinal cord injury, tetraplegia, and cranial nerve deficits, and they often have significant hemodynamic instability as a result of lower brainstem dysfunction. Diagnosing such an injury can be difficult, even with a high index of suspicion, with previously reported "missed diagnoses" on initial radiographic evaluation in up to 75% of patients experiencing trauma [9, 10]. Most recently, the use of the condylar-C1 interval (CCI) in adults with cutoffs of 1.5 mm was found to have the highest sensitivity and specificity for diagnosing atlanto-occipital dislocation (AOD) [11]; the CCI was devised originally for use in evaluating children for AOD.

In rare scenarios, avulsion-type fracture of the occipital condyle may lead to instability at the cranial-cervical junction. This is due to the association between avulsion fractures, type III condyle fractures, and a rotational mechanism of injury [12].

For cases of cranial-cervical instability, surgical treatment at O-C1 may be undertaken; however, additional instability from disruption of the alar ligaments, tectorial membrane, and transverse-atlantal ligament resulting in C1-2 rotational and translational instability [8, 13, 14] is seen in up to 55% of patients. Thus, O-C1-C2 fixation/fusion is the most commonly used surgical fixation technique for traumatic dislocation [15–17]. Early surgical treatment with stabilization is key for optimizing neurological recovery [9, 18].

Systemic Causes of Cranial-Cervical Instability

Patients with systemic causes of instability often present with progressive myelopathy, lower cranial nerve (CN) dysfunction (CN IX, X, XI, XII), neck pain, and obvious deformities of the cranial-cervical region [5, 7, 8]. The symptoms are more gradual in onset because of the natural history and progression of the systemic illness.

Rheumatoid arthritis (RA) is the inflammatory disease that most often affects the cranial-cervical junction [8]. RA is a chronic inflammatory process characterized by anti-cyclic citrullinated peptide and rheumatoid factor. Whereas the cause of RA is unknown, its downstream effects are well characterized by an immune response that causes destruction of the joints, capsules, and ligaments. Specific to the cervical spine, patients with RA are prone to progressive development of a rheumatic pannus or inflamed granulation tissue within the synovial joints capable of producing collagenases and enzymes that may destroy adjacent bone, tendons, and joints. Patients with RA presenting with cervical spine issues are often elderly and cachectic. Other inflammatory arthropathies that may also affect the cranial-cervical junction by a similar mechanism include Reiter syndrome, psoriatic arthritis, inflammatory bowel disease-associated arthritis, and calcium pyrophosphate deposition disease [19].

O-C1 instability may occur with RA, but atlantoaxial and subaxial instability are more common. Additionally, cranial settling and/or subaxial subluxation – often resulting in debilitating pain, spinal cord compression, and neurological dysfunction – may occur. Although cervical involvement of RA is common because of the large number of synovial joints, early intervention and advancements in disease-modifying antirheumatic drugs such as biologic response modifiers have reduced the potential for debilitating neurological deficit and the need for surgical intervention. Still, RA patients with cranial-cervical instability who are treated conservatively may have a grave prognosis, with a large number of patients becoming bedridden and dying of their systemic disease [8]; the mortality rate at 8 years has been reported to be as high as 100% [20, 21]. Surgery with fusion for stabilization has been reported to promote a twofold increase in 5-year survival rate; most patients were afforded improvement in survival, pain reduction, and myelopathy with an increased long-term functional outcome [22, 23].

Infection, tumor burden, and postoperative instability after foramen magnum decompression (Chiari operation) or upper cervical spine decompression are additional causes for cranial-cervical instability [24, 25]. Surgical stabilization may be necessary in these cases, but given the erosive nature of infection and tumor, specifically osteolytic lesions, the amount of bone available may be unsuitable for screw placement [8]. Fusion to the occiput can often be performed in these cases, specifically if there is irreducible subluxation of C1 on C2, when the lateral masses of C1 are not suitable for placement of hardware or if there has been an anterior pannus resection ventral to C1-C2 [19, 26].

The embryological development of the cranial-cervical junction is complex [27]; as a result, there are numerous congenital conditions and developmental anomalies of the cranial-cervical junction that can lead to instability. The most common congenital cause of occipitocervical instability is Down syndrome; if marked instability is seen in dynamic imaging in these patients, then fusion is typically required at a young age [28].

Preoperative Considerations

Radiographic Measurements

There are several standard radiographic measurements that can be used in diagnosing cranial-cervical instability. In 1979, Powers [29] developed a ratio for diagnosis of AOD (Fig. 3.1). This method is sensitive for the evaluation and diagnosis of anterior AOD [30], but a posterior dissociation or vertical distraction injury could result in a normal value causing misdiagnosis.

The atlantodental interval (ADI) is a standard measurement used to evaluate the atlantoaxial relationship. As originally described by [31], normal values are <3 mm in men and <2.5 mm in women on plain X-rays (Fig. 3.2); more recently, a threshold of <2 mm on computed tomography (CT) imaging has been described [29].

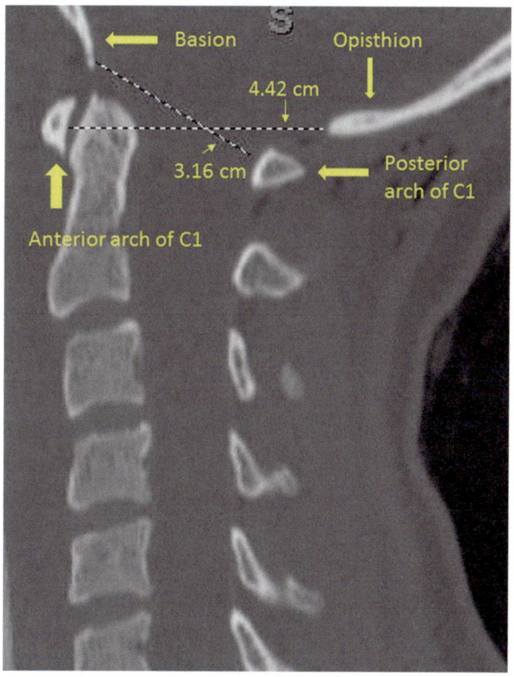

Fig. 3.1 Sagittal CT of the cervical spine without contrast demonstrating the measurement of the Powers ratio (calculated by dividing the measurement between the tip of the basion to the spinolaminar line by the measurement from the tip of the opisthion to the midpoint of the posterior aspect of the anterior arch of C1). In the patient shown here, the calculation would be 3.16/4.42 = 0.71. A ratio > 1.0 suggests cranial-cervical instability

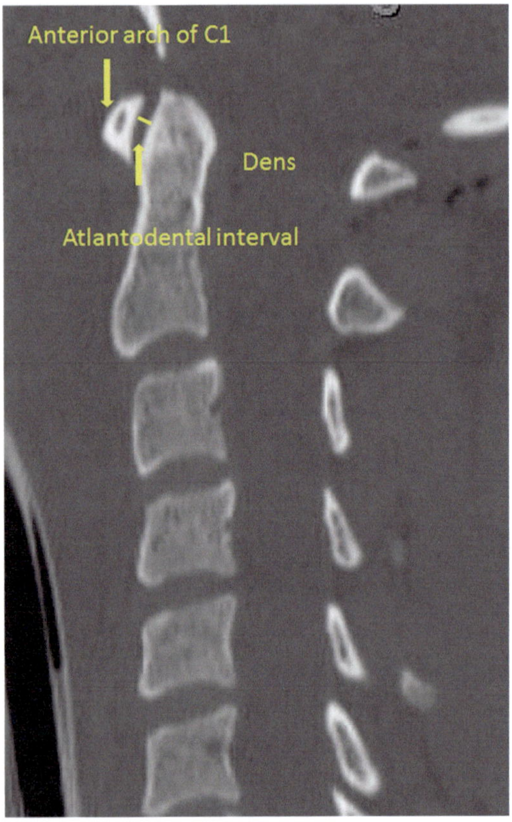

Fig. 3.2 Sagittal CT of the cranial-cervical junction demonstrating the measurement of the atlantodental interval (ADI) which is measured by drawing a line from the posterior aspect of the anterior arch of C1 to the most anterior aspect of the odontoid, preferably at the midpoint of the thickness of the arch in craniocaudal dimension. On X-rays, an ADI <3 mm is considered normal in men and an ADI <2.5 mm is considered normal in women. On CT, an ADI <2 mm is considered normal in all patients

Harris et al. [32, 33] described the use of the basion-dens interval (BDI), originally devised by [34], and the basion-axial interval (BAI) for diagnosing instability. They demonstrated that >95% of adults in a normal study population had a BDI and a BAI <12 mm. These measurements were considered to be at the upper threshold of a normal measurement, as described by [30] who found that CT measurement of the BDI yielded a normal value of <8.5. In Fig. 3.3, we demonstrate the use of the BDI and BAI in diagnosing cranial-cervical instability. The original conception of the aforementioned measurements was made on plain radiographs, but [30] demonstrated the value of using these measures on CT imaging which is the most common method of screening patients for traumatic dislocation. The use of any measurements for diagnosis is typically supplemented by the use of magnetic resonance imaging if available and tolerable by the patient.

Restoring cervical alignment to an anatomic and physiological position is important in treating patients with occipitocervical instability. The craniovertebral angle, which is the angle formed by a horizontal line drawn through the spinous process of C7 and a line joining the spinous process of C7 with the tragus [35, 36], can be a reliable indicator of head and neck posture [36]. Patients with a smaller craniovertebral angle may have forward head posture and resulting disability.

Transoral Decompression (Odontoidectomy)

Some cranial-cervical pathological conditions may require further decompression from an anterior approach. These can include ventral spinal cord compression from a degenerative or inflammatory pannus, from ventral spinal cord compression due to intra- or extradural tumor, or in the setting of irreducible atlantoaxial subluxation with myelopathy and spinal cord compression [37]. This approach can afford access to the area from the top of C1 to the C2-3 disc space. This approach should only be used in patients who are free of dental or oral pathology and have a minimum of 2.5–3.0 cm of dental clearance to allow adequate exposure for resection of the odontoid [38]. Perioperative considerations include airway edema, swallowing dysfunction, oral hygiene, and injury to the oral cavity (soft palate, tongue).

Although large studies regarding outcomes after transoral odontoid resection are lacking, Menezes and VanGilder [39] presented a 10-year review of 72 patients treated via a transoral-transpharyngeal approach to the anterior cranial-cervical junction. They reported two postoperative deaths and one pharyngeal infection requiring a revision operation. All patients in this series, however, had improvement in their overall neurological function [39]. Recent literature has

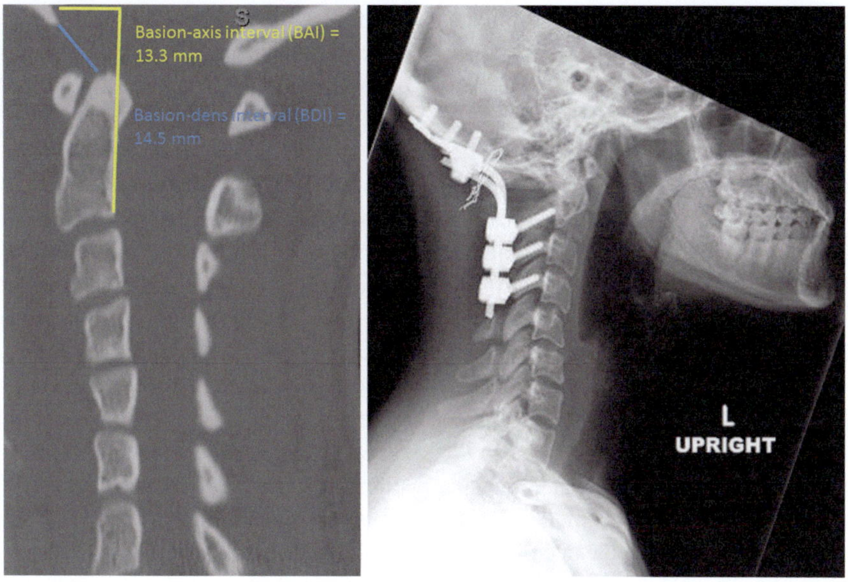

Fig. 3.3 (**a**) Sagittal CT demonstrating the basion-axial interval (BAI) and basion-dens interval (BDI). The BAI is measured by drawing a line along the posterior cortex of the body of the axis and extended cranially. The BAI is the distance between the basion and this line (*yellow*). A normal value is <12 mm on plain X-ray. The BDI is the distance from the most inferior portion of the basion to the closest portion of the superior aspect of the odontoid (*blue*). A normal value is <12 mm on plain X-ray or <8.5 mm on CT imaging. (**b**) Postoperative CT in a grossly unstable (both BAI and BDI >12 mm) patient who underwent an occipital-C4 posterior spinal fusion

questioned the use of the transoral approach for odontoid resection; for instance, Goel [40] proposed that anomalies once requiring transoral surgical decompression may be treated with atlantoaxial facetal distraction spacers. However, the transoral procedure remains a viable option in the treatment of cranial-cervical instability with spinal cord compression.

Surgical Management of Cranial-Cervical Instability

Occipitocervical fusion (OCF) is performed to correct joint instability caused by trauma, rheumatologic conditions, infection, neoplasm, or congenital conditions [41]. Although nonrigid constructs have previously been described in the setting of OCF, rigid fixation involving screws with plate or rods is biomechanically superior to external immobilization in conjunction with sublaminar wiring and bone grafting [42–45].

Occipitocervical Fixation

In the early twentieth century, instability at the cranial-cervical junction was considered inoperable and was often fatal [8]. To this day, stabilization of the mobile cranial-cervical junction presents a surgical challenge and has been associated with high complication rates. The first surgical fusion of the cranial-cervical junction was performed by Förster in 1927 [46] using a fibular strut graft. Early techniques used stand-alone onlay bone grafting with or without wiring to secure the graft. This technique required the use of postoperative halo fixation which caused discomfort and can be associated with significant complications [47]. Since then, significant advances have been made for fixation to the occiput. Wire-based techniques for OCF were found to be biomechanically inferior to screw-based fixation [8]. This is especially true with respect to resistance of cranial settling and axial rotation; additionally, significant neurologic morbidity may occur with previous graft and wire-based methods [43, 48, 49].

Modern techniques now allow for rigid fixation of the cranial-cervical junction with a high rate of fusion success [7, 50]. Fusion rates after primary rigid posterior fixation for OCF have been reported to be between 70% and 100% [5, 51–55]. Current constructs used for OCF include polyaxial screws heads with either 3.5- or 4.0-mm rods, which are bent depending on screw trajectories and the native and desired occipitocervical angle [8]. Most current systems allow for placement of cervical hardware and occipital hardware independently, which can later be linked using the rod/plate construct. The use of occipital plates adds pullout strength to the construct; occipital plates are applied most often to the occipital keel in the midline [8]. This thick midline keel provides the highest resistance to pullout and is attached to the atlantoaxial screws in the modern, modular OCF construct [8, 56]. Some plates provide an option between fixation in the midline, which is superior for axial rotation movements and lateral fixation which may improve resistance to lateral bending [57] (Fig. 3.4). With the development of larger, more versatile occipital plating, however, there can be a loss of bony surface area for fusion medium, so careful attention should be paid to ensuring the presence of adequate bony contact to promote arthrodesis [8]. The ease of use of the modular systems in OCF have made fixation more successful, with an associated increased fusion rate; an additional advantage includes the reduced need for rigid cervical collars after surgery [5, 58].

Surgical Technique: Occipital Plate

Presurgical workup includes high-resolution CT with coronal and sagittal reconstructions to verify and confirm the bony anatomy. The thickness of the occipital keel is of interest while placing the occipital plate. Preoperative traction may be necessary to distract the patient into anatomic alignment.

Patient positioning is crucial in achieving optimal alignment. The patient's head should be secured with rigid cranial fixation – either with pin fixation or using a halo ring. The patient is gently placed into the prone position; neurophysiologic monitoring can be useful, especially in patients with highly unstable injuries, severe myelopathy, or cranial-cervical compression [59, 60]. Prepositioning baseline monitoring can provide a useful reference. The head is then positioned in a neutral position with a slight military tuck [8]; exaggeration of the tuck can lead to postoperative dysphagia and chronic muscular neck pain. If the head is too extended, the patient may have difficulty with mechanical down gaze. It is crucial to verify patient positioning by using

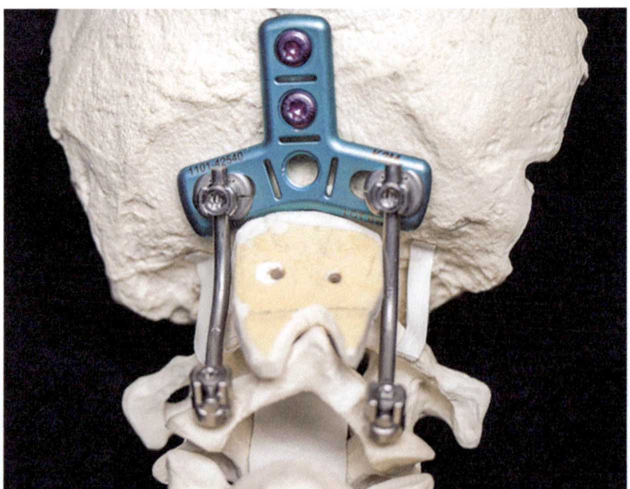

Fig. 3.4 Sawbone model depicting the use an occipital plate (Figure reproduced with permission from [80])

lateral X-ray or C-arm fluoroscopy to ensure the lateral masses align and the ears are parallel to the floor. To improve venous drainage, the patient is placed into slight reverse Trendelenburg position with the patient's back and legs elevated.

Antibiotics are routinely administered preoperatively. The planned incision is typically infiltrated with local anesthetic with epinephrine (1% lidocaine with epinephrine 1:100,000), which can aid with hemostasis. For transarticular screw placement, the trajectory of the screws necessitates a separate stab incision; thus, the sterile field should be made large enough to accommodate this [61]. The incision should extend from the inion, which is palpable along the skull, to the level of the C3 spinous process or lower depending on the operative plan. The incision is carried through the fascia to the spinous processes of C1, C2, C3, and lower if necessary. Then, a subperiosteal dissection is performed to expose C1, C2, C3, and lower if necessary. An additional horizontal incision can be made in the fascia 2 cm inferior to the inion to access the occiput; a muscular cuff aids in fascial closure and coverage of the occipital plate and the associated hardware [8]. Careful dissection of the C1 lateral mass around the C2 nerve root is necessary to access the entry point for the C1 screw. Careful dissection with bipolar cautery is used to avoid manipulation and injury to the vertebral artery.

Once the cervical instrumentation has been placed (see below), attention can be turned to the occipital plate. Several occipital plates are available and approved for use, but a construct and design with midline screw placement into the bony keel in the midline is best for fixation given the thickness of the keel. Any irregularities along the surface of the occipital bone can be evened using a high-speed drill. The plate is commonly positioned 1 cm below the inion. Typically, the most superior screw is placed first. A power drill with associated drill guide is prepared and set to a depth of 6 mm; drilling depth is increased in 2-mm increments until the ventral cortex is penetrated [8]; the hole is probed to ensure the dura mater is not penetrated. After the entire depth of the hole has been tapped, a 4.5-mm blunt cortical screw is placed. Depending on the design of the plate, an additional one or two screws can be placed using the same technique.

Once the plate is secured, 3.5-mm rods are contoured to fit the screw heads and plate. Additional dissection around the C1 arch or C2 lamina may be necessary to facilitate Songer cable placement that can be utilized for interpositional bone graft placement. It is important to decorticate all bony surfaces prior to graft placement to enhance and promote arthrodesis. An additional screw can be placed through the superior end of the graft into the occiput.

C2 Fixation

There are few reports of cranial-cervical fixation involving direct fusion of the occiput to C1. It can be achieved by using atlanto-occipital transarticular screws placed through an anterior corridor with a plate attached to the clivus and the anterior portion of C2 as an adjunct; however, the generalized use of this technique has not been adopted [14, 62, 63]. The choice for fixation in OCF is an O-C1-C2 construct if possible; however, O-C2 is used if there is insufficient bone at C1 [5]. Depending on bone quality and the degree of instability, the fusion constructs can extend to C3, C4, or C5 utilizing lateral mass screws and may need to extend to the cervicothoracic junction in cases of severe instability.

There are four screw-based fixation methods at C2: transarticular, translaminar, pars, and pedicle screws (Table 3.2 and Fig. 3.5a, b). Transarticular screw fixation, introduced by Magerl and Seeman [64], can be used for fixation of the atlantoaxial joint. The screws can then be connected to the rostral or occipital end of the construct with plates or rods [8]. This technique is an improvement biomechanically over the previous rod and wire constructs and carries a fusion rate that nears 100% [43, 44, 50, 65]. Transarticular screw fixation can be technically challenging because of the risk of vertebral artery injury and the need to achieve complete reduction prior to screw placement [8]. Up to 23% of patients may have unfavorable vertebral artery anatomy that precludes the use of transarticular screws [66–69]. The

Table 3.2 Fixation strategies to C2 in cranial-cervical instability

Technique	Patients with unfavorable anatomy (%)	Complications/pitfalls
Transarticular (C1-C2)	23	Vertebral artery injury
C2 pedicle/pars	9 (pedicle)	Canal violation, vertebral artery injury
C2 translaminar screws	Not reported	Spinal cord injury (dorsal columns), decreased surface area for fusion

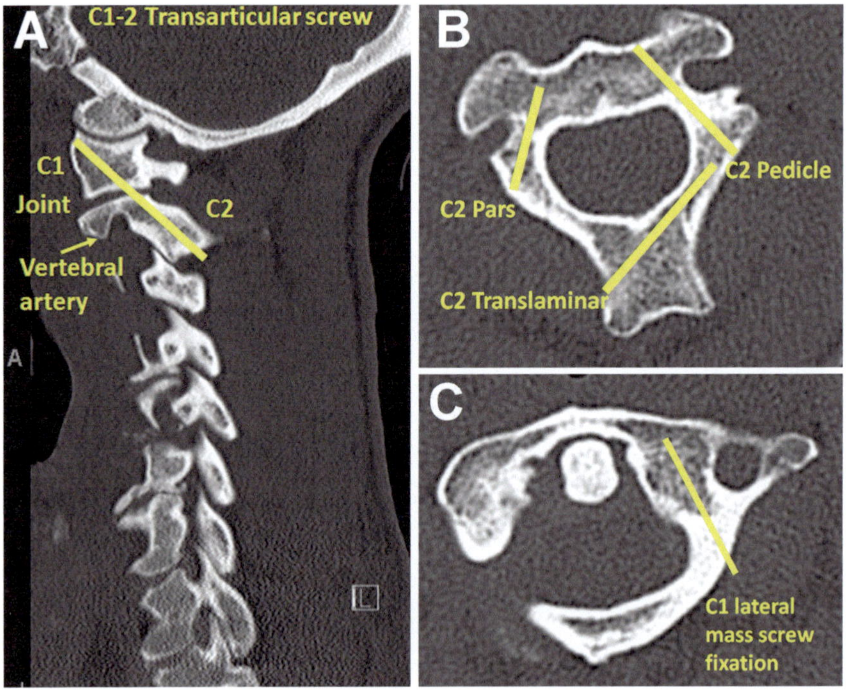

Fig. 3.5 (**a**) Axial CT image cut through C2 with representative lines depicting the trajectory for each of the screw types (pars, pedicle, and translaminar). (**b**) Sagittal CT image depicting the trajectory for a C1-2 transarticular screw. (**c**) Axial CT image representative of placement and trajectory of a C1 lateral mass screw. A C1 pedicle screw (not shown) may also be utilized with a similar trajectory with a higher starting point on the arch of C1

transarticular screw entry point is 3–4 mm rostral and 3–4 mm lateral to the medial portion of the C2–3 facet joint. A K-wire is passed 15° medially oriented with the superior angle aimed at the C1 anterior tubercle (60°) [70].

Fixation can also be achieved through the placement of a Goel-Harms construct – C1 lateral mass screws in combination with C2 pars or pedicle screws [58, 71]. This technique is advantageous when the vertebral artery anatomy is not favorable for placement of transarticular screws. Its other advantages are the ability to perform reduction maneuvers after screw placement and the technical ease of placing C2 pars screws [8]. Biomechanically, this construct has been shown to be of similar strength to the transarticular screw construct in cadaveric studies of cranial-cervical instability [72]; however, the use of pedicle screws at C2 may not be safe in approximately 9% of patients [73]. C1 lateral mass screws are placed by palpating the C1 lateral mass with a Penfield 4. A pilot hole is made with a 3-mm drill bit at the center of the C1 lateral mass. The trajectory for the screw is typically 10° medial angulation and aimed at the anterior tubercle of C1 on lateral fluoroscopy (Fig. 3.5c).

The typical length of a C1 lateral mass screw is 34–36 mm [71, 74].

C2 pars screws are placed in a trajectory that is similar to that of C1-2 transarticular screws but much shorter. The entry point is 3 mm rostral and 3 mm lateral to the inferior medial aspect of the inferior articular surface of C2. The screw follows a steep trajectory (45–60° with 10–15° medial angulation). Screws are typically 16–18 mm in length [71, 74].

The entry point for a C2 pedicle screw is located in the pars of C2, lateral to the superior margin of the C2 lamina, which is 2 mm lateral and 2 mm superior to the C2 pars screw entry point. C2 pedicle screws require medial angulation of 15° with an upward trajectory of 20°. Many patients may have narrow pedicles at C2 that are unsuitable for screw placement; thus, careful study of preoperative imaging (CT) is necessary.

Translaminar screws can be placed across the lamina of C2 in a crossed trajectory and subsequently connected by rods to the lateral mass screws at C1 [5]. This can be used as a primary method of fixation or a salvage technique with an advantage of limited risk of injury to the vertebral artery; an additional risk, however, is possible spinal cord injury from ventral puncture through the lamina which may lead to cerebrospinal fluid (CSF) leak and dorsal column injury. Placing C2 laminar screws is technically less demanding than placing C1-C2 transarticular screws or C2-pars/pedicle screws because the C2 lamina (the largest in the cervical spine) provides adequate space and visualization, thus obviating the need for navigation [8]. The entry point is at the junction of the spinous process and lamina, with the trajectory meeting the slope of the lamina while aiming dorsally to avoid canal breach. Bone graft is often placed into the C1-2 facet joint.

Translaminar screws attached to C1 lateral mass screws are biomechanically equivalent to the Harm-Goels construct but inferior to the occipital-transarticular screw construct and the occipital-C2 pedicle screw construct [72, 75]. An additional drawback of the translaminar screw technique is the screw head placement and loss of surface area of bone to promote a fusion mass [8].

Allograft Versus Autograft

Historically, the use of autograft was favored for promotion of fusion in patients with significant cranial-cervical instability because of the natural trophic factors present in native bone. However, bicortical allograft may provide the same osteoconductive conduit for bony fusion as traditional autograft [76], with similar biomechanical properties [77]. Similar use of allograft for successful arthrodesis has been demonstrated in anterior cervical fusion [78] and posterior C1-2 fusion [79]. Godzik et al. [80] found that patients with symptomatic cranial-cervical instability can be safely and successfully treated with a one-stage OCF with bicortical iliac allograft, with no difference in fusion rate between allograft and autograft groups at 12 months of follow-up (≥95% bony fusion in each group). The use of autograft can be complicated by donor-site morbidity, mostly pain, which has been reported to be as high as 49%. Furthermore, the array of available configurations for allograft allows for adaptable use (strips, cubes, wedges, and matrices) [80].

Postoperative Management and Care

The use of cervical collar is controversial, thus is at the choice of the surgeon. Patients with systemic causes of cranial-cervical instability that have adequate screw purchase and do not suffer from osteoporosis or osteopenia and do not take chronic immunosuppressive therapy are typically may not be prescribed a rigid cervical orthosis, based on surgeon preference. On the other hand, patients with post-traumatic or post-surgical cranial-cervical instability are typically managed with rigid cervical orthoses, and in severe cases of poor nutrition and bone quality, a halo adjunct may be used [8]. More than just a promotion of fusion and alignment, a collar may be used to serve as a reminder to patients of the severity of the cranial-cervical instability [8].

Illustrative Case

History Fourty-three-year-old male was involved in a moped accident in Bermuda. He had significant neck pain on admission to the hospital.

Physical Exam Posterior cervical spine tenderness. Neurologically intact.

Radiographic Imaging. Initial cervical spine CT demonstrated ankylosing spondylitis, acute type II displaced odontoid fracture and C6-C7 fracture dislocation (Fig. 3.6).

Initial Treatment The patient underwent anterior cervical fusion and plating at C6-C7 with multi-level posterior lateral mass fixation. Cranial-cervical instability was evident within 24 h with increasing basion-dental interval (>12 mm) (Fig. 3.7).

Cranial-Cervical Treatment The patient underwent occipitocervical to upper thoracic fixation and fusion to stabilize the instability both at the occipitocervical region as well as the C6-C7 level in the context of ankylosing spondylitis (Fig. 3.8).

Outcome The patient used a Miami J collar for 3 months and remained neurologically intact in follow-up (Fig. 3.9).

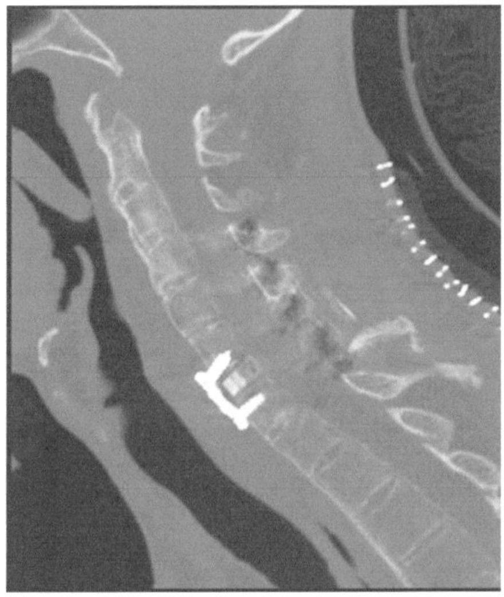

Fig. 3.7 Following anterior-posterior fusion for the C6-C7 injury, craniospinal instability was demonstrated by an increased basion-dental interval

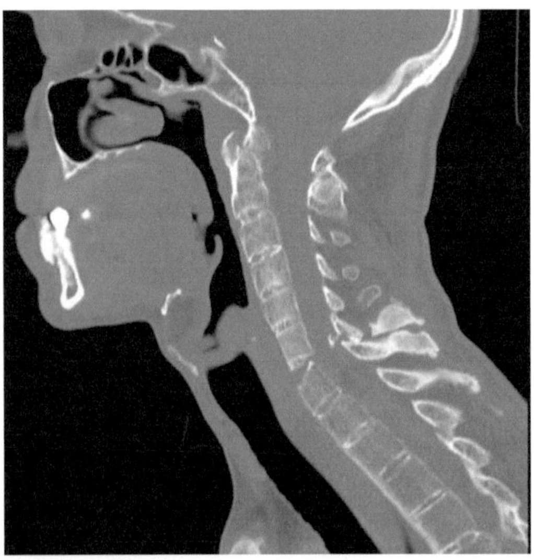

Fig. 3.6 Sagittal CT scan demonstrating C6-C7 fracture dislocation and Type II odontoid fracture in a 43-year-old male following a moped accident

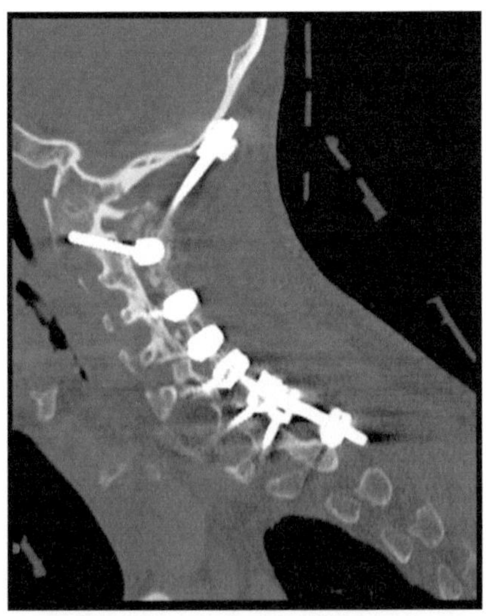

Fig. 3.8 Sagittal CT following stabilization of the craniospinal instability using occipital fixation

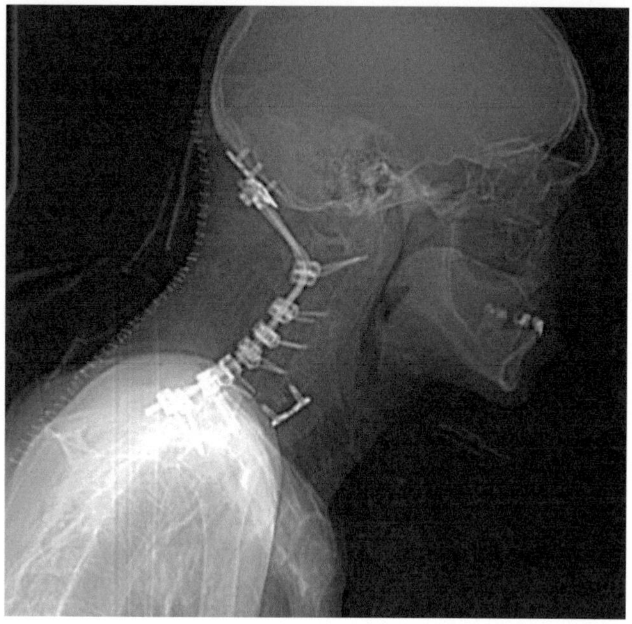

Fig. 3.9 Postoperative lateral radiograph demonstrating occipital-thoracic fusion

Technical Pearls

- Careful study of preoperative imaging and bone morphology can be useful in placement and choice of cervical screw type and location, specifically for the occipital condyle.
- Because cervical hardware (C1-2 transarticular screws, C2 pars/pedicle screws) placement can be more difficult than the more straightforward occipital plate/screw placement, it should be undertaken first for patient safety.
- Vertebral artery injuries may occur during exposure or hardware placement. If vertebral artery injury occurs during placement of the first screw, the ipsilateral hardware should be placed, and the contralateral side should be abandoned to avoid bilateral injury.
- Alignment should be verified both by visual inspection and with fluoroscopy prior to final fixation.

Complications and Strategies for Avoidance

Complication rates for both major and minor complications during occipitocervical surgery range from 12% to 30% [5, 7]. Potential complications include, but are not limited to, wound infection, CSF leak, intracranial traumatic hemorrhage (epidural, subdural hematoma), hardware failure, nonunion requiring reoperation, and fixation in a suboptimal, nonanatomic position [5, 7]. Exposure is done through a midline incision and subsequent subperiosteal dissection to expose the occipital bone and dorsal spinal column. Careful retraction with self-retaining devices is used but should be done with little tension to avoid injury/irritation of the occipital nerve and its branches. Preservation of the fascia at the inion can allow for coverage of the occipital plate with tissue, which can help avoid hardware prominence and discomfort. Blunt dissection of the arch of C1, rather than Bovie electrocautery, is recommended to avoid injury to the vertebral artery in the sulcus arteriosus.

The most severe complication that can occur during exposure or while fixating C1-2 results from vertebral artery injury. Depending on the patient's circulation and vertebral artery dominance, a unilateral injury or occlusion may be asymptomatic, but a bilateral injury can result in brainstem infarction and death. After a unilateral injury, the screw should usually be placed to tamponade the bleeding; hardware should not be placed on the contralateral side to avoid bilateral injury. Additional care and consideration should be given to dural violation and cord injury. If CSF leak is encountered while placing the occipital screw, placement of the screw should provide a permanent solution in most cases. If a CSF leak cannot be repaired primarily, CSF diversion (lumbar drain) should be considered. If a high cervical cord injury is suspected intraoperatively, the patient's clinical and neurological status should be assessed with all tools available, including neurological monitoring, blood pressure augmentation, and in severe cases abortion of the procedure followed by a neurological examination.

Conclusion

There are many potential causes of cranial-cervical instability, and thus, there are multiple surgical options for fixation of this complex biomechanical area. The screw-based techniques have been proven to be the most biomechanically sound and have increased fusion rates to nearly 100%. Although surgery for cranial-cervical instability may be technically challenging, thorough knowledge of the anatomy, both bony and vascular, and surgical constructs available for the task can improve the outcome of the operation and provide the patient with successful arthrodesis.

References

1. Ishii T, Mukai Y, Hosono N, et al. Kinematics of the upper cervical spine in rotation: in vivo three-dimensional analysis. Spine (Phila Pa 1976). 2004; 29(7):E139–44.
2. Panjabi M, Dvorak J, Duranceau J, et al. Three-dimensional movements of the upper cervical spine. Spine (Phila Pa 1976). 1988;13(7):726–30.
3. White AA 3rd, Panjabi MM. The clinical biomechanics of the occipitoatlantoaxial complex. Orthop Clin North Am. 1978;9(4):867–78.
4. Lipscomb PR. Cervico-occipital fusion for congenital and post-traumatic anomalies of the atlas and axis. J Bone Joint Surg Am. 1957;39-A(6):1289–301.
5. Nockels RP, Shaffrey CI, Kanter AS, et al. Occipitocervical fusion with rigid internal fixation: long-term follow-up data in 69 patients. J Neurosurg Spine. 2007;7(2):117–23.
6. Singh SK, Rickards L, Apfelbaum RI, et al. Occipitocervical reconstruction with the Ohio Medical instruments loop: results of a multicenter evaluation in 30 cases. J Neurosurg. 2003;98(3 Suppl):239–46.
7. Deutsch H, Haid RW Jr, Rodts GE Jr, et al. Occipitocervical fixation: long-term results. Spine (Phila Pa 1976). 2005;30(5):530–5.
8. Finn MA, Bishop FS, Dailey AT. Surgical treatment of occipitocervical instability. Neurosurgery. 2008;63(5):961–8. discussion 8–9.
9. Bellabarba C, Mirza SK, West GA, et al. Diagnosis and treatment of craniocervical dislocation in a series of 17 consecutive survivors during an 8-year period. J Neurosurg Spine. 2006;4(6):429–40.
10. Bono CM, Vaccaro AR, Fehlings M, et al. Measurement techniques for upper cervical spine injuries: consensus statement of the Spine Trauma Study Group. Spine (Phila Pa 1976). 2007;32(5):593–600.
11. Martinez-Del-Campo E, Kalb S, Soriano-Baron H, et al. Computed tomography parameters for atlantooccipital dislocation in adult patients: the occipital condyle-C1 interval. J Neurosurg Spine. 2016;24(4):535–45.
12. Hanson JA, Deliganis AV, Baxter AB, et al. Radiologic and clinical spectrum of occipital condyle fractures: retrospective review of 107 consecutive fractures in 95 patients. AJR Am J Roentgenol. 2002;178(5):1261–8.
13. Dvorak J, Panjabi M, Gerber M, et al. CT-functional diagnostics of the rotatory instability of upper cervical spine. 1. An experimental study on cadavers. Spine (Phila Pa 1976). 1987;12(3):197–205.
14. Feiz-Erfan I, Gonzalez LF, Dickman CA. Atlantooccipital transarticular screw fixation for the treatment of traumatic occipitoatlantal dislocation. Technical note. J Neurosurg Spine. 2005;2(3):381–5.
15. Horn EM, Feiz-Erfan I, Lekovic GP, et al. Survivors of occipitoatlantal dislocation injuries: imaging and clinical correlates. J Neurosurg Spine. 2007;6(2):113–20.
16. Hosono N, Yonenobu K, Kawagoe K, et al. Traumatic anterior atlanto-occipital dislocation. A case report with survival. Spine (Phila Pa 1976). 1993;18(6):786–90.
17. Papadopoulos SM, Dickman CA, Sonntag VK, et al. Traumatic atlantooccipital dislocation with survival. Neurosurgery. 1991;28(4):574–9.
18. Diagnosis and management of traumatic atlanto-occipital dislocation injuries. Neurosurgery. 2002;50 (3 Suppl):S105–13.
19. Menezes A. Acquired abnormalities of the craniocervical junction. In: Winn H, editor. Youman's neurological surgery. 5th ed. Philadelphia: Saunders; 2004. p. 4569–85.
20. Marks JS, Sharp J. Rheumatoid cervical myelopathy. Q J Med. 1981;50(199):307–19.
21. Matsunaga S, Sakou T, Onishi T, et al. Prognosis of patients with upper cervical lesions caused by rheumatoid arthritis: comparison of occipitocervical fusion between c1 laminectomy and nonsurgical management. Spine (Phila Pa 1976). 2003;28(14):1581–7. discussion 7.
22. Matsunaga S, Ijiri K, Koga H. Results of a longer than 10-year follow-up of patients with rheumatoid

arthritis treated by occipitocervical fusion. Spine (Phila Pa 1976). 2000;25(14):1749–53.
23. Moskovich R, Crockard HA, Shott S, et al. Occipitocervical stabilization for myelopathy in patients with rheumatoid arthritis. Implications of not bone-grafting. J Bone Joint Surg Am. 2000;82(3):349–65.
24. Arunkumar MJ, Rajshekhar V. Outcome in neurologically impaired patients with craniovertebral junction tuberculosis: results of combined anteroposterior surgery. J Neurosurg. 2002;97(2 Suppl):166–71.
25. Sanpakit S, Mansfield TL, Liebsch J. Role of onlay grafting with minimal internal fixation for occipitocervical fusion in oncologic patients. J Spinal Disord. 2000;13(5):382–90.
26. Menezes AH, VanGilder JC, Clark CR, et al. Odontoid upward migration in rheumatoid arthritis. An analysis of 45 patients with "cranial settling". J Neurosurg. 1985;63(4):500–9.
27. Brockmeyer D. Common pathological conditions of the pediatric craniovertebral junction and cervical spine. In: Brockmeyer D, editor. Advanced Pediatric Craniocervical surgery. New York: Thieme; 2006. p. 43–54.
28. Brockmeyer D. Down syndrome and craniovertebral instability. Topic review and treatment recommendations. Pediatr Neurosurg. 1999;31(2):71–7.
29. Powers B, Miller MD, Kramer RS, et al. Traumatic anterior atlanto-occipital dislocation. Neurosurgery. 1979;4(1):12–7.
30. Rojas CA, Bertozzi JC, Martinez CR, et al. Reassessment of the craniocervical junction: normal values on CT. AJNR Am J Neuroradiol. 2007; 28(9):1819–23.
31. Hinck VC, Hopkins CE. Measurement of the atlanto-dental interval in the adult. Am J Roentgenol Radium Therapy, Nucl Med. 1960;84:945–51.
32. Harris JH Jr, Carson GC, Wagner LK. Radiologic diagnosis of traumatic occipitovertebral dissociation: 1. Normal occipitovertebral relationships on lateral radiographs of supine subjects. AJR Am J Roentgenol. 1994;162(4):881–6.
33. Harris JH Jr, Carson GC, Wagner LK, et al. Radiologic diagnosis of traumatic occipitovertebral dissociation: 2. Comparison of three methods of detecting occipito-vertebral relationships on lateral radiographs of supine subjects. AJR Am J Roentgenol. 1994;162(4):887–92.
34. Wholey MH, Bruwer AJ, Baker HL Jr. The lateral roentgenogram of the neck; with comments on the atlanto-odontoid-basion relationship. Radiology. 1958;71(3):350–6.
35. Watson DH, Trott PH. Cervical headache: an investigation of natural head posture and upper cervical flexor muscle performance. Cephalalgia. 1993;13(4):272–84. discussion 32.
36. Yip CH, Chiu TT, Poon AT. The relationship between head posture and severity and disability of patients with neck pain. Man Ther. 2008;13(2):148–54.
37. Mendoza N, Crockard HA. Anterior transoral procedures. In: An H, Riley III L, editors. An atlas of surgery of the spine. London: Martin Dunitz; 1998. p. 55–69.
38. Mummaneni PV, Haid RW. Transoral odontoidectomy. Neurosurgery. 2005;56(5):1045–50; discussion-50.
39. Menezes AH, VanGilder JC. Transoral-transpharyngeal approach to the anterior craniocervical junction. Ten-year experience with 72 patients. J Neurosurg. 1988;69(6):895–903.
40. Goel A. Atlantoaxial facetal distraction spacers: indications and techniques. J Craniovertebr Junction Spine. 2016;7(3):127–8.
41. Garrido BJ, Sasso RC. Occipitocervical fusion. Orthop Clin North Am. 2012;43(1):1–9. vii.
42. Grubb MR, Currier BL, Stone J, et al. Biomechanical evaluation of posterior cervical stabilization after a wide laminectomy. Spine (Phila Pa 1976). 1997;22(17):1948–54.
43. Hurlbert RJ, Crawford NR, Choi WG, et al. A biomechanical evaluation of occipitocervical instrumentation: screw compared with wire fixation. J Neurosurg. 1999;90(1 Suppl):84–90.
44. Oda I, Abumi K, Sell LC, et al. Biomechanical evaluation of five different occipito-atlanto-axial fixation techniques. Spine (Phila Pa 1976). 1999;24(22):2377–82.
45. Winegar CD, Lawrence JP, Friel BC, et al. A systematic review of occipital cervical fusion: techniques and outcomes. J Neurosurg Spine. 2010;13(1):5–16.
46. Förster O. Pain pathways and the surgical treatment of pain syndromes [German]. Berlin: Urban and Schwarzenberg; 1927.
47. Glaser JA, Whitehill R, Stamp WG, et al. Complications associated with the halo-vest. A review of 245 cases. J Neurosurg. 1986;65(6):762–9.
48. MacKenzie AI, Uttley D, Marsh HT, et al. Craniocervical stabilization using Luque/Hartshill rectangles. Neurosurgery. 1990;26(1):32–6.
49. Sudo H, Abumi K, Ito M, et al. Spinal cord compression by multistrand cables after solid posterior atlantoaxial fusion. Report of three cases. J Neurosurg. 2002;97(3 Suppl):359–61.
50. Sasso RC, Jeanneret B, Fischer K, et al. Occipitocervical fusion with posterior plate and screw instrumentation. A long-term follow-up study. Spine (Phila Pa 1976). 1994;19(20):2364–8.
51. Bhatia R, Desouza RM, Bull J, et al. Rigid occipitocervical fixation: indications, outcomes, and complications in the modern era. J Neurosurg Spine. 2013;18(4):333–9.
52. Grob D, Schutz U, Plotz G. Occipitocervical fusion in patients with rheumatoid arthritis. Clin Orthop Relat Res. 1999;366:46–53.
53. Lee SC, Chen JF, Lee ST. Clinical experience with rigid occipitocervical fusion in the management of traumatic upper cervical spinal instability. J Clin Neurosci. 2006;13(2):193–8.
54. Sandhu FA, Pait TG, Benzel E, et al. Occipitocervical fusion for rheumatoid arthritis using the inside-outside stabilization technique. Spine (Phila Pa 1976). 2003;28(4):414–9.

55. Vale FL, Oliver M, Cahill DW. Rigid occipitocervical fusion. J Neurosurg. 1999;91(2 Suppl):144–50.
56. Roberts DA, Doherty BJ, Heggeness MH. Quantitative anatomy of the occiput and the biomechanics of occipital screw fixation. Spine (Phila Pa 1976). 1998;23(10):1100–7. discussion 7–8.
57. Anderson PA, Oza AL, Puschak TJ, et al. Biomechanics of occipitocervical fixation. Spine (Phila Pa 1976). 2006;31(7):755–61.
58. Goel A, Laheri V. Plate and screw fixation for atlanto-axial subluxation. Acta Neurochir. 1994;129(1–2):47–53.
59. Hilibrand AS, Schwartz DM, Sethuraman V, et al. Comparison of transcranial electric motor and somatosensory evoked potential monitoring during cervical spine surgery. J Bone Joint Surg Am. 2004;86-A(6):1248–53.
60. Lee JY, Hilibrand AS, Lim MR, et al. Characterization of neurophysiologic alerts during anterior cervical spine surgery. Spine (Phila Pa 1976). 2006;31(17):1916–22.
61. Apfelbaum RI. Posterior transarticular C1-2 screw fixation for atlantoaxial instability. Aesculap Scientific Information. 1994;25:1–4.
62. de Andrade JR, Macnab I. Anterior occipito-cervical fusion using an extra-pharyngeal exposure. J Bone Joint Surg Am. 1969;51(8):1621–6.
63. Dvorak MF, Fisher C, Boyd M, et al. Anterior occiput-to-axis screw fixation: part I: a case report, description of a new technique, and anatomical feasibility analysis. Spine (Phila Pa 1976). 2003;28(3):E54–60.
64. Magerl F, Seeman P. Stable posterior fusion of the atlas and axis by transarticular screw fixation. In: Kehr I, Weidner A, editors. Cervical spine I. New York: Springer; 1986. p. 322–7.
65. Puttlitz CM, Goel VK, Traynelis VC, et al. A finite element investigation of upper cervical instrumentation. Spine (Phila Pa 1976). 2001;26(22):2449–55.
66. Bloch O, Holly LT, Park J, et al. Effect of frameless stereotaxy on the accuracy of C1-2 transarticular screw placement. J Neurosurg. 2001;95(1 Suppl):74–9.
67. Gluf WM, Schmidt MH, Apfelbaum RI. Atlantoaxial transarticular screw fixation: a review of surgical indications, fusion rate, complications, and lessons learned in 191 adult patients. J Neurosurg Spine. 2005;2(2):155–63.
68. Madawi AA, Casey AT, Solanki GA, et al. Radiological and anatomical evaluation of the atlantoaxial transarticular screw fixation technique. J Neurosurg. 1997;86(6):961–8.
69. Paramore CG, Dickman CA, Sonntag VK. The anatomical suitability of the C1-2 complex for transarticular screw fixation. J Neurosurg. 1996;85(2):221–4.
70. Finn MA, Apfelbaum RI. Atlantoaxial transarticular screw fixation: update on technique and outcomes in 269 patients. Neurosurgery. 2010;66(3 Suppl):184–92.
71. Harms J, Melcher RP. Posterior C1-C2 fusion with polyaxial screw and rod fixation. Spine (Phila Pa 1976). 2001;26(22):2467–71.
72. Finn MA, Fassett DR, McCall TD, et al. The cervical end of an occipitocervical fusion: a biomechanical evaluation of 3 constructs. Laboratory investigation J Neurosurg Spine. 2008;9(3):296–300.
73. Resnick DK, Lapsiwala S, Trost GR. Anatomic suitability of the C1-C2 complex for pedicle screw fixation. Spine (Phila Pa 1976). 2002;27(14):1494–8.
74. Goel A, Kulkarni AG, Sharma P. Reduction of fixed atlantoaxial dislocation in 24 cases: technical note. J Neurosurg Spine. 2005;2(4):505–9.
75. Gorek J, Acaroglu E, Berven S, et al. Constructs incorporating intralaminar C2 screws provide rigid stability for atlantoaxial fixation. Spine (Phila Pa 1976). 2005;30(13):1513–8.
76. Sawin PD, Traynelis VC, Menezes AH. A comparative analysis of fusion rates and donor-site morbidity for autogeneic rib and iliac crest bone grafts in posterior cervical fusions. J Neurosurg. 1998;88(2):255–65.
77. Ryu SI, Lim JT, Kim SM, et al. Comparison of the biomechanical stability of dense cancellous allograft with tricortical iliac autograft and fibular allograft for cervical interbody fusion. Eur Spine J. 2006;15(9):1339–45.
78. Miller LE, Block JE. Safety and effectiveness of bone allografts in anterior cervical discectomy and fusion surgery. Spine (Phila Pa 1976). 2011;36(24):2045–50.
79. Hillard VH, Fassett DR, Finn MA, et al. Use of allograft bone for posterior C1-2 fusion. J Neurosurg Spine. 2009;11(4):396–401.
80. Godzik J, Ravindra VM, Ray WZ, et al. Comparison of structural allograft and traditional autograft technique in occipitocervical fusion: radiological and clinical outcomes from a single institution. J Neurosurg Spine. 2015;23(2):144–52.

4 Anterior Atlantoaxial Fusion

Andrew Z. Mo and Darren R. Lebl

Introduction

Fusion of the atlantoaxial complex has been achieved for decades through various techniques, predominantly through a midline posterior approach. As described below, improvements in implant technology have permitted an evolution of posterior techniques over the past several decades. Anterior transoral surgery has been described for indications such as periodontoid pannus decompression/odontoid resection and release of irreducible atlantoaxial dislocation [1–3]. Ventral craniocervical techniques and upper cervical plating through a transoral approach may be associated with wound complications, transoral contamination, and potential infection. In contrast, anterior approaches for transarticular screws have also been described [4, 5]. Approach of the anterior cervical spine by the Smith–Robinson approach has a long track record of good clinical outcomes and low associated infection and complication rates for commonly performed procedures such as anterior cervical discectomy and fusion (ACDF) and odontoid screw fixation [6, 7]. An anterior approach for rigid atlantoaxial joint fusion has the benefit of avoiding occipital nerve exposure and manipulation and avoiding the potential for postoperative C2 neuralgia [8, 9]. It also provides another safe technique to the spine surgeons' armamentarium for use in patients with anatomy unfavorable for posterior instrumentation [10–14].

Posterior atlantoaxial fixation techniques can be broadly categorized into various types including wiring, interlaminar clamps, atlantoaxial transarticular screws, screw–plate system fixation, screw–rod system fixation, and hook–screw system fixation techniques [15]. Gallie first reported the use of sublaminar wires for atlantoaxial fixation in 1939 [16]. Early techniques for C1–C2 fixation described by Gallie and Brooks and Jenkins utilized laminar wiring with concomitant on lay bone graft [17, 18]. Transarticular screw (TAS) fixation later demonstrated superior biomechanical strength [19] and higher rates of fusion [19, 20]. Magerl and Seemann first introduced C1–C2 transarticular screw (TAS) fixation in 1979 [21]. The technique described by Jeanneret and Magerl involves placing a transarticular screw through the C1–C2 articular surfaces [22]. This technique has been used effectively in the stabilization of AAI from a variety of causes. Despite reliable stability and high fusion rates, enthusiasm for TAS has decreased in some reports due to

A.Z. Mo, MD
Lenox Hill Hospital, 130 East 77th Street, New York, NY 10075, USA

D.R. Lebl, MD, MBA (✉)
Hospital for Special Surgery,
523 E 72nd St., New York, NY 10010, USA
e-mail: drlebl@gmail.com

L.T. Holly, P.A. Anderson (eds.), *Essentials of Spinal Stabilization*,
DOI 10.1007/978-3-319-59713-3_4

potential risk of vertebral artery injury [23]. Initially described by Goel et al. [24] and Goel and Laheri [25] and later popularized by Harms and Melcher [8], C1 lateral mass screw (C1 LMS) and C2 pedicle screw (C2PS) posterior fixation demonstrated biomechanical stability comparable to TAS techniques [26]. A consecutive series of 319 patients reported by Wang et al. has reported a low rate of screw misplacement and no clinical manifestation of vascular injury with the C1 LMS–C2PS technique [27]. Certain anatomic variations such as a "high-riding" vertebral artery may preclude safe C2PS placement [11, 12]. Other techniques for fixation of the atlantoaxial joint include the Wright C1 lateral mass–C2 translaminar (C1LM–C2TL) screw construct and the C1 lateral mass–C2 (C1LM–C2) pars screw construct [8, 24, 28–33]. C2 translaminar screws provide an alternative technique for posterior instrumentation [34]. There are limitations that may preclude the use of this technique, however, such as limited biomechanical strength of the lamina, previous C2 laminectomy, and certain morphologies of the lamina [35].

Indications and Patient Selection

The most common indication for atlantoaxial fusion is atlantoaxial instability (AAI). AAI is a clinical condition with symptoms ranging from axial neck pain to life-threatening neurologic injury caused by neural compression [36]. AAI is characterized by excessive motion at the atlantoaxial joint with potential for neurovascular compromise. The atlantoaxial articulation has complex biomechanical properties. The anatomy is unique in the sense that this motion segment lacks an intervertebral disk between the C1 and C2 vertebrae. The stability is provided primarily by the transverse, alar, and apical ligaments in association with the joints' articular and osseous structures [22]. AAI can arise from trauma, rheumatoid arthritis (RA), osteoarthritis, infection, Down syndrome, congenital anomalies, tumor, and iatrogenic destabilization [37]. In adults, degenerative (RA) and trauma are the most common causes of AAI, whereas in children congenital conditions such as Down syndrome are more common. One study found that approximately 13% of patients with Down syndrome have asymptomatic AAI, while up to 1.5% exhibit neurologic symptoms stemming from instability [19]. The results of one biomechanical study found that AAI may be associated with an anterior atlantodental distance of greater than 3.5 mm due to laxity or incompetence of the transverse atlantal ligament [38]. Instability of the atlantoaxial articulation may result in catastrophic neurological compromise. Instrumentation and fusion of the C1–C2 joint is indicated in the setting of clinical or biomechanical instability.

The goals of surgery are to provide stability with fixation and bone grafting for biological fusion. This may include reduction of the atlantoaxial motion segment for improvement of alignment and decompression of the neuroanatomy. The indications for anterior atlantoaxial fusion are similar to posterior atlantoaxial fusion and include failure of nonoperative treatments, severe refractory arthritis of the atlantoaxial joint, unstable os odontoideum, and progressive neurological deficit [9, 39].

Anterior transarticular screw fixation may also be a more favorable surgical option in patients where posterior fixation is challenged by anomalous vascular anatomy which may preclude safe posterior exposure and fixation [8, 40–42]. For example, various studies estimate 20–22% of patients are noted to demonstrate a high-riding transverse foramen on at least one side [10, 14, 43, 44]. Hypoplastic lamina of C2 may also preclude C2 translaminar fixation. An inter-transverse branch of the vertebral artery may occur which may make posterior C1 lateral mass fixation a less desirable option. Findings of a narrow C2 isthmus are seen in 10% of patients [13]. Posterior transarticular screw placement should not be attempted in patients with high-riding foramina and ectatic vertebral arteries and in patients in which the C2 isthmus will not accommodate a 3.5-mm screw, or other associated anomalies. The authors recommend meticulous study of reformatted fine-cut cervical spine CT images, potentially including multiplanar reformatted images that can allow visualization of each screw starting point and trajectory. Abnormalities on CT cuts of the foramen transversarium or other bony elements may suggest vertebral artery anomaly in which case a CT angiogram may help further characterize the vascular anatomy.

The advantages of anterior transarticular screws include surgical access through the commonly performed anterior approach with preservation of the posterior cervical musculature (dynamic stabilizers), reduction of anterior dislocation of C1 by the patient's head and neck extension in a prone position, and potentially a more predictable screw trajectory in relation to the vertebral artery, decreasing risk of injury [45]. Additional benefits of the anterior Smith–Robinson approach include a lower risk of postoperative infection by avoiding posterior approaches to the cervical spine [7]. Posterior transarticular screw fixations have been associated with a complication rate as high as 10% in the form of superficial infections and occipital nerve injury [46–48]. The avoidance of exposure of the C1–C2 joint from the posterior aspect may also decrease occipital neuralgia [49]. Posterior approaches to C1–C2 may not be suitable in the setting of revision posterior surgery, anomalous vascular anatomy, hypoplastic bone morphology, or deficit.

Anterior transarticular screw fixation is contraindicated in cases of fixed rotatory atlantoaxial subluxation and cases in which spinal cord decompression is necessary. Rotatory C1–C2 subluxation is a relative contraindication unless it is possible to obtain intraoperative reduction with cervical traction or by direct manipulation of the C1–C2 articulations. In patients with craniocervical malformations and anatomic conditions that result in an extremely deep and narrow surgical field (e.g., platybasia, basilar invagination, and low mandible projection), posterior fixation may be considered [50]. Fixed cervical kyphotic deformities or other unfavorable body habitus (barrel-chested patients) may prohibit anterior C1–C2 exposure as well. Traumatic injuries involving intra-articular extension into the C1–C2 joints and severe osteoporosis may make anterior C1–C2 fixation a suboptimal procedure.

Preoperative Considerations

Prior to any atlantoaxial procedure, the authors recommend meticulous study of reformatted fine-cut cervical spine CT images. Multiplanar reformatted images may be aligned along the direction of the C2 pedicle, for instance, and allow visualization of each screw starting point and trajectory. Abnormalities on CT or MRI imaging of the foramen transversarium or other bony elements may suggest vertebral artery anomaly in which case a CT angiogram may help further characterize the vascular anatomy.

Preoperative patient evaluation includes inspection of body habitus, range of motion of the cervical spine, and any previous anterior cervical surgery. In considering anterior cervical approach that is contralateral to a previous neck dissection, direct laryngoscopy may be undertaken to assess vocal cord mobility and function of the recurrent laryngeal nerve.

Surgical Technique

The patient is positioned supine with the neck in slight extension and the shoulders securely taped to the patient's sides with all appropriate pressure points padded. Gardner–Wells tongs are placed in routine fashion with approximately 10 pounds of axial traction for stabilization throughout the procedure. A radiolucent operating room table such as a Jackson table will permit essential intraoperative imaging. The author's preferred technique involves AP and lateral fluoroscopy; however, intraoperative navigation may augment the technique. Neuromonitoring is performed on all cervical spine procedures at our institution. The open-mouth odontoid view can be enhanced with the aid of a towel or cork in between the patient's teeth and is checked prior to prepping and draping the patient to ensure adequate visualization of the C1–C2 articulation. Use of a radiolucent endotracheal tube by the anesthesia team facilitates high-quality intraoperative fluoroscopic visualization of the upper cervical spine. Dental implants may also prohibit optimal intraoperative radiographic visualization and can be assessed preoperatively.

Prior to prepping and draping the patient, it is essential that adequate AP and lateral images of the C1–C2 articulation are obtained. Also, a guide wire or radiopaque wire may be placed on the patient's chest and visualized on lateral fluoroscopy to visualize the trajectory of the implants and mark out the level of the appropriate skin incision. The author's experience is that the skin incision may be transverse at a level similar to a routine ACDF approach given the significant cranial angulation of the implant trajectory. It may be necessary to put the patient's cervical spine in neutral alignment or even slight flexion to obtain the proper trajectory. In the case of any compressive pathology, this should be done while checking with neuromonitoring repeatedly.

Routine left-sided Smith–Robinson anterior cervical approach is performed to expose the anterior cervical spine. Gentle peanut dissection is performed cranially along the anterior aspect of the cervical spine to the C2 vertebrae. A radiolucent retractor may be placed on the anterior arch of the atlas (Fig. 4.1a). A small-angled curette can be placed into the C1–C2 articulation to decorticate the atlantoaxial joint articular surface and prepare an adequate fusion bed. Iliac crest can be harvested and packed into the articulation with a Penfield instrument. An awl or a matchstick burr can be used at the base of the C2 vertebrae (with care taken to preserve the C2–C3 disk) for a 1–2-mm pilot hole. The starting point can be visualized on AP radiography in the medial one-third of the C1–C2 articulation (Fig. 4.2). A threaded Kirschner wire (k-wire) with protective drill sleeve is advanced through the body of C2 in a cranial and lateral trajectory. Resistance is felt at the C1–C2 articulation at which point a "high-speed light touch" technique

Fig. 4.1 (**a**) Placement of a radiolucent retractor on the anterior arch of the atlas. (**b**) Coronal view of threaded Kirschner wire placement. (**c**) Sagittal view of threaded Kirschner wire placement

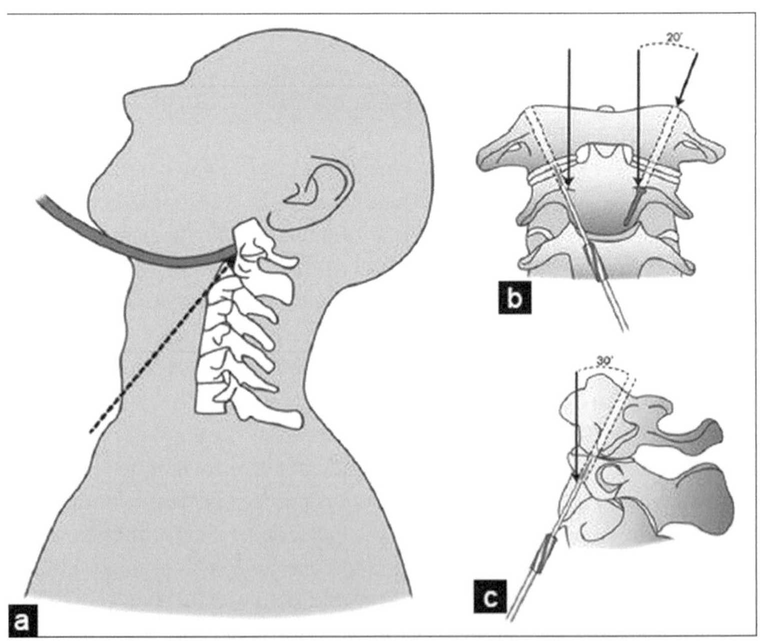

will allow the guidewire to be advanced under lateral fluoroscopy into the C1 lateral mass. The authors prefer to use cannulated stainless steel screws of 3.5 mm or 4.0 mm diameter depending on the patient's size and anatomy. The threaded portion of the screw needs to be placed into the C1 lateral mass to permit lag technique compression across the C1–C2 articulation. A self-cutting cannulated partially threaded cortical screw is advanced from medial-to-lateral and anterior-to-posterior along threaded Kirschner wires under image intensification (Figs. 4.1b, c and 4.3). Care should be taken to avoid screw advancement too far into the occipitocervical articulation.

Most patients can be managed in a cervical collar for 6 weeks. Postoperative halo vest is rarely used by the authors after anterior atlanto-axial fusion; however, it may be appropriate if

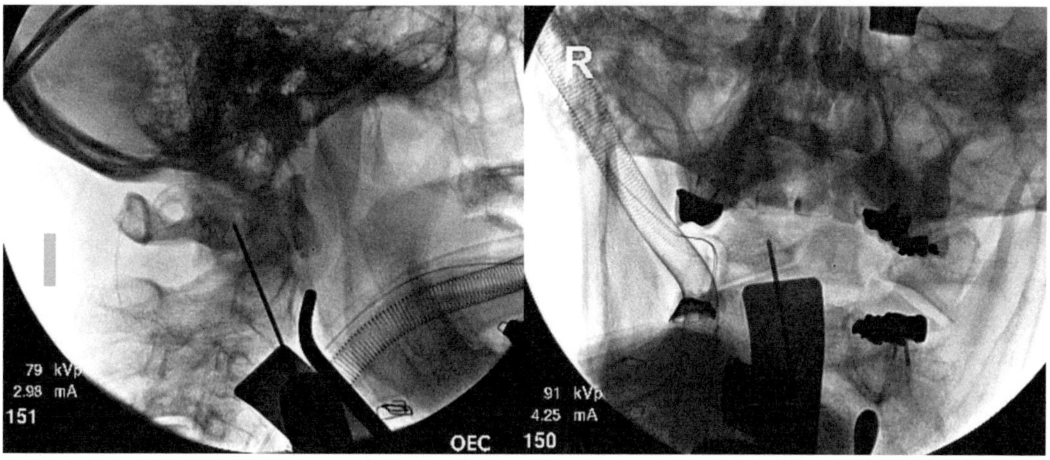

Fig. 4.2 Lateral and AP intraoperative fluoroscopy demonstrating starting point and trajectory of threaded k-wire inserted from the base of C2, through the C2 vertebral body, across the C1–C2 articular surface, and into the C1 lateral mass

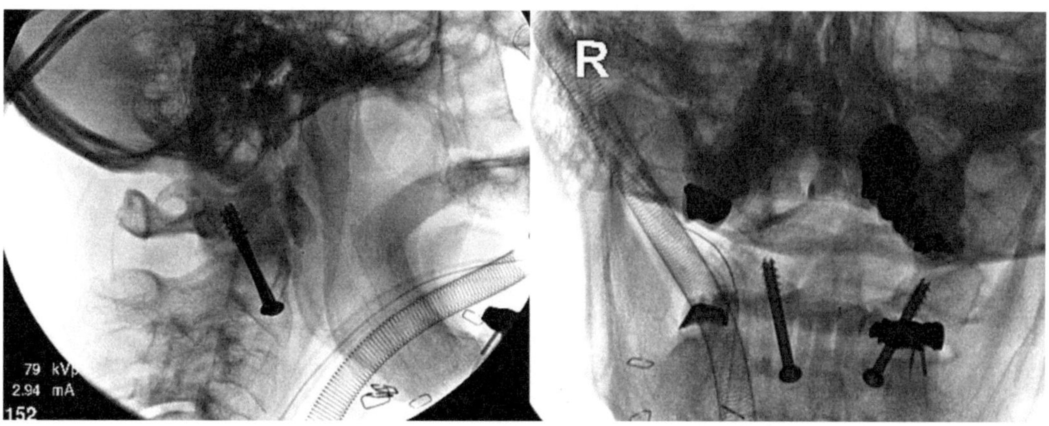

Fig. 4.3 Lateral and AP intraoperative fluoroscopy demonstrating partially threaded screw fixation across the C1–C2 articulation

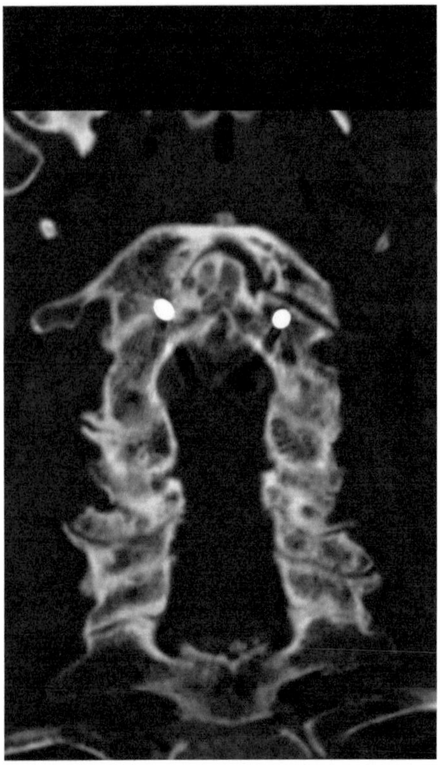

Fig. 4.4 Representative coronal CT image demonstrating fusion of right C1–C2 articulation 1 year postoperatively after C1–C2 anterior screw fixation

fixation is suboptimal or bone quality is poor and the patient can tolerate halo vest fixation. Inpatient postoperative CT scan may be obtained to visualize implant position and to obtain a baseline for subsequent imaging to determine biological fusion. Postoperative CT scan to visualize fusion as an outpatient may be obtained prior to advancing the patient's activity level (Fig. 4.4).

Case Illustration

History A 34-year-old male patient presented with a diagnosis of chronic atlantoaxial instability secondary to an os odontoideum. He complained of neck stiffness and denied numbness or weakness.

Physical Examination On examination, the patient was neurologically intact and had full range of motion of the cervical spine in flexion, extension, lateral bending, and axial rotation.

Imaging CT and plain radiographs demonstrated an os odontoideum. On flexion and extension radiographs, he had significant atlantoaxial displacement (Fig. 4.5). MRI of the brain showed

Fig. 4.5 Atlantoaxial instability of os odontoid on flexion/extension and lateral plain radiography

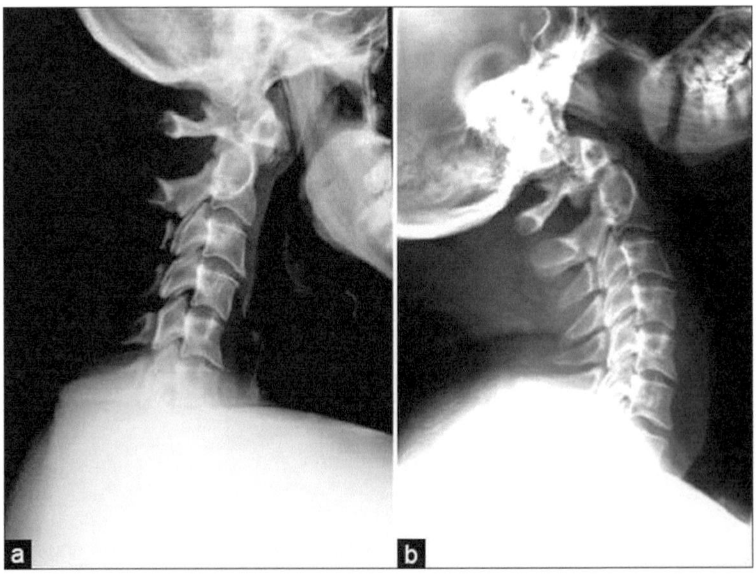

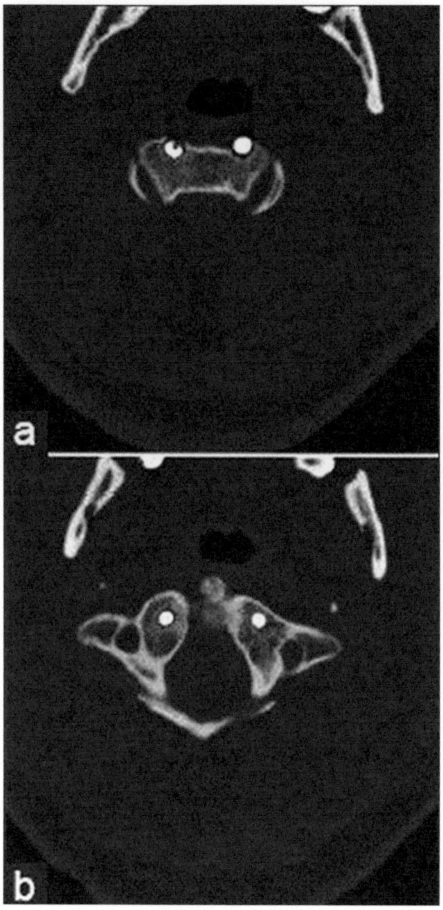

Fig. 4.6 (**a**) Postoperative axial computed tomography (CT) demonstrating anterior atlantoaxial screw position in the axis. (**b**) Postoperative axial CT showing tip of screw in atlas

cerebellar infarct with confirmation on CT angiogram of bilateral vertebral artery occlusions between C2 and C3, collateral reconstitution from the right occipital artery, and bridging anastomoses on the left.

Treatment Significant instability at C1–C2 warranted surgical fusion and an anterior approach was selected due to anomalous vascular anatomy, which precluded a safe posterior exposure and fixation by C1 LMS–C2PS. The patient was treated with anterior transarticular C1–C2 instrumentation and fusion. Postoperative CT scans confirmed acceptable screw placement in the axial (Fig. 4.6a, b), sagittal (Fig. 4.7), and coronal (Fig. 4.8a, b) planes.

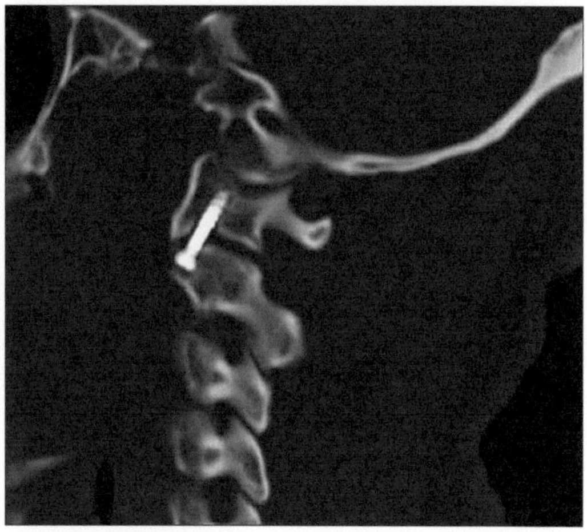

Fig. 4.7 Postoperative sagittal computed tomography showing anterior atlantoaxial screw position across the C1–C2 articulation

Outcome At 16-month follow-up, the patient maintained painless range of motion of the cervical spine with stable fixation and fusion without sensorimotor deficit.

Technical Pearls

- Prior to prepping and draping, AP and lateral radiography are essential to visualize the C1–C2 lateral mass. Cervical spine alignment may be adjusted (with neuromonitoring) to obtain the desired alignment for visualized implant trajectory.
- Careful study of preoperative imaging study will help determine candidates for C1–C2 anterior transarticular fusion. Multiplanar reformatted images can help visualize screw trajectory, and any suspicion of aberrant vascular anatomy may require CT angiography for evaluation.
- Careful intraoperative visualization of the guidewire is essential during screw fixation to avoid unwanted k-wire advancement.
- Threaded portion of screws should not traverse C1–C2 joint to allow lag fixation.
- A curette may carefully be passed into the C1–C2 joint for decortication and subsequent bone grafting. A Penfield retractor may be placed laterally to avoid injury to the vertebral artery.

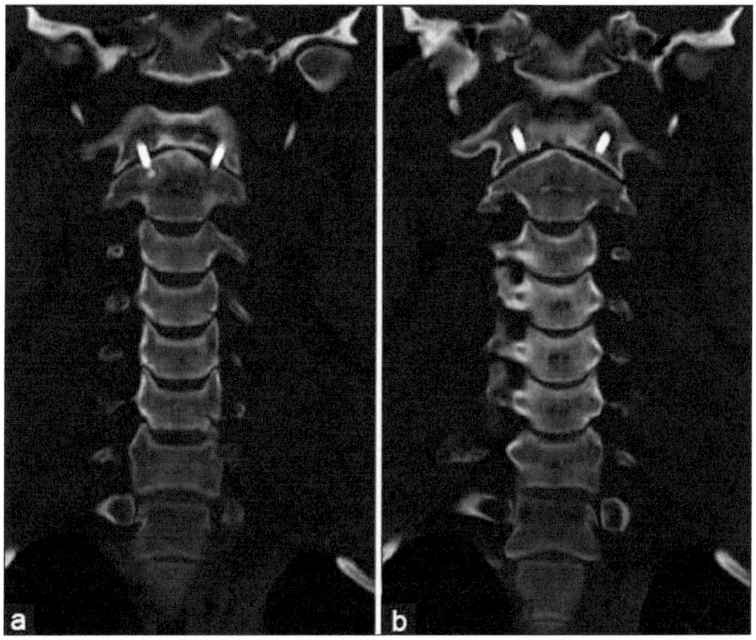

Fig. 4.8 (**a**) Postoperative coronal computed tomography (CT) demonstrating screw placement through the axis. (**b**) Postoperative coronal CT showing screw placement into the atlas

Complications and Strategies for Avoidance

Anterior transarticular screw fixation is not as widely utilized as posterior fixation techniques. With limited clinical data of outcomes in anterior transarticular screw fixation, the literature is thus far promising. Polli and Li reported successful outcomes without complications in 14 and 8 patients, respectively [50, 51].

Possible complications include infection, failure of fixation, and those known to the Smith–Robinson approach including but not limited to injuries of the superior and recurrent laryngeal nerve, carotid artery, esophagus, and trachea [52–54]. Risks of dysphagia and dysphonia are likely to be similar in incidence to that seen after odontoid screw fixation.

A study investigating the risk to the vertebral artery between anterior and posterior transarticular screws found no violation using anterior transarticular screws and risk associated with 19.2% of posteriorly placed transarticular screws [55]. Lu et al. reported in a biomechanical study that an anterior transarticular atlantoaxial screw 15–25 mm long can be inserted with a lateral angulation of 5–25° relative to the sagittal plane and a posterior angulation of 10–25° relative to the coronal plane [56].

Conclusion

While posterior techniques for atlantoaxial fixation have undergone a significant evolution and improvements, posterior Goel–Harms techniques may be associated with C2 neuropathy, extensive muscular dissection, and a relatively high infection rate. The Smith–Robinson approach provides a well-vascularized approach to the high anterior cervical spine with minimal muscular dissection and low associated infection rate. Anterior C1–C2 transarticular fixation is a viable technique for atlantoaxial fusion in select patients. Multiplanar reformatted images can help visualize screw trajectory, and any suspicion of aberrant vascular anatomy may require CT angiography for evaluation. Screw trajectory is determined by patient's individual morphology of the C1–C2 complex. An "up and out" trajectory allows k-wire placement under image guidance and lag-screw fixation of the C1–C2 joint. Decortication and grafting are essential to obtaining biological fusion.

References

1. Crockard H, Pozo J, Ransford A, Stevens J, Kendall B, Essigman W. Transoral decompression and posterior fusion for rheumatoid atlanto-axial subluxation. Bone Joint J. 1986;68-B(3):350–6.
2. Goel A, Karapurkar AP. Transoral plate and screw fixation of the craniovertebral region–a preliminary report. Br J Neurosurg. 1994;8(6):743–5. doi:10.3109/02688699409101191.
3. Kandziora F, Pflugmacher R, Ludwig K, Duda G, Mittlmeier T, Haas NP. Biomechanical comparison of four anterior atlantoaxial plate systems. J Neurosurg Spine. 2002;96(3):313–20. doi:10.3171/spi.2002.96.3.0313.
4. Koller H, Kammermeier V, Ulbricht D, et al. Anterior retropharyngeal fixation C1-2 for stabilization of atlantoaxial instabilities: study of feasibility, technical description and preliminary results. Eur Spine J. 2006;15(9):1326–38. doi:10.1007/s00586-006-0103-2.
5. Apfelbaum RI, Lonser RR, Veres R, Casey A. Direct anterior screw fixation for recent and remote odontoid fractures. J Neurosurg Spine. 2000;93(2):227–36. doi:10.3171/spi.2000.93.2.0227.
6. Olsen MA, Nepple JJ, Riew KD, et al. Risk factors for surgical site infection following orthopaedic spinal operations. J Bone Joint Surg Am. 2008;90(1):62–9. doi:10.2106/JBJS.F.01515.
7. Memtsoudis SG, Hughes A, Ma Y, Chiu YL, Sama AA, Girardi FP. Increased in-hospital complications after primary posterior versus primary anterior cervical fusion. Clin Orthop Relat Res. 2011;469(3):649–57. doi:10.1007/s11999-010-1549-4.
8. Harms J, Melcher RP. Posterior C1-C2 fusion with polyaxial screw and rod fixation. Spine (Phila Pa 1976). 2001;26(22):2467–71. doi:10.1097/00007632-200111150-00014.
9. Stulik J, Vyskocil T, Sebesta P, Kryl J. Atlantoaxial fixation using the polyaxial screw-rod system. Eur Spine J. 2007;16(4):479–84. doi:10.1007/s00586-006-0241-6.
10. Abou Madawi A, Solanki G, Casey AT, Crockard HA. Variation of the groove in the axis vertebra for the vertebral artery. Implications for instrumentation. J Bone Joint Surg Br. 1997;79(5):820–3. http://www.ncbi.nlm.nih.gov/pubmed/9331044. Accessed 21 Aug 2016.
11. Mueller C-A, Roesseler L, Podlogar M, Kovacs A, Kristof RA. Accuracy and complications of transpedicular C2 screw placement without the use of spinal navigation. Eur Spine J. 2010;19(5):809–14. doi:10.1007/s00586-010-1291-3.
12. Ebraheim N, Rollins JR, Xu R, Jackson WT. Anatomic consideration of C2 pedicle screw placement. Spine (Phila Pa 1976). 1996;21(6):691–5. http://www.ncbi.nlm.nih.gov/pubmed/8882690. Accessed 21 Aug 2016.
13. Mandel IM, Kambach BJ, Petersilge CA, Johnstone B, Yoo JU. Morphologic considerations of C2 isthmus dimensions for the placement of transarticular screws. Spine (Phila Pa 1976). 2000;25(12):1542–7. http://www.ncbi.nlm.nih.gov/pubmed/10851104. Accessed 21 Aug 2016.
14. Paramore CG, Dickman CA, Sonntag VK. The anatomical suitability of the C1-2 complex for transarticular screw fixation. J Neurosurg. 1996;85(2):221–4. doi:10.3171/jns.1996.85.2.0221.
15. Huang D-G, Hao D-J, He B-R, et al. Posterior atlantoaxial fixation: a review of all techniques. Spine J. 2015;15(10):2271–81. doi:10.1016/j.spinee.2015.07.008.
16. Gallie WE. Fractures and dislocations of the cervical spine. Am J Surg. 1939;46(3):495–9.
17. Brooks AL, Jenkins EB. Atlanto-axial arthrodesis by the wedge compression method. J Bone Joint Surg Am. 1978;60(3):279–84. http://www.ncbi.nlm.nih.gov/pubmed/348703. Accessed 21 Aug 2016.
18. Gallie WE. Skeletal traction in the treatment of fractures and dislocations of the cervical spine. Ann Surg. 1937;106(4):770–6. http://www.ncbi.nlm.nih.gov/pubmed/17857077. Accessed 21 Aug 2016.
19. Naderi S, Crawford NR, Song GS, Sonntag VK, Dickman CA. Biomechanical comparison of C1-C2 posterior fixations. Cable, graft, and screw combinations. Spine (Phila Pa 1976). 1998;23(18):1946–55. http://www.ncbi.nlm.nih.gov/pubmed/9779526. Accessed 21 Aug 2016.
20. Coyne TJ, Fehlings MG, Wallace MC, Bernstein M, Tator CH. C1-C2 posterior cervical fusion: long-term evaluation of results and efficacy. Neurosurgery. 1995;37(4):688-92-3. http://www.ncbi.nlm.nih.gov/pubmed/8559297. Accessed 21 Aug 2016.
21. Magerl F, Magerl F. Stable posterior fusion of the atlas and axis by transarticular screw fixation. Cerv Spine I. 1987;1:322–7.
22. Du JY, Aichmair A, Kueper J, Wright T, Lebl DR. Biomechanical analysis of screw constructs for atlantoaxial fixation in cadavers: a systematic review and meta-analysis. J Neurosurg Spine. 2015;22(2):151–61. doi:10.3171/2014.10.SPINE13805.
23. Jones EL, Heller JG, Silcox DH, Hutton WC. Cervical pedicle screws versus lateral mass screws. Anatomic feasibility and biomechanical comparison. Spine (Phila Pa 1976). 1997;22(9):977–82. http://www.ncbi.nlm.nih.gov/pubmed/9152447. Accessed 21 Aug 2016.
24. Goel A, Laheri V. Plate and screw fixation for atlanto-axial subluxation. Acta Neurochir. 1994;129(1–2):47–53. doi:10.1007/BF01400872.
25. Goel A, Desai KI, Muzumdar DP. Atlantoaxial fixation using plate and screw method: a report of 160 treated patients. Neurosurgery. 2002;51(6):1351-6-7. http://www.ncbi.nlm.nih.gov/pubmed/12445339. Accessed 21 Aug 2016.

26. Kuroki H, Rengachary SS, Goel VK, Holekamp SA, Pitkänen V, Ebraheim NA. Biomechanical comparison of two stabilization techniques of the atlantoaxial joints: transarticular screw fixation versus screw and rod fixation. Neurosurgery. 2005;56(1 Suppl):151-9-9. http://www.ncbi.nlm.nih.gov/pubmed/15799804. Accessed 21 Aug 2016.
27. Wang S, Wang C, Wood KB, Yan M, Zhou H. Radiographic evaluation of the technique for C1 lateral mass and C2 pedicle screw fixation in three hundred nineteen cases. Spine (Phila Pa 1976). 2011;36(1): 3–8. doi:10.1097/BRS.0b013e3181c97dc7.
28. Bransford RJ, Lee MJ, Reis A. Posterior fixation of the upper cervical spine: contemporary techniques. J Am Acad Orthop Surg. 2011;19(2):63–71. http://www.ncbi.nlm.nih.gov/pubmed/21292929. Accessed 21 Aug 2016.
29. Inoue S, Moriyama T, Tachibana T, et al. Cervical lateral mass screw fixation without fluoroscopic control: analysis of risk factors for complications associated with screw insertion. Arch Orthop Trauma Surg. 2012;132(7):947–53. doi:10.1007/s00402-012-1507-6.
30. Lehman RA, Dmitriev AE, Helgeson MD, Sasso RC, Kuklo TR, Riew KD. Salvage of C2 pedicle and pars screws using the intralaminar technique. Spine (Phila Pa 1976). 2008;33(9):960–5. doi:10.1097/BRS.0b013e31816c915b.
31. Mummaneni P, Haid R. Atlantoaxial fixation: overview of all techniques. Neurol India. 2005;53(4):408. doi:10.4103/0028-3886.22606.
32. Vender JR, Rekito AJ, Harrison SJ, McDonnell DE. Evolution of posterior cervical and occipitocervical fusion and instrumentation. Neurosurg Focus. 2004;16(1):1–15. doi:10.3171/foc.2004.16.1.10.
33. Wright NM. Translaminar rigid screw fixation of the axis. J Neurosurg Spine. 2005;3(5):409–14. doi:10.3171/spi.2005.3.5.0409.
34. Leonard JR, Wright NM. Pediatric atlantoaxial fixation with bilateral, crossing C-2 translaminar screws. Technical note. J Neurosurg. 2006;104(1 Suppl):59–63. doi:10.3171/ped.2006.104.1.59.
35. Wang MY. C2 crossing laminar screws: cadaveric morphometric analysis. Neurosurgery. 2006;59(1 Suppl 1):ONS84–8; discussion ONS84–8. doi:10.1227/01.NEU.0000219900.24467.32.
36. Kandziora F, Kerschbaumer F, Starker M, Mittlmeier T. Biomechanical assessment of transoral plate fixation for atlantoaxial instability. Spine (Phila Pa 1976). 2000;25(12):1555–61. http://www.ncbi.nlm.nih.gov/pubmed/10851106. Accessed 21 Aug 2016.
37. Haid RW, Subach BR, McLaughlin MR, Rodts GE, Wahlig JB. C1-C2 transarticular screw fixation for atlantoaxial instability: a 6-year experience. Neurosurgery. 2001;49(1):65-8-70. http://www.ncbi.nlm.nih.gov/pubmed/11440461. Accessed 11 June 2016.
38. White AA, Johnson RM, Panjabi MM, Southwick WO. Biomechanical analysis of clinical stability in the cervical spine. Clin Orthop Relat Res. 1975;(109): 85–96. http://www.ncbi.nlm.nih.gov/pubmed/1132209. Accessed 11 June 2016.
39. Gluf WM, Schmidt MH, Apfelbaum RI. Atlantoaxial transarticular screw fixation: a review of surgical indications, fusion rate, complications, and lessons learned in 191 adult patients. J Neurosurg Spine. 2005;2(2):155–63. doi:10.3171/spi.2005.2.2.0155.
40. Campanelli M, Kattner KA, Stroink A, Gupta K, West S. Posterior C1-C2 transarticular screw fixation in the treatment of displaced type II odontoid fractures in the geriatric population – review of seven cases. Surg Neurol. 1999;51(6):596-600-1. http://www.ncbi.nlm.nih.gov/pubmed/10369225. Accessed 6 Sept 2016.
41. Farey ID, Nadkarni S, Smith N. Modified Gallie technique versus transarticular screw fixation in C1-C2 fusion. Clin Orthop Relat Res. 1999;359:126–35. http://www.ncbi.nlm.nih.gov/pubmed/10078135. Accessed 6 Sept 2016.
42. Goel A, Gupta S. Vertebral artery injury with transarticular screws. J Neurosurg. 1999;90(2):376–77. http://www.ncbi.nlm.nih.gov/pubmed/9950517. Accessed 6 Sept 2016.
43. Madawi AA, Casey AT, Solanki GA, Tuite G, Veres R, Crockard HA. Radiological and anatomical evaluation of the atlantoaxial transarticular screw fixation technique. J Neurosurg. 1997;86(6):961–8. doi:10.3171/jns.1997.86.6.0961.
44. Jun BY. Anatomic study for ideal and safe posterior C1-C2 transarticular screw fixation. Spine (Phila Pa 1976). 1998;23(15):1703–7. http://www.ncbi.nlm.nih.gov/pubmed/9704379. Accessed 6 Sept 2016.
45. Krzysztof. Rheumatoid atlantoaxial instability treated by anterior transarticular C1-C2 fixation. Case report. Neurochir Pol. 2013;47(3):290–5. doi:10.5114/ninp.2013.35487.
46. Grob D, Jeanneret B, Aebi M, Markwalder TM. Atlanto-axial fusion with transarticular screw fixation. J Bone Joint Surg Br. 1991;73(6):972–6. http://www.ncbi.nlm.nih.gov/pubmed/1955447. Accessed 24 Oct 2016.
47. Statham P, O'Sullivan M, Russell T. The Halifax Interlaminar clamp for posterior cervical fusion: initial experience in the United Kingdom. Neurosurgery. 1993;32(3):396-8-9. http://www.ncbi.nlm.nih.gov/pubmed/8455764. Accessed 24 Oct 2016.
48. Stillerman CB, Wilson JA. Atlanto-axial stabilization with posterior transarticular screw fixation: technical description and report of 22 cases. Neurosurgery. 1993;32(6):948-54-5. http://www.ncbi.nlm.nih.gov/pubmed/8327097. Accessed 24 Oct 2016.
49. Gunnarsson T, Massicotte EM, Govender PV, Raja Rampersaud Y, Fehlings MG. The use of C1 lateral mass screws in complex cervical spine surgery: indications, techniques, and outcome in a

prospective consecutive series of 25 cases. J Spinal Disord Tech. 2007;20(4):308–16. doi:10.1097/01.bsd.0000211291.21766.4d.
50. Polli FM, Miscusi M, Forcato S, Raco A. Atlantoaxial anterior transarticular screw fixation: a case series and reappraisal of the technique. Spine J. 2015;15(1):185–93. doi:10.1016/j.spinee.2014.09.019.
51. Li WL, Chi YL, Xu HZ, et al. Percutaneous anterior transarticular screw fixation for atlantoaxial instability: a case series 2010;92(4):545–549. doi:10.1302/0301-620X.92B4.22790.
52. Tew JM, Mayfield FH. Complications of surgery of the anterior cervical spine. Clin Neurosurg. 1976;23:424–34. http://www.ncbi.nlm.nih.gov/pubmed/975693. Accessed 25 Oct 2016.
53. Bertalanffy H, Eggert H-R. Complications of anterior cervical discectomy without fusion in 450 consecutive patients. Acta Neurochir. 1989;99(1–2):41–50. doi:10.1007/BF01407775.
54. Fountas KN, Kapsalaki EZ, Nikolakakos LG, et al. Anterior cervical discectomy and fusion associated complications. Spine (Phila Pa 1976). 2007;32(21):2310–7. doi:10.1097/BRS.0b013e318154c57e.
55. Xu H, Chi YL, Wang XY, et al. Comparison of the anatomic risk for vertebral artery injury associated with percutaneous atlantoaxial anterior and posterior transarticular screws. Spine J. 2012;12(8):656–62. doi:10.1016/j.spinee.2012.05.010.
56. Lu J, Ebraheim NA, Yang H, Heck BE, Yeasting RA. Anatomic considerations of anterior transarticular screw fixation for atlantoaxial instability. Spine (Phila Pa 1976). 1998;23(11):1229–35; discussion 1236. http://www.ncbi.nlm.nih.gov/pubmed/9636976. Accessed 26 Oct 2016.

5 Posterior Atlantoaxial Fusion

Oliver Tannous, Naveed Nabizadeh, and R. Todd Allen

Introduction

The anatomy of the atlas and the axis is unique and complex. The odontoid process of the axis lies between the anterior atlantal arch and the transverse atlantal ligament. These are the major contributors to atlantoaxial stability. Any disruption in the integrity of these structures can result in C1-C2 instability [1]. Secondary stabilizers include the alar ligaments and their attachments to the occiput. The complex anatomy of the atlantoaxial region, particularly its proximity to the vertebral arteries, spinal cord, and internal carotid arteries, differentiates it from the remainder of the cervical spine. Therefore, surgical procedures in this region are technically demanding and require a deep understanding of the surrounding anatomy [2, 3].

Atlantoaxial fusion may be performed in a wide variety of settings including odontoid fracture, atlantoaxial instability, basilar invagination, severe degenerative arthrosis, or neoplasm of the atlantoaxial region [2]. Although there is controversy with regard to surgical interventions in the setting of an asymptomatic patient, a consensus exists for surgical fixation of patients with symptomatic or progressive instability [1, 4].

Multiple surgical techniques have been described for posterior C1-C2 stabilization including wire fixation, C1-2 interlaminar clamps, C1-2 transarticular screws, and C1-C2 screw-rod constructs, including C2 pedicle, pars, or translaminar screws [2, 5]. The aim of this chapter is to describe the surgical indications, varying fixation techniques, and perioperative pearls and pitfalls associated with posterior atlantoaxial fusion.

O. Tannous, MD
Georgetown University Department of Orthopaedics, Washington, DC, USA
e-mail: otannous@gmail.com

N. Nabizadeh, MD • R.T. Allen, MD (✉)
UCSD Department of Orthopaedics, San Diego, CA, USA
e-mail: nnabizadeh@ucsd.edu; rtallen@ucsd.edu

Indications

Congenital, traumatic, and inflammatory conditions can lead to atlantoaxial instability with or without subsequent neurologic impairment. The most common diseases include rheumatoid arthritis, odontoid fractures, Down syndrome, C1-C2 rotatory subluxation, basilar invagination, Klippel-Feil syndrome, osteogenesis imperfecta, and neurofibromatosis [6–8]. The general indications for surgical intervention in patients with atlantoaxial instability include intractable pain, progressive myelopathy, and progressive radiologic or neurologic instability [9, 10].

Rheumatoid Arthritis Atlantoaxial instability represents the most common manifestation of

L.T. Holly, P.A. Anderson (eds.), *Essentials of Spinal Stabilization*,
DOI 10.1007/978-3-319-59713-3_5

rheumatoid involvement of the spine [10, 11]. The inflammatory changes result in destruction of ligaments, cartilage, and subchondral bone [12]. Clinical manifestation varies from a compressive myelopathy due to a retrodental pannus, to a reducible anterior atlantoaxial subluxation, and ultimately to an irreducible anterior and vertical atlantoaxial subluxation [10]. The retrodental hypertrophic pannus is a reaction to the instability of the C1-C2 segment, not a direct consequence of the inflammatory process [10, 13]. As such, the pannus generally disappears after posterior surgical stabilization. Transoral surgery is reserved for cases with a large compressive pannus, irreducible dislocation, or basilar invagination [10, 14–16].

Odontoid Fractures Odontoid fractures occur with a bimodal distribution and considerable controversy exists with regard to the optimal treatment of type II fractures. Nonoperative treatment for geriatric type II odontoid fractures is associated with high rates of nonunion and mortality [13]. A stable, asymptomatic pseudarthrosis can often be treated with observation, but atlantoaxial fusion becomes indicated when instability or neurologic decline occur.

Down Syndrome Approximately 15% of patients with Down syndrome are affected by atlantoaxial instability secondary to aplasia or hypoplasia of the odontoid process, laxity of the transverse atlantal ligament, or assimilation of the atlas. Although they are mostly asymptomatic, the instability can progress with rapid neurologic decline due to minor trauma. There are no data from which to predict which asymptomatic patients will progress or develop symptoms [17, 18].

Atlantoaxial Rotatory Subluxation Rotatory subluxation has been reported to varying degrees following upper respiratory infection or traumatic events, particularly in the pediatric population. The initial treatment consists of cervical traction for 2–3 weeks and is often sufficient to correct the deformity [19]. If traction fails, posterior C1-C2 fusion becomes indicated.

Basilar Invagination Several congenital, traumatic, inflammatory, or connective tissue disorders can result in basilar invagination (upward migration of the odontoid process into the foramen magnum). In patients who are symptomatic or at risk of progression, anterior decompression by transoral odontoidectomy followed by posterior occipitocervical or atlantoaxial fixation is often the treatment of choice [10, 20].

Skeletal Dysplasia Patients with spondyloepiphyseal dysplasia, achondroplasia, pseudoachondroplasia, Kniest syndrome, and Morquio syndrome are at high risk for upper cervical spine instability and subsequent spinal cord compression. These patients may require posterior stabilization and fusion when the instability progresses or becomes symptomatic [21].

Atlantoaxial Arthrosis The atlantoaxial articulation lacks an intervertebral disc and all loads are transmitted through the articular surfaces. In addition, there is a high degree of sensory input to this articulation so that atlantoaxial movement can be tracked precisely presumably to aid in coordination of visual fields. When osteoarthritis with or without instability occurs, patients may experience disabling suboccipital and occipital pain and difficulty with head rotation. This disease process is likely associated with calcium pyrophosphate disease and a destructive arthropathy. Treatment is highly successful with atlantoaxial arthrodesis.

Preoperative Considerations

Prior to considering a posterior atlantoaxial fusion, it is critical to evaluate the patient's anatomy using plain radiography, computed tomography (CT), and sometimes magnetic resonance imaging (MRI). Radiography is typically sufficient to diagnose atlantoaxial instability on standard open-mouth and lateral flexion and extension views [22].

Open-Mouth View C1-C2 rotatory subluxation is represented by asymmetry or lateral displacement of the atlas on the axis by more than 2 mm. Traumatic rupture of the transverse atlantal ligament should be suspected if combined overhang of the lateral masses of C1 on C2 exceeds 8 mm [23].

Anterior Atlantodens Interval (ADI) The ADI is identified on the lateral view as the distance between the anterior odontoid process and the anterior arch of C1. The normal ADI is less than 3 mm in adults and less than 4 mm in children [24, 25], whereas an ADI greater than 4–5 mm indicates atlantoaxial instability. Occult instability can be identified on the flexion-extension views [26]. When the ADI exceeds 8–10 mm, surgery is recommended, as this value suggests total rupture of the transverse and alar ligaments [25].

Posterior ADI This is the distance from the posterior border of the odontoid to the posterior arch of C1, which represents the space available for the upper cervical spinal cord. The spinal cord becomes threatened when the space available for the cord (SAC) is less than 14 mm [27]. In rheumatoid patients, an ADI less than this value represents a poor prognosis as many will develop neurologic deficits.

Computed Tomography Fine-cut CT images with axial, sagittal, and coronal reformatting is the best modality for evaluating the bony anatomy of C1 and C2. It is especially critical to study the CT images prior to attempting placement of C1 and C2 instrumentation since a ponticulus posticus may be present on the C1 arch in up to 15.5% of patients [28]. Understanding this anatomic variation is important in order to avoid injuring the vertebral artery. CT can additionally be helpful in evaluating rotatory atlantoaxial displacement [29].

Magnetic Resonance Imaging (MRI) MRI is the study of choice to evaluate the integrity of the spinal cord and surrounding soft tissues. It is especially useful to diagnose transverse atlantal ligament rupture in equivocal cases and to evaluate the epidural space in rheumatoid patients with a retrodental pannus [30, 31]. Dynamic MRI in flexion and extension is valuable in patients with clinical signs of myelopathy or cervical pain but without radiological changes on flexion and extension radiographs or neutral MRI [32, 33].

CT Angiography (CTA) Careful preoperative evaluation of the vertebral artery (VA) is mandatory to help prevent iatrogenic VA injury and avoid postoperative neurologic sequelae. The incidence of VA anomalies at the cranio-vertebral junction is increased in patients with osseous anomalies like Down syndrome. Two common VA anomalies are the "C2 segmental type of VA" and "fenestration" of the VA. In the former case, the VA enters the spinal canal between C1 and C2 without passing through the C1 transverse foramen. In the latter case, the VA bifurcates after exiting the C2 transverse foramen – one branch follows the typical anatomic course, whereas the other branch enters the spinal canal between C1 and C2, subsequently joining the other branch at the cranial aspect of C1. Therefore, preoperative CTA in patients with Down syndrome or other bony anomalies can minimize the risk of intraoperative VA injury [34].

Additionally, the narrow isthmus caused by a high-riding vertebral artery can jeopardize the VA when performing the Magerl technique, and many authors recommend that C1-C2 transarticular fixation be abandoned if the isthmus is too narrow [35]. Furthermore, the risk of VA injury is higher in patients with isolated C2 fractures, particularly in type III dens fractures, presence of intraforaminal fragment, or comminuted transverse foramen fractures with intraforaminal fragments greater than 1 mm [36]. Finally, in patients with systemic diseases like rheumatoid arthritis, anatomical variations of the VA and C1 lateral mass deformation may increase the risk of VA injury [37]. Therefore, preoperative evaluation of VA anatomy via CT angiography can help to reduce the complication rate related to the VA injury.

Surgical Technique

Positioning After endotracheal anesthesia, the surgeon places Mayfield tongs to secure the occiput. The neurophysiologic monitoring needles are secured in the appropriate areas, and the patient is rotated prone over a draw sheet with the arms secured to the side. The surgeon must coordinate with the anesthesiologist in order to stand at the head of the bed and hold the Mayfield tongs during the turning process. It is best to keep a cervical collar in place, if present. Once the Mayfield device is secured to the table, the collar is removed and the chin is flexed and retracted to properly align the cervical spine and optimize surgical exposure. The posterior occiput must generally be at the same horizontal level as the apex of the thoracic spine (in the absence of a deformity).

The craniocervical ligament and atlantoaxial reduction is checked using biplanar fluoroscopy. Correct rotation of the head is checked by assuring that the ears are located horizontally and parallel to the thorax. A fluoroscopic image may be used to show that the mandible is in neutral rotation indicating correct head rotation. Reduction, if required, is achieved by translation and angulation using the Mayfield device. In general, a small amount of space between the occiput posterior arch of C1 and C2 should be present on lateral images.

Care is taken to assure adequate padding of the chest, iliac crests, proximal hips, knees, and elbows. The patient's hair is shaved to the level of the external occipital protuberance, and the skin is prepped with chlorhexidine and alcohol.

Exposure A midline incision approximately 75 mm long from the base of the occiput to the level of the C3 spinous process is performed. The dissection is carried down with monopolar cautery through the subcutaneous tissues to the level of the fascia. Using the spinous processes as landmarks, the ligamentum nuchae is dissected down its midline with monopolar cautery in order to remain within the relatively avascular plane and avoid undue bleeding. At this point, the most prominent cephalad spinous process is C2. Care is taken to preserve the attachments of the semispinalis cervicis muscle on the caudal aspect of the C2 spinous process. If the landmarks are not clear, it is prudent to place a clamp on the presumed spinous process of C2 to verify the correct operative level.

The dissection is then carried cephalad along the midline to identify the C1 tubercle and the base of the foramen magnum. Doing so will facilitate lateral exposure. Care must be taken not to violate the thin atlanto-occipital and atlantoaxial membranes. Subperiosteal dissection is then carried laterally along the C1 arch, taking care to remain on the inferior aspect of the arch as the vertebral arteries take a sinusoidal path along its cephalad border. The safe zone of the C1 arch is within 1.5 cm from the tubercle as this is the point where the vertebral arteries ascend into the foramen magnum. Next, subperiosteal exposure of C2 is continued to the lateral edge of the C2 lateral masses, taking care not to violate the C2-C3 facet joint. The subperiosteal dissection for this portion of the exposure is carried out bluntly with a periosteal elevator or Penfield elevator, particularly around the C1 arch and lateral pars of C2, as this minimizes the risk of VA injury that could otherwise occur with electrocautery dissection.

If C1 lateral mass screws are to be inserted, the C2 nerve root must either be retracted caudally or resected. Some authors, including Goel, who first described this technique in 1988, advocate transection of the C2 nerve to facilitate exposure of the C1 lateral mass and C1-C2 facet joint [38], since sacrifice of the C2 ganglion results in suboccipital numbness that is typically inconsequential for the patient and rarely results in postoperative neuralgic pain [39]. Nevertheless, it is our preference to preserve the C2 ganglion and work rostral to it. At this point, significant bleeding from the C2 venous plexus will be encountered. This can be controlled with the use of bipolar electrocautery, thrombin-soaked gel foam, and fibrillar collagen. Workflow can be optimized by working back and forth bilaterally and allowing adequate time for hemostasis of the venous plexuses.

Instrumentation

Many methods of atlantoaxial fixation have been described. Wire techniques provide less fixation strength and usually require a postoperative halo vest. Although wiring methods have fallen out of favor since the popularization of screw-rod constructs, they may still be useful in patients with unfavorable VA anatomy. The two most common fixation methods currently used, however, are C1 lateral mass screws with C2 screws and C1-2 transarticular screws which will be described separately.

Posterior Wiring Techniques Several posterior wiring methods have been described in the literature. Gallie, in 1939, described C1-C2 sublaminar steel wire fixation [40]. In his method, an iliac crest bone graft is notched inferiorly and fitted over the spinous process of C2 below and leaned against the posterior arch of C1 above. The steel wire is passed under the C1 lamina, then dorsal to the iliac crest graft, and tightened around the spinous process of C2. Sonntag described a modification of this technique in 1991 [41], where the bone graft is fitted along the caudal surface of the C1 posterior arch, as apposed to leaning it on the dorsal surface of the C1 posterior arch. This modification, which utilizes the same wiring technique, but instead applies a "press-fit" wedging of the graft, resulted in significantly high fusion rates (up to 97%). Brooks and Jenkins, in 1978, described another wiring method [42] where two separate iliac crest grafts are beveled and wedged between the posterior C1 arch, and C2 lamina. These are secured with two sublaminar wires, one on each side of the midline, passed underneath the laminae of C1 and C2, and wrapped around each graft, respectively. They reported a 93% fusion rate with this technique.

The disadvantage of these wiring techniques includes risk of dural or neurologic injury, as well as weaker rotational strength than screw-rod constructs. In addition, they usually require postoperative immobilization with a halo-vest device.

C1 Lateral and C2 Screws The use of C1 lateral mass and C2 pedicle screws was initially described by Goel in 1988 [38] and popularized by Harms in 2001 [43]. Both reports describe a 100% fusion rate with this technique, which has prompted widespread adoption of this screw-rod construct for atlantoaxial arthrodesis.

C1 Lateral Mass Screw Once exposure is complete, the dorsal root ganglion of C2 is retracted caudally to expose the start point for the C1 lateral mass screw, which is the midpoint of the inferior lateral mass at its junction with the posterior arch (Fig. 5.1a). An alternative start point for the C1 lateral mass screw can be on the dorsal C1 arch, with advancement of the drill, tap, and screw through the pedicle analog of C1 (the height of the posterior arch at the groove for the VA). The advantage of this modification is avoidance of the venous plexus surrounding the C2 ganglion; however, meticulous preoperative measurement is needed to ensure that the height of the pedicle analog exceeds 4 mm at the level of the groove of the VA [44]. This minimum height is absent in 19.2% of patients, which would preclude safe use of the alternative start point [44].

The start point is marked with a 2-mm high-speed burr (Fig. 5.1a). The screw track is prepared with a 2.5-mm drill medialized 15–20° and with a sagittal trajectory toward the inferior half of the anterior C1 arch (Fig. 5.1b, c). It is the author's preference to confirm the sagittal trajectory with fluoroscopic imaging. The drill is advanced to the posterior aspect of the anterior atlantal arch as lying more anterior is the carotid artery. Following drilling and tapping, a 3.5-mm polyaxial screw is placed. The length of the screw track within the lateral mass is typically 16–18 mm; however, the base of the screw contains an additional 10-mm unthreaded portion, which allows the screw head and tulip to line up with the C2 screw and minimizes irritation of the C2 nerve root [45]. There is variability in the dimensions of the C1 lateral masses, and preoperative screw measurement is important. The usual total screw length is 30–35 mm.

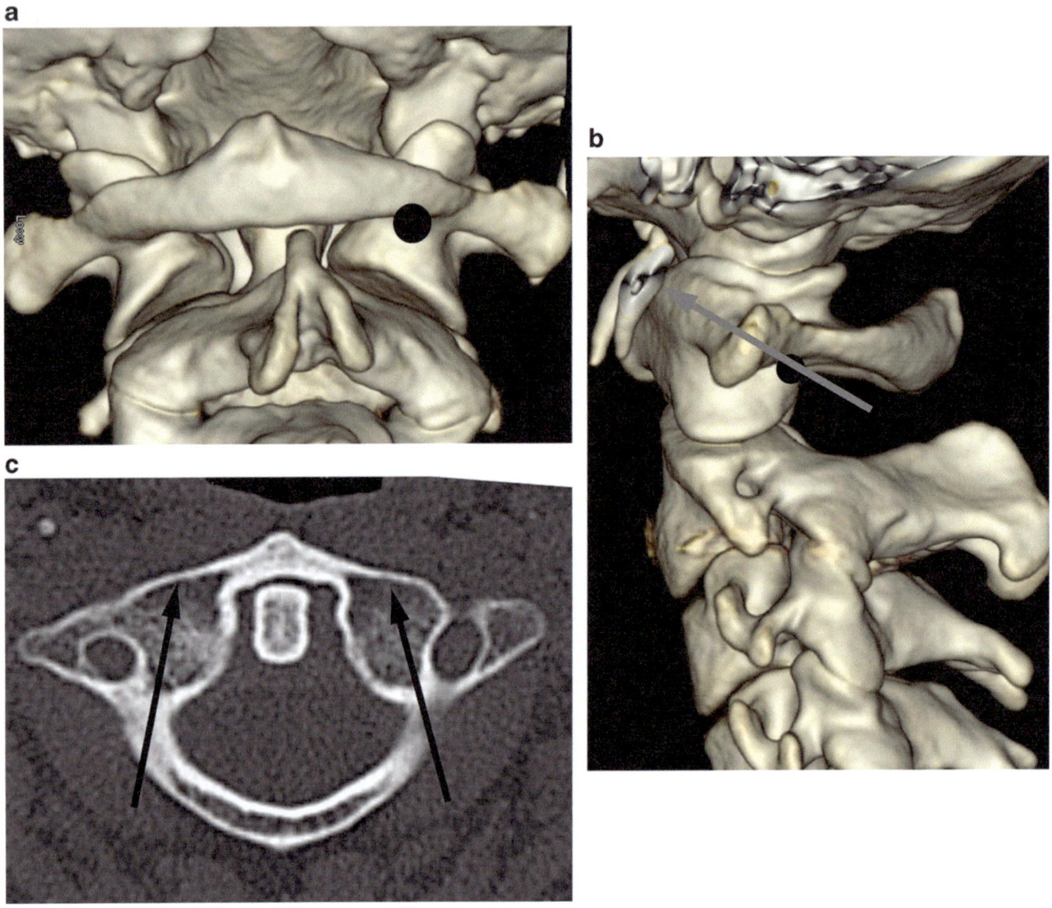

Fig. 5.1 (**a**) Dorsal view showing starting point (*circle*) for C1 lateral mass screw. (**b**) Lateral view demonstrating C1 lateral mass screw orientation (*arrow*). The screw should aim at the superior aspect of the C1 anterior arch. (**c**) *Arrows* show the slight medial orientation(*arrows*) of C1 lateral mass screws

C2 Pedicle Screw The C2 pedicle is defined as the portion of bone beneath the superior facet and anteromedial to the transverse foramen [46]. Prior to attempting a C2 pedicle screw, the CT images must be carefully examined to assure adequate width of the C2 pedicle. This is best measured on the axial images, which allows one to measure the distance between the medial aspect of the vertebral foramen and medial aspect of the pedicle, which must be a minimum of 4 mm to safely place a pedicle screw. The start point of the pedicle screw is within the superior medial quadrant of the C2 pars and is marked with a 2-mm high-speed burr (Fig. 5.2a). The medial border of the pedicle is defined with a Penfield 4, which is used as a reference point while drilling. The screw track is formed with a 2.5-mm hand drill directed 20–30° medial and cephalad, taking care to hug the medial pedicle wall, as the vertebral foramen is at risk laterally. The position of the drill is verified on lateral fluoroscopic imaging and should lie just below the bony isthmus (Fig. 5.2b, c). The track is then verified with a blunt-tipped probe, which is clamped at the entry point to obtain an accurate length, followed by tapping and placement of the appropriate length 3.5- or 4-mm polyaxial screw, typically 22–26 mm in length.

C2 Pars Screw In cases where the C2 pedicle is too narrow to safely place a screw, an excellent alternative is the pars screw. The pars (or isthmus)

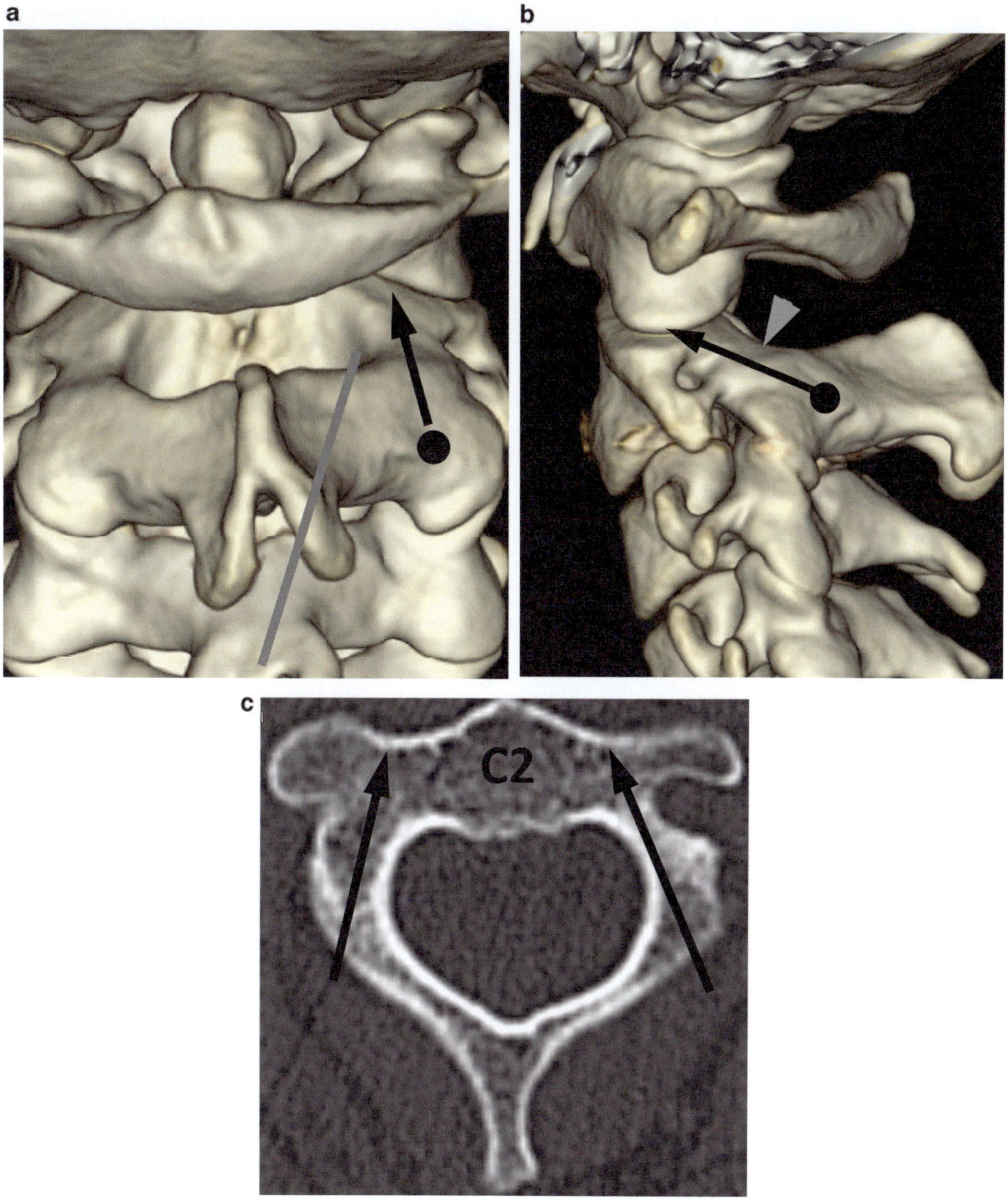

Fig. 5.2 (**a**) Dorsal view of C2. The medial edge of the right pedicle is identified by a Penfield elevator (*gray line*). The starting point for screw insertion (*circle*) is just lateral to the medial edge of the pedicle and is marked by a burr. It is located 3–5 mm above the C2-3 facet joint. The screw is oriented slightly medial (*arrow*) (**b**) (Lateral view showing the screw position just below the upper edge of the pedicle (*gray arrowhead*). (**c**) On the axial CT, the screw direction is slightly medial. On the *left side*, there is a medial position of the vertebral artery with therefore a high risk of vertebral artery injury

of C2 is defined as the narrow portion of bone between the superior and inferior articular facets [46]. The start point is typically on the inferior quarter of the vertical bisector of the pars, immediately caudal to a ridge that is often present. The trajectory for the screw is directed 10–15° toward the medial border of the pedicle, with a steeper angle than the C2 pedicle screw, and directed toward the C1 anterior tubercle. The trajectory must be measured on preoperative CT imaging, as the screw must stop short of the vertebral foramen (typically 16 mm in length). The same steps for marking the start point and preparing the screw track are used, except a high-speed drill with a drill stop can be used. The typical length of a C2 pars screw is 14–18 mm.

C2 Translaminar Screws This technique, described by Wright in 2004, is an excellent and relatively safe option in patients with aberrant vertebral artery anatomy or with failed pedicle or pars screws [47]. The risk of vertebral artery injury is essentially eliminated, however, the risk of spinal cord injury is still present if the inner laminar cortex is breached. Prior to considering this technique, the C2 laminae must be measured on axial CT imaging to verify that a 3.5- or 4-mm screw can be accommodated. After exposure of the posterior elements, a 2.0-mm high-speed burr is used to create an entry point at the spinolaminar junction. One screw will have a rostral entry point and the other a caudal entry point on the contralateral spinolaminar junction; this is to ensure that the screws' tracks will not cross. Next, a cervical pedicle finder is used to cannulate the contralateral lamina, taking care not to breach the inner cortex. After tapping and probing the track, a polyaxial screw is placed (typically 3.5 × 30 mm). A modified technique includes creating a cortical "exit" window at the junction of the C2 facet and lamina, which allows the surgeon to confirm the lack of inner cortex breach, measure an accurate screw length, and obtain bicortical purchase [48].

After C1 and C2 screw placement, appropriate length rods are placed and set screws tightened to proper torque. A crosslink can be placed to increase the torsional strength of the construct, which may be advantageous in the trauma setting. Bone grafting is performed as described below.

C1-C2 Transarticular Screw This technique was first described by Magerl et al. in 1979 for the treatment of odontoid fracture [49]. Prior to considering the C1-C2 transarticular screw, one must carefully study the CT images to verify that the C2 pedicle is wide enough to accommodate a 3.5- or 4-mm screw. Once the patient is positioned, a lateral fluoroscopic image is obtained to confirm that the C1-C2 joint is reduced. A malreduced joint may increase the risk of vertebral artery injury significantly [50]. Another image is obtained with a guide wire lateral to the neck which allows the surgeon to visualize the trajectory needed for the screw, plan the entry point for the percutaneous cannula, and make positioning adjustments prior to draping. The skin preparation must extend to the upper thoracic spine as the percutaneous entry point for the drill is typically at the cervicothoracic junction.

The start point is similar to that of the pars screw, but the trajectory must be steeper in order to cross the C1-C2 joint and reach the anterior border of C1 at the level of the arch (Fig. 5.3a, b). Once C1 and C2 are exposed, the start point is marked with a high-speed burr. The starting point is just lateral to the medial edge of the C2 pedicle which is palpated and 5–7 mm above the C2-3 facet joint. A stab incision in the skin and fascia is made 1–2 cm from the midline at the cervicothoracic junction. A guide tube is passed percutaneously and docked onto the start point followed by the passage of a guide wire. The guide wire is medialized 10–15° while visualizing the medial border of the pedicle with a Penfield 4. The sagittal angle is confirmed with a lateral image to ensure the proper trajectory. The tip of the wire is placed a few millimeters short of the anterior C1 tubercle to avoid penetration into the retropharyngeal space. Next, a cannulated drill is advanced over the wire, taking care not to bind the wire or breach the anterior C1 cortex. The drill is removed while maintaining the guide wire position; the track is prepared with a cannulated tap, followed by advancing the appropriate length 3.5- or 4-mm cannulated screw.

Decortication Decortication is ideally done after screw track tapping and prior to screw placement, as the polyaxial screw tulips can interfere with exposure. It is best to use a cutting burr; however, one must be careful not to weaken the screw tracks or injure neurovascular structures. It is safe to decorticate the middle third of the C1 arch; however, the lateral two-thirds must be decorticated with care to avoid injury to the

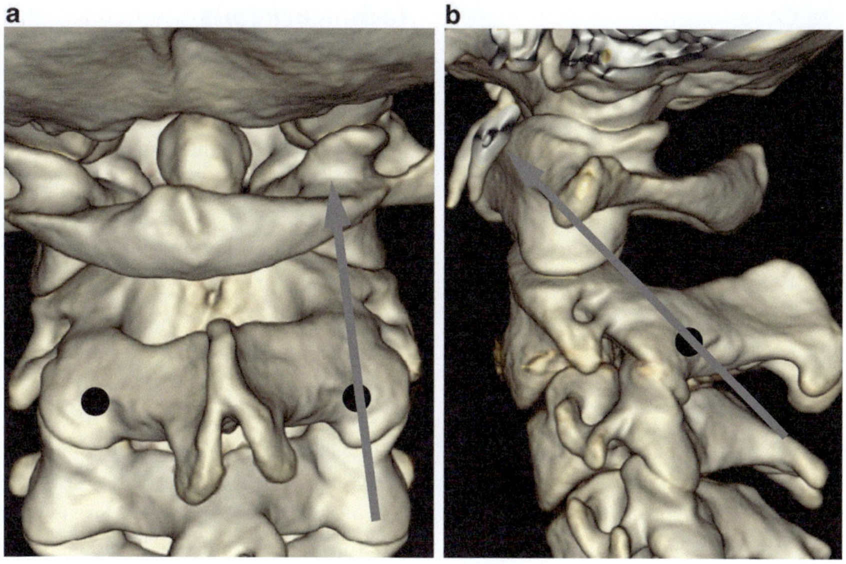

Fig. 5.3 (**a**) The starting point for C1-2 transarticular screw insertion is 3 mm above the C2-3 facet in a line just lateral to medial edge of the pedicle. The screw is oriented to aim towards the center of the C1-2 articulation (*arrow*). (**b**) The *arrow* identifies the screw orientation from the starting point (*circle*) in C2, across the C1-2 articulation and into the C1 lateral mass. The screw tip should appear to be angled end near the superior aspect of the anterior arch of C1 (*arrow*)

nearby C2 nerve roots and vertebral arteries. Again, it is critical to study the preoperative advanced imaging and assess the course of the vertebral artery.

Bone Graft Although iliac crest bone grafting is the gold standard for posterior fusion, this is associated with a high potential for donor site morbidity. In patients who are biologically compromised (smokers, diabetics, immunosuppressed, etc.), it may be prudent to harvest autograft bone from the iliac crest.

Biomechanics There are many studies evaluating the biomechanical outcomes of the different atlantoaxial fusion techniques [51]. Melcher et al. compared the biomechanical properties of C1-C2 transarticular screws with Gallie wiring to those of C1 lateral mass-C2 pedicle screw and rod instrumentation [52]. They found no statistically significant difference between the two constructs in flexion/extension, lateral bending, or axial rotation. Du et al. performed a systematic review and meta-analysis of studies evaluating the biomechanical stability of various instrumentation constructs for atlantoaxial fusion, including C1 lateral mass-C2 pedicle screws, C1 lateral mass-C2 pars screws, C1 lateral mass-C2 translaminar screws, and C1-2 transarticular screws [53]. Their meta-analysis showed that all constructs provided significant stabilization in all axes of rotation, except for the C1 lateral mass-C2 translaminar construct in lateral bending.

Elliott et al. performed a meta-analysis comparing the clinical and radiographic outcomes of patients treated with transarticular screws versus C1-C2 screw-rod constructs for atlantoaxial fusion [54]. They found no difference in 30-day mortality or neurologic injury between the techniques. However, there was a higher incidence of vertebral artery injury (4.1% vs. 2%) and malpositioned screws (7.1% vs. 2.4%) and a lower rate of fusion (97.5% vs. 94.6%) with the transarticular screw technique.

Illustrative Case

History

This is a 66-year-old female pedestrian who was struck by a vehicle. She sustained a type II odontoid fracture in addition to multiple rib fractures, bilateral pneumothoraces, and a clavicle fracture. She was initially treated at an outside institution, and her cervical spine was stabilized with a hard cervical collar. She presented to our institution 2 months later with severe, intolerable neck pain that was exacerbated by neck motion and alleviated by immobilization. She had no previous history of neck pain. She is a non-smoker and nondiabetic and exercised daily prior to her injury.

Physical Examination

Her examination on presentation revealed a normal neurologic exam but significant pain in her upper neck with cervical range of motion.

Imaging

Initial radiographic and CT, and MRI imaging (Fig. 5.4a–c) demonstrated a nonunion of her odontoid fracture with no compromise of her spinal canal or spinal cord.

Treatment

The C2 pedicles were closely examined on CT imaging prior to planning the pedicle screws (Figure 5.2c). She underwent a C1-C2 fusion with a C1 lateral mass-C2 pedicle screw/rod construct and iliac crest autograft. (Fig. 5.4d and 5.4e).

Postoperative Course

Postoperatively, she noted resolution of her neck pain once her surgical pain resolved and achieved a solid C1-C2 fusion, which was noted at 9-month clinical and radiographic follow-up.

Technical Pearls

- Preoperative planning

Preoperative evaluation of the CT is critical as there is significant variability in the C2 pedicle anatomy as well as the course of the vertebral artery. It is not uncommon to encounter C2 pedicles that are too narrow to safely insert a pedicle screw in which case C2 pars or translaminar screws are an excellent backup option.

Evaluating for the presence of a ponticulus posticus (osseous arch on the superior aspect of the C1 lamina that contains the vertebral artery) preoperatively is important as this can be confused with the C1 lamina. Vertebral artery injury can occur if this structure is not appreciated preoperatively.

- Positioning Pearls

Prior to positioning, a roll of gauze is placed in the patient's mouth to allow for adequate open-mouth view shots during the procedure.

The chin is tucked to flex the base of the skull away from the posterior arch of C1; this facilitates the exposure and placement of the C1 lateral mass screws.

- C1 Lateral Mass Fixation

Placement of C1 lateral mass screws requires adequate exposure. This is associated with significant bleeding from the surrounding venous plexus. Using hemostatic agents such as thrombin-soaked gel foam or fibrillar collagen and alternating from side to side can optimize the workflow.

The optimal start point for the C1 screw is at the junction of the inferior lateral mass and the C1 arch. In patients with an overhanging arch, the start point can be exposed by burring the caudal aspect of the arch. Alternatively, in patients with an arch thick enough to accommodate a 3.5-mm screw, the start point can be created directly on the arch.

- C2 Pedicle Screws

When placing C2 pedicle or transarticular screws, it is critical to visualize the medial aspect of the C2 pedicle which is typically done with a

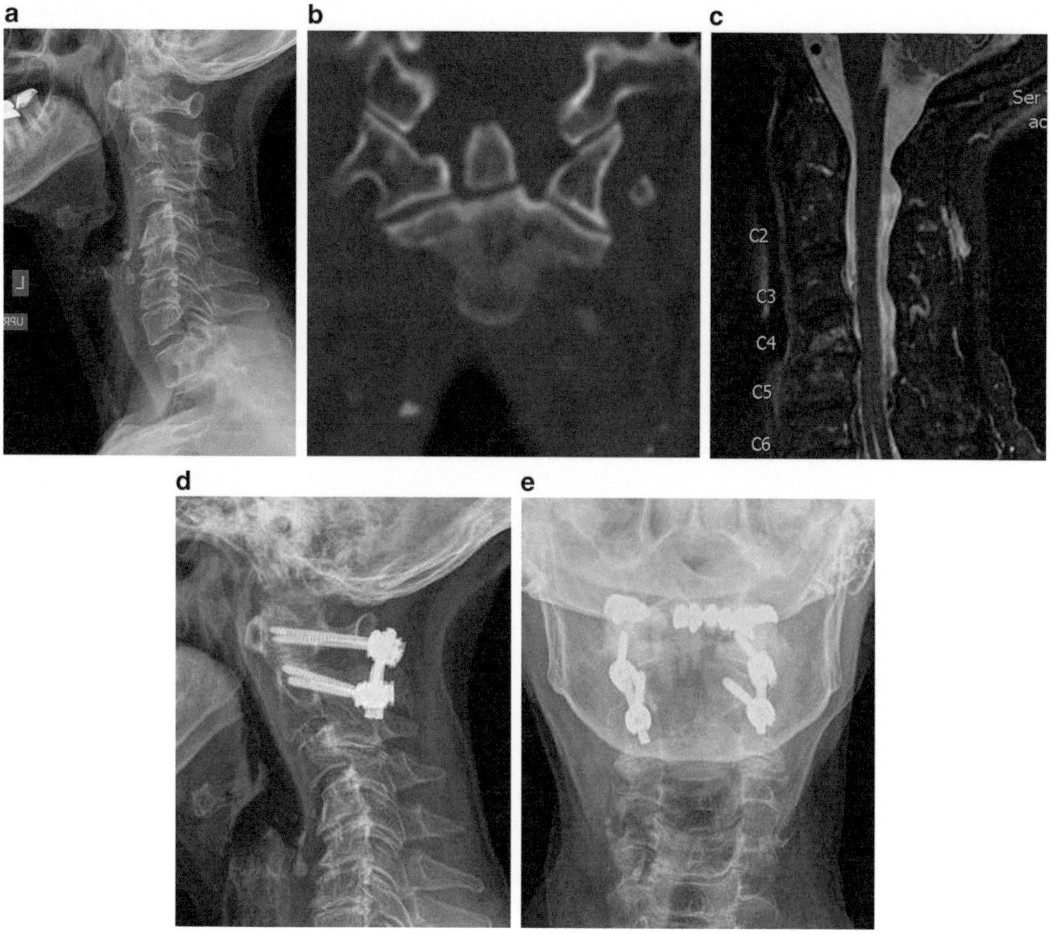

Fig. 5.4 (**a**) Initial lateral radiograph of 66-year-old female with non-displaced type II dens fracture. (**b**) Coronal CT shows nonunion of dens fracture. (**c**) Sagittal T2-weighted MRI demonstrates increased signal in nonunion of dens fracture. No spinal cord compression is present. (**d**) Postoperative lateral radiographs following C1-2 posterior fusion using C1 lateral mass screws and C2 pedicle screws. (**e**) Postoperative open-mouth radiograph following posterior C1-2 fusion

Penfield 4. This landmark allows the surgeon to safely medialize the screw trajectory while avoiding the vertebral artery laterally and the spinal cord medially. This step is also helpful while placing a C2 pars screw.

Complications and Strategies for Avoidance

Vertebral Artery Injury (VAI)

Approximately 20% of patients have a vertebral artery with an anomalous course at the level of C1 and C2 [49, 53]. It is critical to scrutinize the bony anatomy of the atlas and axis on CT imaging; furthermore, one should consider a CT or MR angiogram if any doubt is present with regard to the vertebral artery anatomy. The reported rate of vertebral artery injury is up to 5.8% during C1 lateral mass screw placement and up to 8.2% with C1-C2 transarticular screws [55, 56]. Madawi et al. showed that VAI risk increases significantly when C1 and C2 are not completely reduced [50].

Neo et al. performed a retrospective survey that included 5641 cervical spine surgeries and eight cases of VAI with C1-C2 transarticular screw fixation [52]. When VAI occurred in the screw hole, hemostasis was obtained by tamponade or screw insertion. In contrast, VAI in the "open space" resulted in uncontrolled bleeding and necessitated embolization. The authors reported no deaths or postoperative neurologic sequelae in this study; they recommend prompt consultation with an endovascular team if hemostasis cannot be achieved.

Internal Carotid Artery (ICA) Injury

The internal carotid arteries traverse anterior to the lateral masses of C1. Atlantoaxial fusion puts this structure at risk since the ideal exit point for a bicortical C1-C2 transarticular screws and C1 lateral mass screws is the center of the C1 lateral mass. Currier et al. performed an anatomic study using computed tomography to evaluate the relationship of the ICA to the ideal exit point of a bicortical screw through the C1 lateral mass [57]. They found the mean distance of the ICA to the anterior cortex of C1 to be approximately 2.9 mm and the ICA lumen medial to the foramen transversarium of C1 in nearly 85% of cases. They concluded that the proximity of the ICA to the anterior arch of C1 posed a moderate risk of injury in 46% of cases and a high risk in 12% of cases. In such cases, they advise using unicortical fixation in order to mitigate the risk of injury.

Conclusion

There are multiple posterior fixation options for C1-C2 pathology and each with its advantages and disadvantages. Pedicle screw-rod constructs have gained widespread popularity due to the increased biomechanical rigidity and low risk of VA injury in the hands of experienced surgeons who have a complete understanding of the atlantoaxial anatomy as well as the morphometric and vascular variations. Preoperative planning and evaluation of CT imaging is critical when approaching these procedures. CT angiography is especially important when aberrant vertebral anatomy is suspected. It is our preference to perform C1 lateral mass-C2 pedicle screw-rod instrumentation when possible; however, older wiring/arthrodesis methods have proven invaluable in our practice with regard to revision cases or patients with unfavorable anatomy or history of vertebral artery injury.

References

1. Wang S, Wang C, et al. Novel surgical classification and treatment strategy for Atlantoaxial dislocations. Spine. 2013;38(21):E1348–56.
2. Derman PB, Lampe LP. Atlantoaxial fusion: sixteen years of epidemiology, indications, and complications in New York state. Spine. 2016; Publish Ahead of Print. doi: 10.1097/BRS.0000000000001603.
3. Mummaneni PV, Haid RW. Atlantoaxial fixation: overview of all techniques. Neurol India. 2005;53:408–15.
4. Burke SW, French HG, Roberts JM, Johnston CE, White-cloud TS, Edmunds JO. Chronic atlantoaxial instability in children. J Bone Joint Surg Am. 1985;67:1356–60.
5. Henriques T, Cunningham BW, Olerud C, et al. Biomechanical comparison of five different atlantoaxial posterior fixation techniques. Spine. 2000;25:2877–83.
6. Crockard HA, Stevens JM. Craniovertebral junction anomalies in inherited disorders: part of the syndrome or caused by the disorder? Eur J Pediatr. 1995;154:504–12.
7. Isu T, Miyasaka K, Abe H, et al. Atlantoaxial dislocation associated with neurofibromatosis. Report of three cases. J Neurosurg. 1983;58:451–3.
8. Bouchaud-Chabot A, Liote F. Cervical spine involvement in rheumatoid arthritis. A review. Joint Bone Spine. 2002;69:141–54.
9. Nagaria J, Kelleher MO, et al. C1-C2 transarticular screw fixation for atlantoaxial instability due to rheumatoid arthritis: a seven-year analysis of Outcome. Spine. 2009;34(26):2880–5.
10. Grob D, Grauer W, et al. Fusion and retrodental pannus in rheumatoid arthritis. Spine. 1997;22(14):1580–15832.
11. Davis FW, Markley HE. Rheumatoid arthritis with death from medullary compression. Ann Intern Med. 1951;35:451–61.
12. Boden SC, Dodge LD, Bohlmann HH, Rechtine GL. Rheumatoid arthritis of the cervical spine: long term analysis with predictors of paralysis and recovery. J Bone Joint Surg Am. 1993;75:1282–97.
13. Smith JS, Kepler CK, et al. Effect of type II odontoid fracture nonunion on outcome among elderly patients treated without surgery: based on the AOSpine North America geriatric odontoid fracture study. Spine. 2013;38(26):2240–6.
14. Clark CR, Goetz DD, Menezes AH. Arthrodesis of the cervical spine in rheumatoid arthritis. J Bone Joint Surg Am. 1989;71:381–91.
15. Crockard HA, Calder I, Ransford A. One-stage transoral decompression and posterior fixation in rheuma-

toid atlantoaxial subluxation. J Bone Joint Surg (Br). 1990;72:682–5.
16. Grob D, Jeanneret B, Aebi M, Markwalder T. Atlantoaxial fusion with transarticular screw-fixation. J Bone Joint Surg (Br). 1991;73:972–6.
17. Platter P, Vécsei V, et al. Posterior atlanto-axial arthrodesis for fixation of odontoid nonunions. Spine. 2008;33(6):624–30.
18. Chen Q, Yang X, et al. Anterior retropharyngeal reduction and sequential posterior fusion for atlantoaxial rotatory fixation with locked C1–C2 lateral facet. Spine. 2015;40(21):E1121–7.
19. Goel A. Progressive basilar invagination after transoral odontoidectomy: treatment by atlantoaxial facet distraction and craniovertebral realignment. Spine. 2005;30(18):E551–5.
20. Ain MC, Chaichana KL, et al. Retrospective study of cervical arthrodesis in patients with various types of skeletal dysplasia. Spine. 2006;31(6):E169–74.
21. Kulkarni AG, Goel AH. Vertical atlantoaxial index: a new craniovertebral radiographic index. J Spinal Disord Tech. 2008;21(1):4–10.
22. Heller JG, Viroslav S, Hudson T. Jefferson fractures: the role of magnification artifact in assessing transverse ligament integrity. J Spinal Disord. 1993;6(5):392–6.
23. Menezes AH, van Gilder JC, Clark CR, et al. Odontoid upward migration in rheumatoid arthritis. J Neurosurg. 1985;63:500–9.
24. Boden SD, Dodge LD, Bohlman HH, et al. Rheumatoid arthritis of the cervical spine. J Bone Joint Surg. 1993;75A:1282–97.
25. Mallory GW, Halasz SR, Clarke MJ. Advances in the treatment of cervical rheumatoid: less and less morbidity. World J Orthop. 2014;5(3):292–303.
26. Bland JH. Rheumatoid arthritis of the cervical spine. Bull Rheum Dis. 1967;8:471–6.
27. Young JP, Young PH, Ackermann MJ, Anderson PA, Riew KD. The ponticulus posticus: implications for screw insertion into the first cervical lateral mass. J Bone Joint Surg Am. 2005;87(11):2495–8.
28. Ilkko E, Tikkakoski T, Pyhtinen J. The helical three-dimensional CT in the diagnosis of torticollis with occipitocondylar hypoplasia. Eur J Radiol. 1998;29(1):55–60.
29. Stiskal MA, Neuhold A, Szolar DH, Saeed M, Czerny C, Leeb B, et al. Rheumatoid arthritis of the craniocervical region by MR imaging: detection and characterization. AJR Am J Roentgenol. 1995;165:585–92.
30. Younes M, Belghali S, Kriâa S, Zrour S, Bejia I, Touzi M, et al. Compared imaging of the rheumatoid cervical spine: prevalence study and associated factors. Joint Bone Spine. 2009;76:361–8.
31. Reijnierse M, Breedveld FC, Kroon HM, Hansen B, Pope TL, Bloem JL. Are magnetic resonance flexion views useful in evaluating the cervical spine of patients with rheumatoid arthritis? Skelet Radiol. 2000;29:85–9.
32. Bundschuh C, Modic MT, Kearney F, Morris R, Deal C. Rheumatoid arthritis of the cervical spine: surface-coil MR imaging. AJR Am J Roentgenol. 1988;151:181–7.
33. Yamazaki M, Okawa A, et al. Fenestration of vertebral artery at the craniovertebral junction in down syndrome: a case report. Spine. 2004;29(23):E551–4.
34. Neo M, Matsushita M, et al. Atlantoaxial transarticular screw fixation for a high-riding vertebral artery. Spine. 2003;28(7):666–70.
35. Durand D, Wu X, Kalra VB, et al. Predictors of vertebral artery injury in isolated C2 fractures based on fracture morphology using CT angiography. Spine. 2015;40(12):E713–8.
36. Paik S-C, Chun H-J, et al. Unilateral C1 lateral mass and C2 pedicle screw fixation for Atlantoaxial instability in rheumatoid arthritis patients: comparison with the bilateral method. J Korean Neurosurg Soc. 2015;57(6):460–4.
37. Goel A, Laheri V. Plate and screw fixation for atlantoaxial subluxation. Acta Neurochir. 1994;129:47–53.
38. Goel A. C2 ganglion resection for lateral mass fixation techniques. J Craniovertebr Junction Spine. 2015;6(1):10–1.
39. Gallie WE. Fractures and dislocations of cervical spine. Am J Surg. 1939;46:495–9.
40. Dickman CA, Sonntag VK, Papadopoulos SM, Hadley MN. The interspinous method of posterior atlantoaxial arthrodesis. J Neurosurg. 1991;74(2):190–8.
41. Brooks AL, Jenkins EB. Atlanto-axial arthrodesis by the wedge compression method. J Bone Joint Surg Am. 1978;60(3):279–84.
42. Harms J, Melcher P. Posterior C1-C2 fusion with Polyaxial screw and rod fixation. Spine. 2001;26(22):2467–71.
43. Christensen DM, Eastlack RK, Lynch JJ, Yaszemski MJ, Currier BL. C1 anatomy and dimensions relative to lateral mass screw placement. Spine (Phila Pa 1976). 2007;32(8):844–8.
44. Tan M, Wang H, Wang Y, Zhang G, Yi P, Li Z, Wei H, Yang F. Morphometric evaluation of screw fixation in atlas via posterior arch and lateral mass. Spine (Phila Pa 1976). 2003;28(9):888–95.
45. Ebraheim NA, Fow J, Xu R, Yeasting RA. The location of the pedicle and pars interarticularis in the axis. Spine (Phila Pa 1976). 2001;26(4):E34–7.
46. Wright NM. Posterior C2 fixation using bilateral, crossing C2 laminar screws: case series and technical note. J Spinal Disord Tech. 2004;17:158–62.
47. Dmitriev AE, Lehman RA Jr, et al. Acute and long-term stability of atlantoaxial fixation methods: a biomechanical comparison of pars, pedicle, and intralaminar fixation in an intact and odontoid fracture model. Spine (Phila Pa 1976). 2009; 34(4):365–70.
48. Jeanneret B, Magerl F. Primary posterior fusion C1/2 in odontoid fractures: indications, technique, and results of transarticular screw fixation. J Spinal Disord. 1992;5:464–75.
49. Madawi AA, et al. Radiological and anatomical evaluation of the atlantoaxial transarticular screw fixation technique. J Neurosurg. 1997;86(6):961–8.

50. Jea A, Sheth RN, Vanni S, Green BA, Levi AD. Modification of Wright's technique for placement of bilateral crossing C2 translaminar screws: technical note. Spine J. 2008;8(4):656–60.
51. Melcher RP, Puttlitz CM, Kleinstueck FS, Lotz JC, Harms J, Bradford DS. Biomechanical testing of posterior atlantoaxial fixation techniques. Spine (Phila Pa 1976). 2002;27(22):2435–40.
52. Du JY, Aichmair A, Kueper J, Wright T, Lebl DR. Biomechanical analysis of screw constructs for atlantoaxial fixation in cadavers: a systematic review and meta-analysis. J Neurosurg Spine. 2015;22(2):151–61.
53. Elliott RE, Tanweer O, Boah A, Morsi A, Ma T, Frempong-Boadu A, Smith ML. Outcome comparison of atlantoaxial fusion with transarticular screws and screw-rod constructs: meta-analysis and review of literature. J Spinal Disord Tech. 2014;27(1):11–28.
54. Neo M, et al. Vertebral artery injury during cervical spine surgery: a survey of more than 5600 operations. Spine. 2008;33(7):779–85.
55. Yoshida M, et al. Comparison of the anatomical risk for vertebral artery injury associated with the C2-pedicle screw and atlantoaxial transarticular screw. Spine. 2006;31(15):E513–7.
56. Currier BL, Maus TP, Eck JC, Larson DR, Yaszemski MJ. Relationship of the internal carotid artery to the anterior aspect of the C1 vertebra: implications for C1-C2 transarticular and C1 lateral mass fixation. Spine (Phila Pa 1976). 2008;33(6):635–9.
57. Paramore CG, Dickman CA, Sonnag VK. The anatomical suitability of the C1–2 complex for transarticular screw fixation. J Neurosurg. 1996;85:221–4.
58. Doyle JS, Lauerman W, et al. Long-term outcome of upper cervical spine arthrodesis in patients with down syndrome. Spine. 1996;21(10):1223–31.

Odontoid Screw Fixation

6

Mark Benjamin Frenkel and David J. Hart

Introduction

Anderson and D'Alonzo [1] published their categorization of fractures of the odontoid process of the axis in 1974 recognizing the unique challenges of managing type II odontoid fractures. Their series described the outcomes of both those treated nonoperatively in tong traction for 6 weeks and those treated with posterior wiring and fusion, and they advocated for the use of operative fixation in these patients. While there have been significant developments in both nonoperative immobilization and operative fixation since that time, operative fixation remains the mainstay of treatment for type II odontoid fractures today. In fact, the 2013 *Neurosurgery* Spinal Trauma Guidelines concluded that "Surgical stabilization and fusion of Type II and Type III odontoid fractures with dens displacement ≥5 mm, comminution of the odontoid fracture, and/or inability to achieve or maintain fracture alignment with external immobilization are recommended" [2]. In this chapter, we discuss the role of anterior odontoid screw fixation for management of odontoid fractures, its indications, and how the procedure is performed. We also provide a number of technical pearls and strategies for complication avoidance.

Direct anterior fixation of a fracture of the odontoid process or odontoid screw fixation was first reported independently by both Bohler [3] and Nakanishi in 1982. In the years since, there have been many refinements to their techniques and new instrumentation developed specifically for this procedure. While a number of different systems exist, we prefer to use a currently available system which allows for the insertion of non-cannulated screws through an all-in-one drill/tap/screw guide tube for reasons which will be discussed later in the chapter. The procedure below will be described using this system, although the technique may be generalized and applied to other systems.

There is controversy in the literature over the optimal management of acute type II odontoid fractures, especially in regard to rates of nonunion between operative and conservative management. Some authors [4–6] consider the concept of a stable fibrous union which can be defined as a lack of motion on flexion-extension radiographs, despite the lack of definitive evidence of bony fusion in an asymptomatic patient to be a satisfactory outcome. However, this "stable fibrous union" concept is not universally accepted. This has a significant impact on reported success rates of any management strategy. For example, a retrospective study by

M.B. Frenkel, MD, MA • D.J. Hart, MD (✉)
Department of Neurosurgery, Wake Forest Baptist Medical Center, 1 Medical Center Blvd, Winston Salem, NC 27157, USA
e-mail: mfrenkel@wakehealth.edu; djhart@wakehealth.edu

L.T. Holly, P.A. Anderson (eds.), *Essentials of Spinal Stabilization*,
DOI 10.1007/978-3-319-59713-3_6

Koech et al. [6] examined patients aged 65 years or older with type II odontoid fractures treated nonoperatively, including 10 who were treated in cervical collars alone and 32 in halo braces. While only 50% of those in collars and 37.5% of those in halo braces had evidence of bony fusion at follow-up, all patients except one treated in a collar appeared to have developed a stable fibrous union. We consider the primary goals of anterior odontoid fixation to be stabilization of the fracture fragment on flexion-extension radiographs and relief of clinical symptoms.

The atlantoaxial interface plays a unique biomechanical role among vertebrae as it is responsible for approximately one-third of the total rotation of the cervical spine [7]. As compared to other methods of atlantoaxial fixation, odontoid screw fixation may offer the benefits of preserving this motion [8], being less painful than posterior fusion techniques, decreasing risk of vertebral artery injury, and having no need for bone graft harvest.

Indications and Patient Selection

The ideal candidates for odontoid screw placement are patients with acute or subacute type II odontoid fractures and selected patients with shallow type III odontoid fractures [9], Table 6.1. In regard to type II fractures, Grauer et al. [10] proposed three subtypes which can be used to determine optimal management based on several characteristics of the fracture. They suggest that type IIa, transverse fractures without comminution or displacement, may be successfully managed with external immobilization. Further, while type IIb, displaced transverse fractures or fractures that pass from anterosuperior to posteroinferior, may be optimally treated with odontoid screw fixation, they recommend a posterior approach for type IIc, fractures passing from anteroinferior to posterosuperior or significantly comminuted fractures.

Table 6.1 Indications and contraindications for odontoid screw fixation

Indications	
	Acute or subacute type II fractures
	Shallow type III fractures
Contraindications	
	Comminuted fractures
	Severe medical comorbidities
	Body habitus (barrel chest) or severe kyphosis preventing appropriate trajectory
	Pathologic fractures
	Associated transverse ligament injury
	Chronic nonunion (>6 months)
	Irreducible subluxation/translation of dens fragment by >5 mm

Patient age plays an important role in determining the optimal management of type II odontoid fractures. While young, healthy patients may be treated with external immobilization, Lennarson et al. [11] examined 33 type II odontoid fractures treated with halo vest immobilization and found that patients above the age of 50 had a risk of bony nonunion 21 times higher than younger patients. In addition, halo vest immobilization in elderly patients with odontoid fractures has been associated with increased morbidity and mortality [12].

In 1989, Hadley et al. [13] examined 68 patients of various ages with acute type II odontoid fractures treated with nonoperative immobilization and found an overall nonunion rate of 28%. Furthermore, they found that a dens dislocation of 6 mm or greater had a 78% nonunion rate with nonoperative immobilization compared with only 10% in those with dens dislocations less than 6 mm. It is further discussed in the *Neurosurgery* spine trauma guidelines [2] that a greater degree of fracture displacement should warrant consideration for operative fixation.

Absolute contraindications to anterior odontoid screw placement include comminuted and pathologic fractures of the C2 vertebral body, as well as other general contraindications to spine surgery such as active infection, anticoagulation, etc. Injury to the transverse atlantal ligament (TAL) complex is also an absolute contraindication as the C1-C2 complex would remain unstable despite screw fixation of the odontoid fracture.

Furthermore, there are also several relative contraindications such as an anterior oblique fracture, extreme osteoporosis, patient anatomy, and fracture age. While Grauer et al. [10] suggest that an anterior obliquely oriented fracture is a relative contraindication as the screw may cause fracture displacement with tightening, we find that in some cases, shallow, minimally displaced anterior oblique fractures can be successfully stabilized with a regular non-lag screw.

Chronic fractures are also considered to be a relative contraindication for odontoid screw placement because the presence of fibrous tissue prevents reapproximation, and poor bony fusion rates have been reported. Some authors have described good outcomes in fractures up to 6 months old by using a specialized technique in which a long-tipped right-angle curette is inserted into the fracture gap and used to curette out any fibrous tissue which has formed [9]. While good results have been reported using this technique, it is an advanced maneuver which requires specialized instruments and it has not been widely adopted. In patients with symptomatic/unstable chronic odontoid fractures, we recommend posterior C1-C2 arthrodesis.

There are situations in which the patient's anatomy makes an anterior approach difficult or even impossible. In individuals with a barrel chest, severe thoracic kyphosis or lower cervical kyphosis may prevent the correct screw trajectory. In some patients, it may be impossible to accurately determine whether the trajectory can be reached until they are positioned in the operating room with fluoroscopy. Patients with possible anatomic obstacles should be counseled preoperatively about the possibility of needing to convert to a posterior approach.

Dysphagia in the elderly is a well-described complication of any anterior cervical approach. Dailey et al. [4] reported a 35% incidence of dysphagia requiring diet modification and an 11% incidence of aspiration pneumonia after odontoid screw fixation in an elderly population. Other studies [14] have found as high as a 60% rate of dysphagia after anterior approaches to the cervical spine. While this is not a true contraindication in the majority of patients, it should be discussed with the patient preoperatively, and a posterior approach may be considered in those who have preexisting moderate to severe dysphagia.

Preoperative Considerations

Patients with acute type II odontoid fractures should be maintained in external immobilization prior to surgical treatment. Generally, a hard collar is appropriate and preferred to halo orthosis, especially in elderly patients. As with other invasive procedures, anticoagulation should be held, if possible, and coagulopathies corrected prior to surgery.

In any acute fracture, adequate and appropriate imaging and trauma survey should be performed. Some authors had previously considered preoperative MRI for evaluation of transverse atlantal ligament (TAL) injury to be mandatory before odontoid screw placement; however, more recent literature [15] suggests that concomitant odontoid fracture and TAL injury is a rare event, and MRI for this purpose should be reserved for those with neurologic deficits or ADI (atlanto-dental interval) widening. However, owing to the routine technique of hyperextending the patient's head and neck during intraoperative positioning for odontoid screw placement (which is necessary to obtain the correct trajectory), we believe there is benefit in obtaining a cervical spine MRI preoperatively in order to rule out any potential sources of neurologic compression which may not be imaged well on plain radiograph or CT scan. Many elderly patients with odontoid fractures will have pre-injury degenerative spondylosis, stenosis, and/or mid- or lower cervical spinal cord compression that could cause neurological deterioration with intraoperative positioning maneuvers if not otherwise recognized with preoperative MRI. Based on local practices, we do not routinely obtain preoperative flexion/extension films in acute fractures because of potential concern for additional fracture fragment displacement causing neurologic deficit.

Surgical Technique

Anesthesia Considerations

While awake fiberoptic intubation is commonly employed for unstable cervical spine injuries, the spacious spinal canal at the level of C1-C2 usually does not necessitate such strict precautions. Intubation techniques requiring hyperextension should be avoided, and the goal of minimizing spine movement should be discussed preoperatively with the anesthesiology team, but there are a number of modern intubation techniques such as video laryngoscopy which may be used with minimal risk to the patient. In cases with greater than average displacement of the odontoid fracture and/or preoperative spinal cord compromise, this may not apply.

We do not believe that there is great benefit to the use of intraoperative electrophysiologic monitoring during screw placement as, with the exception of rare, obvious complications such as a K-wire placed too deep or severe retropulsion of a fragment, there is little risk of intraoperative neurologic injury during this procedure, and it is unclear whether monitoring would change an outcome associated with these types of complications. We also position the patient under active fluoroscopic control, minimizing the chances of neurologic injury during the positioning process (see below).

Patient Positioning

The patient is positioned supine on a flat-top Jackson table with a large roll placed transversely beneath the shoulders. A standard operating table is also appropriate, although there can be difficulties with metal pieces of the table obscuring the open-mouth fluoroscopy views depending on the angle of the patient's head. The cervical spine is then carefully extended and the head supported on a gel or foam donut. Arms are tucked at the patient's side with pressure points appropriately padded. We then apply light (5–10 pounds) cervical traction, typically via a soft, padded occipito-mandibular traction sling, although many surgeons prefer Gardner-Wells tongs. In this often elderly, frail patient population, we prefer to avoid the additional, although minor, risk of pin-site complications.

The use of fluoroscopy is necessary during positioning in order to optimize trajectory and to ensure that positioning has not caused further displacement of the dens. We typically do not extend the patient's neck until lateral C-arm fluoroscopy is in place and images can be obtained as the spine is positioned. Any undesired subluxation can be immediately identified before fully placing the patient into hyperextension. We believe this is safer than simply obtaining a post-positioning image after the patient is fully hyperextended. In patients with a posteriorly dislocated dens, alignment can be improved by extending the head with an axis of rotation at the atlanto-occipital interface while maintaining extension of the cervical spine. Conversely, anteriorly displaced fragments can be realigned by flexing the head without flexing the cervical spine. Once optimal alignment is achieved, light traction is applied as described above, more to maintain position rather than to achieve any sort of distraction of the spine.

A radiolucent bite block should be used to hold the patient's jaw open in order to obtain an open-mouth odontoid view with fluoroscopy. A working view of the dens, fracture line, and body of C2 without obstruction from the teeth is crucial. The bite block should be placed with care so as not to risk dislocation of the jaw, as anesthetized patients cannot guard themselves against this. Preoperative assessment of the patient's jaw opening can be helpful, although difficult to do in a hard cervical collar. For our bite block, we typically use a wine cork, trimmed to an appropriate height just short of the patient's maximal jaw opening, with V-shaped notches carved in each end for upper and lower teeth (or gums, if edentulous).

The use of intraoperative navigation has been described for the placement of odontoid screws [16]; however, as of this writing, there is no universally accepted technique for its use. Our technique (described below) allows for manipulation of the fracture fragment intraoperatively if desired, which would immediately compromise the accuracy of navigation based on any intraoperative imaging obtained prior to such fracture manipulation. Should advances in technology one day be able to compensate for this, intraoperative navigation could play an important role in reducing the amount of radiation exposure to the patient and operator associated with fluoroscopy.

Instrumentation System

A unique advantage of the non-cannulated system compared to K-wire-based systems is the ability to directly manipulate the C2 vertebral body relative to the dens which often allows fine tuning of the alignment between the dens and the body of C2 during screw placement (see below). In our experience, this cannot be achieved with cannulated K-wire-based systems and is a large part of the basis for why we use a non-cannulated system. Additionally, non-cannulated screws have stronger resistance to fatigue fracture.

Exposure

After positioning the patient, we place a K-wire alongside the patient's neck in line with the optimal screw trajectory, viewed on lateral C-arm fluoroscopy. We will then plan a transverse incision at the area where the wire crosses the anterior surface of the neck. If a skin crease is present within a few millimeters of this location, we will adjust accordingly for cosmetic purposes. In addition, this maneuver has the benefit of confirming that the patient's anatomy is conducive to odontoid screw placement. This is the point in the case at which a final decision is made whether odontoid screw placement will be feasible or if the procedure will need to be converted to a posterior fusion. In our experience, only in rare cases have we been forced to convert to a posterior fusion prior to incision because a barrel chest or thoracic kyphosis made the optimal trajectory impossible to achieve. In some cases, preoperative imaging will strongly indicate the feasibility of obtaining correct trajectory (either for or against) well before entering the operating room, but in many cases, it can be questionable, with the final determination only possible once the patient is safely positioned in cervical extension in the operating room. In our practice, even in cases where we feel quite confident of our chances of obtaining the correct trajectory, we still discuss the possibility of needing to abort the anterior screw and proceed with posterior arthrodesis with every patient/family prior to the procedure. We reassure them that this decision will be made prior to a skin incision being made.

Once successfully positioned, the patient is then prepped and draped in a sterile fashion and local anesthetic is injected. A skin incision is made in the previously determined location (typically around the C5-C6 disc space level, but we base it on our intraoperative localization), and a plane is dissected out over the platysma with Metzenbaum scissors. We prefer to make a transverse incision through the platysma using electrocautery so that the two edges are easy to find and re-approximate at the end of the case.

A standard Cloward-type approach to the anterior cervical spine is carried out as one would perform for anterior cervical discectomy surgery, with dissection down along the medial border of the sternocleidomastoid muscle and between the carotid sheath and trachea, down to the prevertebral fascia. The longus colli muscle is then elevated from the midline so that medial and lateral retractor blades may be inserted beneath them and connected to the retractor holder.

Retraction

A special angled retractor is then inserted from caudal to cephalad into the prevertebral fascial plane after it is dissected up to the level of C1 using a Kittner dissector. The retractor should at least extend past the fracture line on lateral fluoroscopy. This retractor blade is then connected to the medial-lateral self-retaining retractor and is used to protect the soft tissues anterior to C2 (Fig. 6.1). Subsequent steps are all performed under biplanar fluoroscopy.

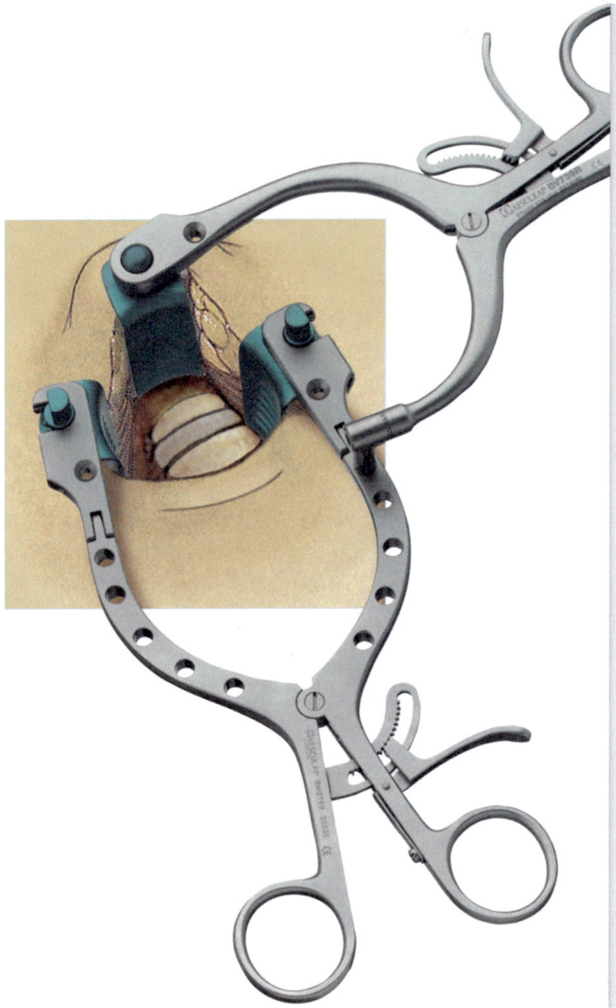

Fig. 6.1 Incision with retractor blades in place (Courtesy Aesculap)

Screw Insertion

A K-wire is inserted at an appropriate trajectory and entry point in the inferior endplate of C2. This generally will penetrate the anterior-most part of the C2-C3 disc space (Fig. 6.2). The optimal location of this is approximately 2 mm posterior from the anterior surface of the body (even 1–2 mm further posterior than what is shown in Fig. 6.2, ideally) and either midline or 3–4 mm lateral to the midline if one or two screws are to be used, respectively. The K-wire should be impacted approximately 4 mm into the bone. It is critical that this initial wire enters the inferior endplate of C2 and not the anterior cortex of the vertebral body as the cortical bone of the endplate is stronger and denser than the usually very thin anterior cortex. Failure to ensure entry into the inferior endplate will often result in postoperative construct failure with the screw(s) cutting out through the anterior vertebral body of C2 when the patient extends his/her neck.

Once the K-wire is inserted, a cannulated 7-mm-fluted-twist drill/rasp is then inserted over it and used to rasp a trough in the anterosuperior aspect of C3 and the C2-C3 annulus (Fig. 6.3).

The drill guide is then assembled and passed over the K-wire. The distal end of this drill guide has anchoring spikes that are "walked" along the ventral spine until the guide is appropriately positioned over the C3 vertebral body (Fig. 6.4). An impactor sleeve is then placed over the handle assembly (which requires cutting the free end of the K-wire) and is tapped with a mallet to impact

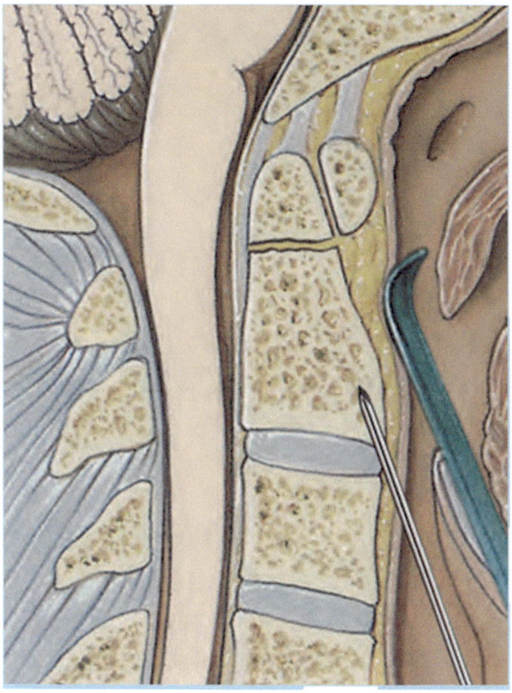

Fig. 6.2 Illustration showing K-wire entry point in the inferior endplate of C2. The authors would suggest an entry point even 1–2 mm posterior to that shown, if feasible (see text) (Courtesy Aesculap)

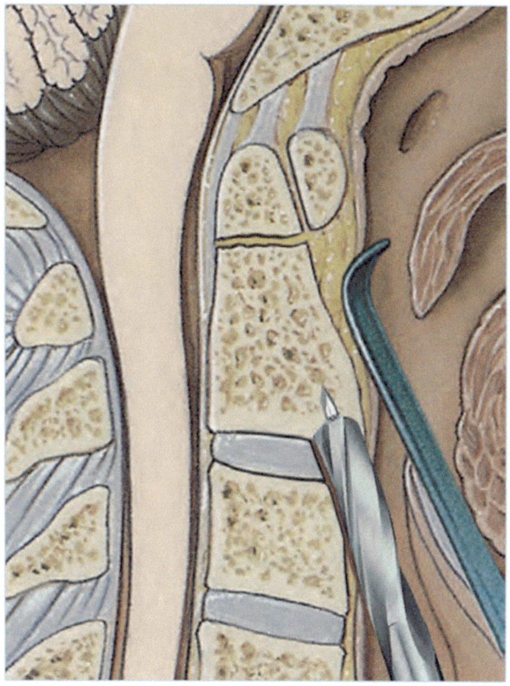

Fig. 6.3 The fluted drill is inserted over the K-wire and a rasp is used to create a trough in the anterosuperior aspect of C3 and the C2-C3 annulus (Courtesy Aesculap)

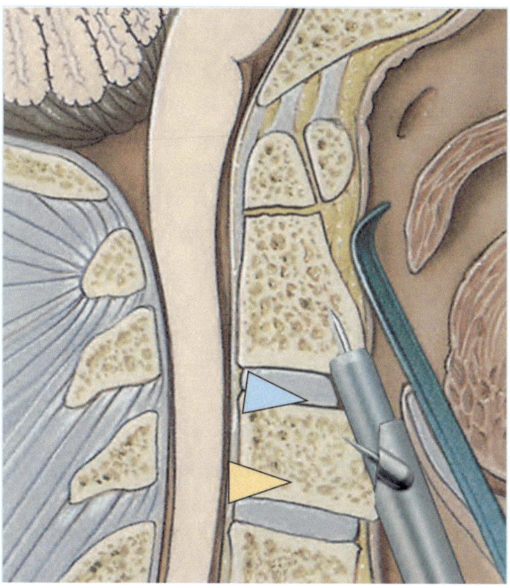

Fig. 6.4 The drill guide is impacted into the anterior C3 vertebral body (*yellow arrowhead*) before the K-wire is removed and replaced with the drill. The inner guide tube is advanced to the inferior endplate of C2 before commencing drilling (*blue arrowhead*) (Courtesy Aesculap)

the spikes into the C3 vertebra, thus firmly securing the drill guide to the body of C3. This represents a sort of "point of no return," and before impacting the drill guide into position, biplanar fluoroscopy images should confirm correct trajectory in both planes. At this point, the inner guide tube is then advanced forward so that it contacts the inferior endplate of C2 and the K-wire is removed. From this point forward until final screw placement, a firm grasp should be maintained on the drill guide with the nondominant hand, not allowing it to move throughout subsequent steps of drilling, tapping, and screw placement. This is critical to the use of the non-K-wire-based system. As previously mentioned, the impacted drill guide can be used to fine-tune the alignment of the odontoid fragment relative to C2, a feature that cannot be accomplished with K-wire-based systems. After ensuring the drill guide is firmly seated in C3, one proceeds to drill into the C2 vertebral body stopping just before the fracture line is reached. Then, if the dens is posteriorly dislocated, gentle downward (toward the floor or dorsal) pressure on the drill guide will

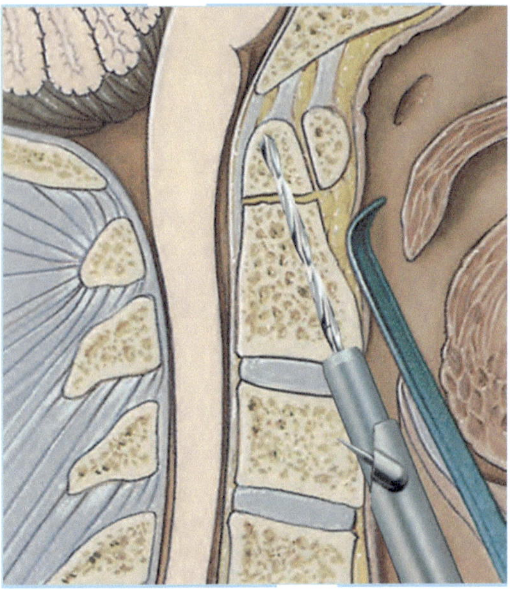

Fig. 6.5 A pilot hole is drilled through the C2 body and fracture line and into the dens. It is important to drill through the distal cortex of the dens (1–2 mm beyond what is shown in this illustration) to achieve bicortical screw purchase (Courtesy Aesculap)

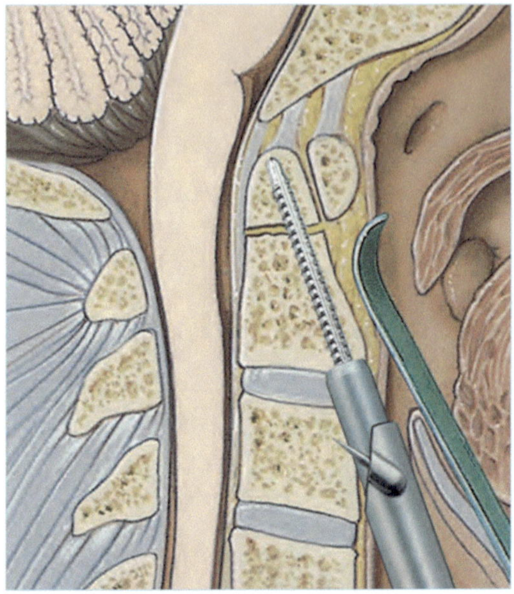

Fig. 6.6 The drill is removed and replaced with the tap which is then used to tap the pilot hole. This should also extend through the distal odontoid cortex, 1–2 mm beyond what is shown in this illustration (Courtesy Aesculap)

usually cause C2 and C3 to move posteriorly, while the dens, C1, and the skull will usually remain fixed, thus aligning the fracture. Maintaining light cervical traction, as described in the patient positioning section, helps with this process. Similarly, if the dens is anteriorly dislocated, the drill guide can be "lifted" (toward the ceiling or ventrally) while carefully maintaining some cephalad pressure to ensure the spikes do not disengage from the C3 vertebra which should bring C2 and C3 into better alignment with the dens. In our experience, these maneuvers can easily correct up to ~3 mm of dislocation. In most cases, with careful patient positioning as described above, the fracture should have less than that amount of dislocation prior to this step. These maneuvers are easier in acute fractures and may be less successful in subacute injuries.

A right-angled drill driver with a depth measurement guide is then inserted through the inner guide tube, and a pilot hole is carefully drilled through C2 and, if no additional realignment is needed (see above), into the odontoid fragment (Fig. 6.5). It is critical to drill through the distal cortex of the odontoid tip so that bicortical purchase can be achieved during screw placement, as the distal tip of the odontoid and the inferior endplate of C2 are the strongest cortical surfaces in C2. The inner guide tube and drill are then withdrawn and a tap is inserted and used to tap the pilot hole (Fig. 6.6). Both the drill and the tap come with calibrated depth markings, although we strongly recommend also measuring screw length on the preoperative CT scans when selecting a screw length. A lag screw is then inserted so that it engages the distal odontoid cortex and approximates the dens to the body of C2 (Fig. 6.7). In the scenario mentioned earlier in which there is an anteriorly oblique fracture, a lag screw should be avoided and a fully threaded screw may be preferable. Once again, throughout the process of drilling, tapping, and screw placement, the drill guide must be maintained in position with a firm grip, also maintaining any anterior or posterior alignment adjustments. In our experience, once familiar with the system, the whole process from drilling to final screw placement can usually be accomplished in about 60–90 s, minimizing fatigue in the hand stabilizing the drill guide.

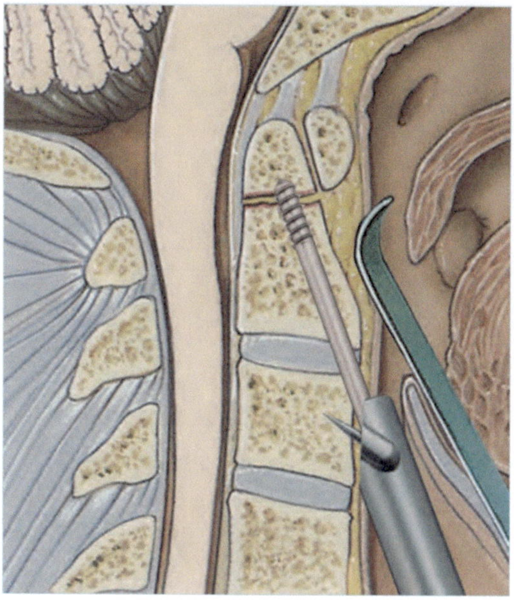

Fig. 6.7 A lag screw is inserted into the previously tapped pilot hole (Courtesy Aesculap)

If two screws are to be used, then the above steps, beginning with K-wire insertion, are repeated on the contralateral side. As the fragment should already be approximated in contact with the C2 body after placing the first lag screw, a fully threaded screw can be used for placement of the second screw.

Closure

The wound is then irrigated, meticulous hemostasis is achieved (the site of spike impaction into the C3 vertebral body often oozes after removing the drill guide, but this can usually be controlled easily with some sort of flowable hemostatic agent and a few seconds of gentle pressure), the retractors are then removed, and the wound is closed in the usual fashion, again similar to the surgeon's preferred techniques for anterior cervical spine surgery.

Postoperative Care

Postoperatively, we do not routinely place patients in a hard collar unless they have very radiolucent bone on radiography or the bone is soft, and minimal insertional torque is experienced during screw placement, both indicators of worse-than-usual osteoporosis or if the patient has had a bone density scan confirming severe osteoporosis. Even in the elderly population, this is only rarely necessary, but many other surgeons routinely use postoperative orthoses and this is per surgeon's discretion.

Illustrative Case

An 82-year-old female with no relevant past medical history presented to the emergency room after a ground-level fall at home. She complained of neck pain but was found to be neurologically intact on examination. A CT scan of her cervical spine was obtained (Fig. 6.8) which showed an acute type II odontoid fracture. After discussion with the patient about management options, she elected to proceed with anterior odontoid screw fixation. The patient was maintained in a Miami J cervical collar until she was taken to the operating theater the following day. The procedure was performed as previously described and two screws were placed (Fig. 6.9). The patient did well postoperatively and tolerated a regular diet with no evidence of dysphagia. Postoperative CT scan (Fig. 6.10) demonstrated satisfactory screw placement with bicortical purchase. The screws in this case ended up longer than they needed to be by about 4 mm, but they remain extradural, causing no harm, and this has no known consequence to the patient. Contrarily, leaving the screws too short to engage the cortical odontoid tip will usually result in screw backout and construct failure; thus, it is preferable to overestimate, rather than underestimate, screw length if any error is to be made.

Technical Pearls

- It is important to achieve bicortical purchase of the inferior endplate of C2 and the distal odontoid tip with the screw. The inferior endplate has much thicker cortical bone than the anterior cortex of C2, and thus it is important for initial K-wire placement to be in the infe-

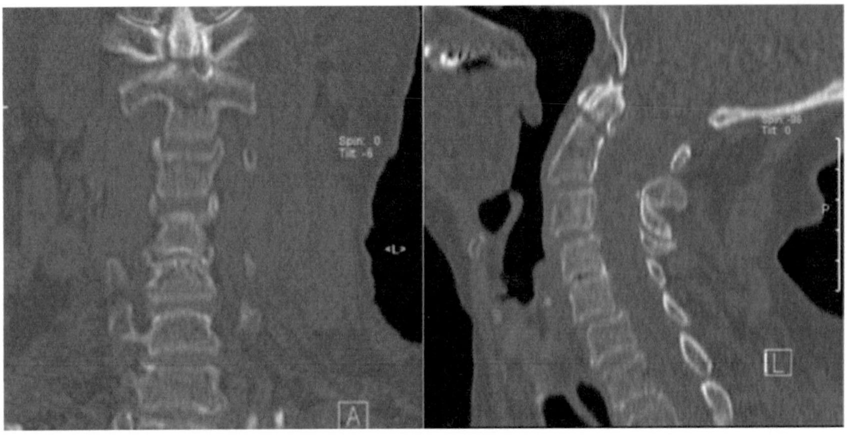

Fig. 6.8 Preoperative coronal (*left*) and sagittal (*right*) CT imaging showing an acute type II odontoid fracture

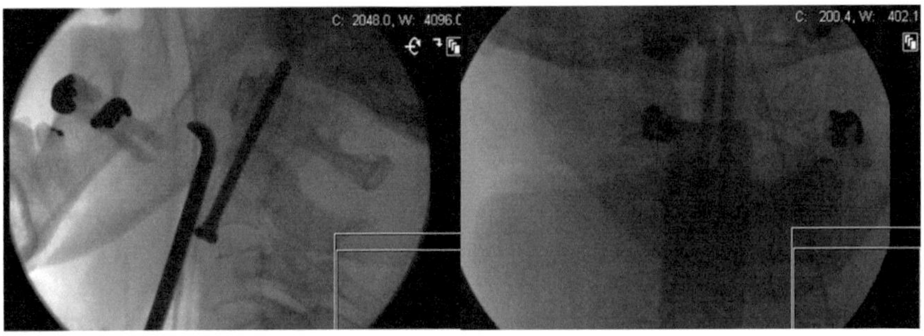

Fig. 6.9 Intraoperative lateral (*left*) and AP (*right*) fluoroscopy views showing the retractor blade elevating the soft tissues and the final placement of the screws. Note the trough rasped in the anterosuperior aspect of the C3 body and the distal cortical purchase of the screws

rior endplate, approximately 2–3 mm posterior from the anterior cortex. In order to achieve distal cortical purchase in the tip of the odontoid, the initial drilling and tapping should penetrate through the distal cortex.

- We do not advocate the use of a cannulated K-wire system for a number of reasons. These include the inherently weaker structure of a cannulated compared to a non-cannulated screw and an inability to manipulate the relation of the odontoid fragment to C2 intraoperatively with the impacted guide tube as described above. In addition, it is important to recognize the potential for neurologic injury if a drilling K-wire is inserted too far past the tip of the odontoid process. Anecdotally, we have heard of unpublished cases where a wire has been inserted into the brainstem and caused severe neurological and vascular arterial compromise.
- There is controversy surrounding the use of either one or two screws for fixation. Two case series have been published which compared rates of successful stabilization between those patients with either one or two screws placed. One of these studies [5] included patients of all ages and found no significant difference between the groups. The other study [4] focused solely on an elderly population and found an increase in successful healing from 56% to 96% with the use of two screws. A biomechanical study [17] found no difference in shear or torsional stiffness between one and two screw constructs. If the patient's anatomy is favorable, i.e., if the narrowest portion of the dens is wide enough to accommodate two

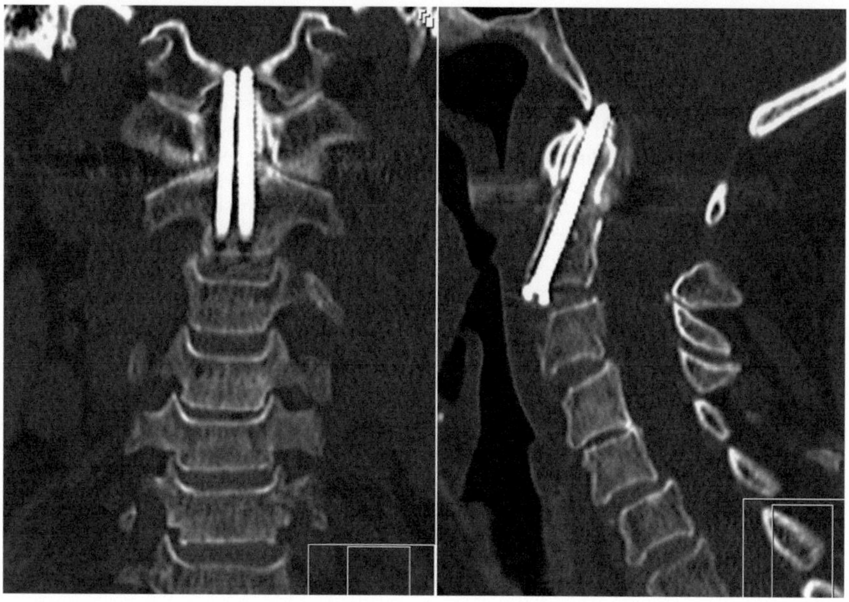

Fig. 6.10 Postoperative coronal (*left*) and sagittal (*right*) CT imaging showing the final positioning of both screws with good distal cortical purchase, although ideal screw lengths would have been about 4 mm shorter (see text)

screws side by side (4 mm needed for each screw, so at least 8–9 mm width preferred), we will routinely place two screws in patients over the age of 70.

Complications and Strategies for Avoidance

We recommend manually flexing and extending the patient's head under fluoroscopy at the completion of the case to detect any instability as a result of previously undetected injury to the TAL. In very rare circumstances, previously undetected gross instability between C1 and C2 despite good fixation across the fracture line has been observed which necessitated posterior atlantoaxial fusion with the patient still under general anesthesia. While this type of injury is best diagnosed preoperatively, this simple maneuver at the end of the case can confirm stability at C1-C2 quickly and easily.

The elderly are at an inherently higher risk for dysphagia with any anterior cervical procedure, and this should be taken into account when determining a management strategy for a patient's fracture. Intraoperatively, this risk can be slightly reduced with gentle dissection of the prevertebral fascia and being careful not to elevate or manipulate the hypopharynx more than necessary with the superior retractor blade. Minimizing operative time and only opening the medial-lateral retractor blades as far as necessary both may help reduce dysphagia, although this is based on extrapolation from studies on ACDF (anterior cervical discectomy and fusion) surgery and has not been directly studied in odontoid screw fixation cases. Postoperatively, our nursing staff routinely performs a simple bedside swallow test before resuming a diet.

It is important to accurately measure the screw length prior to placement. A longer screw has the potential to either protrude too far in front of the C2-C3 disc space which could lead to erosion of the disc and hardware failure or extend past the distal cortex of the dens and cause neurologic or vascular injury. This will generally not occur unless the screw is much too long (by a centimeter or more) or is angulated much too posteriorly and breaches the posterior wall of the dens rather than emerging from the tip. The latter would represent more of a trajectory error than a screw length error. Too short of a screw could lead to poor engagement of the distal cortical bone at the odontoid tip and most commonly will lead to screw backout with failure of fixation.

References

1. Anderson LD, D'Alonzo RT. Fractures of the odontoid process of the axis. J Bone Joint Surg Am. 1974;56(8):1663–74.
2. Ryken TC, Hadley MN, Aarabi B, Dhall SS, Gelb DE, Hurlbert RJ, et al. Management of isolated fractures of the axis in adults. Neurosurgery. 2013;72(Suppl 2):132–50.
3. Böhler J. Anterior stabilization for acute fractures and non-unions of the dens. J Bone Joint Surg Am. 1982;64(1):18–27.
4. Dailey AT, Hart D, Finn MA, Schmidt MH, Apfelbaum RI. Anterior fixation of odontoid fractures in an elderly population. J Neurosurg Spine. 2010;12(1):1–8.
5. Jenkins JD, Coric D, Branch CL. A clinical comparison of one- and two-screw odontoid fixation. J Neurosurg. 1998;89(3):366–70.
6. Koech F, Ackland HM, Varma DK, Williamson OD, Malham GM. Nonoperative management of type II odontoid fractures in the elderly. Spine. 2008;33(26):2881–6.
7. Lopez AJ, Scheer JK, Leibl KE, Smith ZA, Dlouhy BJ, Dahdaleh NS. Anatomy and biomechanics of the craniovertebral junction. Neurosurg Focus. 2015;38(4):E2.
8. Ivancic PC, Beauchman NN, Mo F, Lawrence BD. Biomechanics of halo-vest and dens screw fixation for type II odontoid fracture. Spine. 2009;34(5):484–90.
9. Apfelbaum RI, Lonser RR, Veres R, Casey A. Direct anterior screw fixation for recent and remote odontoid fractures. J Neurosurg. 2000;93(2 Suppl):227–36.
10. Grauer JN, Shafi B, Hilibrand AS, Harrop JS, Kwon BK, Beiner JM, et al. Proposal of a modified, treatment-oriented classification of odontoid fractures. Spine J. 2005;5(2):123–9.
11. Lennarson PJ, Mostafavi H, Traynelis VC, Walters BC. Management of type II dens fractures: a case-control study. Spine. 2000;25(10):1234–7.
12. Tashjian RZ, Majercik S, Biffl WL, Palumbo MA, Cioffi WG. Halo-vest immobilization increases early morbidity and mortality in elderly odontoid fractures. J Trauma. 2006;60(1):199–203.
13. Hadley MN, Dickman CA, Browner CM, Sonntag VK. Acute axis fractures: a review of 229 cases. J Neurosurg. 1989;71(5 Pt 1):642–7.
14. Winslow CP, Winslow TJ, Wax MK. Dysphonia and dysphagia following the anterior approach to the cervical spine. Arch Otolaryngol Head Neck Surg. 2001;127(1):51–5.
15. Sayama CM, Fassett DR, Apfelbaum RI. The utility of MRI in the evaluation of odontoid fractures. J Spinal Disord Tech. 2008;21(7):524–6.
16. Zou D, Zhang K, Ren Y, Wu Y, Yang Y, Li Y. Three-dimensional image navigation system-assisted anterior cervical screw fixation for treatment of acute odontoid fracture. Int J Clin Exp Med. 2014;7(11):4332–6.
17. Feng G, Wendlandt R, Spuck S, Schulz AP. One-screw fixation provides similar stability to that of two-screw fixation for type II dens fractures. Clin Orthop Relat Res. 2012;470(7):2021–8.

Anterior Cervical Decompression and Fusion

7

Vincent J. Alentado and Thomas E. Mroz

Introduction

Cervical spondylosis refers to age-related degenerative changes of the cervical spine. Over time, cervical spondylosis may lead to progressive axial neck pain, upper extremity radiculopathy, and/or cervical myelopathy. These clinical entities may result from any of a variety of degenerative changes including disc degeneration, disc herniation, facet arthrosis, and osteophyte formation. Anterior cervical decompression and fusion (ACDF) is a commonly utilized surgical treatment option for patients experiencing radiculopathy and/or myelopathy secondary to cervical spondylosis that is refractory to nonsurgical management. Cervical corpectomy, another type of anterior decompression, of one or several levels can be performed for degenerative conditions, neoplasia, and infection.

Anterior cervical decompression was first described in 1955 by Robinson and Smith for the treatment of degenerative disc disease [1]. Since that time, this approach has been modified and improved to treat multiple cervical spinal pathologies including radiculopathy and myelopathy. The primary aim of ACDF is physical decompression of neurologic structures, restoration of cervical alignment, and achievement of bony fusion. Excellent results can be achieved through careful patient selection and operative technique. The current literature suggests that over 90% of patients experience relief of symptoms following ACDF when radiculopathy is the primary indication for surgery [2, 3]. Furthermore, patients suffering from cervical myelopathy also demonstrate favorable results postoperatively [2]. The purpose of this chapter is to discuss the surgical indications and techniques for anterior cervical decompressive and fusion surgery. Options for optimizing results and avoiding complications will also be discussed.

Indications and Patient Selection

Appropriate patient selection is essential to achieving successful outcomes following ACDF. The decision to decompress anteriorly as opposed to posteriorly depends not only on surgeon expertise but also on the location of neural compression, alignment of the cervical spine, and the number of levels involved. In patients with lesions posterior to the spinal cord, such as from hypertrophy of the ligamentum flavum, ACDF will not relieve the offending lesion. ACDF is

V.J. Alentado, MD
Indiana University, Department of Neurological Surgery, Indianapolis, IN, USA

T.E. Mroz, MD (✉)
Departments of Orthopaedic and Neurological Surgery, Cleveland Clinic, 9500 Euclid Avenue, S-40, Cleveland, Ohio 44195, USA
e-mail: mrozt@ccf.org

L.T. Holly, P.A. Anderson (eds.), *Essentials of Spinal Stabilization*,
DOI 10.1007/978-3-319-59713-3_7

suitable for patients with one- to three-level disease with neurologic compression at the level of the disc space and in patients with kyphotic, neutral, or lordotic alignment.

Corpectomy is indicated for patients who have cord compression behind the vertebral body proper that cannot be addressed through an ACDF. This can be due to spondylosis, neoplasia, and infection. It is suitable for patients with two- or more level disease due to advanced spondylosis with large vertebral body posterior osteophytes that extend away from the disc space proper and toward the vertebral body. In such cases, performing a complete neurological decompression using an ACDF approach can result in substantial removal of the intervening vertebral body due to the size of the posterior osteophytes. It is often preferred to instead perform a corpectomy to avoid this scenario.

The number of surgical levels and patient-specific factors (i.e., risks for nonunion) should be considered carefully when deciding between ACDF and corpectomy in patients that have compression localized to the disc space proper. There is no ambiguity in the literature that rates of pseudarthrosis increase with the number of fusion surfaces. For example, a three-level ACDF has six fusion surfaces, whereas a two-level corpectomy only has two fusion surfaces. In this example, the three-level ACDF will be expected to have a higher chance of pseudarthrosis. Like the association of surgical levels and pseudarthrosis, there is also little ambiguity about worse clinical outcomes with pseudarthrosis in the anterior cervical spine. Therefore, it is incumbent on the surgeon to carefully weigh all variables (type of graft substrate, type of interbody cage, history of smoking, steroids, or antimetabolites) when deciding the proper surgery for a particular patient.

Patients presenting with radiculopathy without myelopathy should be considered for ACDF if their symptoms fail to improve after a trial of nonoperative management and if advanced imaging modalities demonstrate neural compression in the neuroforamen of the index level. Surgery may also be considered for patients with progressive muscular weakness. Patients with symptoms consistent with progressive myelopathy or myeloradiculopathy are also candidates for ACDF. Other indications for ACDF include cervical discitis, anterior cervical epidural abscess, cervical spondylolisthesis, and traumatic cervical instability. However, ACDF or corpectomy with fusion is not a reliable surgical option for the treatment of axial neck pain secondary to degenerative disc disease. Furthermore, history of previous cervical radiation, radical neck dissection, tracheostomy, severe osteoporosis, vocal cord dysfunction, esophageal injury, or preexisting dysphagia is relative contraindications to ventral surgery.

Preoperative Considerations

A complete history and physical examination should be performed on any patient presenting with possible cervical radiculopathy or myelopathy. The patient should be asked about symptoms related to myelopathy such as difficulty with buttoning shirts or problems with gait and balance. The patient should also be questioned about any nonoperative treatment modalities that have been trialed, any recent falls or trauma, problems with bowel or bladder function, and any history of neck surgery or radiation. In cases of radiculopathy, it is important to ascertain the type and severity of the arm pain. Patients with a C6 or C7 radiculopathy may present with pain radiating into the ipsilateral trapezius muscle region and/or the periscapular or subscapular region. In some instances, this will be the sole presenting complaint (i.e., the patient will not have radicular arm pain). It is imperative in such patients to perform a complete shoulder examination to ensure such pain is not due to shoulder or shoulder girdle pathology. In such cases, an anesthetic selective nerve root block is often helpful as a diagnostic maneuver.

A careful observation of the patient is key. Ability to use the arms to rise out of a chair can offer important clues about pain level and strength. Patients with severe radicular arm pain sometimes will hold their shoulder in an abducted position in order to relieve tension on the affected nerve root and, hence, diminish their pain.

Observe the cervical alignment and global sagittal alignment and note range of forward flexion, extension, left and right rotation, and lateral bending. A Spurling's maneuver (a maneuver in which the patient extends their neck and turns to the symptomatic side before axial compression is performed) should be implemented on all patients suspected of having a cervical radiculopathy. A neuromuscular examination of the upper and lower extremities should be performed. Asymmetric motor weakness along with dermatomal sensory changes can help localize the level of nerve root compression. Biceps, brachioradialis, and triceps reflexes should be tested on both upper extremities. Patients with radiculopathy often have decreased deep tendon reflexes correlating to the site of compression, whereas patients with myelopathy may have hyperactive reflexes with possible presence of a Hoffmann sign and/or inverted radial reflex(es). Lower extremity reflexes should also be assessed for hyperreflexia, presence of Babinski sign(s), increased tone, and sustained or asymmetrical non-sustained clonus as these are potential indicators of myelopathy. Gait analysis, including tandem gait and balance, should also be assessed in patients who are able to ambulate.

Most patients with a cervical radiculopathy do not need imaging to make the diagnosis or initiate treatment. If imaging is warranted, initial imaging studies include standing anteroposterior, lateral, flexion, and extension radiographs of the cervical spine. These images will provide information about spinal alignment, stability, and presence of bony pathology. If further imaging is desired, magnetic resonance imaging (MRI) is the preferred modality. MRI allows for visualization of the soft tissues, neural elements, intervertebral discs, and the vertebral artery. MRI can also allow for visualization of myelomalacia or spinal cord edema. If the patient is unable to undergo MRI or if better assessment of bony structures is required, then computed tomography (CT) myelography is a suitable alternative. This imaging modality allows visualization of both neural elements and bony structures.

Patients with known anatomical anomalies, especially of the vertebral arteries, or a history of previous anterior cervical surgical procedures, including carotid artery and thyroid surgeries, should undergo more extensive preoperative planning. Notably, 2.7% of cadaveric specimens were found to have tortuous vertebral arteries [4]. Therefore, axial images should be reviewed intently on every operative case to ensure there are no abnormalities of the vertebral artery, specifically medialization. Previous surgical treatments may also lead to a more difficult approach with less definitive anatomic planes or altered anatomy. Furthermore, these patients should be considered for preoperative evaluation by an otolaryngologist for assessment of vocal cord dysfunction secondary to recurrent laryngeal nerve injury. If a patient had previous neck surgery and the vocal cords are functioning normally based on laryngoscopy, then the approach should be on the contralateral side. Conversely, if the vocal cords are not functioning normally on the side of a previous surgery, then the approach should be from the same side to avoid damage to the normal vocal cord. Finally, patients with a history of carotid bruit or carotid artery stenosis should be approached opposite the side of the carotid artery pathology to minimize the risk of an intraoperative stroke [5].

Surgical Technique

Positioning and Approach

Anterior cervical discectomy and fusion is performed in the supine position under general anesthesia with endotracheal intubation. Manipulation of the neck should be done with caution in patients with myelopathy. If the patient cannot safely extend the neck without pain or neurologic symptoms preoperatively, then fiberoptic assistance may be needed to facilitate the intubation. The endotracheal tube should be taped at the corner of the mouth opposite the side of the planned approach. A bump or gel roll is placed transversely under the scapulae to facilitate cervical lordosis, but it is important to not exceed the degree of extension that the patient can tolerate while awake, prior to neurological decompression. The occiput should be placed on a foam doughnut with the cervical spine placed in acceptable alignment. It is often advantageous to place multiple towels under the head for patients with cervical kyphosis if the goal of the surgery is to also improve alignment. After the decompression(s) have been performed, the towel can be sequentially removed to allow the head and neck to gently assume a more lordotic posture. This is a very controlled situation and aids in the deformity correction. The reconstruction then proceeds per protocol.

The bed should be placed in approximately 20° of reverse Trendelenburg to allow for venous drainage and to allow the shoulders to move inferiorly to afford better radiographic visualization. The elbows and wrists should be padded with foam to prevent compression neuropathy. The arms should then be tucked at the patient's sides. The shoulders should be taped with downward traction to improve visualization of the neck and allow for improved exposure of lateral intraoperative imaging by moving the shoulders caudally. If an iliac crest autograft is planned, a pillow should be placed underneath the ipsilateral buttock to elevate the iliac crest. An 8-cm oblique line is then drawn 6 cm lateral to the anterior superior iliac spine.

Currently, there is no conclusive evidence demonstrating improved outcomes or reduced complication rates with either a left- or right-sided anterior cervical approach [6]. An advantage of the left-sided approach includes the more predictable and medial course of the recurrent laryngeal nerve on the left side [7]. In contrast, the right-sided approach is more comfortable for the right-handed surgeon and avoids the thoracic duct which is at risk during left-sided exposures of C7–T1. Furthermore, there is a theoretically decreased risk to the esophagus which lies slightly to the left side.

The anatomic landmarks for surgical incision are as follows: C3, hyoid bone; C4 to C5, thyroid cartilage; and C6, cricoid cartilage. Transverse incisions are more cosmetically appealing and can be utilized for procedures of any level. For surgery of three or more levels, the incision can be extended to or past the midline, as well as further laterally, and followed by a more extensive release above and below the platysma to improve access. If a skin crease is present near the desired location for incision, then the incision should be made within the skin crease, as this is more cosmetically appealing. If a transverse incision is planned, it should lie between the medial border of the sternocleidomastoid (SCM) muscle and the midline. Vertical incisions should be made 1 cm medial to the border of the SCM. Once the incision is marked, the operative field should be isolated with circumferential adhesive drapes. Local anesthetic is then injected into the incision site.

Adequate exposure is an important part of ACDF and corpectomy surgery. The skin should be incised with a scalpel to the subcutaneous layer. The skin edges can then be elevated with small self-retaining retractors. The subcutaneous tissue is dissected until the longitudinal muscle fibers of the platysma are visible. The platysma muscle can be divided either vertically or horizontally with sharp dissection or electrocautery. The anterior jugular venous system development varies from person to person. It may be seen deep to the platysma muscle, although it is typically located closer to the midline. If encountered, this vein may be ligated or retracted. The loose areolar tissue deep to the platysma should be dissected with blunt and sharp dissection to facilitate better exposure and retraction. Once this layer is developed, the medial border of the SCM and lateral border of the strap muscles are easily identified.

At this point, it is important to identify the carotid sheath by digital palpation and visual inspection. The middle cervical fascia must be bluntly or sharply dissected medial to the sheath and just lateral to the strap muscles. Be mindful that the development of the middle cervical fascia varies, and, in patients with a well-developed fascial layer, sharp dissection is often an easier technique. As one progresses through the anterior exposure, it is critical to develop all planes equally, as this will afford excellent visualization and require less soft tissue retraction while performing work on the spine. The carotid sheath should be retracted laterally with a handheld retractor to ensure that dissection is carried medial to it, thereby decreasing risk of injury. Another retractor should be utilized to mobilize and protect the infrahyoid muscles, trachea, and esophagus medially. By retracting these structures medially, the risk of injury to the recurrent laryngeal nerve is minimized.

The pretracheal fascia should be penetrated bluntly along the medial border of the SCM to avoid injury to the thyroid vessels or laryngeal nerves. This can be done using Metzenbaum scissors in a spreading fashion. In procedures involving the C5 or C6 level, the omohyoid muscle can be divided to improve visualization. Once this layer is developed, the spine can be palpated and the esophagus and trachea retracted. If the esophagus and trachea cannot be easily mobilized, the esophagus may be adherent to the prevertebral fascia or the neck may be overextended. If adherent, the esophagus must be slowly dissected away from the prevertebral fascia by using peanut dissector sponges, which minimizes the risk of esophageal injury.

At this point, the vertebral level should be verified by using a marker and a lateral radiograph. It is critical to properly and meticulously mark the intended, correct level of surgery in a manner consistent with the operating surgeon. The authors use a *blue* marker *and* a physical electrocautery burn mark into the operative disc(s). Careful examination of preoperative radiographs may reveal anterior osteophytes that can help in identification of the correct level. A radiographic marker can be placed into the vertebral body, as this has been suggested to decrease the chance of unintended disc degeneration at nonsurgical levels. Placement of a needle within a disc space at a non-fused level has been associated with a three-fold increased risk of developing degenerative changes postoperatively [8].

Once the level is confirmed, the longus colli muscles and anterior longitudinal ligament are dissected with electrocautery to the uncovertebral joints bilaterally. The authors will intentionally decrease the power on the electrocautery at this point to decrease the thermal injury to the soft tissues, thereby theoretically decreasing soft tissue edema postoperatively. The longus coli muscles should then be elevated on both sides with self-retaining retractors with or without teeth. Efforts need to be made to ensure the retractors do not migrate from underneath the longus coli as this can injure the sympathetic chain, esophagus, trachea, or carotid artery. Ideally the longus colli muscles should not be divided transversely, as the sympathetic chain is located on the anterolateral aspect of both muscles.

ACDF and Instrumentation

At this point, Caspar pins are placed into the midline of the cranial and caudal vertebral bodies in a parallel manner into the operative level, and distraction across the interspace is performed. Another option for distraction is intraoperative cervical traction. While this will not provide as much as focal traction at the surgical level as Caspar pins, cervical traction can be useful for maintaining alignment during surgery and increased distraction. One other option to consider for traction is the use of two Caspar pins per vertebral body and bilateral distractors. This is a very powerful method to distract across a disc space, and careful attention during distraction is necessary to avoid over-distraction or pin pullout from the bone. Finally, after the discectomy is performed, one may also employ interspace distractors to achieve the amount of desired distraction. After the vertebral body and disc are completely exposed, the anterior lip of the inferior end plate of the cranial vertebral body should be removed using a high-speed burr, rongeur, or Kerrison rongeur. Removal of this lip allows the surgeon an improved visualization of the posterior disc space during discectomy and allows for possible foraminotomy and/ or posterior longitudinal ligament (PLL) resection, if desired. Surgeons may use loupe magnification or the operating microscope. It is the authors' preference to use loupes for the approach with a quick transition to the operating microscope after the final retractors are placed.

Next, the discectomy should be performed. The anterior longitudinal ligament and the ventral portion of the annulus should be incised with a 15-blade scalpel to create a 10–12-mm rectangular opening to the uncovertebral joints. The blade should be held 90° to the axis of the spine such that the sharp end never faces the carotid artery. Following incision of the annulus, the ventral portion of the disc is removed using a pituitary rongeur. Next, disc material and cartilaginous endplates should be removed using a combination of 2–3-mm straight and angled curettes, 1–3-mm Kerrison rongeurs, and a pituitary rongeur.

A high-speed burr is used to remove any posterior osteophytes and prepare the endplates for graft placement. The burden of the posterior osteophytes varies considerably depending on the extent of spondylosis. A high-speed burr is used to remove the osteophytes parallel to the endplates to the level of the PLL. This can be done safely using an operative microscope. Flattening the surface of both endplates allows for maximal bony contact with the graft which encourages fusion. The inferior endplate of the rostral vertebral body may require more preparation due to the increased concavity of inferior endplates. The cortical bone should be removed to the deepest layer of the natural concavity to create a flat surface and preserve cortical bone. The cortical bone must be preserved unless required for adequate decompression or graft subsidence is more likely to occur. Multiple punches should be made in the endplates with a small angled curette to cause bleeding which may increase the likelihood of a successful fusion.

The PLL should be inspected for any defects through which disc material may have extruded. In all cases of myelopathy, the PLL should be resected to directly visualize the dura and achieve an adequate decompression. In cases of radiculopathy, it is the surgeon's discretion as to resect the PLL. Some argue that it affords an easier access into the foramen, while others maintain that an adequate direct foraminal decompression can be performed without resection of the ligament. When PLL resection is indicated, a 2-mm Kerrison rongeur should be used to create a window in the PLL that is large enough to visualize the dura and remove any disc fragments from the spinal canal. Neuroforaminal decompression can be achieved indirectly through restoration of the intervertebral disc height. However, a direct anterior foraminotomy should also be performed. The landmark that defines the extent of an anterior or posterior foraminotomy is the caudal pedicle of the surgical level. The medial portion of the uncinate process can be thinned using a high-speed burr. It is important at the same time to visualize the ventral uncovertebral joint which was exposed with longus coli elevation because this gives the surgeon a clear understanding of how far drilling can progress laterally without putting the vertebral artery at risk. The termination of the foraminotomy is palpation of the caudal pedicle using a micro nerve hook. The authors' preference is to utilize the Rhoton microinstrument set for this part of the procedure. A Kerrison rongeur or microcurette is also used to remove any osteophytes on the lateral border of the foramen. If decompression is adequate, a 1- or 2-mm Kerrison rongeur should fit within the foramen anterior to the exiting nerve root. Larger Kerrison use is discouraged in order to prevent iatrogenic nerve root injury.

Interbody grafts provide structural support and allow for formation of a solid fusion. Graft options include tricortical autogenous bone, cortical allogeneic bone, and a variety of synthetic cages. Graft size should be determined using trial spacers. The spacers should be tamped into place gently with the use of a mallet while the disc space is still under distraction. The correctly sized spacer should fit snugly within the distracted disc space. When using tricortical autograft, the bone should be shaped with the anterior height 1–2 mm taller than the posterior height to facilitate lordosis of the cervical spine and help avoid posterior retropulsion of the graft into the spinal cord. Once the graft is selected or created, it should be tamped to a position approximately 4 mm anterior to the dura and 2 mm posterior to the anterior lip of the vertebral endplates. Once the graft position is adequate, distraction should be released. The graft should then be tested for stability within the disc space using a right-angled probe. Pinhole sites should be covered with bone wax. A lateral radiograph should be taken to confirm proper graft placement.

Although a single-level ACDF procedure can be performed without instrumentation, a plate provides additional stability, increased fusion rates, and prevents segmental kyphosis in patients who develop nonunion. The anterior plate needs to fit flush on the cervical spine. If the plate rocks prior to placement of screws, it will be tilted in the final position and this can increase dysphagia postoperatively. It must be long enough to allow screw placement in both the superior and inferior vertebral bodies, but not too long that it overrides the adjacent disc, potentially contributing to adjacent segment disease. Plates that are within 5 mm of the adjacent discs have been demonstrated to increase adjacent-level ossification after ACDF [9]. Ideally, the prepared endplates should be just visible through the screw holes of the plate. Once properly positioned, the plate can be secured using 14–16-mm screws. Proper angulation of the screws is important as screws that violate adjacent disc spaces may contribute to the development of adjacent segment disease postoperatively. Lateral and anteroposterior radiographs can be taken to ensure proper placement of instrumentation.

Corpectomy

The surgical approach for a corpectomy and ACDF is identical, as are the techniques for plate placement. Once the approach is complete and the intended surgical levels are confirmed, then the Caspar pins are placed above and below the body of interest. As an example, if the intended corpectomy is C6, then Caspar pins should be placed into C5 and C7. After gentle distraction is performed, discectomies above and below the intended level proceed in an identical manner as an ACDF previously described. It is very important to have exposed the anterior uncus bilaterally at both levels as this is the "lighthouse" of this procedure. That is, this important landmark will verify throughout the surgery the midline as well as the lateral extent of the corpectomy trough. One of the major complications of this procedure is drilling too far laterally, typically onto the contralateral side, which will put the vertebral artery at risk.

After the discectomies are performed, a high-speed bur is then used to complete a *vertical* trough from the superior uncus to the inferior uncus, and this should be done bilaterally. As the trough progresses dorsally, a rongeur should be used to remove the intervening vertebral body as it is a prime source of autogenous bone graft. This series of drilling and vertebral body removal continues until the posterior longitudinal ligament is encountered. Of note, some bone is highly vascular, and it is sometimes necessary to revert to a diamond tip bur as this will decreased the amount of bleeding. However, use of a diamond tip will add time to the drilling and bone removal. Another option for the bleeding bone wax, but this should be minimized on biological surfaces as it can interfere with graft consolidation. Once all of the bone has been removed, the PLL is then resected with a Kerrison rongeur to completely expose and decompress the dura. It is not uncommon to encounter areas of PLL-dural adhesions and care should be taken to avoid a durotomy. The Rhoton instrument set is ideal for management of these adhesions. If no plane between the dura and PLL is achievable, it is acceptable to "float" this region of PLL by removing all of the PLL around it.

The typical trough length (left to right) in an adult should be approximately 16–18 mm. The authors rely on the measurement, but also will assess adequacy of the decompression by visualizing the equator of the dura on both the right and left side along the entire superior-inferior extent of the decompression. After the dimensions of the decompression are measured, the authors typically use fibular allograft packed with autogenous bone for reconstruction followed by the placement of a plate as previously described. Such allograft is preferred due to this ability to consolidate, as well as its favorable biomechanical properties and cost. There are other options for reconstruction, however, that one may consider. These include structural iliac crest bone graft and synthetic (e.g., polyetheretherketone) or metallic cages which can be expandable or static. Unlike allograft or iliac crest bone graft, synthetic or metallic cages have no potential for osseous integration, and this should be considered carefully when choosing a cage type.

Proper placement of the strut graft, or cage, is critical. The endplates superiorly and inferiorly should be flat and the graft/cage contact with the endplate should be optimized to maximize fusion and minimize graft/cage migration. A helpful technique is to gently distract with the Caspar pins, then place the graft/cage, and then release distraction. This will afford an acceptable interference fit. Placement of the plate should proceed as previously described. It is particularly important that the plate is flush against the cranial and caudal vertebral bodies and that screw length is optimal to maximize rigidity of the construct. Morselized allograft or autogenous bone graft can then be applied to the lateral aspects of the strut graft/cage if there is enough space.

Hybrid ACDF and Corpectomy

In some instances employing a combination ACDF and corpectomy may be necessary depending on the pattern of compression. For example, consider a patient with cord compression behind the vertebral body of C5 but also a herniated disc with neural compression at C6–C7. In this scenario, performing a C5 corpectomy and ACDF at C6–C7 will address both issues. If pathology allows, the authors design a hybrid construct with the ACDF inferiorly because it provides four points of fixation inferiorly, which can be a biomechanically vulnerable aspect of the construct depending on global sagittal alignment, bone quality, and construct integrity.

Prior to closure, hemostasis should be achieved with electrocautery and procoagulants. The platysma muscle can be closed with 3–0 absorbable sutures. The skin is closed with subcuticular absorbable sutures and the incision should be cleaned and dressed in standard fashion. The use of drains for anterior cervical surgery is controversial, and the literature has not demonstrated definitively that drain usage prevents symptomatic postoperative hematomas. Their use is typically relegated to surgeon preference. The authors, however, use 1/8th inch Davol drains routinely for anterior surgery. The drain is brought through the main incision, and the layered closure is performed around the drain which is pulled typically on the first or second postoperative day. The use of rigid external orthoses (braces) after anterior cervical fusion is also controversial, and there is insufficient evidence in the literature to support their routine use to enhance fusion or clinical outcome. Activity following anterior cervical fusion is restricted to the activity of daily living for 6 weeks. Thereafter, routine patients can slowly resume more activity. Patients that want to resume contact activity should be further restricted until there is radiographic evidence of mature arthrodesis and only after a careful discussion with the surgeon about the potential risks with such activity.

Illustrative Case

History A 63-year-old right-handed male presents with complaints of numbness and tingling in his right arm and right leg over the past 3 years. His symptoms have been stable since onset and do not vary with activities. However, he did notice increasing difficulty grasping and opening objects with his right hand. He denies any weakness or numbness in the left upper or lower extremity and denies any balance or gait issues. His symptoms have failed to improve despite several months of physical therapy and multiple medications. He denies changes in bowel or bladder function.

Physical Examination The patient is able to perform reciprocal heel-to-toe walking with slight ataxia. The cervical spine appears lordotic without tenderness to palpation or paraspinal atrophy. He is able to flex his chin to his anterior chest without pain. However, extension is limited, but also painless. Spurling's test is negative bilaterally. Neuromuscular exam is significant only for diminished strength and sensation in the right upper extremity and right lower extremity.

Radiographic Imaging Plain radiographs including flexion/extension views demonstrated multilevel spondylosis with a stable retrolisthesis of C5 on C6 (Figs. 7.1 and 7.2).

MRI of the cervical spine demonstrates spinal cord compression with myelomalacia at C5–C6 due to spondylotic changes (Figs. 7.3 and 7.4). There is also severe foraminal stenosis at C5–C6 and C6–C7 on the right side.

Given the clinical findings and confirmatory imaging findings, the patient was offered ACDF at C5–C6 and C6–C7. His perioperative course was uneventful and his preoperative symptoms resolved postoperatively. Postoperative imaging demonstrated improvement in cervical alignment (Fig. 7.5).

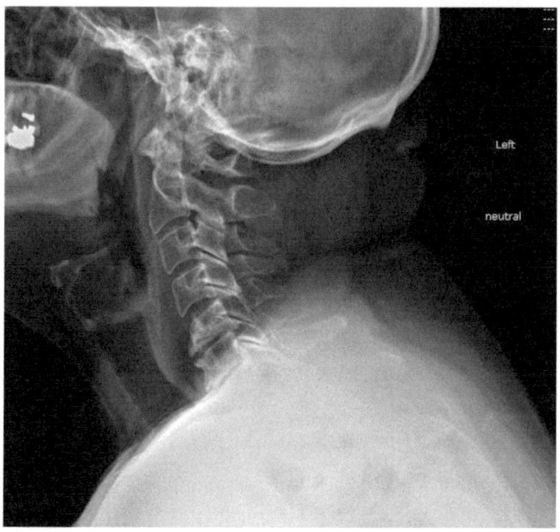

Fig. 7.1 Sagittal plain radiograph demonstrating multilevel cervical spondylosis, most advanced at C5–C6 and C6–C7, with grade I retrolisthesis of C5 on C6

Technical Pearls

- When the patient has a history or imaging findings consistent with myelopathy, pre- and post-intubation and pre-and post-positioning neuromonitoring can be considered.
- Postoperatively, the patient should be kept upright to at least 45° to help minimize fluid accumulation and edema in the prevertebral space.
- Be meticulous when localizing to a specific level, and do not accept a suboptimal radiograph or fluoroscopic image during the localization process.
- The use of an operating microscope is preferred by the authors as it has superior optics and light source.
- Expose the anterior uncus bilaterally for ACDF and corpectomy as it defines the midline and lateral extent of decompression.
- Once the pedicle is palpated during the foraminotomy, then the decompression is complete. Rarely is there ever anything compressive lateral to the pedicle in a degenerative case.

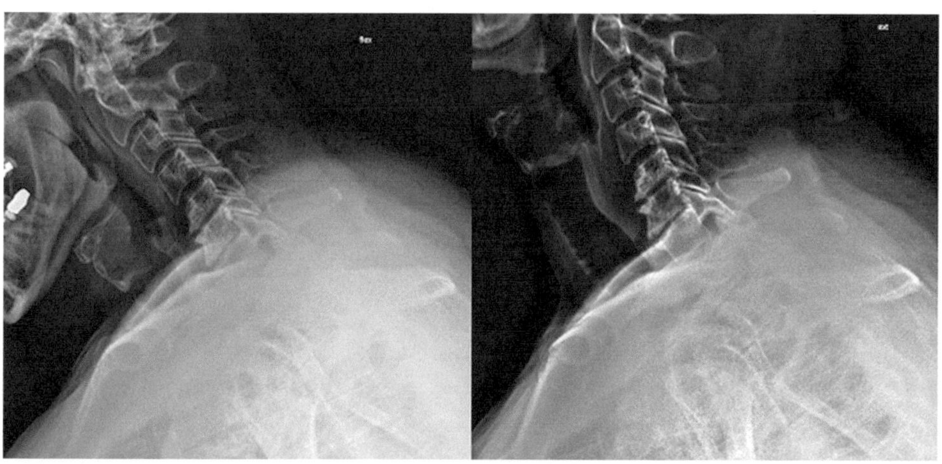

Fig. 7.2 Flexion/extension radiographs demonstrating stable appearance of spondylolisthesis

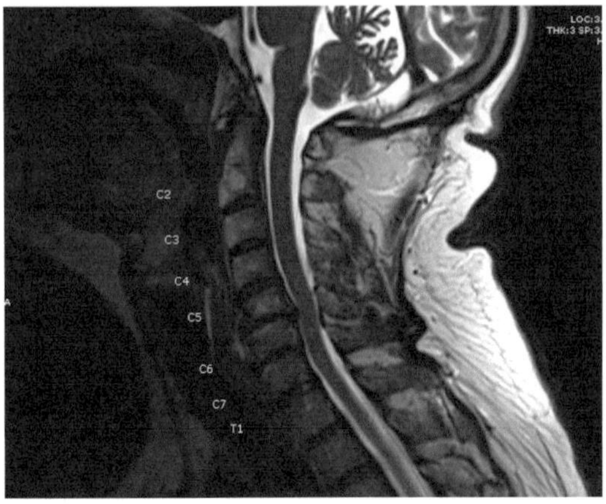

Fig. 7.3 T2-weighted MRI demonstrating multilevel degenerative changes with suspected early myelomalacia and/ or edema

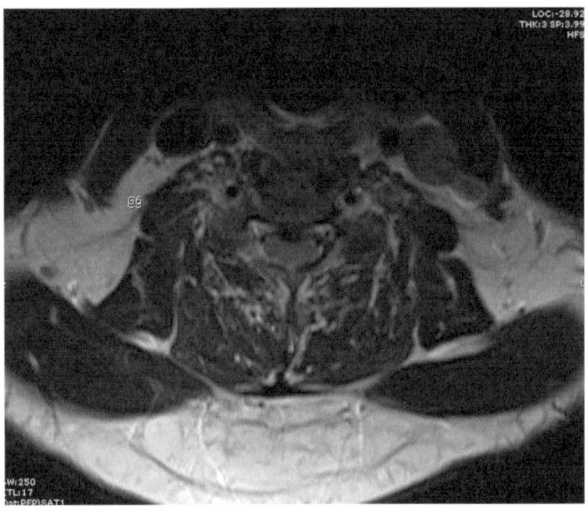

Fig. 7.4 Axial MRI demonstrating severe spinal canal stenosis at the C5–C6 level

corpectomy and reconstruction. It is equally important that the plate and screw placement is ideal for optimal stability.

Complications and Strategies for Avoidance

Nearly all patients experience some dysphagia after ACDF. The dysphagia is usually not clinically significant and improves within the first 3 weeks postoperatively. Chronic dysphagia is uncommon, occurring in approximately 4% of patients receiving ACDF [10]. Potential causes of delayed-onset dysphagia include plate or screw dislodgement causing esophageal obstruction.

Dysphonia may be present in some patients postoperatively due to postsurgical swelling. If the dysphonia does not improve within 2–3 days postoperatively, consider laryngeal nerve injury. Most laryngeal nerve injuries are secondary to retraction and should recover within 3–6 months. However, persistent hoarseness necessitates evaluation by an otolaryngologist. Injury to the superior laryngeal nerve can lead to recurrent aspiration, whereas injury to the recurrent laryngeal nerve usually manifests as hoarseness, but can lead to airway obstruction [10, 11].

A hematoma may also develop postoperatively. Usually this occurs within 12 h of the operation. If a hematoma is visible or palpable in the anterior neck and the patient is experiencing

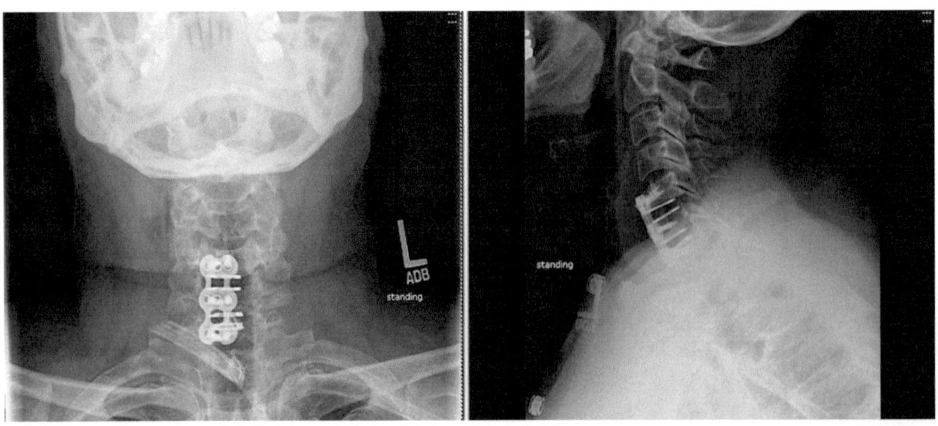

Fig. 7.5 Anteroposterior and lateral radiographs demonstrating anatomic position and alignment of the cervical spine following a two-level ACDF

dyspnea, the incision should be opened immediately. A hematoma can be prevented with placement of a drain at the end of the operation.

Postoperative fluid collection may be secondary to CSF leak or esophageal injury, both of which may lead to devastating consequences for the patient, and therefore require urgent surgical re-exploration. CSF leak can be avoided by watertight closure of incidental durotomies encountered during the procedure. Esophageal injuries can be minimized with careful use of blunt dissection along with gentle retraction of the esophagus.

Symptomatic pseudarthrosis may occur postoperatively. It can be treated with revision ACDF or with posterior cervical fusion. Use of plating instrumentation decreases the rate of pseudarthrosis, especially in multilevel ACDFs. However, plating may increase the risk of adjacent segment disease over time.

Delayed-onset neurologic deterioration may result from epidural abscess, graft dislocation, subluxation, or intervertebral collapse, all of which would require urgent surgical treatment.

Conclusion

ACDF and corpectomy with fusion are common techniques to adequately treat neurological compression with correlative clinical syndromes that are not responsive to nonsurgical treatment. In general, the surgical approach and techniques used to decompress and fuse the anterior cervical spine are safe with very low complication rates. It is imperative, however, to maintain attention to detail and to carefully consider the various factors that influence patient outcomes when selecting a particular surgery, a type of implant, and the graft substrate. Typically, the outcomes following anterior surgery for radiculopathy, myelopathy, and myeloradiculopathy are very favorable and predictable.

References

1. Robinson RA, Smith GW. Anterolateral cervical disc removal and interbody fusion for the cervical disc syndrome. Bull Johns Hopkins Hosp. 1955;96:223–4.
2. Kienapfel H, Koller M, Hinder D, Georg C, Pfeiffer M, Klose KJ, et al. Integrated outcome assessment after anterior cervical discectomy and fusion: myelocompression but not adjacent instability affect patient-reported quality of life and cervical spine symptoms. Spine. 2004;29(22):2501–9.
3. Xie J, Hurlbert RJ. Discectomy versus discectomy with fusion versus discectomy with fusion and instrumentation: a prospective randomized study. Neurosurgery. 2007;61(1):107–16; discussion 116–7.
4. Curylo LJ, Mason HC, Bohlman HH, Yoo JU. Tortuous course of the vertebral artery and anterior cervical decompression: a cadaveric and clinical case study. Spine. 2000;25(22):2860–4.
5. Chozick BS, Watson P, Greenblatt SH. Internal carotid artery thrombosis after cervical corpectomy. Spine. 1994;19(19):2230–2.
6. Beutler WJ, Sweeney CA, Connolly PJ. Recurrent laryngeal nerve injury with anterior cervical spine surgery risk with laterality of surgical approach. Spine. 2001;26(12):1337–42.
7. Ebraheim NA, Lu J, Skie M, Heck BE, Yeasting RA. Vulnerability of the recurrent laryngeal nerve in the anterior approach to the lower cervical spine. Spine. 1997;22(22):2664–7.
8. Nassr A, Lee JY, Bashir RS, Rihn JA, Eck JC, Kang JD, et al. Does incorrect level needle localization during anterior cervical discectomy and fusion lead to accelerated disc degeneration? Spine. 2009;34(2):189–92.
9. Park J-B, Cho Y-S, Riew KD. Development of adjacent-level ossification in patients with an anterior cervical plate. J Bone Joint Surg Am. 2005;87(3):558–63.
10. Frempong-Boadu A, Houten JK, Osborn B, Opulencia J, Kells L, Guida DD, et al. Swallowing and speech dysfunction in patients undergoing anterior cervical discectomy and fusion: a prospective, objective preoperative and postoperative assessment. J Spinal Disord Tech. 2002;15(5):362–8.
11. Dimopoulos VG, Chung I, Lee GP, Johnston KW, Kapsalakis IZ, Smisson HF, et al. Quantitative estimation of the recurrent laryngeal nerve irritation by employing spontaneous intraoperative electromyographic monitoring during anterior cervical discectomy and fusion. J Spinal Disord Tech. 2009;22(1):1–7.

8 Cervical Arthroplasty

Jau-Ching Wu, Michael S. Virk, and Praveen V. Mummaneni

Introduction

Cervical disc arthroplasty (CDA) has become a widely accepted option for surgical management of cervical spondylosis and degenerative disc disease (DDD).Unlike the standard anterior cervical discectomy and fusion (ACDF) that aims at arthrodesis of the diseased spinal segments, CDA allows maintenance of segmental motion at the indexed levels [1–5]. Therefore, CDA not only maintains physiological neck motion after surgery but also has the theoretical advantage to avoid adjacent segment disease (ASD). There have been eight prospective randomized control (RCT) investigational device exemption trials monitored by the United States Food and Drug Administrations (USFDA) of these CDA devices, with 5–8 years of data published [6–12]. These trials demonstrate similar or superior clinical results of CDA to ACDF in the relief of neurological symptoms for one- and two-level spondylosis and DDD [6–8, 13]. The clinical trials also demonstrate that the segmental motion was well preserved by each of these artificial discs with an averaged range of motion of approximately 7–8° during flexion-extension in each level treated by CDA [10, 14–16]. Maintenance of motion was consistently demonstrated in a high percentage of patients during follow-up of these enrolled patients. However, it is still debatable that CDA actually reduced the incidence of ASD which was reported to range from 0.8% to 2.9% per year after ACDF [3, 17].

Currently, available data suggests that, in selected patients, CDA could alleviate neurological symptoms caused by cervical spondylosis and DDD while maintaining the range of motion at the indexed segments after anterior cervical discectomy [5]. Cervical radiculopathy and myelopathy refractory to medical treatment could be managed by CDA with low rates of adverse events and few reoperations. A successful CDA not only decompresses neural tissues but also aims to maintain motion. To achieve optimal functional outcomes and segmental motion, meticulous techniques must be used in performing CDA operations. Theoretically, the surgery for CDA is more demanding than conventional ACDF because of the need to preserve motion. The pros and cons of current CDAs and the best candidates for each specific application remain uncertain. Despite very few studies to date

J.-C. Wu, MD, PhD (✉)
Department of Neurosurgery, Taipei Veterans' General Hospital, Taipei, Taiwan

School of Medicine, National Yang-Ming University, Taipei, Taiwan
e-mail: jauching@gmail.com

M.S. Virk, MD, PhD • P.V. Mummaneni, MD
Department of Neurological Surgery, University of California, San Francisco, CA, USA

L.T. Holly, P.A. Anderson (eds.), *Essentials of Spinal Stabilization*, DOI 10.1007/978-3-319-59713-3_8

comparing these artificial discs, complications and adverse effects of all kinds of CDA devices are reportedly as low as or even lower than conventional ACDF. Most of the implanted artificial discs had few problems and seldom required reoperations. Therefore, as the techniques, materials, and designs of these CDA devices continue to improve, the utilization of CDA is likely to be more prevalent in the future.

Indications and Patient Selection

The accepted indications of CDA are one- or two-level cervical DDD (e.g., disc herniation) or spondylosis from C3 to C7 causing radiculopathy or myelopathy that is not responsive to medical treatment or physical therapy after 6–12 weeks [2, 5, 18]. Candidates for CDA should not have cervical kyphosis, facet arthropathy, instability (i.e., more than 2–3 mm translation/subluxation on dynamic flexion/extension lateral radiographs), ankylosis, or osteoporosis. The best candidate for CDA is a young patient who has radicular symptoms caused by a herniated cervical disc without any facet arthrosis. The CDA replaces the intervertebral disc and preserves segmental motion but cannot correct facet joint disease that frequently coexists with DDD in patients with severe cervical spondylosis. On the other hand, conventional ACDF surgery not only removes the diseased disc, but the graft also increases disc height as well as enlarging the neuroforamen, and is capable of increasing cervical lordosis. By alleviation of segmental motion between fused vertebral bodies, ACDF immobilizes the facets. Therefore, elderly patients (aged over 65 years) with severe spondylosis and those who also have facet degeneration or malalignment of the cervical spine are better candidates for ACDF rather than CDA.

The FDA trials enrolled patients with one- and two-level cervical disc herniation, DDD, or spondylosis and demonstrated similar results for both CDA and ACDF for up to 8 years [6, 8, 10–12, 14–16]. However, these patients with slightly different pathologies and degrees of degeneration might have different outcomes in long-term follow-up. For example, a patient with radicular symptoms from a herniated disc has less degeneration than a patient with an osteophytic spur causing myelopathy [4, 19].

The theoretical advantages of preservation of motion with decompression of the neural tissue by CDA include the decreased risk of ASD and reoperations. Nevertheless, these potential benefits may not be demonstrated in short-term follow-up. This could explain why the ASD rates were very similar among these patients, at least in the short- to midterm reports [6, 7, 20]. However, longer-term studies are showing possible benefits of CDA over ACDF in reoperations. Meta-analyses by Luo et al. and Zhong et al. show significantly lower rates of reoperation at both index and adjacent levels following CDA compared to ACDF [21, 22]. One caution is that while CDA preserves segmental motion at the indexed level, there is also a high chance of continuous facet degeneration. Therefore, facet joint arthropathy and spondylosis at the indexed level, as well as at contiguous levels and ASD, can occur even after the most successful CDA surgery.

Currently available data demonstrate that patients with medically intractable myelopathy or radiculopathy, or both, could be managed with CDA. Nevertheless, patients with osteoporosis, kyphotic deformity, diffuse idiopathic skeletal hyperostosis (DISH), and severe facet disease causing ankyloses (i.e., those whose dynamic radiographs demonstrate a range of motion less than 2–3°) are not considered good candidates for CDA. Also, trauma patients who have ligamentous injuries causing preoperative instability are better suited to ACDF rather than CDA. Because the surgery for CDA only aims to replace the diseased disc, there is little chance of correcting any preexisting deformity, to halt further degeneration or to eliminate pain generators in the facets. Therefore, the promising results should only be expected in selected patients. In cervical spines that are too severely degenerated, CDA is not likely to yield results as good as ACDF because CDA only replaces the disc but leaves other pathologies behind.

Preoperative Considerations

All patients in preparation for CDA should have an MRI for evaluation of stenosis of the spinal canal or neuroforamen. Moreover, reformatted CT scans are suggested for the detection of ossification of the posterior longitudinal ligament (OPLL) and calcified discs or osteophytes. For patients with segmental OPLL or a large calcified disc, anterior discectomy may be associated with the unnecessary risk of durotomy and nerve injury and may therefore be avoided. Preoperative CT scans also provide information about facet arthropathy. There is a low chance of preservation of motion if the facets are severely degenerated or fused preoperatively, even after the most successful CDA.

Lateral dynamic radiographs, including both flexion and extension views, are necessary for evaluation of the segmental range of motion and global alignment of the cervical spine. Patients with preexisting kyphotic deformity, ankylosed joints, diffuse idiopathic skeletal hyperostosis (DISH), or immobile segment (less than 2–3° of motion during flexion/extension) should not undergo CDA [2, 20]. Evaluation of bone quality is also important prior to surgery, because the primary stability of CDA depends largely on the carpentry and bone quality at the interface. Osteoporosis could increase the risk of subsidence or dislodgement of the artificial disc. The adverse effects of cigarette smoking found in arthrodesis (i.e., ACDF) remain uncertain in CDA. Other chronic diseases involving the musculoskeletal system, such as rheumatoid arthritis and seronegative spondyloarthropathies, should be considered with caution. The midsagittal diameter of the segment should be measured to assure that the selected implant system has appropriate sizes.

The FDA trials enrolled diseased discs from C3 to C7 [6–9]. However, the most commonly performed levels of CDA are C5-C6, followed by C4-C5 and C6-C7. It is usually technically feasible to perform CDA in C3-C4, though less commonly encountered. There has been a case report of CDA at C7-T1, but this operation could be limited by the access angle in obese patients or patients with a barrel chest. After positioning of the patient, a lateral fluoroscopy of the cervical spine is necessary prior to the CDA surgery for confirmation of visualization of the index level and that it is properly aligned. A right-sided approach for all levels of subaxial cervical spine CDA is recommended for right-handed surgeons. For patients with prior anterior cervical discectomy or thyroid surgery, a preoperative evaluation of the vocal cord is helpful. An approach from the virgin side is suggested if both vocal cords are functioning normally. The same side approach must be taken when there is unilateral vocal cord palsy in order to avoid the risk of permanent tracheostomy after surgery. General anesthesia (with either a nasal or an oral endotracheal tube) and prophylactic antibiotics are usually recommended for all patients. Both intraoperative neuro-monitoring and perioperative steroids are optional.

Surgical Technique

Proper positioning of the patient's neck is essential for optimal placement of a CDA. The patient should be positioned supine with the neck in neutral or slightly lordotic alignment, Fig. 8.1a. The targeted level of disc space should be well visualized on biplanar fluoroscopy and both endplates should be parallel or slightly lordotic. Shoulder retraction is sometimes useful for CDA at the caudal levels of the subaxial cervical spine. Adequate cushioning underneath the neck and head is also required to maintain the orthogonal position [2]. Prior to incision, biplanar fluoroscopy images are obtained to assure proper patient position and that imaging will be adequate.

Initially, a standard anterior cervical discectomy is performed. A transverse skin incision along one of the preexisting skin creases near the indexed level is good for exposure up to 2 levels of disc spaces. Dissection between the carotid sheath and strap muscles via an avascular plane, which is anterior-medial to the sternocleidomastoid muscle, allows entry to the prevertebral retropharyngeal space. The trachea and esophagus are retracted and protected medially by placement

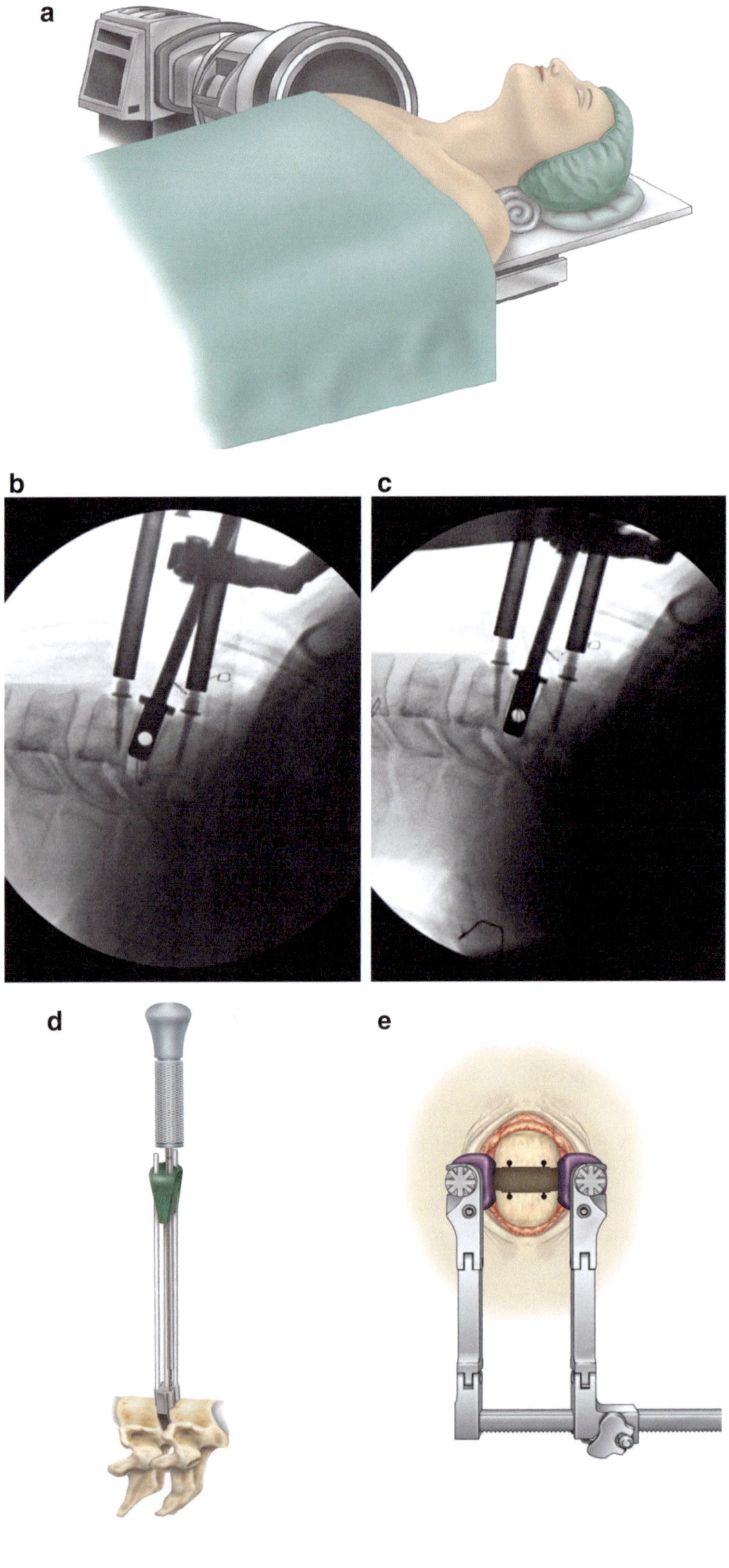

Fig. 8.1 (**a**) The patient is positioned supine with the head in the neutral alignment. It is important to avoid neck extension. A roll is placed behind the neck or shoulders and head stabilized with a doughnut ring. The arms will need to be taped down to allow adequate intraoperative radiographic imaging. A radiolucent table is required that allows biplanar imaging. From Medtronic Sofamor Danek USA, Inc., with permission. After discectomy and foraminal decompression, trials are used to determine implant height and anteroposterior dimensions. (**b**) The *left image* shows a too small implant. (**c**) The *right image* shows maximum footprint and appropriate height. Also the surgeon should place the disc replacement implant in the correct orientation that lies parallel to the endplates. (**d**) When slots for keels are required, the appropriate jig is placed, checked radiographically, and slots created. (**e**) Final anterior view showing complete discectomy and placement of the four rail slots

of the retractor blades underneath the insertion of the collis longus muscles lateral to the anterior vertebral bodies. Caution should be taken during dissection to avoid injury to the superior and recurrent laryngeal nerves which could be associated with postoperative hoarseness and dysphagia. Fluoroscopic confirmation of the indexed level is performed before discectomy. Distraction pins are placed into the vertebral bodies to facilitate anterior cervical discectomy. In the majority of systems, distraction pin placement will control milling operations and final alignment so that care is needed to assure midline placement of the pins. Curettes, Kerrison rongeurs, or high-speed drills are commonly used during decompression. Generous decompression of the spinal canal and bilateral neuroforamen is recommended for each level. We typically remove the posterior longitudinal ligament and both uncovertebral joints to ensure no disc fragments or osteophytes are left. It is essential to balance soft tissue, e.g., if removing the PLL, it needs to be removed symmetrically.

For CDA patients, endplate preparation is more critical than in ACDF because the primary stability of artificial disc devices largely depends on the integration between the interfaces. Caution must be taken not to violate too much the cortical surfaces; otherwise, it could increase the risk of device subsidence or migration. Precise midline placement, appropriate sizing (including both footprint and disc height), and a proper insertion trajectory are extremely important to allow restoration of the physiological range of motion after CDA, Fig. 8.1b. Each of the CDA devices has a specialized fixation mechanism, such as keel, teeth, or dome-shaped designs with screws, requiring meticulous installation, Fig. 8.1c.

The cornerstone of CDA surgery consists of full decompression and good carpentry, Fig. 8.1d. Despite many kinds of artificial discs on the market, which have various biomechanical properties and require different techniques of insertion, they all share a common feature in that thorough decompression including removal of the PLL is absolutely necessary at the index level. Since the devices aim to restore joint function rather than fusion, tailor-made installation of the most-fit artificial disc allows the best chance to maintain mobility for the long term. The accuracy of carpentry in CDA surgery might be related to its long-term outcomes.

Illustrative Case

A 55-year-old male presented with right-sided radiculopathy and mild symptoms of cervical myelopathy that were refractory to medical management for 4 months. MRI demonstrated disc herniations at the C4-C5 and C5-C6 levels. The preoperative CT scan also confirmed the foraminal stenosis at the right C4-C5 and C5-C6 and found no OPLL. The dynamic lateral radiographs demonstrated a normal range of motion of both disc levels prior to the surgery.

The patient underwent a two-level CDA. The symptoms were completely relieved after surgery, and the postoperative radiographs demonstrated good mobility at both levels (Fig. 8.2a, b). The patient has been free of secondary surgery or other cervical spine issues at 2.5 years of follow-up.

Technical Pearls

- Complete decompression of the spinal canal and neuroforamen is crucial.
- Avoid CDA in patients with incompetent facet joints or osteoporosis.
- Resection of bilateral uncovertebral joints and posterior longitudinal ligament in every patient.
- Appropriate sizing and centering of the device is critical.
- Attempts to change the cervical alignment by CDA are rarely effective.

Decompression

The key component of a successful CDA or ACDF remains complete decompression. The importance of decompression cannot be overemphasized in CDA surgery. In conventional ACDF

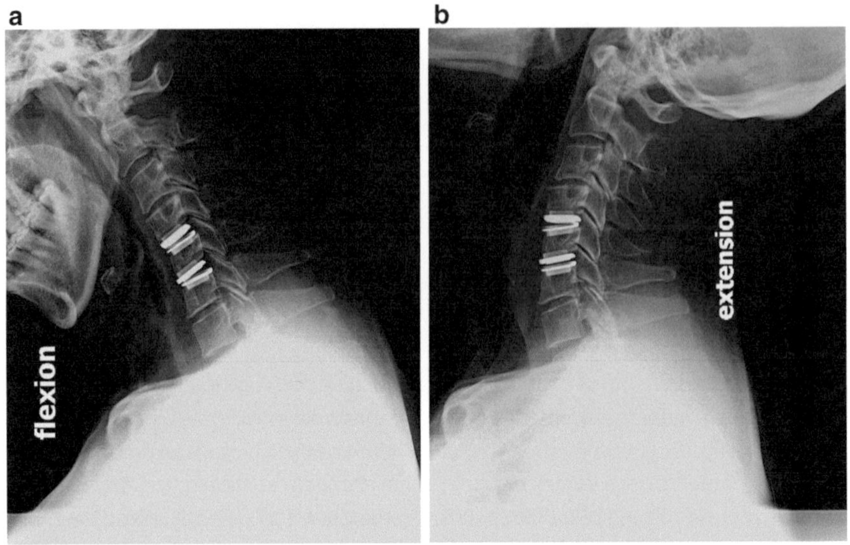

Fig. 8.2 (**a**) Flexion radiographs after C4-C5 and C5-C6 total disc replacement. (**b**) Extension radiographs after C4-C5 and C5-C6 total disc replacement. Excellent motion at both levels is present

surgery, by insertion of a large enough bone graft into the disc space, the effect of indirect decompression automatically increases foraminal height, and radicular symptoms are easily ameliorated. Further remodeling of osteophytes may occur with successful fusion. However, in CDA surgery, complete decompression and resection of uncovertebral joints is essential because there is little advantage to indirect decompression or bony remodeling gained by tall interbody grafts. On the contrary, during extreme neck range of motion (e.g., flexion/extension, axial rotation, and lateral bending), the nerve root might be impinged by osteophytes or residual disc material surrounding the neuroforamen. Therefore, we suggest complete resection of the bilateral uncovertebral joints, including the asymptomatic side. Resection of the posterior longitudinal ligament also assists in visual confirmation of a thoroughly decompressed spinal canal. Copious venous bleeding might be encountered upon decompression of the neuroforamen, and it also indicates proximity to the vertebral artery and nerve root. Excessive epidural venous hemorrhage could be troublesome, but generally it can be controlled by temporary packing with hemostatic agents.

Placement

Proper positioning of the CDA is extremely important for preservation of motion and satisfactory long-term results [23–25]. Only an accurately positioned, suitably sized artificial disc can achieve proper joint kinematics. In lumbar disc replacements as little 3 mm, malposition leads to poor clinical outcomes.

Sagittal Alignment

Each level of CDA also requires a thorough consideration of the indexed and the neighboring segments, since CDA has very little effect on correction of kyphosis. Various choices of implant sizes (including the footprint and height of the artificial discs) should be considered. Excess kyphosis or hyperlordosis may lead to edge impingement and higher rates of wear.

Complications and Strategies for Avoidance

Some retrospective series reported that a substantial portion of patients would develop heterotopic ossification (HO) after CDA [26, 27]. Although the HO did not affect clinical outcomes in 3–4 years of follow-up, the unwanted bone formation might be problematic in the long term. The incidence of HO also varied with the method of detection (by plain radiographs or CT) among studies and different ethnicities. The risk factors for HO might include preexisting degeneration, elderly male patients, Asian ancestry, multilevel DDD, surgical techniques, or design of arthroplasty devices [4, 10, 19, 23–25, 27, 28]. In some trials, attempts to reduce HO by administration of nonsteroidal anti-inflammatory medication were recommended. In our opinion, HO could be regarded as the accelerated consequence of continuous degeneration after CDA and has had few adverse effects on the clinical outcomes according to published studies so far. Given that CDA is unlikely to halt further cervical spine degeneration, the heterogeneity among these CDA patients could cause different outcomes that might require long-term follow-up to demonstrate.

Perioperative management for avoidance of complications in CDA and ACDF surgery is very similar. Both operations use the same anterior cervical approach, so the approach-related complications, such as dysphagia, hoarseness, and swallowing difficulty, are theoretically similar for CDA and ACDF. The potential advantages of CDA over ACDF are less hardware (e.g., no titanium plates and screws are required for most CDA) and thus perhaps a lower chance of dysphagia after surgery [29].

Hardware Failure

The ACDF naturally has the risk of pseudoarthrosis and implant failure (e.g., broken screws). The problems with CDA are dislodgement of the artificial disc and the issue of wear. One distinct difference between CDA and ACDF is the issue of durability. The ACDF has less chance of long-term problems once successful bone fusion is achieved since motion is sacrificed.

Adjacent Segment Degeneration

The most concerning long-term issue regarding ACDF is that of accelerated degeneration of the neighboring disc. CDA was designed to reduce the risk of ASD by preservation of motion at the treated level [3]. Recent reports suggest a reduction of the incidence of ASD by CDA, and all reports have unanimously confirmed the effectiveness of CDA in the preservation of mobility at the index disc level [7]. For patients with multiple-level cervical DDD, preservation of two levels of physiological motion by CDA is theoretically beneficial and definitely noticeable. In order to achieve the goal of preservation of the range of motion, the device in CDA must be properly installed according to its biomechanical design. Therefore, appropriate selection of the size and accurate execution of placement of the device into the optimal position during CDA surgery is crucial. Studies have demonstrated that a large-enough footprint to cover the entire disc area and a tight-enough device height to support but not to over-distract the neutral disc height could lead to less HO formation [23, 24]. Although the most optimal carpentry of these CDA devices varies among each design and is debatable, the aim of CDA remains to restore physiological motion of the disc and maintain cervical spinal alignment.

Keys to Success

The key to success of CDA is appropriate patient selection and accurate execution of surgical techniques [28, 30, 31]. Although it is not possible to reverse the process of aging by CDA, we should always try to halt or slow down the ongoing degeneration in the subaxial cervical spine. Advances in technology would further increase the accuracy of installation and the tailor-made fitness of CDA devices according to each individual's pathology. Of course, CDA cannot treat every patient with cervical DDD or spondylosis, but CDA is indeed superior in motion preservation to ACDF and is a safe and effective option. Long-term follow-up is necessary to determine the true efficacy and efficiency of CDA surgery.

Conclusion

The most commonly accepted indications of CDA include cervical disc herniation and spondylosis that involved one or two levels of subaxial cervical spine. The neurological improvement after CDA is at least non-inferior to the gold standard ACDF surgery. The safety and effectiveness of CDA have been demonstrated by many reports. As the techniques, materials, and designs of these CDA devices continue to improve, the utilization of CDA is likely to be more prevalent in the future.

References

1. Wu JC, Hsieh PC, Mummaneni PV, Wang MY. Spinal motion preservation surgery. Biomed Res Int. 2015;2015:372502.
2. Wu JC, Meyer SA, Gandhoke G, Mummaneni PV. PRESTIGE cervical arthroplasty: past, present, and future. Seminars Spine Surg. 2012;24(1):14–9.
3. Wu JC, Liu L, Wen-Cheng H, Chen YC, Ko CC, Wu CL, et al. The incidence of adjacent segment disease requiring surgery after anterior cervical diskectomy and fusion: estimation using an 11-year comprehensive nationwide database in Taiwan. Neurosurgery. 2012;70(3):594–601.
4. Wu JC, Huang WC, Tu TH, Tsai HW, Ko CC, Wu CL, et al. Differences between soft-disc herniation and spondylosis in cervical arthroplasty: CT-documented heterotopic ossification with minimum 2 years of follow-up. J Neurosurg Spine. 2012;16(2):163–71.
5. Mummaneni PV, Amin BY, Wu JC, Brodt ED, Dettori JR, Sasso RC. Cervical artificial disc replacement versus fusion in the cervical spine: a systematic review comparing long-term follow-up results from two FDA trials. Evid Based Spine-Care J. 2012;3(S1):59–66.
6. Radcliff K, Coric D, Albert T. Five-year clinical results of cervical total disc replacement compared with anterior discectomy and fusion for treatment of 2-level symptomatic degenerative disc disease: a prospective, randomized, controlled, multicenter investigational device exemption clinical trial. J Neurosurg Spine. 2016;25:1–12.
7. Gornet MF, Burkus JK, Shaffrey ME, Argires PJ, Nian H, Harrell FE Jr. Cervical disc arthroplasty with PRESTIGE LP disc versus anterior cervical discectomy and fusion: a prospective, multicenter investigational device exemption study. J Neurosurg Spine. 2015;23:1–16.
8. Burkus JK, Traynelis VC, Haid RW Jr, Mummaneni PV. Clinical and radiographic analysis of an artificial cervical disc: 7-year follow-up from the Prestige prospective randomized controlled clinical trial: clinical article. J Neurosurg Spine. 2014;21(4):516–28.
9. Davis RJ, Kim KD, Hisey MS, Hoffman GA, Bae HW, Gaede SE, et al. Cervical total disc replacement with the Mobi-C cervical artificial disc compared with anterior discectomy and fusion for treatment of 2-level symptomatic degenerative disc disease: a prospective, randomized, controlled multicenter clinical trial: clinical article. J Neurosurg Spine. 2013;19(5):532–45.
10. Upadhyaya CD, Wu JC, Trost G, Haid RW, Traynelis VC, Tay B, et al. Analysis of the three United States Food and Drug Administration investigational device exemption cervical arthroplasty trials. J Neurosurg Spine. 2012;16(3):216–28.
11. Quan GM, Vital JM, Hansen S, Pointillart V. Eight-year clinical and radiological follow-up of the Bryan cervical disc arthroplasty. Spine. 2011;36(8):639–46.
12. Burkus JK, Haid RW, Traynelis VC, Mummaneni PV. Long-term clinical and radiographic outcomes of cervical disc replacement with the Prestige disc: results from a prospective randomized controlled clinical trial. J Neurosurg Spine. 2010;13(3):308–18.
13. Coric D, Kim PK, Clemente JD, Boltes MO, Nussbaum M, James S. Prospective randomized study of cervical arthroplasty and anterior cervical discectomy and fusion with long-term follow-up: results in 74 patients from a single site. J Neurosurg Spine. 2013;18(1):36–42.
14. Murrey D, Janssen M, Delamarter R, Goldstein J, Zigler J, Tay B, et al. Results of the prospective, randomized, controlled multicenter Food and Drug Administration investigational device exemption study of the ProDisc-C total disc replacement versus anterior discectomy and fusion for the treatment of 1-level symptomatic cervical disc disease. Spine J. 2009;9(4):275–86.
15. Heller JG, Sasso RC, Papadopoulos SM, Anderson PA, Fessler RG, Hacker RJ, et al. Comparison of BRYAN cervical disc arthroplasty with anterior cervical decompression and fusion: clinical and radiographic results of a randomized, controlled, clinical trial. Spine. 2009;34(2):101–7.
16. Mummaneni PV, Burkus JK, Haid RW, Traynelis VC, Zdeblick TA. Clinical and radiographic analysis of cervical disc arthroplasty compared with allograft fusion: a randomized controlled clinical trial. J Neurosurg Spine. 2007;6(3):198–209.
17. Hilibrand AS, Carlson GD, Palumbo MA, Jones PK, Bohlman HH. Radiculopathy and myelopathy at segments adjacent to the site of a previous

anterior cervical arthrodesis. J Bone Joint Surg Am. 1999;81(4):519–28.
18. Wu JC. Cervical total disc replacement. Formosan J Surg. 2014;47(2):49–52.
19. Wu JC, Huang WC, Tsai HW, Ko CC, Fay LY, Tu TH, et al. Differences between 1- and 2-level cervical arthroplasty: more heterotopic ossification in 2-level disc replacement: clinical article. J Neurosurg Spine. 2012;16(6):594–600.
20. Fay LY, Huang WC, Tsai TY, Wu JC, Ko CC, Tu TH, et al. Differences between arthroplasty and anterior cervical fusion in two-level cervical degenerative disc disease. Eur Spine J (Official Publication of the European Spine Society, the European Spinal Deformity Society, and the European Section of the Cervical Spine Research Society). 2014;23(3):627–34.
21. Luo J, Gong M, Huang S, Yu T, Zou X. Incidence of adjacent segment degeneration in cervical disc arthroplasty versus anterior cervical decompression and fusion meta-analysis of prospective studies. Arch Orthop Trauma Surg. 2015;135(2):155–60.
22. Zhong ZM, Zhu SY, Zhuang JS, Wu Q, Chen JT. Reoperation after cervical disc arthroplasty versus anterior cervical discectomy and fusion: a meta-analysis. Clin Orthop Relat Res. 2016;474(5):1307–16.
23. Tu TH, Wu JC, Huang WC, Wu CL, Ko CC, Cheng H. The effects of carpentry on heterotopic ossification and mobility in cervical arthroplasty: determination by computed tomography with a minimum 2-year follow-up: clinical article. J Neurosurg Spine. 2012;16(6):601–9.
24. Tu TH, Wu JC, Huang WC, Chang HK, Ko CC, Fay LY, et al. Postoperative nonsteroidal antiinflammatory drugs and the prevention of heterotopic ossification after cervical arthroplasty: analysis using CT and a minimum 2-year follow-up. J Neurosurg Spine. 2015;22(5):447–53.
25. Chang PY, Chang HK, Wu JC, Huang WC, Fay LY, Tu TH, et al. Differences between C3-4 and other subaxial levels of cervical disc arthroplasty: more heterotopic ossification at the 5-year follow-up. J Neurosurg Spine. 2016;24(5):752–9.
26. Tu TH, Wu JC, Huang WC, Guo WY, Wu CL, Shih YH, et al. Heterotopic ossification after cervical total disc replacement: determination by CT and effects on clinical outcomes. J Neurosurg Spine. 2011;14(4):457–65.
27. Wu JC, Huang WC, Tsai TY, Fay LY, Ko CC, Tu TH, et al. Multilevel arthroplasty for cervical spondylosis: more heterotopic ossification at 3 years of follow-up. Spine. 2012;37(20):E1251–9.
28. Fay LY, Huang WC, Wu JC, Chang HK, Tsai TY, Ko CC, et al. Arthroplasty for cervical spondylotic myelopathy: similar results to patients with only radiculopathy at 3 years' follow-up. J Neurosurg Spine. 2014;21(3):400–10.
29. McAfee PC, Cappuccino A, Cunningham BW, Devine JG, Phillips FM, Regan JJ, et al. Lower incidence of dysphagia with cervical arthroplasty compared with ACDF in a prospective randomized clinical trial. J Spinal Disord Tech. 2010;23(1):1–8.
30. Chang HK, Huang WC, Wu JC, Tu TH, Fay LY, Chang PY, et al. Cervical arthroplasty for traumatic disc herniation: an age- and sex-matched comparison with anterior cervical discectomy and fusion. BMC Musculoskelet Disord. 2015;16:228.
31. Chang HK, Huang WC, Wu JC, Chang PY, Tu TH, Fay LY, et al. Should cervical disc arthroplasty be done on patients with increased intramedullary signal intensity on magnetic resonance imaging? World Neurosurg. 2016;89:489–96.

9 Subaxial Posterior Cervical Fusion with Instrumentation

Paul A. Anderson

Introduction

Posterior cervical fusion is a highly successful procedure aimed to achieve arthrodesis and maintain alignment. Modern techniques with lateral mass screws and/or pedicle screw fixation achieve high rates of success with low complication rates. The procedures can be used for a wide range of indications, and lateral mass fixation procedures are relatively easy to master, although pedicle screw fixation is more difficult. In addition, subaxial posterior cervical fixation is extensile and often extended to include atlantoaxial, occiput, and across the cervicothoracic junction.

Fixation may be achieved using various anatomic structures of the posterior elements including the spinous processes, lateral masses, and pedicles. Traditionally, fixation was described using simple wire loops around the spinous processes. Roy-Camille and Magerl developed lateral mass screw-plate techniques that offered more stable fixation, high fusion success, and less postoperative bracing [1]. Variable-angle lateral mass screws and rod fixation are now standard and offer ease of placement over plate methods but are more costly. Pedicle cervical screw fixation has been championed in Asia and improves fixation over lateral mass constructs but increases the risk of injury to the vertebral arteries and neural elements. Regardless of the type of surgery, meticulous techniques are required as fixation is placed in small bony structures in close proximity to neurovascular structures.

This chapter will outline the indications and technique for subaxial posterior cervical fixation. The outcomes and complications will be reviewed and tips to gain excellent results while avoiding complications will be discussed.

Indications

Posterior cervical fusion with instrumentation is as versatile procedure that can be used to treat a variety of conditions, Table 9.1. It has an advantage as being extensile, that is, easily extended cranial and caudally.

Indications for Posterior Surgery in Trauma

Subaxial fixation is commonly used for treatment of unstable spines as a result of trauma. Instability has been defined as the loss of the ability of the spinal column to protect the neural elements from injury, maintain alignment, development of long-term pain, or loss of function. Applying this

P.A. Anderson, MD (✉)
University of Wisconsin, Department of Orthopedic Surgery and Rehabilitation, Madison, WI, USA
e-mail: anderson@ortho.wisc.edu

L.T. Holly, P.A. Anderson (eds.), *Essentials of Spinal Stabilization*,
DOI 10.1007/978-3-319-59713-3_9

Table 9.1 Indication for posterior subaxial cervical fusion

1	Traumatic instability
2	Destructive lesions from tumor, infection, inflammatory disease
3	Degenerative instability
4	Pseudoarthrosis
5	Adjunct to anterior fusion
6	Extension to craniocervical and/ or cervicothoracic junction

definition has proved difficult and therefore numerous classification systems have been developed. More recently quantitative systems grade severity and can aid in surgical decision-making. These include the Subaxial Cervical Spine Injury Classification System (SLIC) and the Cervical Spine Injury Severity Score (CSISS) [2, 3]. In addition an updated AO classification system has been proposed based on injury morphology, facet injury, neurologic status, and case-specific modifiers [4].

A posterior approach can be used for most unstable injury patterns of the subaxial cervical spine. The choice of anterior versus posterior is dependent upon many variables such as comminution, requirement for additional decompression, the goal of minimizing the number of levels fused, bone quality, and reduction. A cohort study by Brodke showed no difference between anterior and posterior fusion for three column injuries when reduction has been achieved prior to surgery [5]. Fracture types where the posterior approach is preferred are fractures in ankylosed spines, fracture dislocations with associated vertebral body fractures, injuries at the cervicothoracic junction, and when reduction of dislocation is required.

Additional Indications for Subaxial Posterior Fusion

The posterior approach is useful as an adjunct to multilevel anterior fusion for degenerative conditions, degenerative spondylolisthesis, subaxial instability associated with inflammatory conditions, and stabilization of destructive processes such as tumors and infections and, when needed, to extend fusions from the craniocervical or cervicothoracic regions. Posterior fusion is more reliable to gain fusion for anterior pseudoarthrosis, although it is not associated with better clinical outcomes than repeat anterior fusion [6].

Preoperative Considerations

Surgical Anatomy

Posterior cervical fixation is obtained by attachments to the spinous processes, lateral masses, and pedicles. The spinous processes are midline posterior projections extending from the lamina and serve as attachments of the nuchal ligaments and multifidus muscles. They are largest in size at C2, C7, and T1 where the nuchal ligaments are firmly attached. The spinous processes from C3–C5 are bifid and may be relatively small which limits fixation opportunities. The C6 spinous process may be larger and may or may not be bifid. The base of the spinous process can be perforated and a hole can be created to allow the passage of wire or cable. At C7, the lamina can be wide enough (mean 5.6 mm) to accept translaminar screws [7].

Lateral Mass Anatomy

The lateral masses form an articular column lateral to the spinal canal. Viewed posteriorly, the lateral masses are square-shaped with the superior and inferior borders being the cranial and caudal facet joints, Fig. 9.1a. The medial border is the valley at the junction of the lamina and the lateral mass and the lateral border is the far edge of the lateral mass. From the side, the lateral masses are parallelogram-shaped with upward and downward projects known as superior and inferior facet articulations. Anterior to the lower half of lateral mass is the exiting nerve root and further anterior is the vertebral artery above C6.

Pedicle Anatomy

The pedicles are small, truncated, cone-like structures that connect the bodies to the lateral masses. The pedicles have a mean transverse diameter of

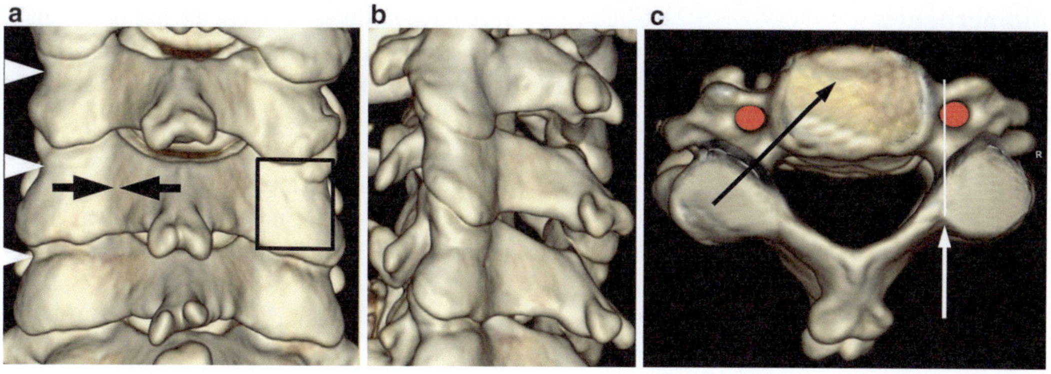

Fig. 9.1 (**a**) Dorsal view of the cervical spine. The lateral notch (*white arrowhead*) is at the sulcus of the pars interarticularis just below the cranial facet joint. The boundaries of the lateral mass (*box*) are the inferior and superior facet joints, the lateral edge of the lateral mass, and the valley at the junction of the lamina and lateral mass. The junction of the lamina and lateral mass is the valley or inflection point (*black arrow* on *left side*). (**b**) On the lateral projection, the lateral mass is parallelogram-shaped bounded by the superior facet cranially and inferior facet caudally. (**c**) Axial view of C5. The junction of the lateral mass and lamina is seen as a valley (*white arrow*). Projected anterior and slightly lateral (*line*) is the vertebral artery (*red circle*). The pedicle is oriented 35–45° medially (*black arrow*)

approximately 5.5–6.5 mm with range 4–8 mm [8]. They are taller in the sagittal plane by 2–3 mm. They are medial deviated when viewed posteriorly from 43° at C3 decreasing caudally to 36° at C7, Fig. 9.1c. In the sagittal plane, the pedicles have upward angulation of about 7° at C2–C3, neutral at C4–C5, and a mean downward angulation of 3–6° at C6 and C7, respectively [9]. The pedicles attach to the vertebral body near the superior end plate anteriorly and at or just below the base of the superior facet joint posteriorly. When viewed posteriorly, a lateral notch can be identified which is a sulcus along the far edge of lateral just below the superior articular facet, Fig. 9.1a. The dorsal projection of the C3–C6 pedicle (which is an essential landmark to identify pedicle screw placement) is located 2 mm medial to the lateral notch [9]. At C7, the pedicle is located 4 mm medial from the lateral notch. There is a wide variation of individual morphology, and each patient's imaging studies should be carefully examined before screw placement is attempted.

Vertebral Artery

The first part of the vertebral artery ascends from its origin off the subclavian artery and passes anterior to the C7 transverse process between the longus colli and anterior scalene muscles. In the second part, the vertebral artery enters the spine between the C6 and C7 transverse processes and ascends upward to C2 in the foramen transversarium. The vertebral artery can be injured by lateral breaches from cervical pedicle screws and insufficient outward angulation or from a too medial starting point of a lateral mass screw.

Nerve Root

The exiting nerve roots lie above each corresponding pedicle in front of the lateral masses. They can be injured by inferiorly placed (insufficient cephalad angle) or too long lateral mass screws or cervical pedicle screws.

Bony Anomalies

Bony anomalies from congenital malformations are frequently accompanied by vascular anomalies. In these cases, a CT angiogram is recommended before screw placement. Similarly, fracture dislocations and fractures involving the foramen transversarium are associated with vertebral artery injury and a CT angiogram is recommended. If there is an arterial injury, then the fixation method with the lowest risk to the functioning artery should be selected.

Biomechanics

Biomechanical studies confirm that cervical pedicle screw fixation offers the greatest flexural, lateral bending, and axial stiffness [10]. However, in most cases lateral mass screws appear to have a sufficient stabilization effect; therefore, the author questions the use of cervical pedicle screws between C3 and C6 except in exceptional cases as the risk of vertebral artery injury is too great. Interspinous wire fixation has a long legacy, is relatively low cost, and requires significant postoperative immobilization to be effective but is the safest form of fixation.

An important biomechanical principle is to match the fixation to the requirements of an individual patient. For example, a stable nonunion of an anterior fusion may be successfully treated by an interspinous wire method. Similarly, a highly unstable fracture with comminution of the bodies and lateral masses or a tumor with similar morphology may best be treated with cervical pedicle screw fixation.

Bone quality is paramount to successful fixation. Many patients, such as those with rheumatoid arthritis, may have osteoporosis or erosions from facet arthritis that limit fixation strength especially when using spinous process wires or lateral mass plates. To gain fixation in such cases, pedicle screws could be considered.

Surgical Technique

Anesthesia and Positioning

Patients requiring posterior fusion frequently have unstable spines and/or spinal cord compression, therefore requiring special consideration during induction and intubation. If cord compression is present, then the mean arterial pressure is maintained at a minimum of 80 mm Hg during the procedure which may require vasopressors. Intubation is performed with a fiberoptic technique that allows the least cervical displacement. Placing a patient prone with an unstable subaxial cervical spine has risks and care must be exercised. If traction has been applied, the use of a turning frame which rotates around the long axis of the operating table can be used while traction is maintained. Other considerations are use of a four-poster frame with the head controlled in a Mayfield device. This is especially useful in patients with significant kyphosis such as ankylosing spondylitis. In unstable conditions, intraoperative radiographs or fluoroscopy should be readily available to check alignment. Patients with more stable conditions can be positioned prone on a Jackson-type table with the head stabilized with a special foam pillow. The arms and sometimes skin are pulled downward to reduce skin folds and allow access for radiographic imaging. Appropriate preoperative antibiotics are given before skin incision.

Exposure

The skin is incised and the nuchal fascia exposed. An incision is made along each spinous process and the multifidus muscle stripped off subperiosteally. The supraspinous and interspinous ligaments are maintained to avoid adjacent segment kyphosis. Dissection is carried out to the far edges of the lateral masses. Radiographic confirmation of the level is performed.

Reduction

If required, facet reduction is performed by manual manipulation of spinous processes or by resection of a portion of the superior facet and use of a small elevator placed into the dislocated facet that acts as a lever to achieve reduction. If kyphosis is present, reduction is easiest by using an interspinous wire or cable. When fixation crosses the cervicothoracic junction, achieving closure between spinous process from C6–7 and C7–T1 can improve sagittal plane alignment. If possible, prior to placement of rods, an interspinous cable is tensioned between C6–7 and or C7–T1 until the spinous processes are compressed, assuming the foramen is not stenotic.

Fixation

The surgeon has several choices available to achieve fixation including monofilament wires, braided wires, cables, screws and plates, and variable angle screws and rods. Selection is dependent on the severity of the condition being treated and bone quality. The author prefers lateral mass fixation from C3–6 and pedicle screws in C2 and C7.

Rod diameter is important since bending stiffness is proportional to the radius^4. Titanium and cobalt-chrome rods have a modulus of elasticity of 110 Gpa and 220 Gpa, respectively, indicating that titanium rods are half as stiff as cobalt-chrome rods. Simply increasing the diameter to 4 mm from 3.5 mm and using cobalt-chrome rods increase stiffness by 3.1 times. However, mixing cobalt-chrome rods with titanium alloy screws may create a potential for galvanic corrosion due to dissimilar metals. However, in vivo both metals produce an oxide layer (self-passivating) that diminishes any battery effect. In the presence of motion, such as between a titanium wire and cobalt-chrome rod, the passivation layers wear off and galvanic corrosion can occur.

Interspinous Wire Fixation

Interspinous wire fixation was described by Hadra in 1890 using silver wire for a fracture dislocation which required a revision but ultimately was a success. Rogers popularized the interspinous wire techniques using stainless steel wire and reported success in 30 of 35 patients with cervical fractures [11]. Bohlman modified the Rogers technique by adding an additional two wires to hold bone grafts along the spinous processes [12]. Since cables composed of stainless steel and titanium became available, they have largely replaced wire fixation. Cables can be tensioned under control and conform to bony contours and have lower risk of fracture. Cables require a crimping mechanism and do not allow adjustment once crimping has been performed. Although polymers have been developed as potential substitutes, they all suffer from creep and potential for loosening over time. Another alternative is to use sublaminar wire fixation which captures the lamina and rods. This provides poor fixation having no resistance to axial loads, is invasive to the spinal canal, and, in the author's opinion, should be avoided.

To place an interspinous cable, a 3-mm hole is placed with a burr on each side of the middle point of the cranial spinous process at its base, Fig. 9.2a. The hole is enlarged with a towel clip or Leween clamp. The cable has a stiff leader and the opposite end has a crimp. The leader is shortened and bent in a curve and is passed through the hole to the opposite side. It is then passed over the spinous process through the interspinous ligament. The leader is then passed back through the hole thus creating a loop around the cranial spinous process. The leader is then passed below the caudal spinous processes and then through the crimp, Fig. 9.2b. The excess length is shortened and the leader passed into the tensioning device. Under careful observation, tension is applied to the cable, usually no more than 30 pounds. The crimp is crushed and excess wire sectioned.

Lateral Mass Fixation

Viewed posteriorly, the square-shaped lateral masses are identified. The superior and inferior borders are the cranial and caudal facet joints, respectively, Fig. 9.1a. The lateral border is the outside edge. The medial border is the valley or inflection point at the junction of the lateral mass and lamina. Deep and anterior to this valley is the vertebral artery, Fig. 9.1c. Thus all lateral mass screws need to start lateral to this point and angle outward. The center of the lateral mass is the summit, its highest point, Figure 9.2a.

The starting point for screw insertion is 1–2 mm medial to the center of the lateral mass, Fig. 9.2a. A starting hole of each lateral mass to be instrumented is placed with a 3-mm burr. These should be oriented in a relatively straight line.

The screw orientation is upward and outward, usually easily identified by laying the drill guide against the next caudal spinous process, Fig. 9.3a. The upward direction is about 20–45° so that it is parallel to the facet joint surfaces,

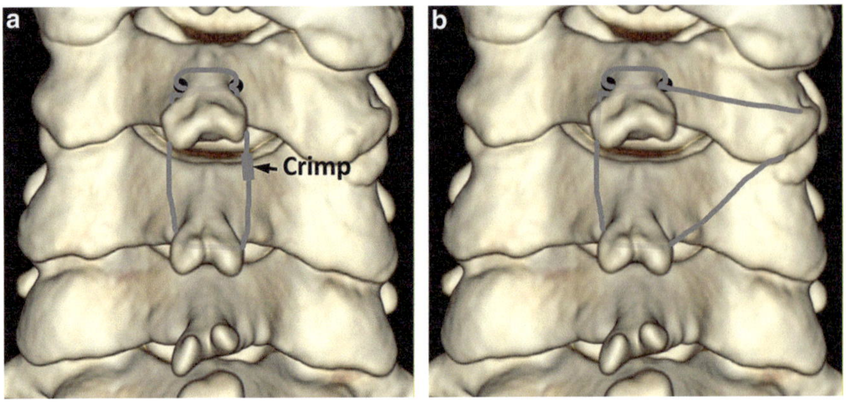

Fig. 9.2 (**a**) Interspinous wire technique with cable. 3-mm holes are placed (*black hole*) in the base of the spinous process. A cable is passed from one side to the other and looped around cranial aspect of spinous process and back through the hole. It then passes under the next caudal spinous process. (**b**) The cable is passed through a crimp and tensioned and then the crimp is compressed

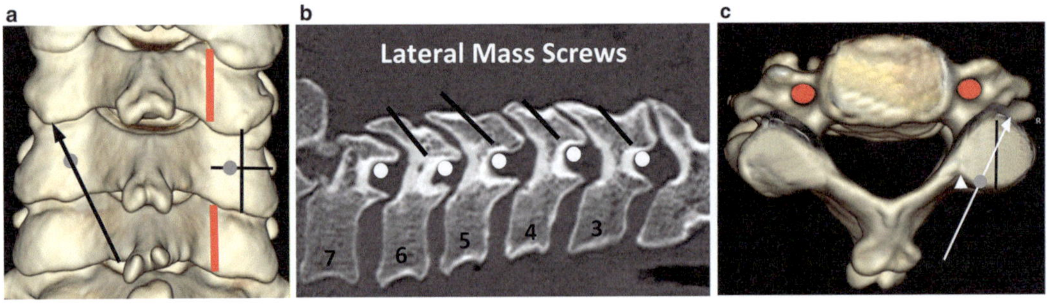

Fig. 9.3 (**a**) The center of the lateral mass is identified on the right lateral mass at the summit (*cross*) of the lateral mass. The starting point is marked with a burr 2 mm medial to the lateral mass center (*circle*). The vertebral artery (*red line*) is located anterior to the medial border of the lateral mass. The screw orientation is upward 30–40° and outward 15–20° on the left lateral mass (*arrow*) away from the vertebral artery. Usually the drill guide will lie against the next caudal spinous process. (**b**) Sagittal view showing the screw orientation (*line*) parallel to the facet articulations. (**c**) Axial view showing orientation of the lateral mass screw outward (*arrow*) angulation away from vertebral artery and starting 2 mm medial from the lateral mass center

Fig. 9.3b. The outward angulation is 15–20° and is limited by abutment of the spinous process, Fig. 9.3c. To place the pilot hole, an adjustable drill is used to avoid inadvertent plunging. The author uses a k-wire as a drill as it is less likely to wrap around a nerve or vessel. Starting at 12–14 mm, a hole is drilled and then checked for perforation. The drill is reset 2 mm and the process repeated until desired length or perforation of the far cortex ensues. Unicortical screws are satisfactory in most cases, but for patients with poorer bone stock or higher degrees of instability, bicortical screws can be placed safely and are more effective.

Lateral mass systems use variable head tulip-like screws and 3.5–4-mm rods. The appropriate length screw is placed maintaining proper orientation. Once the screws are placed, the posterior one-third of the facet joints are decorticated with a burr and packed with local bone or bone graft substitute. Rods of appropriate length are chosen which may require sectioning. Excess rod length should be avoided as it may cause irritation in muscles or impinge on adjacent non-fused bony structures. Lordosis or kyphosis is created with rod contouring as needed. The rods are inserted in the tulips and set screws inserted and tightened to their desired torque. If needed, compression along the rod can be performed but this risks screw loosening. A final lateral radiograph is obtained.

Pedicle Screw

Cervical pedicle screws, except at C7 (in 95% of cases), are at risk for injury to the vertebral artery, and, therefore, complete understanding of the surgical anatomy and identification of landmarks are required. The key landmark is the lateral notch of the lateral mass, Fig. 9.1a. The lateral notch is the most medial part of the pars interarticularis located at a sulcus on the far edge of the lateral mass just below the superior articular facet [9, 13].

For C3–C6 the starting point is 2 mm medial from the lateral notch, Fig. 9.4a. At this point, a 3-mm starting hole is placed with a burr. The pilot hole is orientated medially, the degree being determined from imaging and can range from 25° to 55°. The angulation is greater at C3 than more caudal, Fig. 9.4b [9]. The starting point is more lateral when the medial angle is greater. The sagittal angle is neutral from C3–C6 and upward 7° at C7. The pilot hole can be created using an awl or by a stopped drill technique, checking for perforation as one goes deeper. Usually a 22–25-mm length hole may be placed. CT, navigation, and fluoroscopic aid have all been shown to improve accuracy [14, 15].

Prior to screw placement, the facets are decorticated and bone graft material placed into the joints. The screws are placed, radiographs are obtained to confirm correct positioning, and rods of appropriate length are placed. The set screws are tightened to desired torque.

C7 Fixation

Fixation of C7, like C2, can be safely achieved by several means including interspinous wire and pedicle, lateral mass, or translaminar screws. In general, the author does not recommend stopping fixation of multilevel constructs at C7 and would include fixation to at least T1 with pedicle screws. Combining C7 and T1 pedicle screws provides maximum biomechanical strength with low risk of injury to the vertebral artery. Longer constructs into the thoracic spine are often treated using transition rods which taper from 3.5 mm for cervical fixation to 5.5 mm in the thoracic spine. This taper precludes fixation at one level, which is usually C7 in the author's experience. Cervical fixation can also be combined with more rostral fixation at C2 and even to the occiput. Keeping the points of fixation in a line aids rod placement.

Fixation into C7 can be achieved as described above by translaminar screws as well. Translaminar C7 fixation is achieved by crossing screws and is applicable to C2 and C7 [7]. Computed tomography or MRI should be scrutinized to assess the feasibility of these techniques and will require a minimum of 4-mm inner diameter. The screw length is also judged and is approximately 25 mm.

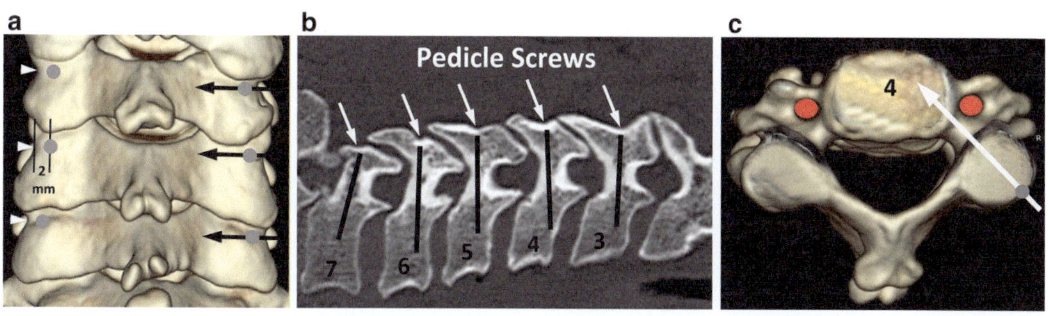

Fig. 9.4 (**a**) The lateral notch is located at the sulcus of the pars interarticularis (*arrowhead*). The starting point for pedicle screw insertion (*circle*) for C3–C6 is 2 mm medial to the lateral notch and is just below the superior facet joint. The orientation is medial 25–45° (*black arrow*). (**b**) The screw is oriented parallel to the superior end plate and is angulated slightly downward more caudally. (**c**) Axial view showing 40° medial angulation required for pedicle screw insertion to avoid the vertebral artery (*red circle*).

A 3-mm burr hole is placed at the base of the spinous process in line with the projection of the opposite lamina. To avoid impingement of opposite screws, the starting point on one side is placed lower and the contralateral slightly higher. Using a pedicle finder or stopped drill technique, the hole is cannulated toward the opposite lamina for approximately 25 mm. During placement the hole is checked for perforation. The screw is inserted and the opposite side is cannulated with the screw placed in similar manner. After screw placement, the appropriate facet joints are decorticated and packed with bone graft material. The lamina and spinous processes should not be decorticated to avoid loss of fixation. Rods are placed and all set screws fully tightened. A final lateral radiograph is obtained to confirm satisfactory screw position.

Extending to Thoracic Spine

Extending the fusion from the cervical to thoracic spine is becoming more common as there is increasing desire to correct sagittal plane deformities which cause cervical kyphosis, dropped head syndrome, and chin-on-chest deformity. The cervical fixation can be placed as described above using lateral mass plates or, if needed, cervical pedicle screws. Thoracic fixation is obtained using pedicle screws. A stiffer rod is required, and transition rods are often utilized, where a 5.5-mm rod tapers to a 3.5-mm rod or is connected by a joint. These transitions take up space and preclude one level from being instrumented, usually C7. The rods require contouring, usually cervical lordosis and thoracic kyphosis. At the cervicothoracic junction, interspinous wires are placed at C7, and T1 if possible, and tensioned to achieve as much lordosis as possible.

Bone Grafting

The ultimate goal of posterior fixation is to obtain arthrodesis. Regardless of the technique, posterior fusion is obtained by decortication and bone grafting. Partially decorticating the facet joints with a burr provides an excellent area for bone union. Decortication can also be performed along the laminae and spinous processes depending upon fixation. Many bone graft materials can be used including autograph, allograft, demineralized bone matrix, and ceramic products. BMP-2 has been used in posterior fusion but is rarely needed as there is a high fusion success in the posterior cervical spine.

Wound Closure

Reattachment of the nuchal ligaments to the spinous processes of C2, C7 and T1 is essential to prevent development of cervical kyphosis. There is a tendency for the multifidus muscle to slide more anteriorly with the spinous processes becoming prominent and loss of the ability to hold the head upward. Thus, proper fascial repair is required. Multiple interrupted sutures are placed through these ligaments and into the periosteum of the spinous processes.

Posterior cervical wounds are at high risk for infection, and placement of 1–2-gm vancomycin powder into muscles at closure has been shown to reduce infection by 80% or more [16].

Since these wound are under tension from shoulder motion, the skin is closed with staples or interrupted nylon.

Postoperative Care

Postoperatively patients with unstable conditions are immobilized in a hard collar, while those with stable type spines (such as pseudoarthrosis repair or in degenerative conditions) may not require immobilization.

Illustrative Case

History A 56-year-old male patient with ankylosing spondylitis sustained a hyperextension injury from a fall and complains of neck pain. He was noted to have a preexisting thoracic kyphotic deformity and stiff spinal column. He is immobilized in a collar.

Physical Examination Neurologic examination shows a Frankel C central cord syndrome.

Radiographical Imaging CT shows preexisting thoracic kyphosis and increased cervical kyphosis. A minimally displaced transverse fracture at C6–C7 is present, Fig. 9.5a. A displaced laminar fracture results in posterior cord compression. Fractures of the superior articular facets with subluxation are seen on parasagittal CT, Fig. 9.5b. The MRI shows a narrow spinal canal and significant stenosis at C6–C7 but absence of epidural hematoma, Fig. 9.5c.

Treatment He underwent immediate posterior decompression of C6–C7, cervicothoracic fusion from C3–T6 using lateral mass screws in the cervical spine, pedicle screws in thoracic, and a transition rod, Fig. 9.5d. Posterior fusion at C6–C7 with allograft was performed. Postoperative CT shows placement of lateral mass screws in C6, Fig. 9.5e. The right screw should have started

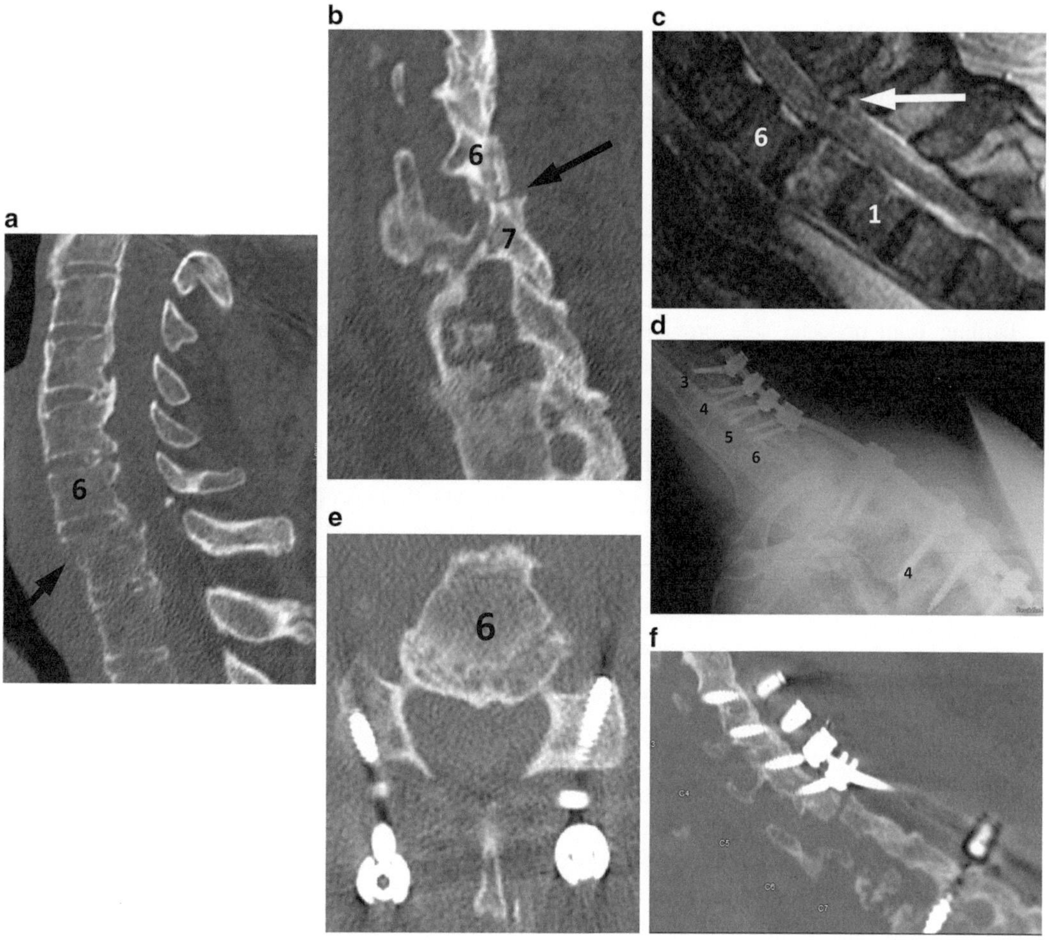

Fig. 9.5 (**a**) Midline sagittal CT of ankylosing spondylitis with extension injury through the body of C7 (*arrow*) and facet joints. There are 3 mm of subluxation and a displaced fracture of the lamina compressing the spinal cord dorsally. (**b**) Sagittal CT through facet joints showing transverse fracture of C7 superior facet with 2–3-mm displacement (*arrow*). (**c**) A fat-suppressed T2 MRI showing spinal canal stenosis caused by subluxation of C6–C7 and a displaced laminar fracture (*arrow*). (**d**) Postoperative lateral radiograph after C3–T6 instrumentation. (**e**) Postoperative axial CT at C6 showing outward direction of lateral mass screws away from the vertebral artery. The right screw should have started 2 mm more medially. (**f**) Postoperative sagittal CT in the plane of the lateral masses demonstrating correct upward angulation of lateral mass screws

1–2 mm more medially but both show outward angulation avoiding risk to the vertebral artery. Sagittal CT shows correct upward angulation of lateral mass screws, Fig. 9.5f.

Outcome He made significant recovery of neurologic function and is now fully ambulatory and has excellent hand function. He complains of chronic spinal pain which is minimally different than prior to injury. His fusion appears healed at 6 months of follow-up.

Technical Pearls

- Adjust relative position of head to neck to optimize alignment and then confirm by radiographs prior to skin incision.
- Maintain midline soft tissue envelope to avoid postoperative kyphosis at adjacent segment.
- Place a small burr hole at the ideal lateral mass starting points prior to drilling.
- Drilling from opposite side provides a more natural trajectory for the screw, but it can be performed from the ipsilateral side if preferred.
- Use adjustable drill guide or pedicle probe.
- Decorticate facets and place bone grafts.

Complications

Surgical Site Infection

Posterior cervical wounds are at high risk for surgical site infections (SSI) with wide ranges from 1.5 to greater than 10% [17]. Using the American College of Surgeons data, Nassr reported a rate of 2.9% in 5441 patients [18]. Others have reported greater than 10% with higher incidences in trauma settings. Risk factors for SSI in posterior cervical surgery are older age, BMI > 35, chronic steroid use, and procedures lasting longer than 3 h [19]. The use of 1 gm of intrawound vancomycin powder in posterior wound has been shown to reduce SSI by 80–100% although not uniformly [17]. Martin found no statistically significant differences in SSI between control (6.9%) and vancomycin (5.2%) [20].

Screw Malposition

Coe reported that screw violation of the foramen transversarium, neuroforamen, and facet joint was 1.5%, 1.0%, and 0.6%, respectively, while no patient had screw malposition into the spinal canal [21]. Yoshihara noted that 1.1% of patients required revision surgery for lateral mass screw malposition [22].

Cervical pedicle screw insertion is more challenging than lateral mass screws with higher rates of malposition. Ghori performed a systematic review of studies and found pedicle screw penetration rates from 6.7% to 30% with two-thirds being lateral penetration toward the vertebral artery [15]. The most important risk factor was operative level with higher rates of perforation occurring more proximally, especially at C3, due to smaller size and more medial angulation. Kast reviewed 94 pedicle screws using CT and found that only 46 were completely within the bone and 20 screws had no more than 1 mm of cortical perforation. [23] Another 20 screws had minor cortical violation (≤25% of screw diameter) and an additional 8 had major violations. The most common penetrations were medially (10.6%) and lateral narrowing of the foramen transversarium (10.6%). Anterior and lateral perforation of the vertebral body was seen in 5.7% of cases and caudal perforation into the neuroforamina occurred in 3.1% of patients. Only two patients had clinically relevant screw malposition. Hojo reviewed 1090 pedicle screws placed using fluoroscopy in multiple centers and found that 14.8% of screws were malpositioned [14]. Four-fifths of screws were laterally misplaced, while one-fifth were medially malpositioned. There is a documented learning curve with more accurate positioning after 10–20 cases. Computer navigation-aided screw insertion reduces malposition by 3–5 times [15].

Neurologic Injury

Neurologic injury is most commonly associated with the procedure and not directly to the internal fixation. Coe reported that 3.9% of patients treated by lateral mass screws had a nerve root injury but only 1.0% were considered to have been caused by the screw placement. Two large case series (Sekhon, Katonis) reported no nerve root injuries in a combined 2688 lateral mass screws.

Cervical pedicle screws similarly have a low rate of neurologic complications. Abumi reported only 2 nerve root injuries in 712 pedicle screws, while Kast had 2 in 96 screws [23, 24]. No spinal cord injuries related directly to screw insertion were noted. Hojo found that only 1% of patients had root injury from misplaced cervical pedicle screws [14].

Fixation Failure

Failure of fixation with loss of lordosis or increased translation occurs more commonly when crossing the cervicothoracic junction or in treatment of more complex conditions such as trauma or tumor reconstruction. Prevention is best achieved by creation of a load-sharing construct using proper anterior reconstruction if possible. Using lateral mass fixation, Yoshihara reported 2.2% and Heller 2.6% of patients had loss of correction [22, 25]. Hojo found that 2.5% of patients treated by pedicle screw fixation had screw loosening, almost exclusively in rheumatoid arthritis patients [14]. Correction of sagittal plane deformity, use of orthosis including the halo vest when needed, and using longer constructs with more points of fixation should be considered to avoid fixation failure.

Poor Screw Purchase

Inadequate screw purchase is not uncommon when placing interspinous wire or lateral mass screws. When the lateral masses are small or eroded from inflammatory diseases, there may be little area for screw purchase. Additionally, obtaining the safest screw orientation, upward and outward, may lead to the screw breaking out during insertion or when the rods are loaded into screw heads. Yoshihara reported in a systematic review that 1.62% had lateral mass fracture during placement [22]. Careful attention to detail during screw insertion and proper rod bending is required to avoid excessive pullout forces on screws. Creating a starting point with a small burr can help to avoid walking of the drill laterally which leads to poor purchase when drilling. When conditions do not allow adequate screw purchase, alternatives include adding longer constructs, pedicle screws, and combined anterior reconstruction, and use of facet cortical grafts should be considered.

Broken Hardware

The rods used in posterior cervical fixation have small diameter (3.5 mm) and usually are made of titanium alloy. Titanium alloy is notch sensitive which occurs during rod bending causing poor fatigue resistance and thus possible breakage. This is particularly common at the craniocervical and cervicothoracic junction. Use of larger rods (4.0 mm) and pre-bent rods will minimize the chance of rod failure. When bending rods, try to contour the rod at multiple points and avoid creating a sharp bend at a single point.

Vertebral Artery Injury

The vertebral artery is at risk when placing lateral mass screws and pedicle screws from C3 to C6. Although theoretically possible, no cases of lateral mass screw placement injuring the vertebral artery have been reported [4, 22]. Lateral breaching of cervical pedicle screws is relatively common when analyzed by CT but does not necessarily result in vertebral artery injury. Abumi reported one case of vertebral artery injury in his first 180 patients treated with cervical pedicle screws [26]. Uehara reported 20% of pedicle screws violated the pedicle with 75% being lateral toward the vertebral artery although no injuries occurred [27]. In a multicenter study, Hojo reported 2 of 283 patients sustained vertebral artery injury after cervical pedicle screw placement using the freehand technique as described, Abumi [14].

Conclusion

Posterior subaxial fusion is commonly performed and can be used for a variety of conditions. The indications are most frequently secondary to instability and as adjuncts for treatment of degenerative conditions. Interspinous wire or cable fixation is less often used but still highly successful. Modern instrumentation using lateral mass screws and rods is highly effective with low rates of complications. Added strength of fixation can be obtained from subaxial pedicle screws with the added risk of vertebral artery injury. Meticulous technique is required as the area for fixation is limited and neurovascular structures are in close approximation. In all cases, proper bone grafting techniques are required to obtain ultimate arthrodesis.

References

1. Denaro V, Di Martino A. Cervical spine surgery: an historical perspective. Clin Orthop Relat Res. 2011;469(3):639–48.
2. Vaccaro AR, Hulbert RJ, Patel AA, Fisher C, Dvorak M, Lehman RA Jr, et al. The subaxial cervical spine injury classification system: a novel approach to recognize the importance of morphology, neurology, and integrity of the disco-ligamentous complex. Spine. 2007;32(21):2365–74.
3. Anderson PA, Moore TA, Davis KW, Molinari RW, Resnick DK, Vaccaro AR, et al. Cervical spine injury severity score. Assessment of reliability. J Bone Joint Surg Am. 2007;89(5):1057–65.
4. Vaccaro AR, Koerner JD, Radcliff KE, Oner FC, Reinhold M, Schnake KJ, et al. AOSpine subaxial cervical spine injury classification system. Eur Spine J (Official Publication of the European Spine Society, the European Spinal Deformity Society, and the European Section of the Cervical Spine Research Society). 2016;25(7):2173–84.
5. Brodke DS, Anderson PA, Newell DW, Grady MS, Chapman JR. Comparison of anterior and posterior approaches in cervical spinal cord injuries. J Spinal Disord Tech. 2003;16(3):229–35.
6. McAnany SJ, Baird EO, Overley SC, Kim JS, Qureshi SA, Anderson PA. A meta-analysis of the clinical and fusion results following treatment of symptomatic cervical pseudarthrosis. Global Spine J. 2015;5(2):148–55.
7. Ilgenfritz RM, Gandhi AA, Fredericks DC, Grosland NM, Smucker JD. Considerations for the use of C7 crossing laminar screws in subaxial and cervicothoracic instrumentation. Spine. 2013;38(4):E199–204.
8. Ludwig SC, Kramer DL, Balderston RA, Vaccaro AR, Foley KF, Albert TJ. Placement of pedicle screws in the human cadaveric cervical spine: comparative accuracy of three techniques. Spine. 2000;25(13):1655–67.
9. Lee DH, Lee SW, Kang SJ, Hwang CJ, Kim NH, Bae JY, et al. Optimal entry points and trajectories for cervical pedicle screw placement into subaxial cervical vertebrae. Eur Spine J (Official Publication of the European Spine Society, the European Spinal Deformity Society, and the European Section of the Cervical Spine Research Society). 2011;20(6):905–11.
10. Kotani Y, Cunningham BW, Abumi K, McAfee PC. Biomechanical analysis of cervical stabilization systems. An assessment of transpedicular screw fixation in the cervical spine. Spine. 1994;19(22):2529–39.
11. Rogers WA. Fractures and dislocations of the cervical spine; an end-result study. J Bone Joint Surg Am. 1957;39-a(2):341–76.
12. Bohlman HH. Surgical management of cervical spine fractures and dislocations. Instr Course Lect. 1985;34:163–87.
13. Karaikovic EE, Kunakornsawat S, Daubs MD, Madsen TW, Gaines RW Jr. Surgical anatomy of the cervical pedicles: landmarks for posterior cervical pedicle entrance localization. J Spinal Disord. 2000;13(1):63–72.
14. Hojo Y, Ito M, Suda K, Oda I, Yoshimoto H, Abumi K. A multicenter study on accuracy and complications of freehand placement of cervical pedicle screws under lateral fluoroscopy in different pathological conditions: CT-based evaluation of more than 1,000 screws. Eur Spine J (Official Publication of the European Spine Society, the European Spinal Deformity Society, and the European Section of the Cervical Spine Research Society). 2014;23(10):2166–74.
15. Ghori A, Le HV, Makanji H, Cha T. Posterior fixation techniques in the subaxial cervical spine. Cureus. 2015;7(10):e338.
16. Pahys JM, Pahys JR, Cho SK, Kang MM, Zebala LP, Hawasli AH, et al. Methods to decrease postoperative infections following posterior cervical spine surgery. J Bone Joint Surg Am. 2013;95(6):549–54.
17. Bakhsheshian J, Dahdaleh NS, Lam SK, Savage JW, Smith ZA. The use of vancomycin powder in modern spine surgery: systematic review and meta-analysis of the clinical evidence. World Neurosurg. 2015;83(5):816–23.
18. Sebastian A, Huddleston P 3rd, Kakar S, Habermann E, Wagie A, Nassr A. Risk factors for surgical site infection after posterior cervical spine surgery: an analysis of 5,441 patients from the ACS NSQIP 2005–2012. Spine J (Official Journal of the North American Spine Society). 2016;16(4):504–9.
19. Sebastian AS, Adair MJ, Morris JM, Khan MH, Arndt CA, Nassr A. Minimally invasive treatment of a painful osteolytic lumbar lesion secondary to epithelioid hemangioendothelioma. Global Spine J. 2015;5(2):135–9.
20. Martin JR, Adogwa O, Brown CR, Kuchibhatla M, Bagley CA, Lad SP, et al. Experience with intrawound vancomycin powder for posterior cervical fusion surgery. J Neurosurg Spine. 2015;22(1):26–33.

21. Coe JD, Vaccaro AR, Dailey AT, Skolasky RL Jr, Sasso RC, Ludwig SC, et al. Lateral mass screw fixation in the cervical spine: a systematic literature review. J Bone Joint Surg Am. 2013;95(23):2136–43.
22. Yoshihara H, Passias PG, Errico TJ. Screw-related complications in the subaxial cervical spine with the use of lateral mass versus cervical pedicle screws: a systematic review. J Neurosurg Spine. 2013;19(5):614–23.
23. Kast E, Mohr K, Richter HP, Borm W. Complications of transpedicular screw fixation in the cervical spine. Eur Spine J (Official Publication of the European Spine Society, the European Spinal Deformity Society, and the European Section of the Cervical Spine Research Society). 2006;15(3):327–34.
24. Abumi K, Kaneda K. Pedicle screw fixation for nontraumatic lesions of the cervical spine. Spine. 1997;22(16):1853–63.
25. Heller JG, Silcox DH 3rd, Sutterlin CE 3rd. Complications of posterior cervical plating. Spine. 1995;20(22):2442–8.
26. Abumi K, Shono Y, Ito M, Taneichi H, Kotani Y, Kaneda K. Complications of pedicle screw fixation in reconstructive surgery of the cervical spine. Spine. 2000;25(8):962–9.
27. Uehara M, Takahashi J, Ikegami S, Mukaiyama K, Kuraishi S, Shimizu M, et al. Screw perforation features in 129 consecutive patients performed computer-guided cervical pedicle screw insertion. Eur Spine J (Official Publication of the European Spine Society, the European Spinal Deformity Society, and the European Section of the Cervical Spine Research Society). 2014;23(10):2189–95.

10 Posterior Cervical Subaxial Spine Fixation: Facet Fusion Techniques

Mena Kerolus and Vincent Traynelis

Introduction

Cervical spondylosis is a common disease process that is increasing in frequency given the longer mean survival age. Individuals with symptomatic cervical spondylosis who have failed to respond to nonoperative therapy are candidates for surgical intervention. The goals of surgery in these cases include decompression of the spinal cord and/or nerve roots while maintaining stability either by limiting surgical destabilization or performing an arthrodesis. In this chapter we discuss the role of the subaxial facet joint in the pathogenesis of cervical spondylosis, a brief overview of the biomechanical and anatomical considerations of the subaxial facet joint, the surgical technique when placing subaxial interfacet spacers, indications, complications, and clinical outcomes when using interfacet spacers for subaxial spine fusion.

Fusion techniques of the cervical spine have been well described and consist of anterior, posterior, or combined anterior and posterior procedures depending on the extent of disease, deformity, and history of prior surgery. Cloward introduced the anterior discectomy and fusion approach in 1958 and it has since gained wide popularity due to its safety and efficacy [1]. Various posterior fusion procedures have been described for the fixation of the subaxial cervical spine including interfacet, spinous process, or sublaminar wiring, lateral mass or pedicle fixation with screw/plate or screw/rod instrumentation, and hook/rod constructs [2, 3]. Recently a technique using cervical interfacet grafts has been added to as another means of achieving stabilization and arthrodesis. The use of the facet joint for fusion has shown promising radiologic and clinical outcomes [4–6].

The pathogenesis of cervical spondylosis has traditionally been thought to be initiated by disc degeneration which translates to changes in other aspects of the spinal functional unit. With age, there is a natural decrease in disc height which triggers a cascade of events which may include thickening and/or buckling of the posterior longitudinal ligament and ligamentum flavum, osteophyte formation, foraminal stenosis, vertebral listhesis, and facet degeneration. Depending on the specific changes and their severity, this degenerative process may also produce deformity and/or segmental instability. Recently, an alternative hypothesis has been suggested by Goel et al. which defines facet degeneration as the origin of the spondylotic process [7]. The facet joint can undergo degenerative changes similar to other synovial joints in the body. Goel

M. Kerolus, MD • V. Traynelis, MD (✉)
Department of Neurosurgery, Rush University Medical Center, 1725 West Harrison Street, Suite 855, 60612 Chicago, IL, USA
e-mail: menakerolus@gmail.com; Vincent_Traynelis@rush.edu

L.T. Holly, P.A. Anderson (eds.), *Essentials of Spinal Stabilization*, DOI 10.1007/978-3-319-59713-3_10

et al. describes a sequence of events that begin with cartilage degeneration and can progress to include a number of other pathological changes. Sclerosis of the facet joint begins to form, the bony pillars of the facet are exposed, and facet osteophyte formation, synovial cyst formation and capsule calcification become evident [4, 6–8]. These changes are thought to subsequently cause disc degeneration and osteophyte formation leading to foraminal and central canal stenosis. Regardless of the etiology, degenerative pathologic changes in the cervical spine may result in stenosis, instability, and structural misalignment, all of which are associated with symptomatic radiculopathy and myelopathy. The radiographic evaluation of facet arthropathy has been reported and graded by computed tomography (CT) as described by Pathria et al. where Grade I corresponds to facet joint space narrowing, Grade II corresponds to facet sclerosis or hypertrophy, and Grade III corresponds to osteophyte formation [9].

The cervical facet has been advocated as a strategic location for fusion given its relatively large size and surface area, biomechanical strength, firmness, and anatomical distance from critical neural structures. The interfacet space provides an effective means for distraction of the spinal segment. The distraction itself will stiffen the segment, and if further stabilization is needed, the articular pillar is a common site for screw purchase [10, 11].

Facet strength was tested in cadavers by Raynor et al. in 1985. In fresh and fixated cadaveric specimens, the facet was able to withstand compressive loads of up to 195 pounds before either dislocation or loss of fixation of the vertebral bodies. Even with 50% of the facet removed, facet fracture required loads of 135lbs [12]. In a separate study Raynor and Carter examined the use of the Roy-Camille lateral mass plates in a human cervical spine facet injury model. When half of the facet was removed, placement of 3.5 mm diameter lateral mass screws resulted in a significant decrease in the load due to failure at the instrumented level. Failure occurred by fracture through the screw holes. These authors concluded that following partial medial facetectomy, use of the lateral mass plate may result in inadequate holding strength, and failure is likely to occur through the screw holes [13]. Frequently a foraminotomy may result in resection of half of the lateral mass which makes screw fixation precarious. Interfacet spacers can open the foramen and preserve bone for screw purchase if that is desired.

Finite element models of the ligamentous cervical spine segments have estimated that the cervical facet joint can be responsible for up to 23% of axial loading [4, 14, 15]. Morphometric and volumetric analysis of the superior facet of the subaxial cervical spine ranges from 7.5 to 12 mm in width and the inferior facet of the subaxial cervical spine ranges from 8 to 15 mm in width. The smallest facet is at C4 [16, 17]. The distance from the inferior facet to the transverse foramen ranges from 5 to 7 mm, the furthest at C3 and closest at C4 in the subaxial spine [17]. The anatomic relationship of the lateral mass to the nerve roots, spinal cord, and vertebral artery is important to understand if one plans to place screws into this structure [18–20].

In 2007, Goel described the use of cervical interfacet spacers as a new method of facet fixation [21]. These facet spacers were composed of titanium alloy spikes on both sides to provide fixation. Multiple holes were made to allow bone arthrodesis. Various sizes of the spacers are used for distraction and adequate graft size placement [6, 7, 21]. These spacers provided indirect neuroforaminal decompression while providing a large osteoconductive surface for fusion. The natural compressive forces applied by the cervical spine on the facet may also increase the rate of fusion [4].

Cervical interfacet spacers assist with an increase in the height and diameter of the cervical intervertebral foramen and a simultaneous increase in the interlaminar distance and intervertebral body height. Goel and Shah reported a mean increase of 2 mm for interspinous distance and an increase of 0.4–1.2 mm in intervertebral body distance when cervical interfacet spacers were used [6]. Tan et al. found that the use of interfacet spacers provide distraction of the foraminal area as high as 18.4% in a cadaver study [4]. Maulucci et al. examined the kinetics and stiffness of the subaxial cervical spine with the use of cervical interfacet spacers. They found that the addition of 2 mm or higher interfacet grafts provided a significant increase in the foraminal area cross-section but did not provide any more significant stiffness compared to an intact spine. However, when using 3 mm or 4 mm spacers without posterior instrumentation, the stiffness of the segment increased along with foraminal height [22]. Siemionow et al. performed an in vivo study and found a significant increase in foraminal area and height with bilateral facet joint cages at a 3-, 6-, and 12-month follow-up. However, foraminal area did decrease from the 6- to the 12-month follow-up, but this was not significant and favorable clinical outcomes remained [23].

Due to the relatively new development of cervical interfacet spacers, clinical outcomes are limited but promising. Goel and Shah reported on his series of 36 patients with placement of cervical interfacet spacers without additional posterior instrumentation with 92% of patients having an excellent or good outcome. Fusion rates were 100% at 6-month follow-up based on flexion and extension radiographs. However, in their series of patients, they reported a non-statistically significant loss of lordosis at the levels treated, especially when longer levels were treated [6]. Tan et al. reported similar results in a series of 64 patients who underwent 154 levels of implanted cervical interfacet spacers. This group did not show any statistically significant loss of cervical lordosis compared to preoperative lordosis. No patients developed kyphosis [14]. Kasliwal et al. reported on a series of 19 patients with symptomatic pseudoarthrosis after anterior cervical decompression and fusion. There was statistically significant improvement in VAS scores for neck pain (83% improved, $p < .004$) and radicular arm pain (72% improved, $p < .007$) after a mean follow-up of 20 months after posterior instrumentation and fusion with facet spacers were used. Also, although a small number of patients were described in this series, 100% of patients fused at the prior levels of pseudoarthrosis. Although not statistically significant, there was an improvement in cervical lordosis but worsening sagittal vertical axis [5].

Indications and Patient Selection

Patients with symptomatic cervical spondylosis treated using the posterior approach who require foraminal enlargement or fusion are candidates for cervical interfacet spacers. MRI or CT myelogram findings of severe compression or foraminal involvement should correlate with the clinical scenario. Cervical interfacet spacers can still be placed after a prior laminectomy or prior fusion as long as the facet is not already fused or compromised. Also, facet interfacet spacers can be placed at the time of laminectomy and fusion for patients have myeloradiculopathy and may be a substitute for direct foraminal decompression in these cases. Patients with anterior cervical hardware that develop symptomatic pseudoarthrosis may benefit from the addition of cervical interspace spacers when addressing the fusion with a posterior cervical approach. Transitioning a straight or kyphotic spine to a lordotic configuration using a posterior strategy can produce or exacerbate foraminal stenosis. The risk of creating iatrogenic foraminal narrowing is minimized or even negated by first placing the cervical interfacet spacers as they increase the foraminal area and height. Interfacet spacers are indicated for patients having degenerative spondylolisthesis secondary to erosive facet remodeling. In these cases, the spacers can provide a reduction force and aid in prevention of reoccurrence of slippage.

Preoperative Considerations

Evaluation of a preoperative MRI or CT myelogram should be carefully examined to determine the desired approach to the cervical spine. If a posterior approach with fusion is needed, cervical interfacet spacers may be used. Preoperative imaging for candidates of cervical interfacet spacers should include plain cervical AP, lateral, and dynamic flexion and extension films. Preoperative C2/C7 lordosis, sagittal vertical axis, and T1 slope should all be measured preoperatively to identify and quantify the degree of deformity (if present) and the amount of correction needed. Dynamic films are important to verify stability. CT may also be used to assess any prior arthrodesis. If there is a solid arthrodesis either anterior or posterior, there is no need to place a cervical interfacet spacer.

If a posterior cervical approach is needed, cervical interfacet spacers may be used prior to or after a cervical laminectomy. CT, MRI, or CT myelogram should be used to assess foraminal height and width. Facet width and length can also be assessed to make sure there is adequate surface area for the 8 × 8 mm spacer. MRI may be used to carefully examine the exiting nerve root and vertebral anatomy. If the desired cervical levels involve the C4/C5 disc space, it may be worthwhile to address this level first as it is a sensitive nerve root.

Each patient will undergo general anesthesia and the operation will be performed in the prone position. The patient will need to be on a Jackson table using a Mayfield clamp for fixation. The patient's arms are placed along the body and well-padded over the elbow and hand. The C-arm can be placed in the operative field and will be used to determine the correct level of surgery.

Surgical Technique

Each patient will be induced using general endotracheal anesthesia. The patient is placed prone on a Jackson table and the head secured with a Mayfield clamp. A midline incision and subperiosteal dissection is utilized to expose the dorsal cervical spine including the lateral masses. Care is taken to avoid detaching the muscle insertions onto the C2 spinous process or dissecting too far lateral to the articular pillars. It is our practice to place the interfacet grafts just after exposure. At this point, the lamina protects the spinal cord and the lateral masses have not been compromised by drilling or the exposure hampered by instrumentation. The intended facet joint is inspected and capsule removed. If needed, removal of osteophytes to gain access to the joint is done using rongeur or high-speed burr. The facet joint is freed of all articular cartilage using customized rasps which are 8 × 8 mm in width and depth and vary in height (2, 3, 4 mm) (Fig. 10.1) (FacetLift, Medtronic, Memphis, TN). Each size is used twice beginning with the 2 mm rasp and increasing to 3 or 4 mm. The rasp also serves to determine the size of the graft. If the 3 mm fits very snugly, then the 4 mm rasp is not used and a 3 mm graft placed. It is best to place at least a 3 mm graft, but in select circumstances only a 2 mm graft will fit. The interfacet spacer is tapped into place and slightly countersunk (Fig. 10.2). It is important not to place the graft too deeply into the joint or it could impinge the nerve root. The C4/C5 level is always addressed first followed by the other cervical levels as we believe this will minimize the likelihood of developing a postoperative C5 palsy. Once the grafts are in position, the decompression and/or lateral mass fixation is performed. Prior to final fixation of the rods to the polyaxial screws, the Mayfield device is released and the neck is manually extended to improve lordosis. Hemostasis is achieved using bipolar cautery, thrombin-soaked Gelfoam, or similar hemostatic agents. The wound is irrigated and closed in layers.

Clinical Case

A 42-year-old female with a history of multiple sclerosis presented to our clinic after a hydraulic door fell on her head. She was suffering from severe right-side neck pain which was exacerbated with activity. She was also experiencing interscapular pain as well as numbness and tingling in the middle three digits of both her hands. On physical examination she had neck discomfort on flexion and extension with tenderness on palpation of her posterior cervical neck. She was full strength on individual motor testing but found to have hypesthesia in the right C4 dermatome. She had normal deep tendon reflexes and

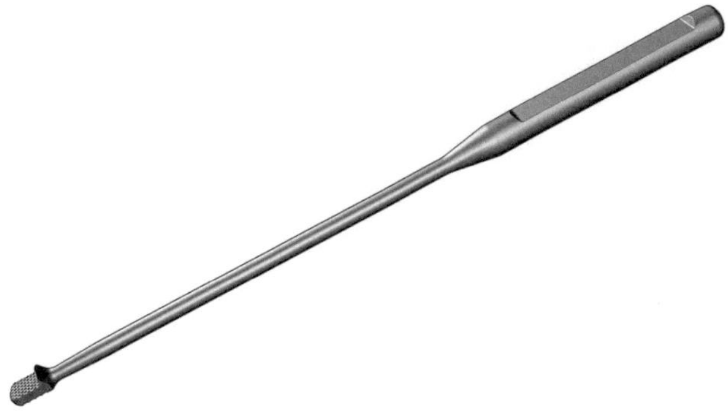

Fig. 10.1 Illustration of a 2 mm rasp. All rasps are 8 × 8 mm in depth and width. The height changes depending on the rasp selected which will help determine the size of the graft

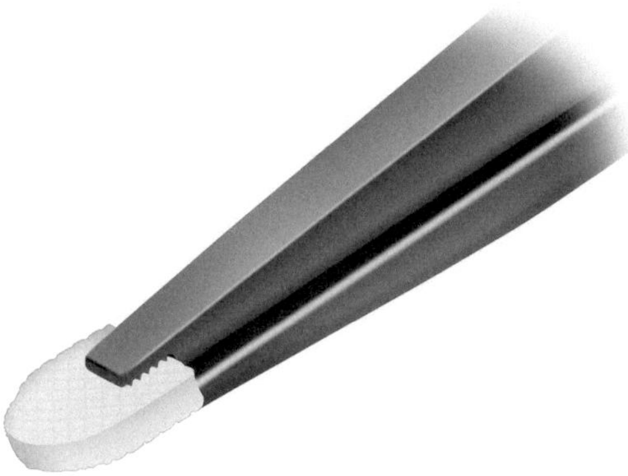

Fig. 10.2 Illustration of a graft holder and interfacet graft which will be lightly tapped into the prepared interfacet space

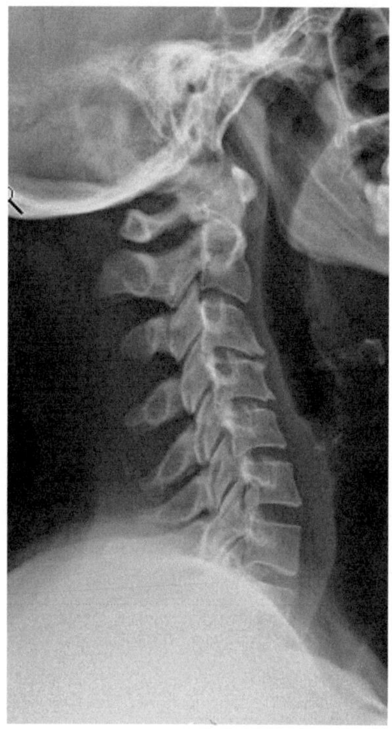

Fig. 10.3 Upright neutral lateral cervical radiograph revealing kyphosis at C3/C4 and loss of lordosis at C4/C5

no Hoffman's reflex. A course of conservative management with physical therapy, NSAIDs, and muscle relaxants was suggested but the neck pain remained.

Her radiographs revealed kyphosis at C3/C4 and loss of lordosis at C4/C5 (Fig. 10.3). Flexion and extension cervical radiographs showed increased disc collapse at C3/C4 and C4/C5. Magnetic resonance imaging (MRI) revealed bilateral C3/C4 and C4/C5 foraminal narrowing and central canal stenosis.

She underwent a C3/C4 and C4/C5 anterior cervical discectomy and fusion (ACDF) which resulted in resolution of her symptoms (Fig. 10.4). Unfortunately she did not fuse at either level and the nonunion was symptomatic. Radiographs revealed a new C3 screw fracture and widening of the C3/C4 and C4/C5 interspinous space with flexion.

She was treated with a posterior fusion using cervical interfacet spacers and lateral mass fixation. The C4/C5 level was addressed first using an 8x8x3mm spacer. At the C3/C4 level, an 8x8x4mm spacer was used. Posterior instrumentation with lateral mass screws and a rod placement was used to secure the reconstruction. Postoperative lateral plain radiographs and sagittal CT revealed good placement of the cervical interfacet spacers and posterior instrumentation

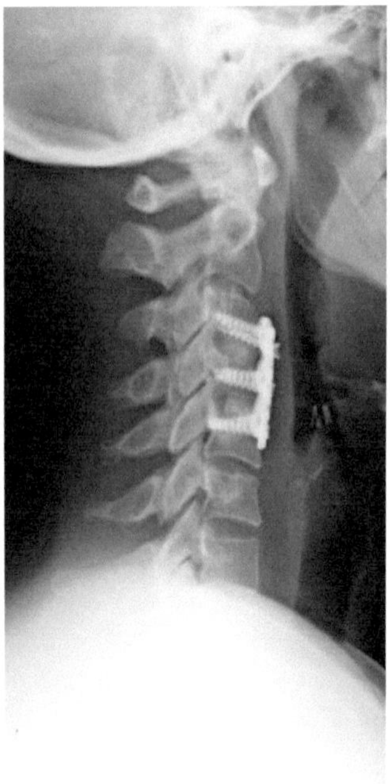

Fig. 10.4 Upright neutral lateral cervical radiograph after undergoing a C3/C4 and C4/C5 anterior cervical discectomy and fusion

(Fig. 10.5a, b). Postoperative coronal CT highlights the placement of the facet spacers in relationship to the central canal (Fig. 10.6). The patient's pain subsequently improved, and at her 1-year follow-up, there was radiographic evidence of successful arthrodesis of the facet and interbody space at C3/C4 and C4/C5 (Fig. 10.7).

Technical Pearls

- Interfacet spacers are placed rather easily, safely, and quickly. They can be utilized with and without supplemental spinal fixation techniques [5, 6]. The "joint hammering technique" for placement of cervical interfacet spacers was first described in atlantoaxial fixation [21] and then applied to the subaxial spine for placement of cervical facet spacers without supplemental hardware [6]. A similar technique has been used and described in

a b

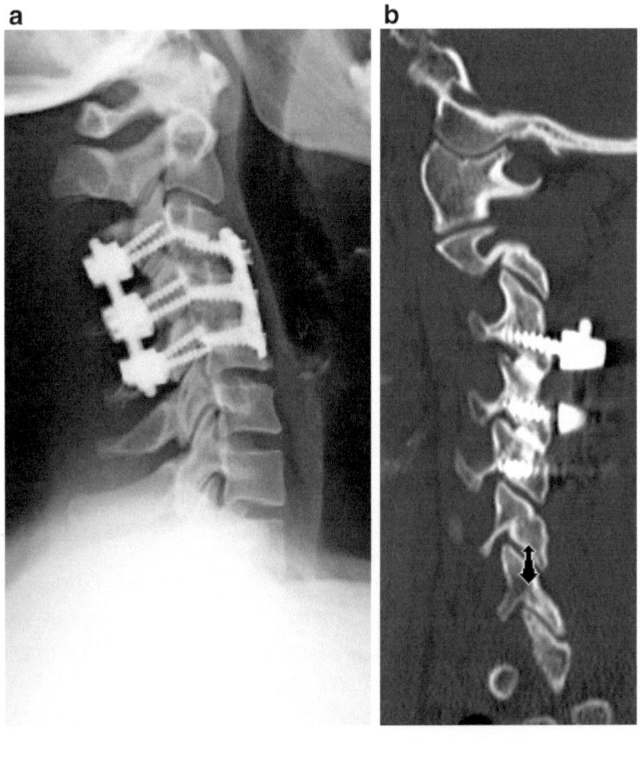

Fig. 10.5 (**a**, **b**) Postoperative neutral lateral radiograph (**a**) and parasagittal cervical computed tomography (**b**) of the same patient after undergoing a C3/C4 and C4/C5 posterior cervical instrumented with interfacet spacers for symptomatic pseudoarthrosis and a fractured C3 screw

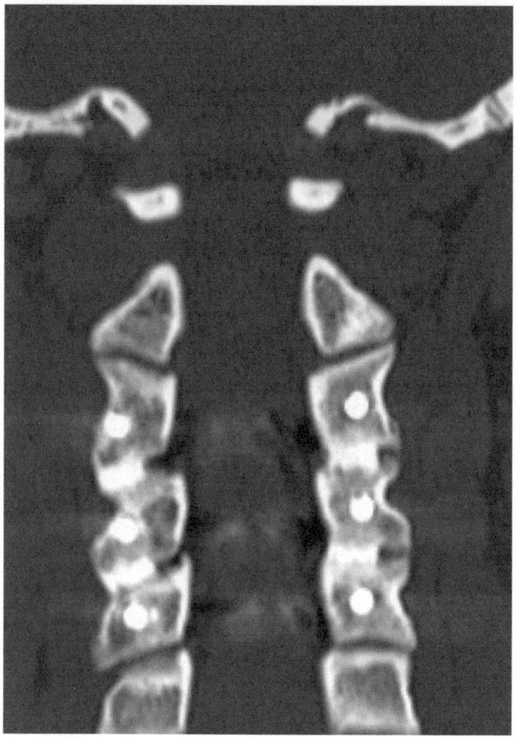

Fig. 10.6 Postoperative coronal cervical computed tomography highlighting bilateral interfacet spacers at C3/C4 and C4/C5 in relationship to the central canal

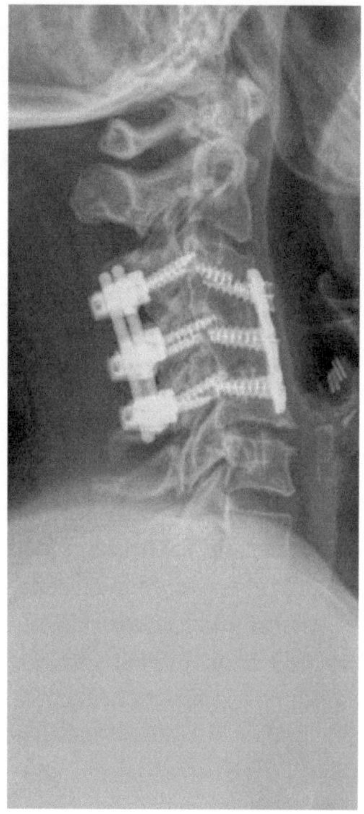

Fig. 10.7 One-year follow-up upright neutral lateral cervical radiograph with evidence of successful arthrodesis of the facet and interbody space at C3/C4 and C4/C5

patients with the addition of posterior cervical instrumentation [5, 14].
- Some caution while impacting the facet spacers should be taken. This may require a fair amount of force. Some surgeons could be alarmed at what is necessary in terms of the degree of impact, but it is totally safe. The key is to prepare the interspace correctly and choose a graft size that mirrors the interspace preparation. Creating a pathway using a burr or rongeur may help placement if osteophytes are present. Occasionally after placement of one graft, the other space seems to be too small. This "teetotaler" effect should be managed by re-rasping the joint in question.
- Concerns regarding iatrogenic loss of lordosis or formation of kyphosis with placement of cervical interfacet spacers have been reported [6]. Tan et al. reported on a series of 64 patients who underwent 154 levels of implanted cervical interfacet spacers. This study demonstrated that there was no statistically significant difference between those patients with spacers and those without in terms of preoperative and postoperative lordosis. No patient in this study developed kyphosis [14]. Goel and Shah reported similar results with mild loss of lordosis with no kyphosis in 36 patients [6]. Kasliwal et al. reported on a series of patients who developed a nonsignificant loss of lordosis but with improved outcome with the use of interfacet spacers and posterior instrumentation after failed anterior instrumentation [5].

Complications and Strategies for Avoidance

Risks involved with the placement of cervical interfacet spacers are similar to that of traditional posterior fixation techniques. Nerve injury, spinal cord injury, or vertebral artery injury is possible. When impacting the interfacet spacer, careful attention to the width of the facet and location of the graft in relationship to the spinal canal will negate this complication. In the summation of all cases of cervical interfacet spacers, there have been no reported vertebral or neurologic injuries directly related to interfacet spacers [5, 6, 14].

Conclusion

Cervical interfacet spacers is a promising adjuvant for the treatment of cervical spondylosis where both fusion and foraminal enlargement is desired. The use of cervical interfacet spacers is a safe technique and adds minimal time compared to traditional posterior fusion techniques.

References

1. Cloward RB. The anterior approach for removal of ruptured cervical disks. J Neurosurg. 1958;15(6):602–17.
2. Chapman JR, Anderson PA, Pepin C, Toomey S, Newell DW, Grady MS. Posterior instrumentation of the unstable cervicothoracic spine. J Neurosurg. 1996;84(4):552–8.
3. Deutsch H, Eichholz KM, Haid RW Jr, Traynelis VC. In: Benzel EC, editor. Spine surgery: techniques, complication avoidance, and management. 3rd ed. Philadelphia: Saunders; 2012. p. 1423.
4. Tan LA, Gerard CS, Anderson PA, Traynelis VC. Effect of machined interfacet allograft spacers on cervical foraminal height and area. J Neurosurg Spine. 2013;20(2):178–82.
5. Kasliwal MK, Corley JA, Traynelis VC. Posterior cervical fusion using cervical interfacet spacers in patients with symptomatic cervical pseudarthrosis. Neurosurgery. 2016;78(5):661–8.
6. Goel A, Shah A. Facetal distraction as treatment for single- and multilevel cervical spondylotic radiculopathy and myelopathy: a preliminary report. J Neurosurg Spine. 2011;14(6):689–96.
7. Goel A. Facet distraction spacers for treatment of degenerative disease of the spine: rationale and an alternative hypothesis of spinal degeneration. J Craniovert Jun Spine. 2010;1(2):65–6.
8. Fujiwara A, Lim TH, An HS, Tanaka N, Jeon CH, Andersson GB, et al. The effect of disc degeneration and facet joint osteoarthritis on the segmental flexibility of the lumbar spine. Spine. 2000;25(23):3036–44.
9. Pathria M, Sartoris DJ, Resnick D. Osteoarthritis of the facet joints: accuracy of oblique radiographic assessment. Radiology. 1987;164(1):227–30.
10. Barrey C, Mertens P, Jund J, Cotton F, Perrin G. Quantitative anatomic evaluation of cervical lateral mass fixation with a comparison of the Roy-Camille and the Magerl screw techniques. Spine. 2005;30(6):E140–7.
11. Stemper BD, Marawar SV, Yoganandan N, Shender BS, Rao RD. Quantitative anatomy of subaxial cervical lateral mass: an analysis of safe screw lengths for Roy-Camille and magerl techniques. Spine. 2008;33(8):893–7.
12. Raynor RB, Pugh J, Shapiro I. Cervical facetectomy and its effect on spine strength. J Neurosurg. 1985;63(2):278–82.
13. Raynor RB, Carter FW. Cervical spine strength after facet injury and spine plate application. Spine. 1991;16(10 Suppl):S558–60.
14. Tan LA, Straus DC, Traynelis VC. Cervical interfacet spacers and maintenance of cervical lordosis. J Neurosurg Spine. 2015;22(5):466–9.
15. Pal GP, Routal RV. A study of weight transmission through the cervical and upper thoracic regions of the vertebral column in man. J Anat. 1986;148:245–61.
16. Abdullah KG, Steinmetz MP, Mroz TE. Morphometric and volumetric analysis of the lateral masses of the lower cervical spine. Spine. 2009;34(14):1476–9.
17. Shah A. Morphometric analysis of the cervical facets and the feasibility, safety, and effectiveness of Goel inter-facet spacer distraction technique. J Craniovert Jun Spine. 2014;5(1):9–14.
18. An HS, Gordin R, Renner K. Anatomic considerations for plate-screw fixation of the cervical spine. Spine. 1991;16(10 Suppl):S548–51.
19. Ebraheim NA, Xu R, Yeasting RA. The location of the vertebral artery foramen and its relation to posterior lateral mass screw fixation. Spine. 1996;21(11):1291–5.
20. Xu R, Haman SP, Ebraheim NA, Yeasting RA. The anatomic relation of lateral mass screws to the spinal nerves. A comparison of the Magerl, Anderson, and an techniques. Spine. 1999;24(19):2057–61.
21. Goel A. Atlantoaxial joint jamming as a treatment for atlantoaxial dislocation: a preliminary report. Technical note. J Neurosurg Spine. 2007;7(1):90–4.
22. Maulucci CM, Sansur CA, Singh V, Cholewczynski A, Shetye SS, McGilvray K, et al. Cortical bone facet spacers for cervical spine decompression: effects on intervertebral kinetics and foraminal area. J Neurosurg Spine. 2016;24(1):69–76.
23. Siemionow K, Janusz P, Glowka P. Cervical cages placed bilaterally in the facet joints from a posterior approach significantly increase foraminal area. Eur Spine J Off Publ Eur Spine Soc Eur Spinal Deform Soc Eur Sect Cerv Spine Res Soc. 2016;25(7):2279–85.

Cervical Laminoplasty

11

Kevin L. Ju, FeiFei Zhou, and John M. Rhee

Introduction

Multilevel cervical stenosis and resultant myelopathy can arise from ventral and/or dorsal compressive structures. Examples of ventral pathology include disc osteophyte complexes, spondylotic bars, or ossification of the posterior longitudinal ligament (OPLL). These pathologies lead to greater cord compression in the setting of congenital stenosis. Dorsal pathology can include hypertrophied or ossified ligamentum flavum. There is a wide variety of surgical options for addressing multilevel cervical stenosis, which can be broadly categorized into anterior, posterior, or combined approaches. Anterior approaches can directly address ventral compressive pathology and include procedures such as anterior cervical discectomy or corpectomy combined with fusion. Posterior options are able to directly address dorsal compressive pathology, but can also achieve indirect cord decompression by allowing the cord to drift posteriorly away from anterior pathology as long as the cervical alignment is not excessively kyphotic. Posterior procedures that have been used to address multilevel stenosis include multilevel laminectomy alone, laminectomy and fusion, laminoplasty, and skip laminectomy.

Multilevel laminectomy without fusion was traditionally used to effect multilevel neurologic decompression, but was complicated by high rates of postoperative kyphosis and is not routinely recommended today [1, 2]. Multilevel laminectomy with fusion minimizes the risk of postoperative kyphosis; however, it does so at the expense of cervical motion, requires more stringent postoperative restrictions, has higher implant costs, has greater risk of complications, and may be associated with the potential for accelerated adjacent segment degeneration (ASD).

Laminoplasty is a posterior method for spinal cord decompression that was originally developed as an alternative to multilevel laminectomy [3]. Laminoplasty achieves decompression of the spinal canal by expanding, but not completely removing, the posterior laminar arch. Laminoplasty achieves decompression from ventral pathology by allowing the spinal cord to

K.L. Ju, MD (✉)
Texas Back Institute, 3164 Horizon Road, Suite 100, Rockwall, TX 75032, USA
e-mail: kevinjumd@gmail.com

F. Zhou, MD
Peking University Third Hospital, Orthopaedics, No.49 North Garden Rd, Beijing 100191, China
e-mail: orthozhou@gmail.com

J.M. Rhee, MD
Emory University, Orthopaedic Surgery, 59 Executive Park South, Suite 3000, Atlanta, GA 30329, USA
e-mail: jmrhee@emory.edu

L.T. Holly, P.A. Anderson (eds.), *Essentials of Spinal Stabilization*,
DOI 10.1007/978-3-319-59713-3_11

drift posteriorly [4]. Laminoplasty affords several advantages over laminectomy alone. First of all, laminoplasty has a much lower rate of postoperative kyphosis and thus potentially less neck pain, deformity, or recurrent myelopathy. Laminoplasty also avoids the development of a post-laminectomy membrane, which can cause recurrent cord compression. Additionally, the preservation of bone stock and covering over the dura can make a revision posterior operation safer and easier to perform than after multilevel laminectomies. Laminoplasty is also a motion-sparing approach that has the advantage of avoiding potential fusion-related complications (e.g., nonunion, implant failure, potential for accelerated ASD), and patients can also be more aggressively rehabilitated in the early postoperative phase.

Skip laminectomy is a newer technique that was developed as a less invasive method of posterior cervical decompression with the aim of minimizing intraoperative damage to the cervical extensor musculature that can come with laminoplasty [5]. This technique involves performing standard laminectomies at appropriate levels along with partial laminectomies of the cephalad half of the laminae at other levels where the muscle attachments are left undisturbed. Using this technique, decompression from C3 to C7 can be accomplished with standard laminectomies of C4 and C6 and partial laminectomies of the cephalad half of the C5 and C7 laminae. A recent systematic review of the skip laminectomy literature showed no difference in postoperative neurological outcome, range of motion, and cervical lordosis when compared to laminoplasty for the treatment of multilevel cervical spondylotic myelopathy [6]. However, patients undergoing skip laminectomy did have a shorter operative time and less blood loss. Most of the studies included in the systematic review did not demonstrate a significant difference in the complication rates between the two techniques. The same systematic review did highlight the fact that almost all of the published studies have had small sample sizes, were not randomized, and had a high risk of bias. Thus, higher-quality, randomized controlled studies are needed to better discern and compare the outcomes following skip laminectomy for the treatment of multilevel cervical spondylotic myelopathy.

The purpose of this chapter will be to discuss the indications, alternatives, risks, and different techniques of cervical laminoplasty.

Indications and Patient Selection

Cervical laminoplasty is ideally indicated for those patients with myelopathy due to multilevel spinal cord compression at three or more motion segments, little to no spondylotic axial neck pain, and preserved cervical lordosis (Table 11.1). Preoperative upright neutral lateral radiograph is necessary for assessing cervical alignment and ensuring there is no significant segmental instability. It is important to determine whether sufficient posterior cord drift can be achieved after posterior decompression by evaluating the K-line. This is a straight line that connects the midpoints of the spinal canal at C2 and C7. If anterior impinging structures, such as OPLL, do not intersect or cross posterior to the K-line, then adequate drift back can likely be achieved with a posterior decompression [4].

Myelopathic patients with significant axial neck pain may have poorer results with lamino-

Table 11.1 Indications and contraindications for cervical laminoplasty

Indications	Contraindications
Cervical myelopathy involving three or more levels	More than 13° of cervical kyphosis
Cervical alignment that is lordotic	Ventral compressive pathology intersects or extends posterior to the K-line
Ventral compressive pathology does not intersect or extend posterior to the K-line	Primary complaint of axial neck pain
	Significant segmental instability

plasty, as this is a motion-preserving procedure and thus not designed to address potential sources of spondylotic axial neck pain such as facet arthrosis or disc degeneration. Patients with concomitant cervical instability may require a fusion procedure, either with a decompressive laminectomy or laminoplasty, to avoid any worsening postoperatively. Rheumatoid arthritis is also a relative contraindication to laminoplasty as these patients may be at higher risk for postoperative instability [7].

Preoperative Considerations

Preoperatively, it is important to check the amount of neck extension and flexion a patient can tolerate without developing any exacerbation of their neurologic symptoms (e.g., increased numbness, Lhermitte's, etc.) and then take great care to never exceed this during the intubation and positioning process, especially in a severely myelopathic patient. Determining the cranial-most level to include in the laminoplasty also has important implications. A laminoplasty of C3 requires detaching some of the extensor muscle attachments along the caudal aspect of C2 in order to get sufficient exposure to allow the opening of C3. Disrupting these C2 muscle insertions has been associated with increased postoperative axial neck pain [8] and a greater loss of cervical lordosis postoperatively [9]. Fortunately, patients with multilevel myelopathy often do not have stenosis at the C2/C3 disc level. This is advantageous because then one can start the laminoplasty at C4, which only requires dissecting the muscle off the inferior portion of C3, allowing all muscle attachments on C2 to remain undisturbed. However, patients with stenosis above the level of the C3/C4 disc (e.g., OPLL behind the C3 vertebral body, stenosis at C2/C3, etc.) may require a C3 laminoplasty, necessitating the detachment of at least some of the muscle insertions on C2. In a study by Michael et al., when the most proximal laminoplasty level was at C3, the average postoperative loss of lordosis was 9° compared to only 3° if the most proximal level was C4 [9].

Surgical Technique

Positioning

Proper patient positioning is critical for facilitating a successful surgery and avoiding potential complications. Mayfield tongs are typically used to immobilize the cervical spine and also prevent any pressure on the eyes and face. The patient is then positioned prone onto longitudinal bolsters on the operative table in order to diminish abdominal pressure, and care is taken to pad the knees and lower legs. The foot of the operative bed is then flexed up, which bends the knees and prevents the patient from sliding caudally as the table is placed into a reverse Trendelenburg position in order to decrease venous pressure at the surgical site. Next, the shoulders are gently pulled caudally and taped in this position to both keep them out of the way for lateral x-ray localization and also to reduce redundant skinfolds along the back of the neck. It is important to not tape the shoulders with excessive force, as this may lead to a brachial plexus neurapraxia. The neck is then placed into a neutral to slightly flexed alignment. Avoiding neck extension during positioning is important for a couple of reasons. First, neck extension generally results in further narrowing of the canal diameter and thus can worsen spinal cord compression. Second, neck extension results in more overlap and shingling between adjacent laminae, making the operation more difficult to perform. Typically, once the neck position is properly set during positioning, it does not need to be changed during the laminoplasty procedure. However, if one is performing a fusion in conjunction with laminoplasty, it will be important to reposition the neck into an appropriate amount of lordosis prior to securing the instrumentation.

Anesthesia

When operating on myelopathic patients, it is important to develop a plan with anesthesia. For these patients having symptomatic spinal cord compression, anesthesiologists need to avoid neck extension more than what the patient could tolerate preoperatively. This may necessitate using a video laryngoscope (e.g., GlideScope) or even a fiber-optic intubation in patients who cannot tolerate much neck extension without developing neurologic symptoms or who have difficult airways. Furthermore, it is important to maintain adequate spinal cord perfusion intraoperatively, being especially mindful during anesthetic induction and when raising the head to place the patient in a reverse Trendelenburg position. There is no consensus on the optimal intraoperative blood pressure, but keeping the mean arterial pressure (MAP) above 80 mmHg is a good guideline. Those patients with significant preoperative hypertension may require a higher MAP goal throughout the surgery. An arterial line can be necessary for those with labile blood pressure or when cuff readings are not reliable.

Neurologic Monitoring

Although there are no absolute accepted guidelines, intraoperative neurophysiological monitoring is generally used during laminoplasty. Even though laminoplasty does not involve deformity correction, monitoring still provides potentially useful information. Baseline readings should be obtained just after positioning to serve as a point of comparison throughout the case. Pre-positioning baselines in the supine position may also be considered in those with severe myelopathy to detect any malpositioning when the patient is turned prone, but we do not routinely find this necessary. Excessive cervical traction or extension can adversely affect neuromonitoring signals due to stretching or increased compression of the spinal cord, respectively. Monitoring can also help detect cord hypoperfusion, which can occur from a drop in blood pressure, oxygenation, or hematocrit. It is also helpful for identifying positioning-related nerve compression in the extremities or excessive traction on the brachial plexus from forcefully taping the shoulders.

Even though motor evoked potentials (MEPs) have generally become the standard of care with deformity surgery due to their high sensitivity in detecting neurologic injury during correction maneuvers, the utility of MEPs during laminoplasty remains unclear. MEPs may be more sensitive than somatosensory evoked potentials (SSEPs), but they are less specific and thus more prone to false-positive results as MEPs tend to be more affected by anesthetic and other factors [10]. Opponents of using MEPs during laminoplasty argue that false-positive results require searching for a possible cause, which can lead to increased operative time and unnecessary maneuvers that can be counterproductive (e.g., removing fixation devices that may not be problematic, converting to a full laminectomy to be certain there is no cord compression under the lamina, or possibly even aborting the surgery). As a result, the authors typically use SSEPs, but not MEPs, during routine laminoplasty.

Exposure

The posterior cervical spine is exposed via a midline longitudinal approach, taking care to stay strictly in the midline raphe in order to minimize muscle damage and bleeding. Once down to the spinous processes, exposure is continued subperiosteally along the lamina laterally to just beyond the lateral mass-laminar junction. During the approach, we do not attempt to preserve the supraspinous or interspinous ligaments as the spinous processes will ultimately be removed. If plate fixation will be used, the central portion of the lateral mass will need to be exposed a little further to accommodate the plate. However, the remainder of the facet joint should be kept intact as much as possible. Also, the muscle attachments to C2 and C7 should be left intact whenever possible in order to help preserve the integrity of the cervical extensor mechanism. After exposure has been obtained and the correct levels verified with an intraoperative radiograph, the interspinous ligaments at the top and bottom of the construct are removed. The ligamentum flavum at both ends of the construct can also be excised at this time with a Kerrison rongeur, or it can be removed after the laminae have been opened.

Creating the Opening Trough

The first step is to create the opening trough. By completing the opening trough first, one is able to lift up on the lamina and serially test the "springiness" of the hinge to guide how deep the hinge trough needs to be burred in the next step. In those patients with purely myelopathic findings, the authors favor opening from the side with greater radiographic compression or clinical symptoms. For patients with concomitant root compression, foraminotomies are easier to perform on the open side, although they can be performed on the hinge side. The opening trough is created at the lateral mass-laminar junction by using a burr to go through the dorsal cortex and cancellous bone and thinning down the ventral laminar cortex until there is only a thin shell of bone remaining. Our personal preference is to use a 3 mm matchstick burr to accomplish this. A curette or small Kerrison rongeur is then used to remove the remaining flake of bone. Sufficiently thinning the bone is important as it allows smaller instruments to be used, minimizing canal intrusion, epidural bleeding, and possible spinal cord injury.

Of note, it is often necessary to focus the burring along the cephalad aspect of each lamina as this is the area that tends to be both thicker and potentially covered by the overhang, or "shingling", of the caudal aspect of the superior lamina. Paradoxically, burring in this cephalad region requires extra caution because, whereas the dura is protected by the ligamentum flavum along the inferior portion of the lamina, there is no protective flavum along the cephalad aspect of the lamina. As the lamina is thinned, it becomes somewhat translucent, and one can appreciate the yellowish hue of the underlying ligamentum along the caudal aspect of the lamina and, along the cephalad aspect, the bluish hue of the underlying dura or the crimson of the longitudinal epidural veins. Once this color change is seen, the bone is sufficiently thin enough to be removed with a curette or small Kerrison rongeur. As the lamina is being thinned, a Penfield 4 or angled micro-curette can also be used to periodically palpate whether the lamina has been completely divided or not.

Creating the Hinge Trough

Next, the hinge trough is created at the contralateral lateral mass-laminar junction. However, this time only the dorsal cortex and the cancellous bone are burred away, leaving the rest of the ventral bone intact to serve as a hinge. For the same reasons as discussed above, deeper burring will be needed along the cephalad portion of each lamina. As the hinge is progressively thinned, it is repeatedly tested for pliability by using a nerve hook or curette to lift dorsally along the cut edge of the lamina created during the opening trough. It is important to not thin the bone excessively in order to maintain a "springy" hinge. However, great care must be taken whenever testing the hinge to ensure that the lamina does not accidentally recoil and slam down onto the dural sac. If the hinge becomes completely incompetent at some point during the procedure, either through excessive burring or hinge fracture, it can be reconstructed with a hinge plate that fixates the lamina to the lateral mass on the hinge side, effectively creating a stable "hinge." However, we have found that hinge plates are generally not necessary if stable fixation can be provided on the open side. We prefer to use plate fixation to keep the laminoplasty open, which typically affords enough stability in the setting of an incompetent hinge to allow the hinge side to heal without the need for a hinge plate.

Opening the Laminae and Application of Fixation

Once the opening and hinge troughs have been created, the laminoplasty is sequentially opened by lifting the lamina dorsally away from the canal one level at a time. The surgeon can accomplish this by using a curette to lift dorsally on the cut edge of the lamina while the assistant places an angled curette or nerve hook along the same cut edge to help hold it open. As the lamina is being held open by the assistant, the ligamentum flavum at each segment along the opening side will come under stretch and is resected with a Kerrison rongeur. Similarly, the ligamentum flavum extending across the interlaminar space at the cranial and caudal ends of the construct should be resected at this time if this has not been done already. As the flavum is excised, epidural bleeding may be encountered and should be controlled with bipolar cautery or thrombin-gelfoam. This bleeding can be quite vigorous at times, but will often subside substantially once the entire length of the construct has been opened and the tourniquet effect on the epidural veins is released.

Once the entire length of the laminoplasty has been opened, fixation is applied to maintain this opened position. There are several different techniques for stabilizing and maintaining the expanded canal, including sutures passed around the base of the spinous process and into the hinge side facet (Hirabayashi technique), bone struts (either spinous process autograft or rib allograft) wedged across the open side from the cut edge of the lamina into the lateral mass, or plate fixation. The authors prefer plate fixation as it affords more secure fixation than the alternative methods and is easy and safe to apply. Typically, each level is instrumented with two screws placed into the lateral mass and either one or two screws into the hemi-lamina on the opening side.

According to Matsumoto et al., premature laminoplasty closure occurs in up to 34% of segments with suture fixation, and bone struts can dislodge into the spinal canal causing neurologic compression [11]. In contrast, a study of 217 laminoplasty levels with plate fixation alone and no supplemental bone graft demonstrated no premature closures, plate dislodgements, or plate failures [12]. In addition, CT scans confirmed that 93% of hinges were healed by stringent criteria at 12 months postoperatively and the remaining 7% had a stable fibrous union that maintained an expanded canal without cord compression.

Foraminotomy

Foraminotomies can be done where necessary. However, there is no conclusive evidence on whether prophylactic C4/C5 foraminotomy decreases the incidence of postoperative C5 root palsy. The authors will generally perform a C4/C5 foraminotomy on the opening side after the plate fixation has been applied. However, if a foraminotomy is needed on the hinge side, it should be performed prior to opening the laminoplasty, as this process limits access to the hinge side to perform the foraminotomy.

Occasionally, lateral mass fusion is performed in conjunction with laminoplasty. The benefit of "laminoplasty and fusion" versus "laminectomy and fusion" is that the former provides a larger surface area for bony fusion. However, this is at the expense of using the laminae for local autograft. Additionally, the sequence of instrumentation needs to be appropriately orchestrated because lateral mass screws need to be inserted prior to opening the laminoplasty. In general, we prefer laminectomy and fusion over laminoplasty and fusion for the reasons above.

French-Door Laminoplasty

French-door laminoplasty is similar to the open-door variant discussed above, but involves creating a midline opening trough through the spinous process and bilateral hinge troughs at the lamina-lateral mass junction. The technique for creating the opening and hinge troughs is identical to those used in the open-door procedure. Once all three troughs are created, the hemi-laminae are then opened bilaterally and a graft or plate is inserted in the midline to keep the two doors open. This technique tends to result in less epidural bleeding than the open-door technique because the epidural veins are generally located along the lateral aspect of the spinal canal.

We generally favor the open-door technique because it is simpler and potentially safer to perform because burring is always performed lateral to the spinal cord, thus minimizing the risk for direct injury to the spinal cord during the creation of either the hinge or opening troughs. The French-door technique involves opening the canal directly dorsal to the spinal cord and thus carries with it the potential for spinal cord compression as instruments are used to create the midline opening.

Open-Door Laminoplasty with Unilateral Muscle-Ligament Complex Preservation

This is a variation of the traditional open-door laminoplasty technique discussed earlier that was introduced by Yoshida et al. with the goal of preserving much of the posterior ligaments and muscle attachments along the hinge side of the cervical laminae [13]. Proponents of this procedure tout its lower incidence of postoperative axial neck pain and better maintenance of postoperative cervical alignment and range of motion [14–16].

With this technique, the paraspinal muscles on the opening side are elevated to expose the hemi-laminae (Fig. 11.1a). An osteotomy is then performed at the base of the spinous process to detach the spinous process from the lamina at each of the operative levels (Fig. 11.1b). A hole is then burred through the spinous process (Fig. 11.1c) so that it can be secured to the opened laminae once the laminoplasty is opened. The spinous processes with the preserved unilateral muscular attachments are then retracted toward the hinge side to facilitate exposure of the contralateral lamina-lateral mass junction (Fig. 11.1d), completing the bilateral exposure to allow the creation of the opening and hinge troughs as discussed earlier in this chapter. Just prior to creating the troughs, the hemi-laminae on the opening side are decorticated with a burr (Fig. 11.2a). Once both troughs are made and the laminoplasty opened, a hole is burred through the ipsilateral hemi-lamina at each level (Fig. 11.2b). The previously osteotomized spinous process, with its preserved muscular attachments, is now secured to the surface of the decorticated hemi-laminae to keep the laminoplasty open (Fig. 11.2c). This is accomplished by passing titanium cables through the drill holes in the spinous process and its corresponding hemi-lamina (Fig. 11.2c). A schematic of the final construct is seen in Fig. 11.2d.

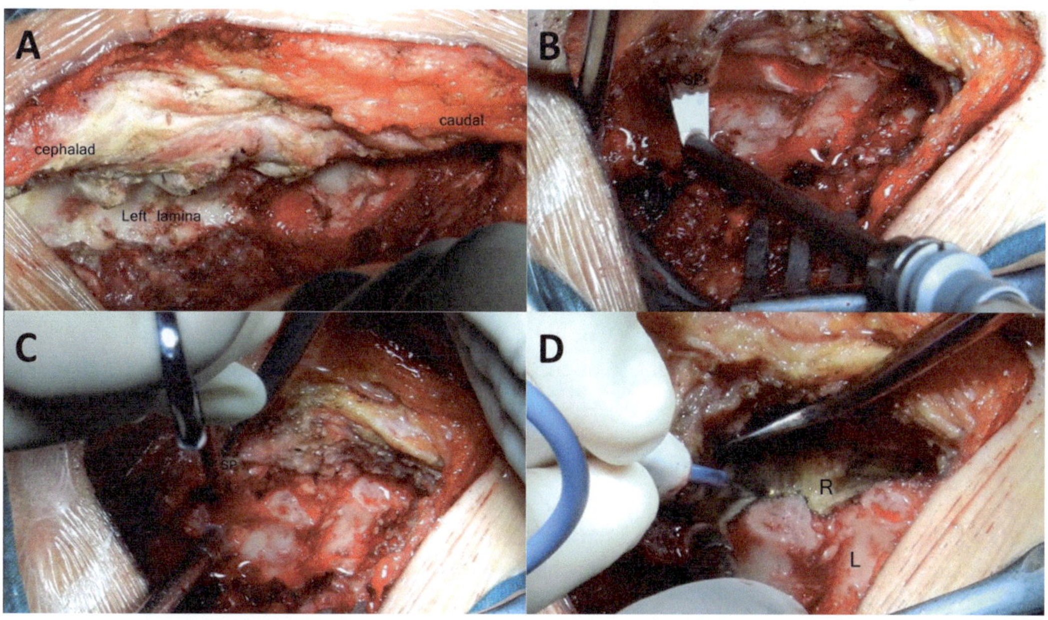

Fig. 11.1 Open-door laminoplasty with unilateral muscle-ligament complex preservation. (**a**) Hemi-laminae on the opening side are exposed. (**b**) Spinous processes are detached at each of the laminoplasty levels. (**c**) A hole is drilled through each detached spinous process for later reattachment to the opened lamina. (**d**) The contralateral hemi-laminae are exposed

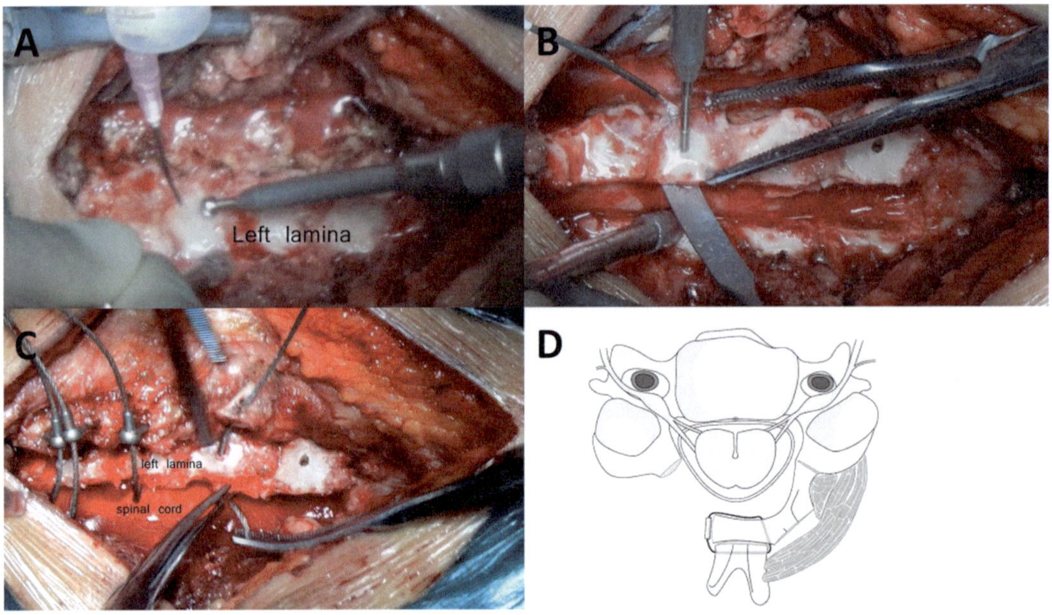

Fig. 11.2 Open-door laminoplasty with unilateral muscle-ligament complex preservation. (**a**) Decortication of the hemi-laminae on the opening side. (**b**) After the opening and hinge troughs are created, a hole is drilled through each hemi-lamina on the opening side. (**c**) At each laminoplasty level, the spinous process is now secured to the previously decorticated hemi-laminae with titanium cable. (**d**) A schematic showing the final laminoplasty construct

Finally, the paraspinal muscles on the opening side are sutured back to the spinous processes and the wound is closed.

Closure

As with any posterior cervical procedure, a layered closure of the muscle, fascia, subcutaneous, and skin layers is important. After a deep drain is placed, the cervical extensor muscles are first reapproximated with Vicryl sutures. This is followed by figure-of-eight stitches to securely close the fascial layer in a watertight fashion. With each interrupted figure-of-eight suture, the fascia is reattached to the underlying muscle. It is important that this fascial layer be accurately identified, especially since it may be retracted laterally by the end of the case when the wound is being closed. The subcutaneous and skin layers are then closed in separate layers and the incision covered with a sterile dressing.

Postoperative Care

Since the goal of laminoplasty is to preserve motion, we do not typically put patients in a cervical collar postoperatively. In fact, we encourage patients to move their necks as tolerated after surgery. Patients are instructed to work on cervical extension as soon as possible and to avoid flexion of the neck. Patients are typically discharged 1–2 days after surgery.

Illustrative Case

History A 78-year-old woman with cervical myelopathy involving the upper and lower extremities. She complained of progressive gait imbalance, hand clumsiness, and numbness and tingling involving the hands. She denied pain, in either the neck or arms.

Physical Exam Preserved strength in the bilateral upper extremities with the exception of 4/5 strength in the bilateral finger flexors and interossei. She has 3+ deep tendon reflexes in the bilateral biceps, brachioradialis, and triceps with a positive Hoffmann's and inverted brachioradialis reflex in both arms.

Radiographical Imaging Preoperative neutral lateral radiograph (Fig. 11.3) demonstrated multilevel spondylosis with preservation of lordosis. Preoperative MRI (Fig. 11.4) showed multilevel cord compression from C3 to C6.

Treatment The patient underwent a C4–C6 open-door laminoplasty and C3 laminectomy without complication (Fig. 11.5).

Outcome Postoperatively, she had rapid improvement in the numbness and tingling in her hands. Over the next several months, her gait gradually improved as did the strength in her finger flexors and interossei. She is over 1 year post-op now and has not had any deterioration in her neurological status.

Technical Pearls

- Positioning the patient with some cervical flexion helps facilitate the operation by decreasing the shingling of the lamina.

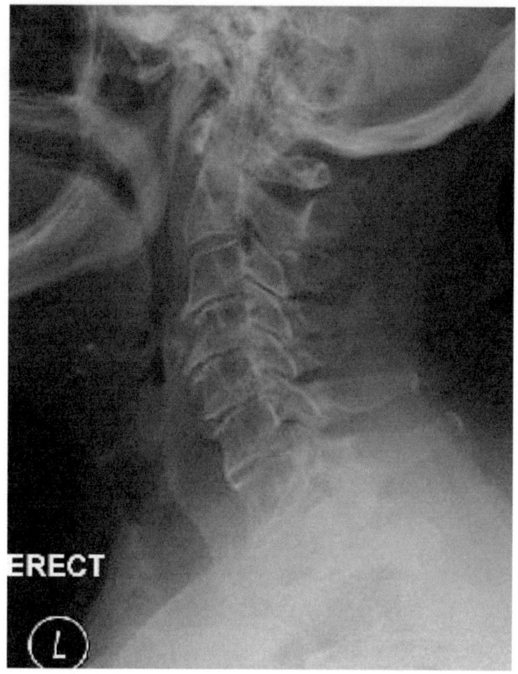

Fig. 11.3 Preoperative neutral lateral cervical radiographg of a 78-year-old woman with progressive cervical myelopathy showing multilevel spondylosis with preservation of lordosis

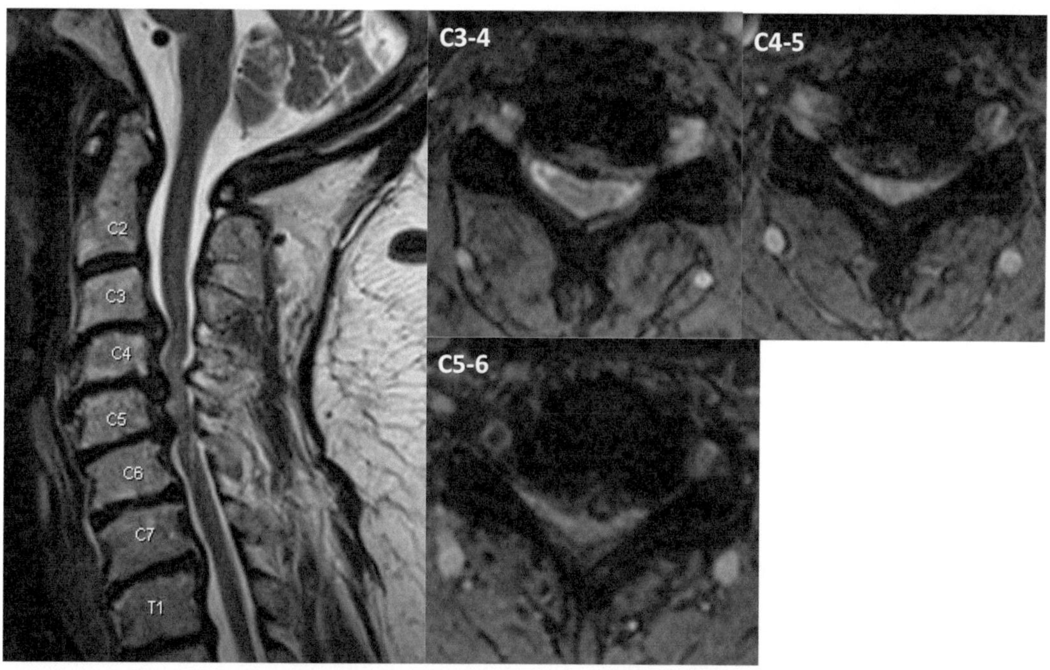

Fig. 11.4 Preoperative cervical MRIg of a 78-year-old woman with progressive cervical myelopathy demonstrating spinal cord compression from C3 to C6

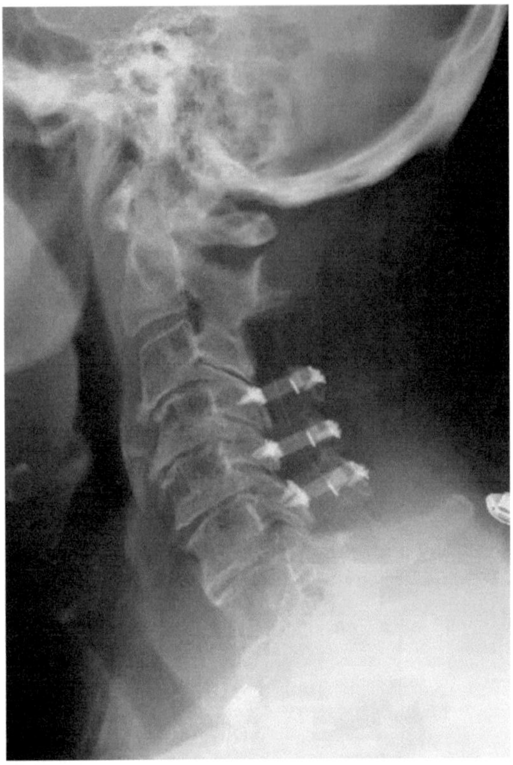

Fig. 11.5 Postoperative neutral lateral cervical radiograph after C3 laminectomy with C4 to C6 open-door laminoplasty

- Keep the patient's blood pressure normotensive and maintain mean arterial blood pressure to a minimum of 80 mm Hg.
- If asymmetric compression is present, it may be beneficial to open the laminoplasty on the more affected side.
- If unilateral foraminotomies are planned, then one should consider making the opening trough on the ipsilateral side as foraminotomies are easier to perform on the opening side of the open-door laminoplasty.
- The cephalad portion of each lamina is thicker and deeper; thus, this region will require more burring than the caudal aspect of the lamina.
- When creating the hinge trough, repeatedly checking how easily the lamina will open is critical for avoiding a hinge that is too stiff on the one hand or too floppy on the other. Be sure that the opening trough is complete before proceeding onto making the hinge; otherwise, it will be impossible to judge how much to thin the hinge bone because the lamina will still be tethered on the opening side.
- To open the laminoplasty, use a curette to lift up on the cut edge of the lamina while the assistant places an angled curette or nerve hook along the same cut edge and holds the lamina open. Repeat this for each level of the laminoplasty.

Complications and Strategies for Avoidance

Axial Neck Pain

Laminoplasty has often been associated with symptomatic postoperative axial neck pain. However, the literature is not clear as to whether this pain is simply a persistence of preoperative spondylotic pain or de novo pain postoperatively. There are mixed reports on this phenomenon as some have published a relatively high rate of new-onset postoperative neck pain [17], while others contend that persistence of preoperative pain is more common [18].

In the authors' experience, appropriate patient selection is the most critical factor to avoiding postoperative axial neck pain. Typically, those who deny significant neck pain preoperatively do not develop long-term axial pain postoperatively, which is why we believe laminoplasty is indicated for patients without significant preoperative spondylosis or axial neck pain. On the other hand, patients with severe preoperative axial neck pain who undergo laminoplasty will likely have a worsening, or at least lack of resolution, of that pain postoperatively. Of note, there is literature to support that preserving the C2 muscle attachments diminishes postoperative axial pain [8].

Loss of Cervical Lordosis

Even though laminoplasty was developed as a means to avoid post-laminectomy kyphosis, some loss of lordosis does occur even with laminoplasty. Fortunately, it is rarely of the catastrophic variety that can be seen with multilevel laminectomy without fusion. According to Suk et al., patients tend to lose approximately 5° of lordosis after C3–C7 open-door laminoplasty, and 11% developed postoperative kyphosis [19]. As discussed earlier, a recent study demonstrated that starting the laminoplasty at C4 results in less loss of lordosis than if the laminoplasty extends up to C3 [9]. Another risk factor for postoperative kyphosis is a preoperative lordosis <10°, which is why we recommend laminoplasty for patients with well-preserved lordosis. Patients with kyphotic cervical spines may be better candidates for laminectomy and fusion, anterior surgery, or combined anterior-posterior surgery.

Wound Complications

Postoperative infection can occur, as with any surgical procedure, and it is well documented that posterior cervical procedures, including laminoplasty, are associated with higher rates of infection (approximately 1–2%) than anterior cervical surgery. Meticulous attention to sterile technique and multilayered closure may be helpful in decreasing infection rates. During closure, the authors routinely use a subfascial drain and approximate the cervical extensor muscles prior to performing a watertight fascial closure to diminish the dead space within the surgical bed.

Neurologic Injury

Fortunately, iatrogenic spinal cord injury is a rare complication during laminoplasty. As emphasized previously, whenever testing the hinge or opening the laminoplasty, great care must be taken to prevent the laminae from recoiling back onto the dura and injuring the spinal cord.

What is more common is the development of a postoperative root palsy, which has a reported incidence of 5–12% after laminoplasty and most commonly affects the C5 root resulting in deltoid and/or biceps weakness [20]. C5 root palsies may also occur with laminectomy, laminectomy and fusion, and even anterior cervical surgery, but direct comparison of rates among the different approaches remains controversial in the current literature. These root palsies tend to be motor-dominant, but sensory dysfunction and radicular pain are also possible. Although this complication can present at any point postoperatively, from immediately to a few weeks after surgery, it typically presents a few days after the procedure. Several theories have been proposed as to its etiology, but it is most likely multifactorial and may involve stretching of the involved root as the cord drifts into the decompressed space. As alluded to previously, the utility of prophylactic foraminotomy in lowering the rate of postoperative root palsy is unclear. Recovery of useful motor function usually occurs over 6–12 months in the majority of patients, though some will be left with residual deficits.

Conclusion

Multilevel cervical stenosis with resultant myelopathy is a problem with several possible solutions. Multilevel anterior cervical discectomy and fusion can effect neurologic decompression, but pseudoarthrosis, dysphagia, and dysphonia are real concerns when multiple levels are being addressed. Additionally, conditions like OPLL can make an anterior approach less desirable. An alternative is multilevel posterior cervical decompression and fusion; however this procedure sacrifices cervical motion and is associated with higher implant costs and the potential for accelerated adjacent segment degeneration. Laminoplasty, on the other hand, is a safe, motion-preserving operation that can effectively decompress the spinal cord in the properly selected multilevel cervical spondylotic myelopathy patient, i.e., those with little to no axial neck pain, no significant cervical instability, and a lordotic cervical alignment.

References

1. Hamanishi C, Tanaka S. Bilateral multilevel laminectomy with or without posterolateral fusion for cervical spondylotic myelopathy: relationship to type of onset and time until operation. J Neurosurg. 1996;85(3):447–51.

2. Herkowitz HN. A comparison of anterior cervical fusion, cervical laminectomy, and cervical laminoplasty for the surgical management of multiple level spondylotic radiculopathy. Spine. 1988;13(7):774–80.
3. Hirabayashi K, Watanabe K, Wakano K. Expansive open-door laminoplasty for cervical spinal stenotic myelopathy. Spine. 1983;8(7):693–9.
4. Fujiyoshi T, Yamazaki M, Kawabe J, Endo T, Furuya T, Koda M, et al. A new concept for making decisions regarding the surgical approach for cervical ossification of the posterior longitudinal ligament: the K-line. Spine. 2008;33(26):E990–3.
5. Shiraishi T. Skip laminectomy—a new treatment for cervical spondylotic myelopathy, preserving bilateral muscular attachments to the spinous processes: a preliminary report. Spine J. 2002;2:108–15.
6. Yuan W, Zhu Y, Liu X, Zhou X, Cui C. Laminoplasty versus skip laminectomy for the treatment of multilevel cervical spondylotic myelopathy: a systematic review. Arch Orthop Trauma Surg. 2014;134(1):1–7.
7. Mukai Y, Hosono N, Sakaura H, Ishii T, Fuchiya T, Fijiwara K, et al. Laminoplasty for cervical myelopathy caused by subaxial lesions in rheumatoid arthritis. J Neurosurg. 2004;100(1 Suppl Spine):7–12.
8. Kato M, Nakamura H, Konishi S, Dohzono S, Toyoda H, Fukushima W, et al. Effect of preserving paraspinal muscles on postoperative axial pain in the selective cervical laminoplasty. Spine. 2008;33(14):E455–9.
9. Michael KW, Neustein TM, Rhee JM. Where should a laminoplasty start? The effect of the proximal level on post-laminoplasty loss of lordosis. Spine J. 2016;16:737–41.
10. Kim DH, Zaremski J, Kwon B, Jenis L, Woodard E. Risk factors for false positive transcranial motor evoked potential monitoring alerts during surgical treatment of cervical myelopathy. Spine. 2007;32:3041–6.
11. Matsumoto M, Watanabe K, Tsuji T, Ishii K, Takaishi H, Nakamura M, et al. Risk factors for closure of lamina after open-door laminoplasty. J Neurosurg Spine. 2008;9(6):530–7.
12. Rhee JM, Register B, Hamasaki T, Franklin B. Plate-only open door laminoplasty maintains stable spinal canal expansion with high rates of hinge union and no plate failures. Spine. 2011;36(1):9–14.
13. Yoshida M, Otani K, Shibasaki K, Ueda S. Expansive laminoplasty with reattachment of spinous process and extensor musculature for cervical myelopathy. Spine. 1992;17(5):491–7.
14. Kotani Y, Abumi K, Ito M, Sudo H, Takahata M, Ohshima S, et al. Minimum 2-year outcome of cervical laminoplasty with deep extensor muscle-preserving approach: impact on cervical spine function and quality of life. Eur Spine J. 2009;18(5):663–71.
15. Takeuchi K, Yokoyama T, Ono A, Numasawa T, Wada K, Kumagai G, et al. Cervical range of motion and alignment after laminoplasty preserving or reattaching the semispinalis cervicis inserted into axis. J Spinal Disord Tech. 2007;20(8):571–6.
16. Sakaura H, Hosono N, Mukai Y, Iwasaki M, Yoshikawa H. Medium-term outcomes of C3-6 laminoplasty for cervical myelopathy: a prospective study with a minimum 5-year follow-up. Eur Spine J. 2011;20(6):928–33.
17. Hosono N, Yonenobu K, Ono K. Neck and shoulder pain after laminoplasty. A noticeable complication. Spine. 1996;21(17):1969–73.
18. Yoshida M, Tamaki T, Kawakami M, Nakatani N, Ando M, Yamada H, et al. Does reconstruction of posterior ligamentous complex with extensor musculature decrease axial symptoms after cervical laminoplasty? Spine. 2002;27(13):1414–8.
19. Suk K-S, Kim K-T, Lee J-H, Lee S-H, Lim Y-J, Kim J-S. Sagittal alignment of the cervical spine after the laminoplasty. Spine. 2007;32(23):E656–60.
20. Uematsu Y, Tokuhashi Y, Matsuzaki H. Radiculopathy after laminoplasty of the cervical spine. Spine. 1998;23:2057–62.

Minimally Invasive Posterior Cervical Fusion Techniques

12

Carolina Gesteira Benjamin
and Anthony Frempong-Boadu

Introduction

Posterior cervical fusion techniques have been employed to address acute as well as chronic pathologies. These techniques can be used in the setting of trauma or instability requiring stabilization of the axial or subaxial spine. Alternatively, it can be used for decompression and stabilization in the setting of cervical spondylotic myelopathy, one of the leading causes of chronic degenerative neurologic decline [1, 2]. Specifically, minimally invasive posterior cervical fusion techniques provide an alternative to traditional open procedures. Minimally invasive techniques were initially limited to decompressive procedures but are now commonly used for instrumentation and fusion as well [3–5].

The safety and efficacy of minimally invasive posterior cervical decompression was initially described by Adamson and then subsequently by Fessler and Khoo [3, 4, 6]. Wang et al. later described the safety and efficacy of minimally invasive posterior cervical fusion techniques. The long-term results of these minimally invasive fusion techniques were described by Wang and Levi, where they found no complications or pseudarthroses at 2 years. Similar findings were again confirmed by Fong and DuPlessis and other series [7–9]. Over the last decade, there has been a noticeable shift toward minimally invasive procedures. This is likely multifactorial, including improvements in the technology of the tubular retractor systems, improvements in intraoperative imaging, and the natural learning curve for surgeons incorporating these techniques into their practice.

With appropriate patient selection and surgical technique, minimally invasive procedures can achieve the same goal as open procedures while minimizing complications.

One of the main advantages to this technique is that it maintains the integrity of the posterior tension band. Additionally, it minimizes muscle dissection, which decreases surgical blood loss and postoperative pain, thus shortening hospital stays [10–13]. Finally, it also decreases prolonged muscle retraction which can lead to devascularization and denervation injury as has been previously described in animal models, as well as in the lumbar spine [14, 15]. The goal of this chapter is to elucidate the process of patient selection for such procedures and to detail the nuances of the surgical technique.

C.G. Benjamin, MD (✉) • A. Frempong-Boadu, MD
Department of Neurosurgery, NYU Langone Medical Center, 530 First Avenue Suite 8R, New York, NY 10016, USA
e-mail: Carolina.benjamin@nyumc.org; Anthony.frempong-boadu@nyumc.org

L.T. Holly, P.A. Anderson (eds.), *Essentials of Spinal Stabilization*,
DOI 10.1007/978-3-319-59713-3_12

Indications and Patient Selection

Patient Selection

The choice of surgical approach is largely determined by the patient's clinical picture as well as image findings. Patients eligible for posterior cervical decompression and fusion include those with progressive symptoms of myelopathy including motor or sensory deficits, gait instability, and bowel or bladder dysfunction. Patients with C1–C2 instability secondary to chronic processes such as rheumatoid arthritis and os odontoideum or more acute processes such as odontoid fractures can also be good candidates for posterior cervical fusion. If cervical pathology extends over several segments, a posterior approach is preferred over an anterior approach by some surgeons [5]. Furthermore, for patients undergoing multi-level anterior decompression, posterior supplementation can be considered to prevent hardware subsidence as bony fusion takes place [16].

Generally, these aforementioned indications are suitable for patients undergoing either open or minimally invasive techniques. One important consideration is that minimally invasive posterior cervical fusions are generally limited to three vertebral levels.

Patients with a rotatory component to their atlantoaxial instability may not be good candidates for minimally invasive procedures as the anatomy can be distorted. Additionally, in order to correct the rotatory component, it may be necessary to release the muscular and ligamentous attachments, thus making a minimally invasive approach not feasible. Patients with a significant kyphotic deformity or sagittal imbalance should not be addressed from a solely posterior approach and are not good candidates for minimally invasive approaches [17]. Finally, the patient's body habitus is also an important consideration as it can make intraoperative visualization of bony landmarks a challenge.

Radiographic Imaging

Imaging studies including MRI and computerized tomography (CT) should be obtained to confirm the presence of cervical compressive pathology. The most common pathologies causing compression of the spinal cord include osteophytes, ossified posterior longitudinal ligament, and hypertrophied ligamentum flavum. This can lead to intrinsic T2 signal change in the spinal cord or myelomalacia if present for prolonged periods of time.

Obtaining a CT scan with sagittal and coronal reconstructions is particularly important for evaluation of the bony anatomy to determine orientation of the facet joints, the size of the lateral masses and pedicles, and the location and course of the vertebral artery within the foramen transversarium. If it appears that the vertebral artery has a tortuous or unconventional course, a CT angiogram can be obtained to evaluate its course. This can be useful for surgical planning in order to avoid intraoperative injury [18].

Flexion-extension plain radiographs should also be part of the diagnostic workup. In the setting of atlantoaxial pathology, flexion-extension radiographs can provide information about the presence and degree of dynamic instability.

Preoperative Considerations

Patient Counseling

The goals of surgery and, specifically, the advantages and disadvantages of a minimally invasive approach must be made clear to the patient. Rather than reverse neurologic damage, the goal of this surgery is to prevent further neurologic decline from compressive pathology or instability. While this approach attempts to minimize complications, there is still the potential for neurologic injury that can be clinically relevant.

These risks include damage to neurologic structures including the spinal cord itself or a nerve root leading to motor deficits, sensory deficits, bowel and bladder dysfunction, or focal weakness such as a deltoid palsy. There is also a possibility of vascular complications such as an epidural hematoma requiring re-operation or a vertebral artery injury that can lead to stroke or death. Additionally, minimally invasive approaches introduce the possibility of cerebral spinal fluid leaks that can be difficult to repair and can lead to fistulas or wound complications in the long term. Delayed complications are similar to that of open procedures and can include hardware breakdown, failure of fusion, or adjacent segment disease.

It is important to counsel patients that if the goals of surgery cannot be adequately achieved through minimally invasive methods, there is always the possibility that the procedure will be converted to an open procedure. Patients must understand prior to surgery that this does not represent a failure of the procedure, but rather a dynamic intraoperative decision made to successfully achieve the goals of surgery while avoiding complications.

Anesthesia and Positioning

Minimally invasive posterior cervical procedures are performed under general anesthesia. In all patients undergoing an operation for cervical stenosis or instability, particular attention must be paid to the alignment of the neck during intubation. Neutral positioning should be maintained at all times. For patients with instability secondary to fractures, a cervical collar must be kept in place during intubation and an asleep fiberoptic intubation should be performed. For patients whose symptoms are exacerbated by gentle motion or with a tenuous neurologic exam, an awake fiberoptic intubation should be considered. The endotracheal tube should be tightly secured using tape. During positioning, the circuit should be disconnected and the anesthesiologist should be aware of the endotracheal tube at all times to prevent unintentional extubation.

An arterial line should be placed in order to monitor mean arterial blood pressure continuously throughout the procedure. The blood pressure should be maintained in the normotensive range and can be increased pharmacologically if there is concern for decreased spinal cord perfusion during a particular portion of the procedure, such as the decompression. A Foley catheter can be placed by the surgical team if deemed necessary. A single dose of prophylactic antibiotics should be given by the anesthesia team within 1 hour of start time.

The eyes should be protected with occlusive bandages to prevent mechanical injury or chemical burns from prep solutions during the time the patient is in the prone position. The head is fixed to a Mayfield three-point fixation device (Integra LifeSciences Corporation, Cincinnati, Ohio). The patient is carefully turned into the prone position on an operating table with two parallel gel rolls. The Mayfield head holder is attached to the operating table. The head is positioned in slight military flexion for fusion procedures of the subaxial spine. The degree of flexion can be increased during positioning for atlantoaxial fusions so as to open up the space between C1 and C2. In the setting of fractures, a hard cervical collar should be in place during the flip, and the head adjustments for final positioning should be done under fluoroscopic guidance in order to reduce and align the fractured segments. If necessary, tape can be used to retract the shoulders caudally and should be secured to the operating table. The feet should be elevated and the operating room table should be placed in reverse Trendelenburg for final positioning. This, along with avoidance of hypotension, helps prevent postoperative visual loss. A fluoroscopy machine should be available for image guidance throughout the entirety of the procedure. Alternatively, three-dimensional fluoroscopy and CT-based image guidance have also been used to increase accuracy of hardware placement [19].

Neurophysiologic Monitoring

Neurophysiologic monitoring should be used during all minimally invasive posterior decompression and fusions. Baseline somatosensory evoked potentials (SSEPs) and motor evoked potentials (MEPs) should be obtained once the patient is asleep. If there are residual paralytics on board after intubation, it may not be possible to obtain baseline signals. In order to obtain reliable signals throughout the case, total intravenous anesthesia must be used.

Any change in neurophysiologic monitoring throughout the case must be taken seriously. A methodical approach should be taken to address this. First, the neurophysiologic monitoring team should ensure that all electrodes are appropriately positioned and connected. Second, the anesthesiologist must ensure that the patient is still under total intravenous anesthesia and that the patient has not received any volatile anesthetics or paralytics. Third, the surgeon should ensure there is no structural compression of the neural structures in the surgical field. It may be necessary to reverse the steps of the operation back to the point where neurophysiologic monitoring was stable. Once all of the above steps have been confirmed, one can consider increasing the mean arterial pressure greater than 85 to increase perfusion to the spinal cord [20]. The patient's core body temperature should also be brought to normal ranges as this can affect neurophysiologic monitoring as well as anesthetic metabolism [21]. Finally, one can consider a wake-up test if none of the aforementioned interventions have worked.

Surgical Technique

MIS Atlantoaxial Fixation

Once the patient is in the appropriate position, the fluoroscopy machine should be brought in to confirm appropriate reduction at C1–C2. The midline is marked and a starting point 2–2.5 cm lateral to the midline is chosen (Fig. 12.1). Alternatively, a slightly larger midline skin incision can be made and taken down to the fascia, and then the fascial incision can be made off midline. The trajectory is defined by inserting a spinal needle parallel to the C2 spinous process under fluoroscopic guidance. This trajectory leads to the C2 lateral mass. The skin is incised sharply at the previously marked incision centered around the spinal needle. Monopolar electrocautery is used to dissect through the subcutaneous tissues until fascia is reached. A small cut is made in the fascia using the monopolar electrocautery, and the smallest dilator from

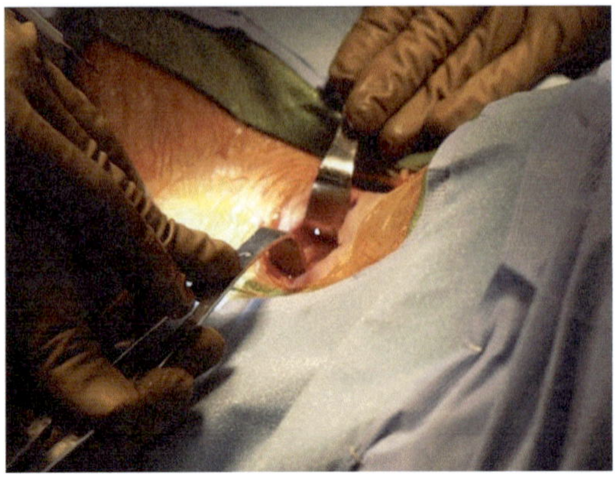

Fig. 12.1 For minimally invasive atlantoaxial fusions, the incision should be made 2–2.5 cm off midline. The spinous process of C2 can be used as a landmark and this can be confirmed with lateral fluoroscopy

the Quadrant retractor set (Medtronic Sofamor Danek, Memphis, TN) is passed down to the lamina of C2. It is important to sharply incise the cervical fascia. It is thick and requires a considerable amount of force to pass the serial dilators which could lead to violation of the canal and spinal cord injury if the fascia is not sharply incised. A working channel is created by passing serial dilators (Fig. 12.2). The retractor is then placed over the dilators and is fixed to the bed using a flexible arm (Fig. 12.3). The retractor is opened superficially with the crank system and then flared out at its depth. The dilators are removed taking care not to dislodge the positioning of the retractor (Fig. 12.4). This provides good exposure from the C1 lateral mass to the C3 lateral mass.

The monopolar is used to complete the subperiosteal dissection for exposure of the C2 lateral mass. The C2 pars is then traced along its superior border until the C1–C2 facet joint is reached. It is then dissected and exposed using bipolar cautery and scissors. The C2 nerve root is coagulated using bipolar electrocautery and cut to allow for better visualization of and access to the C1–C2 facet joint. This is well tolerated with minimal numbness in the C2 dermatome distribution and allows for improved surgical visualization as well as increasing the surface area for decortication and arthrodesis [22]. The dissection is also continued cranially for exposure of the inferior portion of the C1 lateral

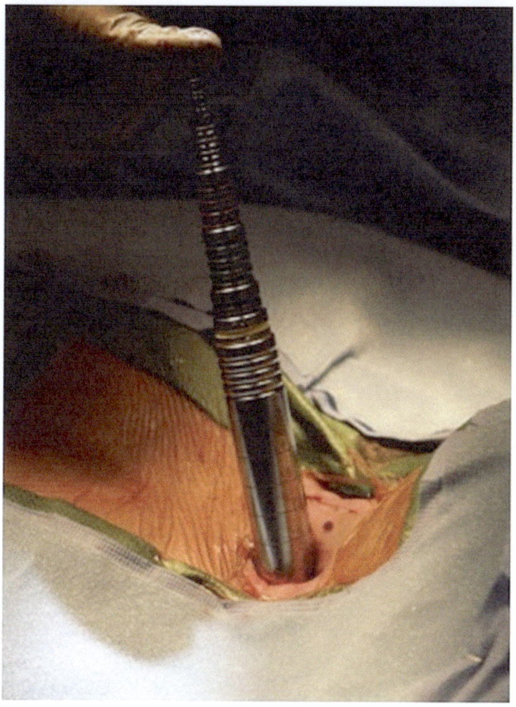

Fig. 12.2 Image that depicts the working channel created by the serial dilators. It is important to sharply incise the thick cervical fascia prior to passing the dilators so as to prevent violation of the canal and injury to neurovascular elements

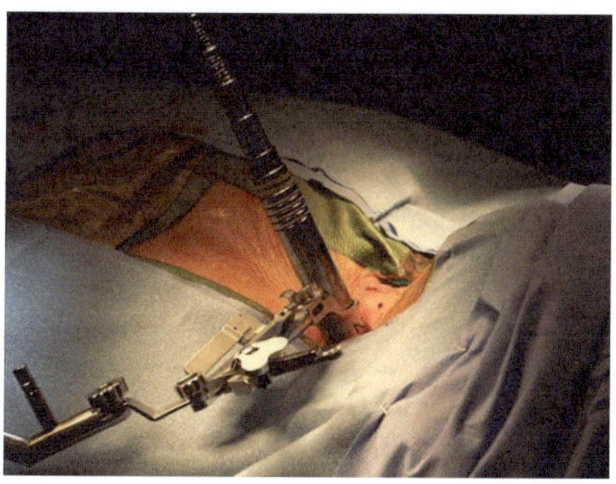

Fig. 12.3 The configuration of the retractor system passed over the dilators and fixed to the bed using a flexible arm. Care must be taken when removing the dilators so as to not dislodge the retractor system

mass. Throughout this dissection, the surgeon must always maintain awareness of the location of the vertebral artery in the sulcus arteriosus on the superior surface of the C1 lamina.

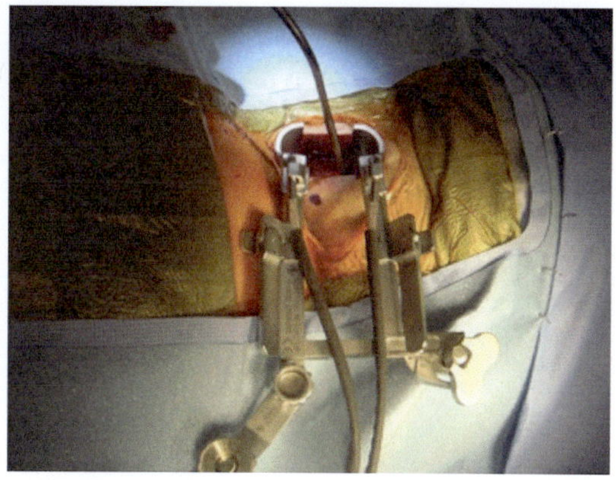

Fig. 12.4 Retractor system in place opened superficially with the crank system and flared out at its depth to allow for adequate visualization from C1 to C3

Once the anatomy is adequately exposed, focus can be shifted to instrumentation and arthrodesis. The C1–C2 facet joint is opened using a small upgoing curette. A micro-facet shaver (Medtronic Cornerstone, Memphis, TN) is used to clean off the C1–C2 facet joint. The articular surface is then decorticated. The facet joint is packed with allograft bone chips mixed with a cancellous matrix, a facet micrograft, or a cervical facet unloading implant. The C1 lateral mass and C2 pedicle screws are placed under fluoroscopic guidance using the trajectory and technique described by Harms and Melcher [23] (Figs. 12.5 and 12.6). A rod is then cut, fit into the polyaxial screw heads, and fixed into place with set screws (Fig. 12.7). This is final tightened using a torque/counter-torque device. The procedure is completed bilaterally. The wounds are copiously irrigated and closed in multiple layers. There is no need for the placement of drains given the small size of the wounds.

Subaxial Fixation

The patient is positioned prone as previously described and lateral fluoroscopy is used throughout the case. A 2–2.5 cm midline skin incision is made with the entry point centered at two spinal segments below the intended level of instrumentation. Monopolar electrocautery is used to dissect through the soft tissues until fascia

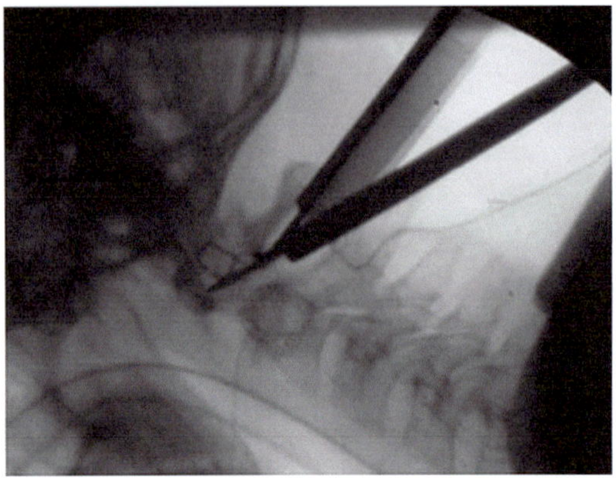

Fig. 12.5 Lateral fluoroscopic image of placement of C1 lateral mass pilot hole through a minimally invasive approach using a tubular retractor system

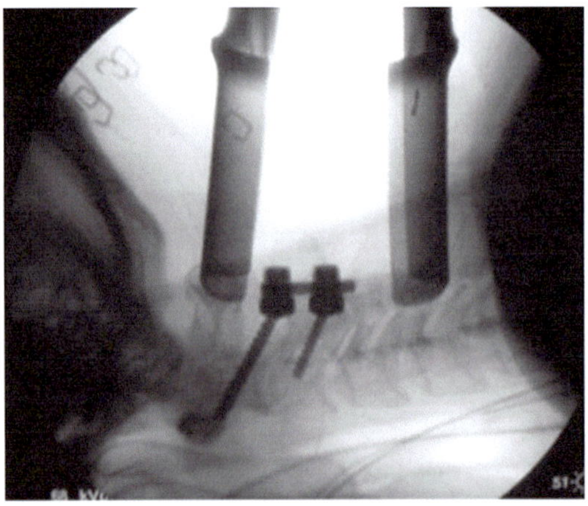

Fig. 12.6 Lateral fluoroscopic image of placement of C1–C2 screw and rod construct placed using a minimally invasive approach

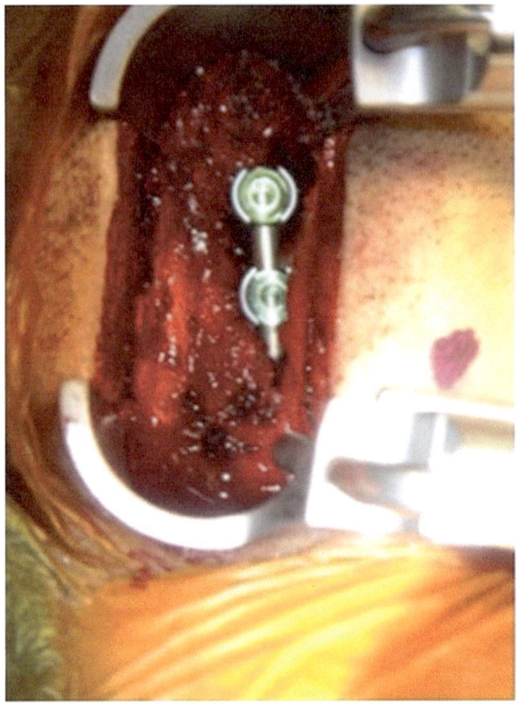

Fig. 12.7 Intraoperative image of the C1–C2 screw and rod construct as visualized through the tubular retractor system

is noted. The fascia is sharply incised using monopolar electrocautery to allow for the passage of the dilators. Serial dilators from the Quadrant retractor set (Medtronic Sofamor Danek, Memphis, TN) are placed in a trajectory that is parallel to the facet joint in the sagittal plane, hence the reason why the entry point must be two levels below the intended level. An expandable tubular retractor is placed over the dilators, directed superolaterally in the intended trajectory of the screw, and then fixed to the bed using a flexible bed-mounted arm. Using the crank system, the retractor is then opened superficially and flared out at the depth of the exposure. Once the retractor is secured into place, monopolar electrocautery is used to clean off the overlying muscle and soft tissue so as to expose the lateral mass. The facet joints are cleaned off using small curettes and are then decorticated to act as a surface for arthrodesis.

At this juncture, attention is paid to screw placement. With the retractor in place, the superior, inferior, medial, and lateral borders of the lateral mass should be identified for the placement of each hole. The pilot hole can be performed with a high-speed drill or an awl and should be placed 1 mm medial and 1mm inferior to the hillock of the lateral mass. Next, a power or hand twist drill set to a fixed depth is used to drill a hole within the lateral mass using the Magerl technique [24, 25]. The drill is aimed 20–30° cranially to avoid the neural foramen and 20 to 30° laterally to avoid the vertebral artery within foramen transversarium.

The hole is then prepared with a 3.5 mm tap, and bicortical cervical polyaxial lateral mass screws measuring either 3.5 or 4 mm in diameter and 14 or 16 mm in length are placed. Slight adjustments of the retractors are made to allow for the placement of the screws at adjacent levels. After the screws are placed on one side, a connecting rod is placed down the retractor lengthwise and then advanced cranially toward the superior polyaxial screw head. The retractor is then adjusted and lifted up slightly in order for the inferior end of the rod to fit into the polyaxial head of the screw at the caudal end of the construct. Locking cap screws are then placed and a torque/counter-torque device is used to final tighten. This same procedure is carried out bilaterally. The wound is copiously irrigated. The fascial incisions are closed and then the midline incision is closed in multiple layers. Again, given the small size of the wound, a drain is not necessary.

Postoperative Management

Given the small incisions and minimal muscle retraction, the postoperative pain that patients experience is minimal compared to open procedures. This is beneficial for purposes of early mobilization which helps prevent deep venous thrombotic complications. Additionally, the blood loss is significantly less during these procedures [9, 11, 13, 26]. The absence of postoperative anemia precludes the need for aggressive resuscitation with intravenous fluids, and this also helps patients mobilize more quickly after minimally invasive procedures. Finally, patients require smaller doses of narcotics which prevent postoperative urinary retention and constipation. All of these factors shorten the length of the hospital stay and allow patients to begin physical and occupational therapy to maximize their functional status.

The decision to use a soft cervical collar, a rigid cervical collar, or no collar at all depends on the patient's preoperative pathology and intraoperative findings. In the setting of instability, patients can be kept in a rigid cervical collar in the acute postoperative setting. Lateral and anteroposterior (AP) cervical spine x-rays are obtained either intraoperatively or postoperatively to evaluate the spinal instrumentation. A CT may be obtained if there is a particular concern about the instrumentation secondary to intraoperative difficulties. There is no need for routine use of steroids postoperatively. Nonsteroidal agents should be avoided for 3 months. The patients should be evaluated at 2 weeks for an initial neurologic and wound check and then followed sequentially with x-rays to inspect the hardware as well as assess for evidence of fusion.

Illustrative Case A 54-year-old male presented to the hospital after a fall while intoxicated complaining of neck pain. A CT of the cervical spine for evaluation of trauma revealed a Type II odontoid fracture. It was also noted on the preoperative CT scan that the patient had a high riding vertebral artery groove and a small C2 isthmus (Fig. 12.8). The patient was neurologically intact at presentation.

He underwent a C1–C3 minimally invasive posterior instrumented fusion. C1 lateral mass screws were successfully placed under fluoroscopic guidance using the technique described by Harms and Melcher [23]. Given the findings on the CT scan, the anatomy prohibited the placement of adequate C2 pedicle screws (Fig. 12.9). Therefore, the decision was made to place short C2 pars screws and extend the construct down to C3 for further supplementation (Fig. 12.10). The patient remained neurologically intact and his neck pain improved after surgery. At his 2-year follow-up, dynamic imaging revealed a stable construct, and the patient continued to do well clinically. It is important to note from this case that a minimally invasive approach does not preclude the ability to extend the construct as needed based on patient-specific anatomy.

Technical Pearls

- Minimally invasive cervical fusions are difficult due to limited access to the anatomic landmarks that are normally available in an open procedure. One of the keys is being able

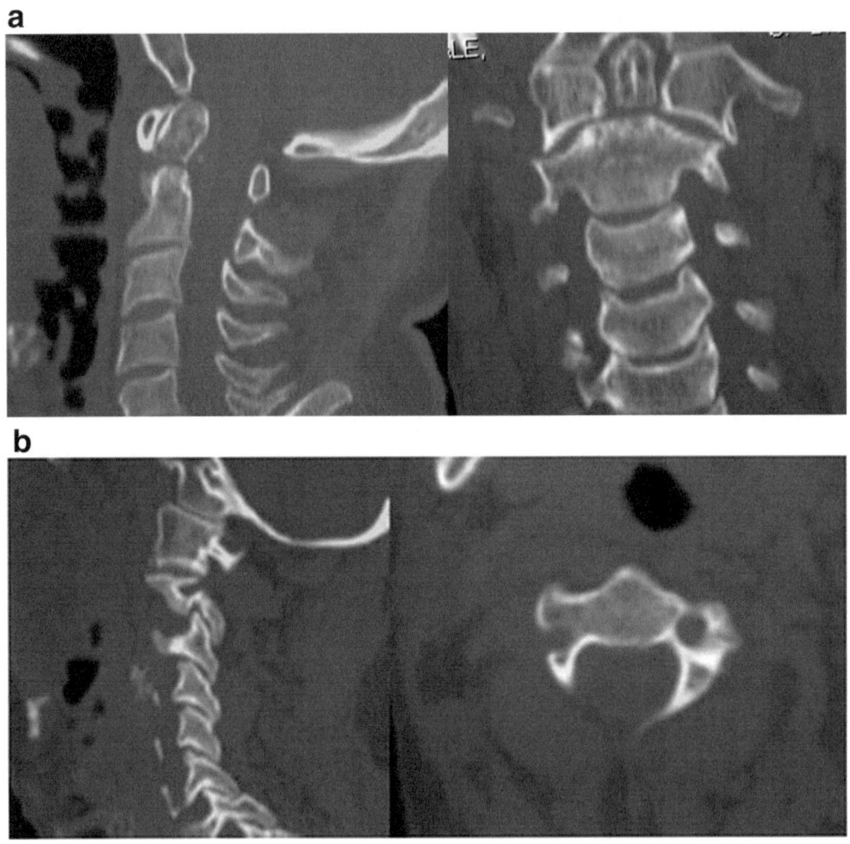

Fig. 12.8 (**a**) Sagittal and coronal computerized tomography (CT) images revealing a Type II odontoid fracture. (**b**) Sagittal and axial computerized tomography (CT) images revealing high riding vertebral artery groove and a small C2 isthmus which precluded the placement of C2 pedicle screws. Consequently, the decision was made preoperatively to extend the construct to C3

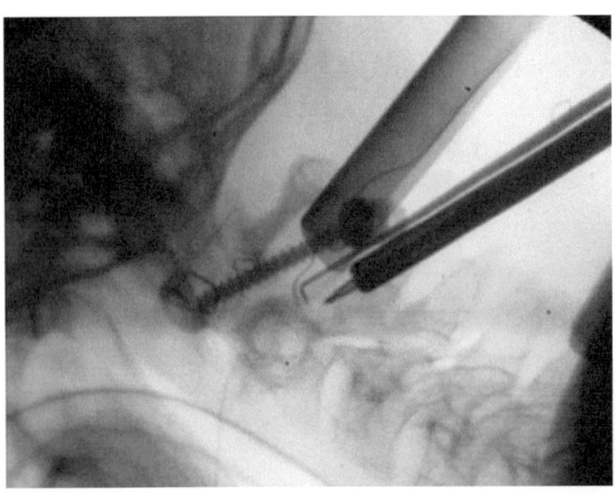

Fig. 12.9 Lateral fluoroscopic image of the placement of C1 lateral mass and short C2 pars screws in a patient whose anatomy was not suitable for placement of C2 pedicle screws

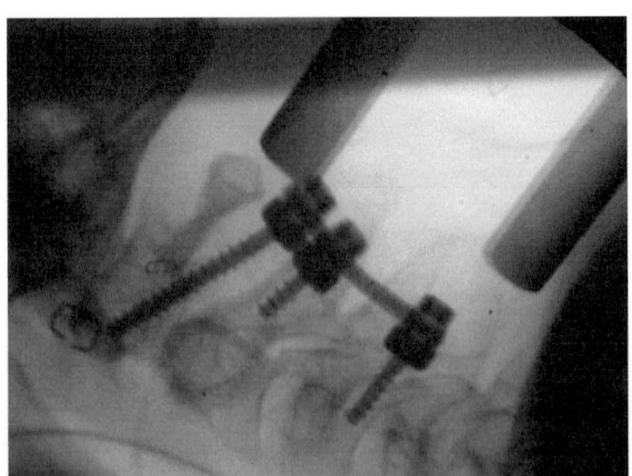

Fig. 12.10 Lateral fluoroscopic image of the C1–C3 construct for the same patient

to use fluoroscopic guidance as an adjunct in order to correctly place the hardware.

- In the case of atlantoaxial fixation, the identification of the C1–C2 facet joint and its orientation is critical not only to identify the starting point for the C1 lateral mass screw but also from an arthrodesis standpoint. Some authors advocate for inferior retraction of the C2 nerve root. However, we feel that sacrificing this nerve root for better visualization of the anatomy is one of keys to success in this procedure and carries minimal consequence.

Complications and Strategies for Avoidance

Given the limited working space in minimally invasive procedures, intraoperative complications can be difficult to manage. Again, as previously mentioned, it is crucial to obtain and interpret fluoroscopic images as a guide to assist in finding the correct anatomic landmarks that dictate the starting point for the instrumentation so as to prevent misplacing hardware. One of the most dangerous complications when performing a minimally invasive atlantoaxial fusion is injury to the vertebral artery. If this occurs, a screw should immediately be placed in the pilot hole to tamponade the bleeding. The case should be aborted at this point and the contralateral screw should not be placed in order to avoid bilateral vertebral artery injuries. If vertebral artery injury occurs during the approach, it may be necessary to hold pressure and convert to an open procedure. The patient will need to have postoperative angiography to assess and treat any intraoperative vertebral artery injuries.

Conclusion

Minimally invasive posterior cervical instrumentation is a valuable technique that should be in the armamentarium of all complex spine surgeons. In the properly selected patient, these techniques reduce approach-related complications, blood loss, and postoperative pain, while preserving the efficacy of open posterior cervical fusions.

References

1. Young WF. Cervical spondylotic myelopathy: a common cause of spinal cord dysfunction in older persons. Am Fam Physician. 2000;62(5):1064–1070, 1073.
2. Emery SE. Cervical spondylotic myelopathy: diagnosis and treatment. J Am Acad Orthop Surg. 2001;9(6):376–88.
3. Fessler RG, Khoo LT. Minimally invasive cervical microendoscopic foraminotomy: an initial clinical experience. Neurosurgery. 2002;51(5 Suppl):S37–45.
4. Adamson TE. Microendoscopic posterior cervical laminoforaminotomy for unilateral radiculopathy: results of a new technique in 100 cases. J Neurosurg. 2001;95(1 Suppl):51–7.
5. Abbas SF, Spurgas MP, Szewczyk BS, Yim B, Ata A, German JW. A comparison of minimally invasive posterior cervical decompression and open anterior cervical decompression and instrumented fusion in the surgical management of degenerative cervical myelopathy. Neurosurg Focus. 2016;40(6):E7.
6. Adamson TE. The impact of minimally invasive cervical spine surgery. Invited submission from the joint section meeting on disorders of the spine and peripheral nerves, March 2004. *Journal of neurosurgery*. Spine. 2004;1(1):43–6.
7. Fong S, Duplessis S. Minimally invasive lateral mass plating in the treatment of posterior cervical trauma: surgical technique. J Spinal Disord Tech. 2005;18(3):224–8.
8. Wang MY, Green BA, Coscarella E, Baskaya MK, Levi AD, Guest JD. Minimally invasive cervical expansile laminoplasty: an initial cadaveric study. Neurosurgery. 2003;52(2):370–3. discussion 373
9. Wang MY, Levi AD. Minimally invasive lateral mass screw fixation in the cervical spine: initial clinical experience with long-term follow-up. Neurosurgery. 2006;58(5):907–12. discussion 907-912
10. Holly LT, Isaacs RE, Frempong-Boadu AK. Minimally invasive atlantoaxial fusion. Neurosurgery. 2010;66(3 Suppl):193–7.
11. Joseffer SS, Post N, Cooper PR, Frempong-Boadu AK. Minimally invasive atlantoaxial fixation with a polyaxial screw-rod construct: technical case report. Neurosurgery. 2006;58(4 Suppl 2):ONS-E375. discussion ONS-E375
12. Mikhael MM, Celestre PC, Wolf CF, Mroz TE, Wang JC. Minimally invasive cervical spine foraminotomy and lateral mass screw placement. Spine. 2012;37(5):E318–22.
13. Taghva A, Attenello FJ, Zada G, Khalessi AA, Hsieh PC. Minimally invasive posterior atlantoaxial fusion: a cadaveric and clinical feasibility study. World Neurosurg. 2013;80(3–4):414–21.
14. Gejo R, Matsui H, Kawaguchi Y, Ishihara H, Tsuji H. Serial changes in trunk muscle performance after posterior lumbar surgery. Spine. 1999;24(10):1023–8.
15. Gejo R, Kawaguchi Y, Kondoh T, et al. Magnetic resonance imaging and histologic evidence of postoperative back muscle injury in rats. Spine. 2000;25(8):941–6.

16. Tetreault L, Tan G, Kopjar B, et al. Clinical and surgical predictors of complications following surgery for the treatment of cervical Spondylotic myelopathy: results from the multicenter, prospective AOSpine international study of 479 patients. Neurosurgery. 2016;79(1):33–44.
17. Sakai K, Yoshii T, Hirai T, et al. Cervical sagittal imbalance is a predictor of Kyphotic deformity after Laminoplasty in cervical Spondylotic myelopathy patients without preoperative Kyphotic alignment. Spine. 2016;41(4):299–305.
18. Yoshida M, Neo M, Fujibayashi S, Nakamura T. Comparison of the anatomical risk for vertebral artery injury associated with the C2-pedicle screw and atlantoaxial transarticular screw. Spine. 2006;31(15):E513–7.
19. Holly LT, Foley KT. Percutaneous placement of posterior cervical screws using three-dimensional fluoroscopy. Spine. 2006;31(5):536–40. discussion 541
20. Vale FL, Burns J, Jackson AB, Hadley MN. Combined medical and surgical treatment after acute spinal cord injury: results of a prospective pilot study to assess the merits of aggressive medical resuscitation and blood pressure management. J Neurosurg. 1997;87(2):239–46.
21. Sutter M, Deletis V, Dvorak J, et al. Current opinions and recommendations on multimodal intraoperative monitoring during spine surgeries. Eur Spine J. 2007;16(Suppl 2):S232–7.
22. Goel A, Desai KI, Muzumdar DP. Atlantoaxial fixation using plate and screw method: a report of 160 treated patients. Neurosurgery. 2002;51(6):1351–6. discussion 1356-1357
23. Harms J, Melcher RP. Posterior C1-C2 fusion with polyaxial screw and rod fixation. Spine. 2001;26(22):2467–71.
24. Barrey C, Mertens P, Rumelhart C, Cotton F, Jund J, Perrin G. Biomechanical evaluation of cervical lateral mass fixation: a comparison of the Roy-Camille and Magerl screw techniques. J Neurosurg. 2004;100(3 Suppl Spine):268–76.
25. Barrey C, Mertens P, Jund J, Cotton F, Perrin G. Quantitative anatomic evaluation of cervical lateral mass fixation with a comparison of the Roy-Camille and the Magerl screw techniques. Spine. 2005;30(6):E140–7.
26. Lu Y, Wang J, Zheng W, Liu J, Huang B. Minimally invasive anterior transarticular screw fixation and fusion for atlantoaxial instability. Zhongguo Xiu Fu Chong Jian Wai Ke Za Zhi. 2012;26(7):769–72.

Correction of Post-laminectomy Kyphosis and Cervical Deformity

13

Melvin C. Makhni and K. Daniel Riew

Introduction

Multilevel laminectomy is commonly performed for patients with cervical stenosis and may lead to cervical kyphosis or swan neck deformity. Up to 47% of patients who have undergone decompression without concurrent fusion develop post-laminectomy kyphosis [1]. Kaptain et al. evaluated patients without sufficient preoperative cervical lordosis and noted that they had significantly higher rates of kyphotic progression postoperatively than those with adequate preoperative alignment [2]. Finite element analysis has shown increased flexion after laminectomy, and in vivo sheep models have confirmed this finding and also shown that endplate chondrocyte apoptosis may be involved in the pathway leading to kyphotic deformity [3, 4]. Because nearly two-thirds of the load in the cervical spine is borne through the posterior column, disruption can predispose to altered biomechanics. However, current evidence suggests that careful laminectomy with meticulous preservation of facets and muscle integrity can be performed without fusion for properly indicated patients with cervical stenosis, predominantly those with sufficient preoperative lordosis [5–9].

M.C. Makhni, MD, MBA (✉) • K.D. Riew, MD
The Spine Hospital, Columbia University Medical Center, 5141 Broadway, 3 Field West - Room 021, New York, NY 10034, USA
e-mail: mcm2225@cumc.columbia.edu; kr2637@cumc.columbia.edu

Van Geest et al. showed an 18% rate of postoperative kyphosis after cervical laminectomy for degenerative spinal cord compression; however, they reported that these cases occurred nearly always in patients who had decreased cervical lordosis preoperatively [7]. Li et al. performed a long-term review of patients who had undergone multilevel laminectomy for cervical spondylotic myelopathy due to stenosis with ligamentum flavum hypertrophy [8]. In patients who initially had cervical lordosis, they showed that at mean follow-up of 12.1 years, the cervical curvature index had significantly decreased; however, despite a decrease in the amount of lordosis, none had experienced neurologic deterioration, and on average they had only mild pain at follow-up.

Cervical deformities present debilitating problems to patients and have significant impact on their quality of life. They can result in not only pain and disability from loss of horizontal gaze but also myelopathy and radiculopathy as the deformity progresses. Severe cases can also result in dysphagia and even chest sores from chin-on-chest deformity. Additionally, they pose difficult challenges to surgeons who seek to safely improve their patients' pain, disability, and deformity. Before attempting to surgically intervene in these cases, it is important to understand the etiology of the deformity and also the various operative and nonoperative treatment options available.

Cervical deformities can have several different etiologies. A clear understanding of the reason for the deformity and the history of any previous

L.T. Holly, P.A. Anderson (eds.), *Essentials of Spinal Stabilization*,
DOI 10.1007/978-3-319-59713-3_13

cervical or other spinal surgeries can help guide treatment options. Cervical kyphotic deformities are the most common types of deformities encountered. Patients can develop cervical kyphosis after laminectomy procedures or as a result of prior fusion (surgically induced or through autofusion, e.g., from ankylosing spondylitis). Scoliosis, tumors, trauma, and compensatory change after thoracolumbar deformity or correction can all be reasons for loss of normal cervical alignment as well.

The goals of surgery must be tailored to each individual patient. In general, one major goal of surgery is pain control. Another major goal is improvement of function which could include restoration of neutral horizontal gaze. Another is decompression of neural elements that might be compromised in progressive deformities. It is crucial to achieve a fixed fusion between vertebral levels which may require adjunct procedures to achieve circumferential fusion. Finally, it may be helpful to focus not only on cervical alignment but also global spinal alignment to achieve regional and global balance.

This chapter will describe various types of cervical deformities and develop a framework of understanding the conditions and how to approach them in a stepwise fashion. First we will discuss indications, patient selection, and other preoperative considerations. Then we will specifically address surgical options for management of post-laminectomy kyphosis and fixed cervical flexion deformities.

Indications and Patient Selection

Before surgical intervention, several factors must be considered about the patient's underlying pathology and clinical situation. The surgeon must elicit what brought the patient to the office, whether that may be neurologic compromise, pain, inability to maintain horizontal gaze, or even cosmesis – or a combination of these. Some may also complain of dysphagia or dysphonia as a result of sufficient deformity.

Then the patient's medical status must be fully evaluated to determine if they are able to tolerate surgery including a full assessment of their comorbidities, especially their cardiac and pulmonary health. Nutritional, vascular, and endocrine workup should also be performed in order to optimize postoperative healing and rule out deep venous thrombosis and osteoporosis. Those with osteoporosis should be considered for treatment with metabolic therapies preoperatively in order to avoid fractures at end vertebrae with deformity correction. Additionally, it is recommended that patients be weaned off narcotics before surgery. Those on significant preoperative doses could require massive doses of narcotics postoperatively, predisposing them to risks such as respiratory depression and pneumonia. Smoking cessation is essential for healing before proceeding with any operation of the magnitude needed to correct cervical deformity.

Preoperative Considerations

Proper preoperative planning hinges on several factors. These help determine whether to approach the spine anteriorly, posteriorly, or circumferentially and also help determine fusion levels:

1. Flexibility of deformity. Surgery for flexible deformities can be performed anteriorly, posteriorly, or circumferentially based on other considerations. Rigid deformities must be treated with osteotomies, regardless of whether the rigidity is due to natural diseases such as ankylosing spondylitis or iatrogenic etiologies as a result of prior fusion. These osteotomies can also be done anteriorly, posteriorly, or circumferentially.
2. Neurologic deficit. Presence of neurologic compromise may help determine approach. An anterior approach may be indicated if there is anterior compression or severe foraminal compromise that requires direct anterior decompression rather than indirect deformity correction. Similarly, posterior soft tissue scarring may more successfully be managed directly.

3. Osteoporosis. Poor bone quality necessitates circumferential fusion rather than a unilateral approach in order to improve the strength and stability of the construct.
4. Other approach-related considerations. The patient's clinical and personal scenario as well as their past medical history should be considered when deciding direction of approach. Patients who are singers and those who have had prior anterior surgery or anterior radical neck dissections may have decreased risk with posterior approach. In contrast, a posterior approach may be more difficult in patients who, for example, have dural ectasia (Fig. 13.1).
5. Severity of deformity. Patients with severe chin-on-chest deformity may be difficult to access anteriorly. They may be best suited for a posterior or circumferential approach.
6. Location of deformity. The location of the deformity helps determine the distal fusion level. In general all laminectomized levels should be instrumented. If the deformity is focal, correcting it locally should be all that is necessary. If the focal deformity is severe, such that a posterior correction would leave a large anterior gap, it may even be necessary to perform an anterior arthrodesis. Anterior arthrodesis should also be considered if posterior fixation is deemed to be inadequate. If the kyphosis is a compensatory phenomenon due to a more distant deformity or otherwise part of a more global deformity, full-length radiographs must be considered to plan the order and extent of correction.

All patients with post-laminectomy kyphosis and cervical deformity should receive routine multiplanar radiographs of the cervical spine, as well as flexion-extension films to assess and reveal the rigidity of the deformity. If the patient has a severe local imbalance or global imbalance, full-length films are necessary. An MRI can help

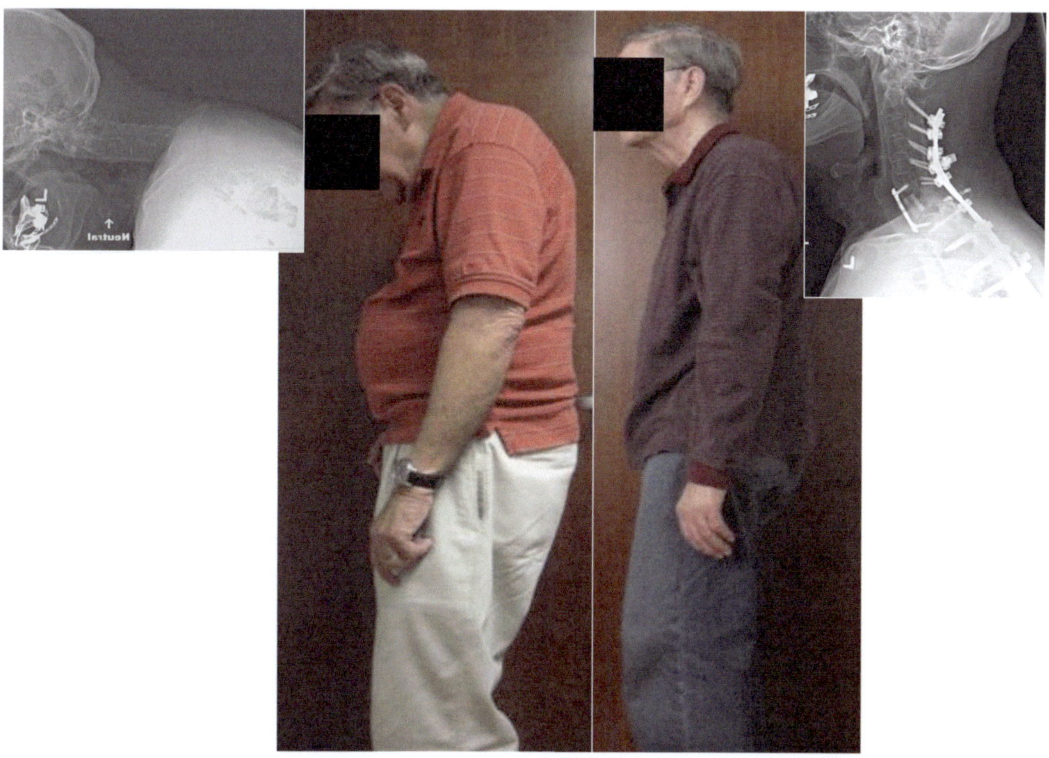

Fig. 13.1 Myelopathic 45-year-old lady status post C4–C6 laminectomy for astrocytoma at age 15. Because of the patulous dura posteriorly, we elected to perform an anterior-only operation. Although the results are not perfect, it is a vast improvement and avoided possible dural complications

identify sites compression in patients with neurologic symptoms, and a CT scan can further assist with preoperative planning due to its enhanced bony resolution. Patients with significant deformity or those undergoing osteotomies may benefit from CT or MR angiogram to better identify the course of the vertebral arteries.

Post-laminectomy Kyphosis

Overview

Patients with iatrogenic post-laminectomy kyphosis can be surgically managed with either anterior-only or circumferential procedures. Anterior compression can be managed with corpectomy and discectomy at the offending levels. If only a single-level corpectomy is required, then an anterior-only approach can be considered in patients with sufficient bone quality. Only in those patients with good bone quality can one consider anterior-only procedures to restore cervical lordosis. Ideally, these patients should also have four to six points of fixation above and below the level of the corpectomy.

Sole reliance on anterior approach for correction of post-laminectomy kyphosis had been associated with high risk of complications of over 60% in patients treated with up to four-level corpectomy within a 2.7-year follow-up period [10]. In these patients without instrumentation, the studies showed a high rate of pseudarthrosis, progressive kyphotic deformity, reoperation, and graft extrusion despite use of halo vests. With instrumentation and adequate immobilization, Herman et al. and Steinmetz et al. showed improvement in neurologic function and kyphosis after performing corpectomies with plate fixation [11, 12]. These were predominantly one- and two-level corpectomies. We recommend circumferential fixation for two or more corpectomy levels in order to minimize graft- and plate-related complications. In patients who have had a laminectomy, the vertebra is divided, and a subsequent corpectomy then separates the vertebra anteriorly producing two halves that are only connected by soft tissues. With multilevel corpectomies, this results in a highly unstable construct, even with anterior instrumentation.

Whenever possible, anterior cervical interbody fusions (ACDF) are preferred over corpectomies, as they have decreased risk of subsidence and graft extrusion. Because ACDFs also allow for segmental fixation, they are inherently more stable than corpectomies. However, if compression located behind the vertebral body necessitates a corpectomy, one should minimize the number of corpectomy levels and perform discectomies whenever possible, with the goal of avoiding long corpectomy segments (Fig. 13.2). One way to avoid a posterior operation in a patient who requires a corpectomy is to perform a hybrid procedure with ACDFs above and below the corpectomy level(s). With an anterior-only construct, we always use at least one ACDF construct at the caudal end which allows for the placement of four screws above and below the ACDF. This provides distal stability which helps to prevent graft-related complications. Park reported 23 cases of this hybrid technique, corpectomy, and ACDF with plate fixation, for correction of post-laminectomy kyphosis [13]. They showed a mean improvement from 20.9° of kyphosis to 9.6° of lordosis at average 4-year follow-up, with significantly improved outcome scores and only one pseudarthrosis at one level.

For most patients, however, it is recommended that circumferential fusions be performed to promote fusion and mitigate instability incurred by removing the anterior column in levels where the posterior elements have previously been removed (Fig. 13.2) [14].

Surgical Technique

Anterior surgical reconstruction can be performed with or without supplemental posterior fixation, according to the criteria outlined above [13, 14]. For the anterior approach, all patients should have appropriate intraoperative motor and somatosensory evoked potential monitoring; these potentials should be monitored at positioning, after application of traction and periodically throughout the case, especially during deformity correction. Gentle retraction of the shoulders with tape, as well as kerlix applied to the wrist and extended distally to the foot of the bed, can be used to help improve visualiza-

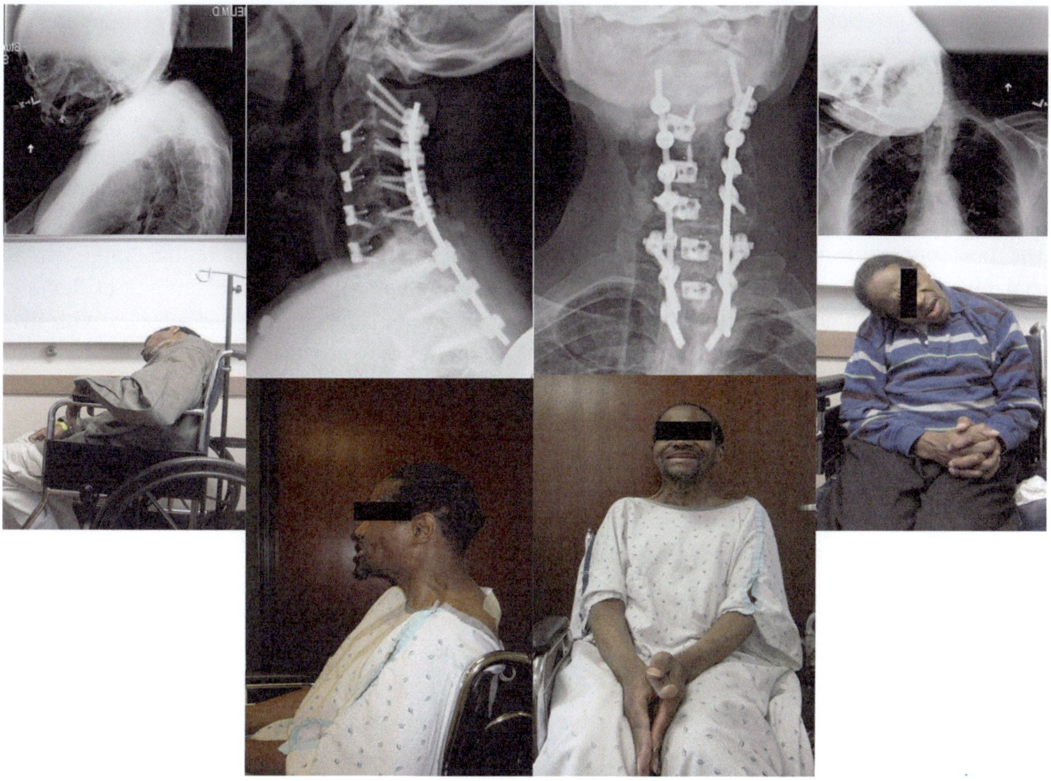

Fig. 13.2 A 20-year-old female presenting with post-laminectomy kyphosis. Circumferential fusion is obtained using hybrid anterior fixation involving a corpectomy and an ACDF

tion especially when offending vertebral levels at the apex of the kyphotic deformity is more distal in the cervical spine. With flexible deformities, it is important to make sure that the neck is positioned in lordosis prior to prepping the skin. A lateral radiograph should be obtained after patient positioning to check alignment. Adjustment, as needed, can then be performed and radiographs rechecked. In cases where the deformity is inflexible, the flexible segments must be placed into hyperlordosis at the outset or the positioning will make correction of the kyphotic segment more difficult.

After a standard preoperative cleansing regimen of alcohol foam and chlorhexidine, standard anterior cervical approach is performed at the levels of interest [15]. We recommend a transverse incision and mobilization of soft tissue that can allow exposure from C2 to T1 in most cases. After radiographic localization, distraction pins are placed into the vertebral bodies of interest. They can be angled to converge anteriorly so as to help achieve more angular correction when distracted. The disc space can be entered with sharp dissection and the disc removed with a pituitary rongeur and curettes. Bony resection can be performed with a burr; dural tears are minimized with constant motion of a side-cutting matchstick burr along the superficial aspect of the PLL. Ossified PLL may be removed to assist in extension of kyphotic deformity.

In patients with osteoporosis or those in which at least one ACDF at the proximal and distal ends of the construct with at least four fixation points above and four to six points of screw fixation below the corpectomy levels is not obtainable, the construct should ideally be supplemented with posterior fixation. Occasionally a single-level corpectomy can be fixed with an anterior-only operation, but for most patients with kyphosis and stenosis, circumferential fusion is required. In most situations anterior plating of the corpectomy site would help prevent graft extrusion; however, in some circumstances (such as in patients with significant dysphagia), posterior fixation without an anterior plate may suffice. The posterior spine must be approached with care, given the revision nature of the surgery. The scar must be meticulously dissected through with awareness of the exposed spinal cord. Sufficient posterior fixation consisting primarily of lateral mass and pedicle screws can then be applied to promote circumferential fusion. Unless there is pathology at the cranio-cervical junction, we try never to include levels cranial to C2. Usually, the highest fixation strength proximally can be achieved at C2.

Following surgery, patients should be placed in rigid cervical collars for 6 weeks. For extensive intubation, consideration should be given to transferring the patient to the ICU intubated postoperatively to prevent airway compromise in the setting of significant soft tissue swelling.

Rigid Flexion Deformity

Overview

Flexion deformities can occur for a variety of reasons aside from loss of posterior support after laminectomy. Rigid flexion deformities must be treated with osteotomies; crucial in planning surgery is an understanding of the degree of extension correction needed. Osteotomies, including posterior column, pedicle subtraction and anterior, as well as combinations of the three, can help improve alignment, pain, and function.

Before deformity correction, the curve should be assessed globally to determine if it is compensatory to, for example, a thoracolumbar sagittal deformity. Examination of the regional and global sagittal alignment, as well as the chin-brow vertical angle to assess horizontal gaze, can help assist with preoperative planning to optimize balance and function postoperatively.

Detailed review of the imaging can confirm the rigidity of the deformity before performing osteotomies. If the curve appears flexible, then the neck can be manually manipulated into appropriate position and fused with either a posterior, anterior, or circumferential approach. If the curve has only a minimal amount of flexibility, a combination of anterior releases with discectomies may provide sufficient mobility. If the spine does prove to be completely ankylosed, osteotomies are the only option to achieving angular correction.

Patients should undergo extensive nonoperative treatment for symptomatic improvement before undergoing a cervical osteotomy, due to the severity of risks inherent in the procedure; this could be expedited or circumvented in the presence of progressive neurologic deterioration. In reality, however, for a fixed deformity, there is no effective nonoperative treatment.

The choice of an anterior or posterior osteotomy is determined by a number of factors. Most deformities are amenable to correction either anteriorly, posteriorly, or with a combination approach [16, 17]. Different surgeons with varying levels of experience and preference can achieve a successful outcome with radically different procedures. In the past, our most common approach to deformity correction was posterior, utilizing a pedicle subtraction osteotomy. We subsequently developed an anterior osteotomy technique that we have found to be as fast or faster than a posterior osteotomy and associated with less blood loss [19].

Anterior Osteotomy

The anterior approach may be physically difficult to access in some circumstances, especially in the apex of a rigid deformity. Often, the depth of the osteotomy is so deep that the burr has to be held at the most distal part of the handle. This makes it difficult to control the tip so only surgeons who

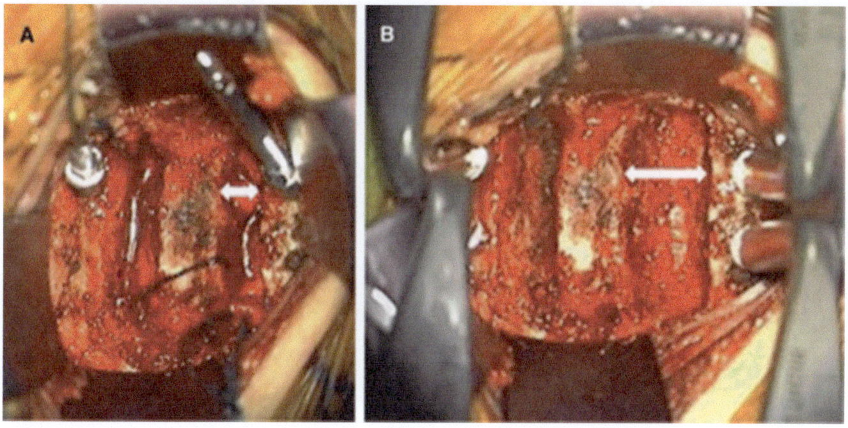

Fig. 13.3 Divergent Caspar pins are placed initially; distraction of the pins introduces lordosis (From Kelly et al. [20] with permission)

are highly experienced and comfortable using a burr should attempt the anterior approach in a severely kyphotic case.

If an anteriorly based osteotomy is to be performed, one must decide which side to approach from. If the patient has undergone prior anterior surgery, recurrent laryngeal nerve function on the previously approached side should be assessed preoperatively. If it remains uninjured, the contralateral approach can be utilized, in order to navigate through normal anatomy rather than scar tissue. If the prior surgery has damaged the recurrent laryngeal nerve on the initial side, the same side must be used in order to preserve the integrity of the contralateral nerve. If more correction than an anterior osteotomy or posterior column osteotomy (PCO) is needed, both can be combined, which has been shown to yield similar angular correction than a single pedicle subtraction osteotomy (PSO) with lower length of stay and operative blood loss [16].

Instead of, or in addition to, a posterior approach, an anterior approach can be utilized for an anterior cervical osteotomy [18, 19]. Positioning may require a setup tailored to the individual in order to cushion the head which may be elevated off the frame due to kyphosis. Gardner-Wells tongs are applied and the head is rested on a foam donut and sheets as needed. When planning to perform osteotomies, 2.2 kg of traction is applied initially with more weight applied at osteotomy closure. A standard Smith-Robinson approach is utilized, with attention to the side of approach as mentioned above if there has been prior anterior cervical surgery. Divergent Caspar distraction pins are placed at kyphotic vertebral segments around the osteotomy site, and then the bone is resected with a burr to correct the planes of deformity present (Fig. 13.3). The bone is resected posteriorly until the posterior longitudinal ligament is reached. Laterally, care is taken to avoid iatrogenic injury to the vertebral artery. Foraminotomies can be performed at these levels prophylactically to prevent neural compromise with extension of the osteotomy.

Then, extension forces can be applied to achieve correction. The padding underneath the patient's head can be removed, and gentle constant pressure can be applied on the patient's forehead. Concurrently, an intervertebral spreader can be used for distraction at the osteotomy site (Fig. 13.4). Traction is increased at this time to 9 or 11.3 kg if needed in order to maintain lordosis. A maximally wide and deep graft is placed with anterior hardware. This can

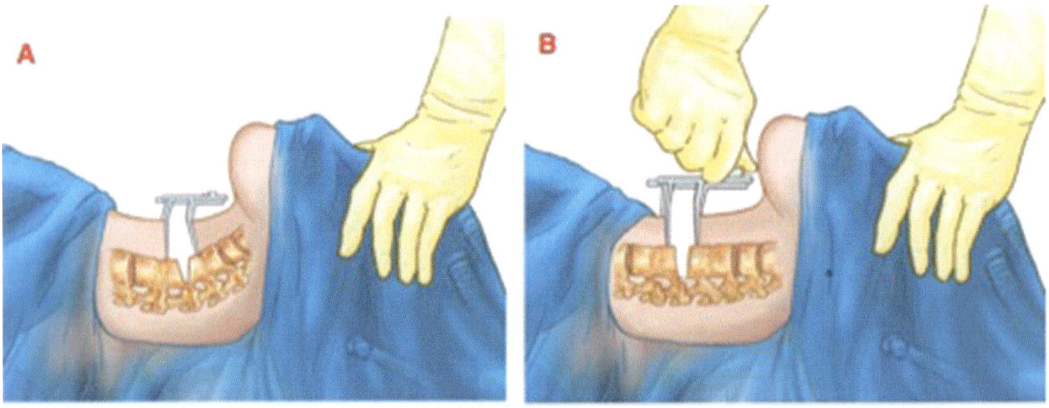

Fig. 13.4 Extension is obtained using an intervertebral spreader as well as pressure on the patient's forehead (From Kelly et al. [20] with permission)

all be performed as an anterior-only procedure or with adjunctive posterior osteotomy or simply instrumentation and fusion for supplemental support (Fig. 13.5). Because the center of rotation with an anterior osteotomy is at the posterior aspect of the vertebral body, there is minimal stretching of the cord or vertebral artery. In our series of 17 patients who underwent anterior osteotomies with the average of 23° of mean angular correction, no patients had intraoperative neuromonitoring changes or neurologic deficits [19]. However, if any of these occur, the neural elements must be carefully inspected to ensure thorough decompression; less correction may be warranted in order to minimize stretch on the spinal cord.

Pedicle Subtraction Osteotomy Surgical Technique

The site of deformity and proposed osteotomy must be planned in context with the direction of approach. Determining how much correction is needed will influence which osteotomy to perform. As in the thoracolumbar spine, pedicle subtraction osteotomies can provide more curve correction than posterior column osteotomies. The principle also remains that more distally based osteotomies allow for larger absolute distances of translation than more proximally based ones.

If a PSO is needed, C7 is the most desirable level for multiple reasons, provided it would be suitable to provide correction to the individual's deformity. This allows for decreased risk to the vertebral artery which usually lies anterior to the foramen transversarium at this level unless it is aberrant. The vertebral foramen is also larger at this level. As mentioned previously, the more distal the osteotomy, the greater the translation of the proximal vertebra.

Posterior column osteotomies can be performed at a single or multiple levels. In a patient with a mobile anterior column, simple Ponte osteotomies can achieve correction. In a patient with an ankylosed spine, however, Smith-Petersen or pedicle subtraction osteotomies must be performed. With both osteotomies, the superior and inferior facets are removed, along with the lamina and ligamentum flavum at that level, as well as part of the adjacent levels, as needed. With a Smith-Petersen osteotomy, one creates an opening wedge that elongates the anterior column. Without adequate posterior fixation, this is more unstable than a pedicle subtraction osteotomy which is a closing wedge osteotomy

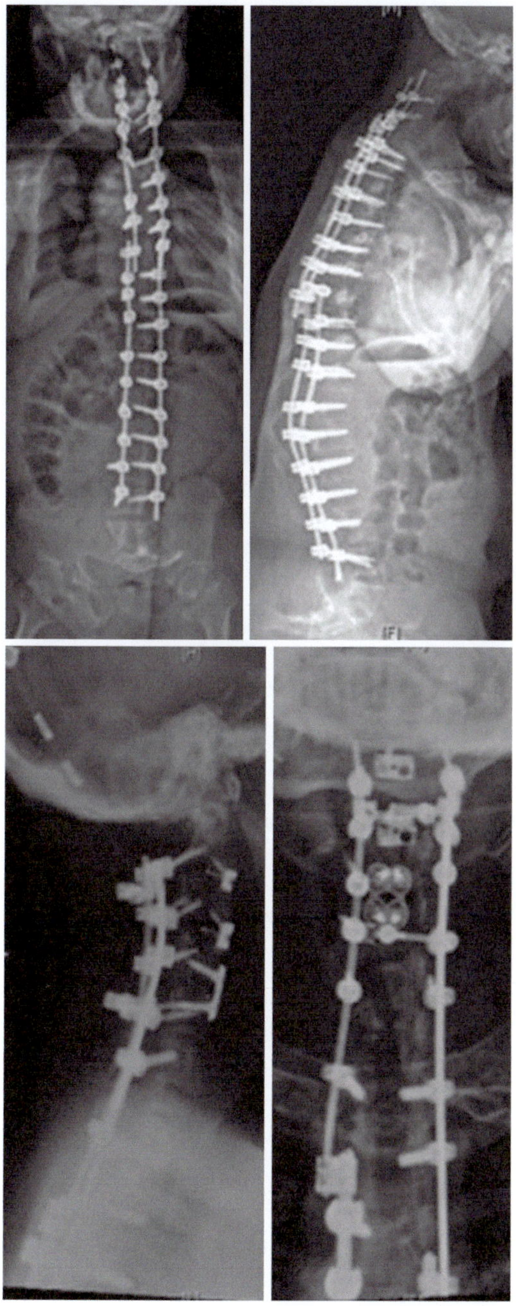

Fig. 13.5 Cervical deformity corrected with anterior cervical osteotomies at C2–C3, C3–C4, and ACDF C4–C5 followed by posterior revision of hardware and revision decompression and fusion C2-T2 with posterior column osteotomies at C2–C3 and C3–C4 for patient with achondroplastic dwarfism and congenital spinal stenosis presenting with myelopathy

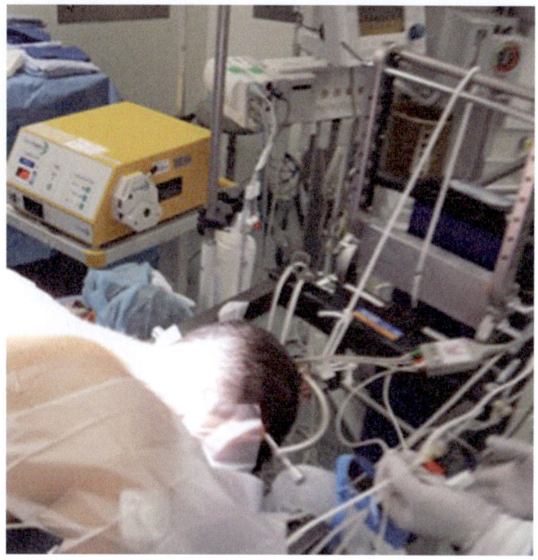

Fig. 13.6 Bivector traction attached to the Gardner-Wells tongs, with one rope pulling in line traction and the other providing an extension moment

with an intact anterior column. In truth, however, when large corrections are performed utilizing a pedicle subtraction osteotomy, often the anterior column opens up. This usually occurs when an inadequate amount of the body is decancellated from the posterior approach.

Positioning

Positioning can be difficult due to the kyphotic deformity. We utilize the OSI Jackson frame with extra padding under the chest which is nearly always necessary to support a kyphotic thoracic spine. The head is suspended with Gardner-Wells tongs with bivector traction (Fig. 13.6) to provide neutral and extension moments. Before the osteotomy, 20 pounds are suspended from the neutral traction rope; after the osteotomy, the weight is transferred to the extension rope.

To prevent infections, we square off a large area with plastic drapes, ideally 10 cm or more past the site of the incision cranially and caudally and as wide laterally as possible. We then spray alcohol foam over the skin and the plastic drapes. After drying, we do a standard prep.

Operative Technique

The exposure is a critical part of the case. A meticulous exposure in the midline avascular and amuscular raphe results in minimal blood loss. A poorly done exposure can result in several 100 ml during the exposure and throughout the case, as the muscles bleed. We dissect down to the spinous processes and then osteotomize the tips of the spinous processes with the muscles attached to them. From C3 to C6, they are usually bifid, so we cut it in the axilla of the bifid process. For lower levels that are monofid, we cut the tips of the spinous processes obliquely with the paraspinal muscles attached. This allows us to close bone to bone at the end of the case, minimizing muscle necrosis from sutures.

With a planned PSO at C7, the posterior aspect of the spine is exposed in the usual fashion. Proximally, the instrumentation is placed at least four to six points above the osteotomy, depending upon the quality of fixation. If the ankylosis extends to C2 or even to the occiput, we will usually go as high as the ankylosed level. This is because, with long-standing ankylosis, the spine becomes very osteoporotic and prone to screw pullout. In addition, patients are at risk for a fracture above the instrumented level. Distally, fixation should be extended preferably to T3, T4, or lower, with a minimum of six points of distal fixation for the construct. One cannot use both C6 and T1 screws, as, after the closure of the osteotomy, they are too close together and interfere with full closure of the osteotomy. With extensive corrections, both C6 and T1 screws have to be skipped. We usually skip the C6 level since, after the closure of the osteotomy, the C6 screws are too close to the T1 screws to be utilizable. Alternatively, one can use the C6 screws and skip the T1 screws, depending upon the fixation points available for a given patient. The proximal and distal fixation levels also are chosen based on the patient's medical condition, as the longer the construct, the longer the operating time. In cases with a chin-on-chest deformity in the prone position, the patient's head is pointed toward the ground. In such a position, a prolonged operation with excessive blood loss increases the risk of postoperative blindness. So the operation must be performed as expeditiously but as safely as possible (Figs. 13.7 and 13.8).

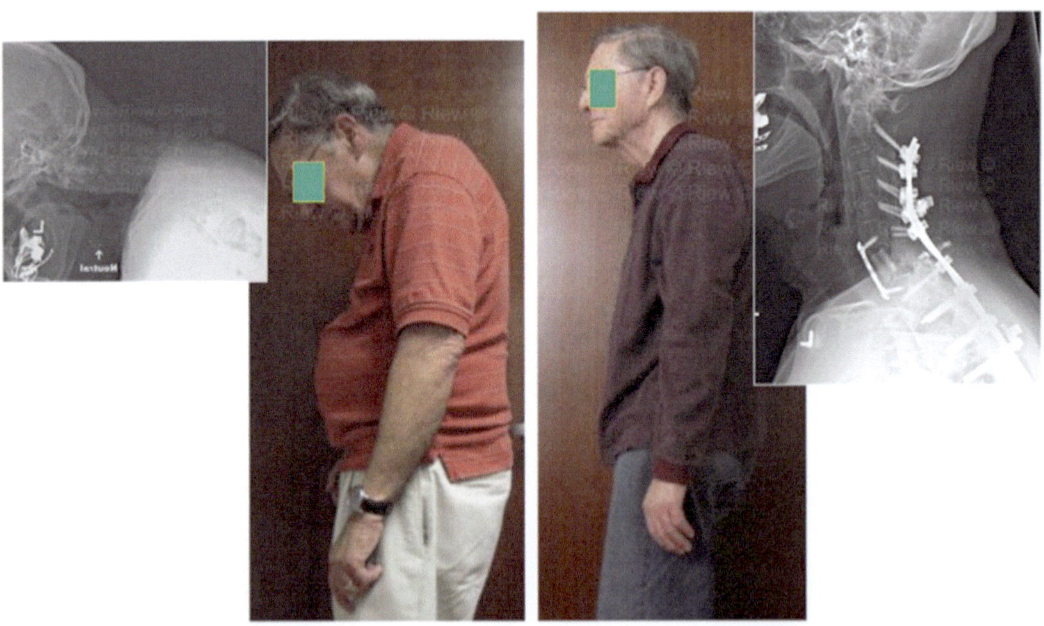

Fig. 13.7 This patient with ankylosing spondylitis had a missed fracture and developed a chin-on-chest deformity, which was corrected with an anterior osteotomy/corpectomy, followed by posterior stabilization

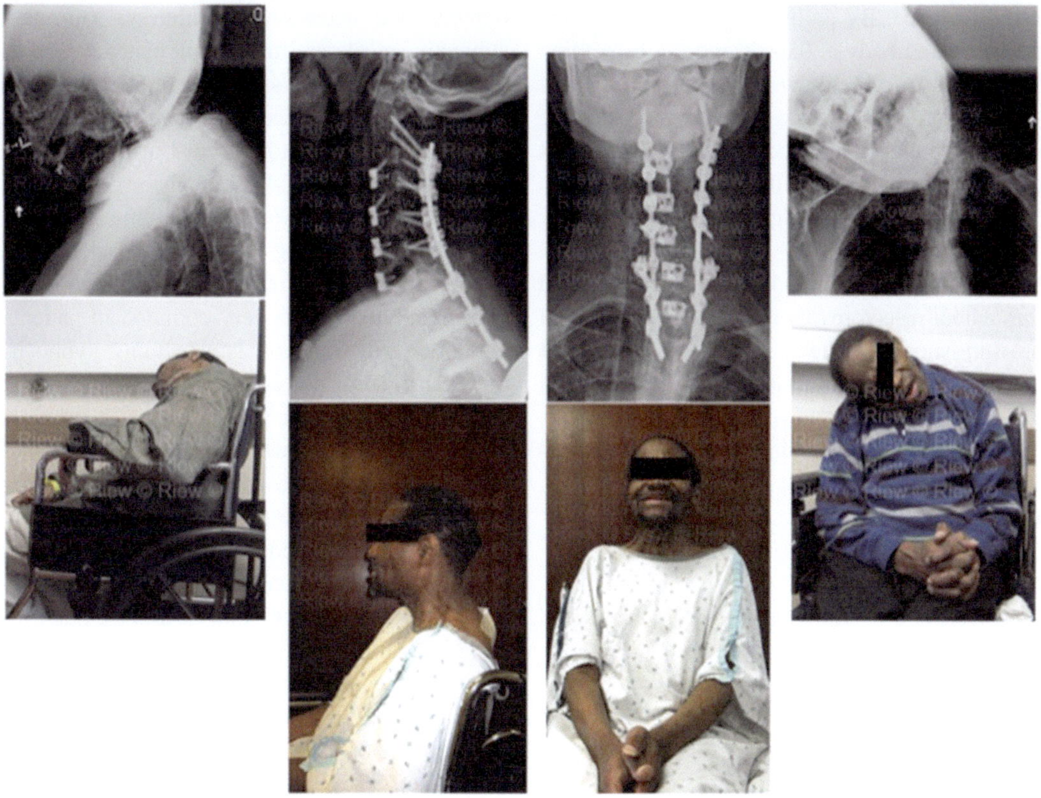

Fig. 13.8 We performed an anterior osteotomy followed by posterior stabilization to correct this ear-on-shoulder and chin-on-chest deformity. The use of stand-alone cages makes it easier to get further posterior correction and is faster than multilevel plate fixation

After complete C7 laminectomy and adjacent removal of the caudal and cranial halves of the C6 and T1 laminae, respectively, the lateral masses of C7 are resected. The inferior portion of the C6 facet and the superior portion of the T1 superior facet are removed as well. The C7 pedicle is then entered with a burr, leaving the walls intact to protect the nerves and cord. Through the pedicle, the body is decancellated, using the burr, reverse angle curettes, and tamps (Fig. 13.9). Then the pedicle walls are thinned and removed and the posterior cortex of the vertebral body is pushed anteriorly.

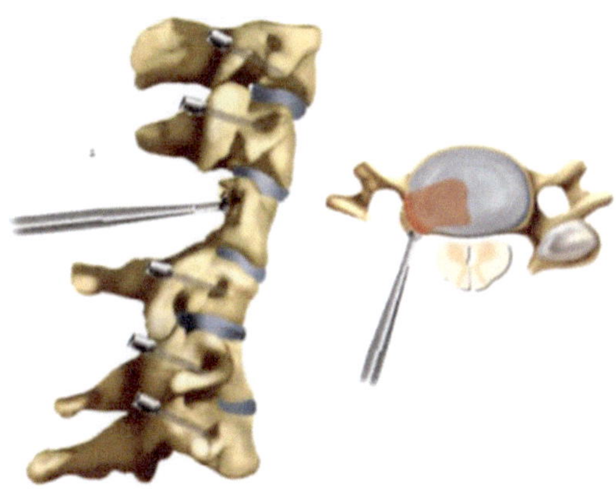

Fig. 13.9 The vertebral body is decancellated after entering the pedicle in a PSO (From Kelly et al. [20] with permission)

At this point, the rods are placed into the screws and the set screws are placed loosely. We prefer to use rods that have an articulation that allows bending, as it is easier than bending the rods. Some of the correction occurs through the articulation, but the rods also have to be able to slide through the screws distal to the osteotomy. The surgeon then holds the Gardner-Wells tongs, and the suspending weight is switched to the extension rope. By pulling up on the tongs, the decancellated body collapses and the osteotomy site begins to close down. Once closed, the set screws are tightened down. The C7 and C8 nerve roots and the cord must be protected throughout the resection as well as the closure in order to confirm that no overhanging facet from C6 or T1 compresses the C7 or C8 nerve roots. Neuromonitoring should also be checked throughout osteotomy closure, and mean arterial pressure should be elevated above 80 mmHg at this time; neurologic status can be confirmed with a wake-up test as needed. Bone graft is added to fuse the spine. One can use the laminectomy bone alone in most cases, as the osteotomized segment usually fuses well.

Closure

Proper closure of the wound is critical to avoid dehiscence and infections. Our infection rate for posterior cervical procedures is less than 0.05%, even including massive osteotomies and occiput to thoracic procedures. Part of this is due to the meticulous dissection described above. We also irrigate frequently. We then place vancomycin powder 1 g in the wound [15], a deep drain, followed by thrombin-soaked Gelfoam on top of the drain. Gelfoam minimizes the postoperative bleeding such that most patients are able to be discharged after an overnight stay. It should not be used if a laminectomy has been performed as it can expand and compress the cord. We then place interrupted sutures every 1 cm using 75–100 sutures to close a C2 to T4 wound. This prevents any dead space where blood can accumulate and act as a nidus for infection. If there is greater than 5 cm of fat, we place a supra-fascial drain also.

Illustrative Case

A 20-year-old female presented with post-laminectomy kyphosis of C3–C6 with axial neck pain, stiffness, and myelopathy due to remote history of C1–C4 laminectomy and radiation treatment for a meningioma (Fig. 13.2). Preoperatively she had numbness in her feet worsened with extension of her neck, difficulty picking up objects, and occasional numbness, pain, and subjective weakness in her right hand, as well as a positive Hoffman's sign. Anterior cervical corpectomy was performed at C4 with ACDF at C5–C6, as well as posterior cervical instrumentation and fusion from C3–C4 with revision decompression C3–C4 to achieve circumferential stabilization. Despite having a "flexible" deformity without any areas of autofusion, she was very stiff and immobile. This is very common in patients with long-standing post-laminectomy kyphosis. Only partial correction could be achieved anteriorly. We then used dynamic screws to allow for greater posterior fixation. However, posteriorly, we found osteoporotic bone and could not achieve further lordosis without risking instrumentation failure. We therefore accepted a suboptimal correction. To avoid this, we recommend using a buttress type of plate with screws into C5 and C6 but with the plate only about 50% of the distance in front of the corpectomy to prevent the graft from kicking out. By not fixing into C3, one can get better posterior correction. The patient did very well postoperatively; at 12-week follow-up, she reported continued resolution of her symptoms and had complete resolution of her neck pain.

Technical Pearls

- Positioning the cervical spine preoperatively can be optimized with traction to achieve optimal correction of deformity, especially when osteotomies are performed. Increasing traction, using an intervertebral spreader, and adjunct manual force can help restore lordosis when anterior, and bivector traction can assist when posterior.
- Anterior osteotomies may be used in addition or instead of posterior osteotomies and may allow for comparable correction with decreased blood loss.
- Divergent Caspar pins can be placed anteriorly in kyphotic deformity; these can then be distracted to become more parallel, which helps restore lordosis.
- In patients with osteoporosis or those in which four to six points of fixation are not achievable

above and below sites of corpectomy (ideally with ACDFs proximally and distally), the construct should be supplemented with posterior fixation.

- In patients with rigid cervical deformity, Smith-Peterson or pedicle subtraction osteotomies must be performed. Proximal fixation should extend throughout the ankylosed levels and at least four to six levels above the osteotomy, while there should be at least six points of distal fixation.
- Meticulous wound closure technique can help decrease infection rates, especially in posterior cervical surgery.

Complications and Strategies for Avoidance

One of the most devastating complications that can result from cervical spine deformity surgery is paralysis. Protection of the neural elements is a primary focus throughout the case. When performing the anterior decompression, a high-speed, side-cutting burr is used; by applying gentle downward pressure with a continuous sweeping motion along the PLL, dural tears are minimized. This step can be especially difficult during anterior approach to rigid flexion deformities, sometimes requiring the surgeon to hold the burr at the tip to use the full depth of the instrument, so surgeon comfort with the burr is a prerequisite. Additionally, nerve root compression can be preemptively avoided by performing foraminotomies before osteotomy closure. Communication with the anesthesia and neuromonitoring teams during osteotomy closure also helps decrease risk of overcorrection and neurologic deterioration; a wake-up test can be employed for further confirmation of neurologic status.

Damage to the vertebral artery can also be life threatening. These should be studied carefully on preoperative imaging to localize and identify any aberrant anatomy so that they can be protected, especially during the osteotomies. Also, anterior decompression occurs widely until the uncinate processes bilaterally; if they are removed, caution must be used to free up and protect the vertebral artery with a Penfield during uncinectomy.

Hardware failure can occur, especially in osteoporotic bone. If insufficient fixation is achievable in both proximal and distal directions, or in the case of osteoporotic bone, circumferential fusion can help strengthen the construct. Larger screws and grafts can also provide additional strength. After an anterior extension osteotomy, graft placement slightly posterior with a small buttress plate or interference screws in the adjacent endplates can be used to prevent graft extrusion. An anterior fracture may result from closure of a posterior osteotomy if too little bone is resected or if the anterior cortex had been perforated during a PSO. If there is adequate fixation posteriorly, then no further intervention may be needed, although our preference is to flip the patient and plate anteriorly with four points of fixation above and below the fracture site. Postoperative use of a rigid cervical collar can also be used to protect fixation, especially in osteoporotic patients and those in which osteotomies were performed.

Meticulous, efficient surgical technique also can help avoid certain complications. Prolonged posterior surgery, especially without appropriate padding, can lead to blindness as a result of pressure on the eyes. Patients with prolonged cervical surgery or increased blood loss should be considered for delayed extubation to avoid airway compromise. Efficient, minimally tissue destructive surgery with decreased blood loss can also decrease the risk of surgical site infection.

References

1. Kato Y, Iwasaki M, Fuji T, Yonenobu K, Ochi T. Long-term follow-up results of laminectomy for cervical myelopathy caused by ossification of the posterior longitudinal ligament. J Neurosurg. 1998;89:217–23.
2. Kaptain GJ, Simmons NE, Replogle RE, Pobereskin L. Incidence and outcome of kyphotic deformity following laminectomy for cervical spondylotic myelopathy. J Neurosurg. 2000;93:199–204.
3. Kode S, Kallemeyn NA, Smucker JD, Fredericks DC, Grosland NM. The effect of multi-level laminoplasty and laminectomy on the biomechanics of the

cervical spine: a finite element study. Iowa Orthop J. 2014;34:150–7.
4. Kong D, Zheng T, Fang J, Li X. Apoptosis of endplate chondrocytes in post-laminectomy cervical kyphotic deformity. An in vivo animal model in sheep. Eur Spine J. 2013;22(7):1576–82.
5. Cabraja M, Abbushi A, Koeppen D, Kroppenstedt S, Woiciechowsky C. Comparison between anterior and posterior decompression with instrumentation for cervical spondylotic myelopathy: sagittal alignment and clinical outcome. Neurosurg Focus. 2010 Mar;28(3):E15.
6. McAllister BD, Rebholz BJ, Wang JC. Is posterior fusion necessary with laminectomy in the cervical spine? Surg Neurol Int. 2012;3(Suppl 3):S225–31.
7. van Geest S, de Vormer AM, Arts MP, Peul WC, Vleggeert-Lankamp CL. Long-term follow-up of clinical and radiological outcome after cervical laminectomy. Eur Spine J. 2015 Apr;24(Suppl 2):229–35.
8. Li Z, Xue Y, et al. Extensive laminectomy for multilevel cervical stenosis with ligamentum flavum hypertrophy: more than 10 years follow-up. Eur Spine J. 2015;24(8):1605–12.
9. Laiginhas AR, Silva PA, Pereira P, Vaz R. Long-term clinical and radiological follow-up after laminectomy for cervical spondylotic myelopathy. Surg Neurol Int. 2015;6:162.
10. Riew KD, Hilibrand AS, Palumbo MA, Bohlman HH. Anterior cervical Corpectomy in patients previously managed with a laminectomy: short-term complications. J Bone Joint Surg Am. 1999;81(7):950–7.
11. Herman JM, Sonntag VK. Cervical corpectomy and plate fixation for postlaminectomy kyphosis. J Neurosurg. 1994;80:963–70.
12. Steinmetz MP, Kager CD, Benzel EC. Ventral correction of postsurgical cervical kyphosis. J Neurosurg. 2003;98(1 Suppl):1–7.
13. Park Y, Riew KD, Cho W. The long-term results of anterior surgical reconstruction in patients with postlaminectomy cervical kyphosis. Spine Journal. 2010;10:380–7.
14. Riew KD, Auerbach JD, Angevine PD. Postoperative deformity of the cervical spine. In: Rothman-Simeone the spine. Philadelphia: Elsevier; 2011.
15. Pahys JM, Pahys JR, Cho SK, Kang MM, Zebala LP, Hawasli AH, Sweet FA, Lee DH, Riew KD. Methods to decrease postoperative infections following posterior cervical spine surgery. J Bone Joint Surg Am. 2013;95(6):549–54.
16. Kim HJ, Piyaskulkaew C, Riew KD. Comparison of Smith-Petersen osteotomy versus pedicle subtraction osteotomy versus anterior-posterior osteotomy types for the correction of cervical spine deformities. Spine. 2015;40(3):143–6.
17. Kim HJ, Nemani VM, Riew KD. Cervical osteotomies for neurologic deformities. Eur Spine J. 2015;24(Suppl 1):S16–22.
18. Nemani VM, Derman PB, Kim HJ. Osteotomies in the cervical spine. Asian Spine Journal. 2016;10(1):184–95.
19. Kim HJ, Piyaskulkaew C, Riew KD. Anterior cervical osteotomy for fixed cervical deformities. Spine. 2014;39(21):1751–7.
20. Kelly MP, Wollowick AL, Riew KD. Cervical osteotomies for kyphosis. In: Rhee J, Wiesel SW, Boden SD, Flynn JM, editors. Operative techniques in spine surgery. Philadelphia: Lippincott Williams and Wilkins; 2013.

14 Considerations for Approaches Crossing the Cervicothoracic Junction

James S. Harrop, Jeff Wilson, and Payman Vahedi

Introduction

The cervicothoracic junction (CTJ) is a challenging region for spine surgeons. Anatomically, it is an area of transition from cervical lordosis to thoracic kyphosis and from medially placed cervical pedicles to more laterally placed thoracic ones, making posterior spinal instrumentation and fusion more technically challenging. Radiologically, conventional radiographic images have historically been difficult to interpret in this area because of the superimposed shadows of nearby bony structures; however, the issue has been resolved to a great extent in recent years with the advent of 3D-reconstructed CT scan and high-resolution MRI. Biomechanically, it is regarded as a high stress zone; crossing from the fairly mobile lordotic lower cervical to the rigid kyphotic upper thoracic spine mandates sophisticated preoperative and intraoperative justifications for any decompressive surgery or instrumentation in this area. Large bending forces are encountered at the CTJ, while only smaller-sized fixation devices may be used or are available to provide resistance. From the surgical standpoint, anterior approaches to this region are confined by the sternum and crowding of neurovascular structures which may pose significant postoperative morbidity.

Two main concerns of operating on the CTJ are adjacent segment disease (ASD) and treatment failure/pseudarthrosis. Several risk factors have been suggested for treatment failure and regional instability following cervicothoracic junction surgery including multilevel corpectomy and laminectomy crossing over the CTJ, history of prior surgery, tobacco use, and surgery for the correction of deformity. Moreover, because of the higher range of flexion/extension movement at the CTJ, posterior constructions terminating near the CTJ area theoretically have higher risk of developing ASD in future [1]. Adjacent level stress is most pronounced in flexion-extension which represents the most likely construct failure mode. Biomechanical data supports rostral and

J.S. Harrop, MD, FACS
Department of Neurological and Orthopedic Surgery, Division of Spine and Peripheral Nerve Surgery, Neurosurgery Director of Delaware Valley SCI Center, Thomas Jefferson University, 909 Walnut Street, Philadelphia, PA 19107, USA

J. Wilson, MD PhD FRCSC
St. Michael's Hospital, University of Toronto, Li Ka Shing Knowledge Institute, 30 Bond Street, Toronto, ON M5W 1W8, Canada
e-mail: WilsonJeff@smh.ca

P. Vahedi, MD (✉)
Department of Neurosurgery at Tehran Medical Sciences Branch, Islamic Azad University, Tehran, Iran

Department of Neurosurgery, Thomas Jefferson University Hospitals, 909 Walnut Street, Philadelphia, PA 19107, USA
e-mail: payman.vahedi@gmail.com; payman.vahedi@jefferson.edu

L.T. Holly, P.A. Anderson (eds.), *Essentials of Spinal Stabilization*, DOI 10.1007/978-3-319-59713-3_14

caudal extension of constructs in some cases, but must be supported by clinical outcomes. The surgeon should take into account added operative time/blood loss, loss of additional motion segments, and potential morbidity of screw placement when considering extending constructs to include C2 and/or T2 in order to offset changes in adjacent level biomechanical stress. Herein, we describe the relevant surgical anatomy, indications for the surgery, techniques, and biomechanical issues any spine surgeon must know before operating on CTJ area.

Biomechanics

The contour of the spine consists of five sagittal curves which include three kyphotic (occiput to C2, T2 to T11, and S1 to coccyx) and two lordotic curves (C2 to T2 and L1 to L5). CTJ is the junction of cervical lordosis to thoracic kyphosis. The normal lordosis of the cervical spine is 14.4°, and the weight-bearing axis is posterior to vertebral bodies. A load transmission of 36% and 64% is divided between anterior and posterior columns, respectively. Loss of posterior tension band after laminectomy in posterior approaches to this area or in traumatic cases with posterior ligamentous injury shifts the weight-bearing axis anteriorly and may gradually proceed to a kyphotic deformity. Muscular fatigue and pain may also exacerbate the deformity and result in spinal cord draping and uncompromised sagittal deformity. It is believed that up to 36% of cervical extension capacity comes from semispinalis capitis only [2] and removal of its attachments on C2 results in cervical loss of alignment and the development of kyphosis [3].

Facets play a pivotal role in the cervicothoracic junction. Although both cervical and upper thoracic vertebrae are coronally oriented, the transition from C6 to T3 vertebrae increases axial rotatory movements while restricting flexion/extension and lateral bending motions. This is mainly because of thoracic attachments to the rib cage.

Two-column injury biomechanical studies on cadavers suggest that posterior instrumentation alone is sufficient to stabilize two-column injury at the CTJ; however, the length of construct is controversial [4, 5]. Nonetheless, three-column injury cadaveric studies suggest that posterior instrumentation alone is insufficient for stabilization of the CTJ and an anterior supplementation in combination with posterior instrumentation restores stability [5]. However, this has not been repeated in clinical studies of injuries at the CTJ.

Adjacent segment disease (ASD) at the rostral or caudal segments of a posterior cervical construct may develop over time. The results of a cadaveric biomechanical study have found that regardless of laminectomy length, marked increases in adjacent level range of motion and intradiscal pressure at both rostral and caudal segments of a C3 to C6 laminectomy model occur with increasing construct length [1].

Surgical Anatomy

The term CTJ denotes the C7 and T1 vertebra with intervertebral disk and ligamentous structures. However, because of biomechanical concerns in surgical procedures on this area, the caudal extent may be considered to be down to T2 or T3. At the cervicothoracic junction area, transition happens from smaller mobile cervical vertebrae to larger thoracic vertebrae supported by the rib cage. Posterior anatomical structures include muscle and bony structures. Major muscles include trapezius, rhomboid, and serratus; the trapezius extends from the spinous processes of C7 to T10 and attaches onto the scapula, acromion, and posterior lateral third of clavicle.

The anatomy of a lower cervical vertebra includes body, thin pedicles and lamina, spinous process, transverse process, and lateral masses (superior and inferior articulating processes). In contrast, lateral masses are absent in the upper thoracic spine, and separate articulations exist between the body and transverse processes with the ribs. Relatively small pedicles allow limited margin of error when placing instrumentation; moreover, intraoperative fluoroscopic imaging is limited to the AP view, as the lateral view is frequently unhelpful due to obscuration from shoulder structures.

Three important parameters in inserting pedicle screws at this area are transverse pedicle angle, transverse pedicle diameter, and pedicle height (sagittal pedicle diameter). The width and height of the pedicle increases from C5 to T1, while the angle between the pedicle and body decreases [6]. It becomes increasingly more difficult to put pedicular screws from T1 to T4 due to gradual decrease in the transverse pedicle diameter [7, 8, 9]. Pedicle height constantly decreases in the thoracic spine from T1 to T12 and superiorly projecting transverse processes at upper thoracic turn to project inferiorly at lower thoracic spine [10].

The vertebral artery is main vascular structure of the posterior approach in the cervical spine which ascends through transverse foramina of C6 to C2. There is a 5% chance for this artery to traverse the C7 transverse foramina. The possibility of this variant anatomy should be considered whenever attempting to put a lateral mass or a pedicle screw into the C7 vertebra.

Major anatomical considerations in an anterior approach are muscular, bony, and critical neurovascular structures. The cricoid cartilage is a landmark for C6 level from which the skin incision usually starts. Anterior bony structures include the sternum, the clavicle, and the first rib. Because of their important muscular attachments, the clavicle and the first rib play a pivotal role in the stability of the shoulder girdle. The thoracic inlet is composed of T1 posteriorly, cartilaginous tissue of the first rib laterally, and the suprasternal notch anteriorly. Surgically, important muscular tissues include platysma, sternocleidomastoid (SCM), scalene, strap, and deep prevertebral (longus colli) muscles. SCM originates from two different sites – the manubrium of sternum and the clavicle – and runs superolaterally to attach to the mastoid process of the temporal bone. It divides the anterolateral surface of the neck into two separate anterior and posterior triangles. The anterior triangle includes the common carotid artery (CCA), internal jugular vein, and the vagus nerve, all within the carotid sheath. The posterior triangle is divided by the inferior belly of omohyoid muscle into supraclavicular and occipital triangles. The external jugular vein crosses obliquely ventral to SCM and drains into the subclavian vein at the base of the posterior triangle. The course of the subclavian vein is ventromedial and runs ventral to the anterior scalene muscle and joins the internal jugular vein on the medial border of this muscle to form the innominate vein. The internal jugular vein runs deep to SCM within the anterior triangle and lateral to the CCA and finally joins the subclavian vein at the posterior sternal end of the clavicle. The surgeon should be very vigilant not to injure the thoracic duct when attempting a left approach to CTJ, because it runs an ascending course to drain into the junction of the left subclavian and internal jugular veins.

The left subclavian artery originates directly from the aortic arch, while the right subclavian artery is branched from the innominate artery. The two arteries run posterior to the sternoclavicular joint and pass within the space between anterior and middle scalene muscles.

The vagus nerve is located posterior to the CCA and internal jugular vein within the carotid sheath and courses back to the sternoclavicular joint to give off the right recurrent laryngeal nerve. This surgically important branch runs anterior to the right subclavian artery and makes a loop around it to ascend to the right tracheoesophageal groove. Excessive traction on this branch will cause paresis of the vocal cord. The left recurrent laryngeal nerve loops around the aortic arch and with respect to choosing the surgical approach shows little anatomical variation from the right side.

The phrenic nerve passes obliquely and ventral to the anterior scalene muscle and then lies on the medial surface of this muscle to enter CTJ. It crosses the subclavian vein at its posterior surface lateral to sternoclavicular joint and enters the mediastinum. Every attempt should be made to protect the phrenic nerve from injury during an anterior approach to CTJ. For this reason, care should be taken to detach this muscle as close as possible to the first rib.

The cervicothoracic (Stellate) ganglion is located within the prevertebral fascia and on the anterior surface of C7 transverse process close to the first rib. Iatrogenic damage to this ganglion leads to Horner syndrome.

Indications and Patient Selection

Main indications for surgery include trauma, tumor, degenerative disease, rheumatological diseases, postsurgical instability, and infection.

Trauma

Two to nine percent of cervical spine trauma occurs at CTJ [11]. The rate of missed lower cervical and upper thoracic spine injuries is high at the CTJ due to the fact that conventional radiographic images usually do not provide enough data in a trauma setting [11]. Further reconstructed CT scan and MRI are usually needed to exclude the possibility in the case of inadequate visualization on plain X-rays [11].

Injuries typically occur as fracture, dislocation, and/or ligamentous injury. Isolated fractures in the posterior bony elements may be treated in a cervicothoracic orthosis (CTO) unless they are associated with ligamentous injury. This can be appreciated by flexion/extension studies, T2-fat suppressed, or STIR-MRI. Neurological compromise occurs with significant instability, burst fractures, or cervical cord contusions. The choice of anterior vs. posterior or combined 360′ approaches is a matter of controversy. Although it is primarily a surgeon's choice based on the characteristics of the injury, biomechanical studies have shown that three-column fractures may mandate a combined anterior and posterior approach for instrumentation and fusion [4, 12].

Tumor

Locally invasive, primary, and metastatic tumors may develop in the CTJ. Pancoast tumor is the most common locally invasive tumor in this area. It mostly involves the soft tissues and rarely affects the vertebral body. Other local tumors, such as thyroid or esophageal tumors, may encroach on the vertebral body [13, 14]. Metastatic tumors are more common than primary tumors and commonly arise from lung, prostate, and breast cancers [13, 14]. Primary tumors involving this region may include angiosarcoma, lymphoma, chordoma, plasmacytoma, schwannoma, osteosarcoma, and giant cell tumor [15].

The surgical approach is usually determined by several factors including the patient's life expectancy (curative vs. palliative surgery), anterior or posterior spinal cord compression, and the presence of instability. Extradural and intradural tumors are usually approached posteriorly, while anterior cord compression by the tumor generally mandates anterior corpectomy and fusion with or without posterior instrumentation. To avoid the morbidity of a sternotomy, tumors affecting vertebral bodies below C7 may be approached by costotransversectomy and transpedicular corpectomy, depending on the specifics of the local anatomy [15].

Infection

Infection can occur de novo or in the postoperative setting, presenting as osteomyelitis and/or epidural abscess. Tuberculosis is one important primary infection which may cause significant kyphotic deformity by destructing the vertebral body [6, 16]. An anterior approach with instrumentation with or without posterior fusion has been shown to be the optimal method to correct the deformity when necessary [16].

Postoperative infection is generally treated with broad-spectrum antibiotics (4–6 weeks), irrigation, and debridement. Usually, there is no need to remove posterior instrumentation. If instability occurs due to vertebral body involvement or failure of an anterior device, anterior reconstruction with an autograft becomes necessary.

Degenerative Disease

CTJ is not a common location for primary degenerative diseases; however, secondary degeneration, namely, adjacent segment disease, may develop over time when the prior surgical fusion construct ends at C7. It mostly presents as C7/T1 disk herniation, and myelopathy is a rare sign [11]. An anterior approach (ACDF) is usually sufficient to address the pathology. Facet degeneration resulting in degenerative spondylolisthesis at C7/T1 is not uncommon. A patient often has fusion to C7 and above. Neurologic complaints may be radicular in the C8 distribution or myelopathic.

Rheumatologic Diseases

Ankylosing spondylitis may involve CTJ with the development of large anterior syndesmophytes/osteophytes, and calcification of ALL may occur. The characteristic disabling "chin to chest" deformity [17], as well as traumatic fracture dislocation, may also be seen in the context. A combined surgical approach (APA) has been recommended to treat "chin to chest" deformity [17]. An anterior release is accomplished first by anterior discectomy and osteophyte(s) resection. The second stage is a posterior approach to perform laminectomy, osteotomy, and posterior instrumentation and fusion. This allows intraoperative correction of the deformity by lifting up the head. The final stage is anterior instrumentation and fusion with iliac crest allograft.

Postsurgical Instability

Iatrogenic instability may occur after anterior multilevel corpectomies or posterior laminectomies crossing CTJ [18, 19]. Because of the aforementioned regional biomechanics, CTJ is subject to instability after laminectomy. More vulnerability to flexion stresses may lead to a progressive kyphotic deformity with stretching myelopathy. It is recommended to use instrumentation after laminectomy across CTJ [20]. Moreover, because it is a transitional zone, extension to upper thoracic vertebrae is also advocated [18]. In an interesting systematic review, Steinmetz et al. defined the risk factors for such iatrogenic instability at the CTJ as laminectomy without instrumentation and multilevel anterior corpectomy and ventral fixation [18]. Prior cervical surgery, especially at CTJ, deformity correction and smoking are also associated with increased failure rate. Also, a trend of fusion failure is seen in patients undergoing tumor resection [18].

Preoperative Considerations

Preoperative evaluation starts with meticulous history taking and neurological examination. Preoperative counseling is of paramount importance. Patients with radiculopathy alone are counseled that numbness may persist even after the surgery and the aim of surgery is to relieve pain. Those with myelopathy and motor weakness should be aware that surgery will not cause prompt recovery in most cases and the aim of surgery is to stop its progression and then wait for recovery. The need for postoperative long-term physical therapy should be discussed with these patients. Smoking cessation should be discussed, as this behavior is associated with an increased risk of pseudoarthrosis. Patients are also advised about the need to wear a cervicothoracic orthosis for 12 weeks postoperatively.

Thorough imaging workup should be done preoperatively. This includes plain radiographs (AP, lateral, and flexion/extension), 3D-reconstructed cervicothoracic CT scan, and MRI. A lateral swimmer view may be needed to visualize the CTJ. Fat-suppressed MRI and STIR-MRI are useful adjuncts in cases of trauma and tumor surgery.

EMG/NCV is not routinely requested preoperatively, but may help to differentiate in equivocal cases. The fibrillation pattern is a hint to distinguish radiculopathy from peripheral neuropathy in appropriate patients.

Other preoperative considerations include life expectancy in planning for metastasis surgery, preoperative cervical traction for trauma and deformity, broad-spectrum antibiotics for infection, and general health issues compatible for protracted anterior and posterior approaches.

Surgical Technique

Anterior Approaches

The anterior approach to CTJ was first described by Fielding and Stillwell [21] in 1976. Although the approach has been simplified over decades, it is still unpopular among spine surgeons due to the deep location of vertebral bodies caused by the thoracic kyphosis, potential risks to vital anatomical structures, and postoperative morbidity. The anterior approach has several advantages including direct neural decompression, corpectomy and discectomy, deformity correction, and anterior column support with appropriate graft and instrumentation. Currently, three anterior approaches are used to access the lesions of CTJ: modified anterior, transthoracic, and sternal splitting (transsternal).

Modified Anterior Approach

The modified anterior approach to CTJ was introduced by Kurz et al. [22] in 1991 and has the advantage of exposing C7 to T4 vertebra without the need for sternotomy.

Intraoperative neuromonitoring is applied. After the induction of general anesthesia, the patient is positioned supine, and a rolled towel is placed between the two scapulae to extend the neck. Adhesive tapes are used to pull the shoulders down. An AP radiograph is taken to determine the lowest intervertebral disk accessible above the sternoclavicular joint. A lateral view is then taken to locate the incision. A left-side approach is chosen, and the head is turned to the right. This is to avoid intraoperative injury to the right recurrent laryngeal nerve due to its inconsistent anatomy. After the surgical field is prepared and draped, a hockey stick incision is made with the transverse limb 2–4 cm above and parallel to the left clavicle extending between the lateral border of SCM and the midline. The vertical limb starts from the medial end of the transverse line and extends over the manubriosternal junction. The platysma is divided, and subcutaneous flaps are made. Internal and external jugular veins are preserved and retracted unless they hinder surgical access to CTJ. Sternal and clavicular heads of SCM are divided and retracted laterally and proximally. Strap muscles are then released from the first rib and retracted medially and proximally. Subperiosteal dissection proceeds to expose the left half of the manubrium and medial third of the clavicle. The clavicle is sectioned with a Gigli or oscillating saw at the junction of its middle and medial third. The medial third is then disarticulated from the sternum and is kept to be used as an autograft at the final stage of the operation. Care must be taken to avoid injuring the left subclavian vein, which runs inferior and posterior to the clavicle. Next, a fascial plane is found proximally and opened between the carotid sheath laterally and the esophagus and trachea medially. Richardson retractors are introduced. The esophagus, trachea, and brachiocephalic vessels are retracted inferolaterally to the patient's right. The carotid sheath and the left brachiocephalic and subclavian veins are retracted inferolaterally to the patient's left. This will expose longus colli muscles descending on two sides of the midline to attach onto the T1, T2, and T3 vertebrae. Because of limited radiographic visualization at this area, these muscles are useful landmarks for the midline orientation, as well as numbering the vertebrae. Prevertebral fascia is opened, and access to the corresponding level is achieved. Corpectomy and discectomy are accomplished in a standard fashion, and reconstruction and stabilization are done with autograft or allograft bone (under cervical traction) or an expandable titanium mesh cage filled with bone grafts. An anterior titanium plate is applied, and the wound is irrigated with copious antibiotic saline. Platysma, subcutaneous tissue, and the skin are then closed in a standard fashion.

Transthoracic Approach

The patient is intubated by a double lumen tracheal tube. This helps to collapse the right lung further during the operation to maximize exposure. The patient is placed in a left lateral decubitus position and tilted toward the surgeon. An incision is made over the third or fourth rib extending from the anterior axillary line to the lateral border of right paravertebral muscles. Trapezius and latissimus dorsi muscles are cut over the rib and retracted. The neurovascular bundle is detached from the costal groove at the inferior margin of the rib with a rib elevator. Then, a long segment of rib is cut anteriorly and posteriorly with a rib cutter. The rib cage spreader is placed, the pleura are opened, a wet sponge is put on the right lung, and the right lung is deflated and ventrally retracted to expose the upper thoracic vertebra. Transthoracic approach is used when exposure down to T4 is required; however, it cannot be used directly with a low cervical anterior dissection. For these patients, a combined transthoracic-transsternal approach may be used through a trapdoor approach best described by Nazzaro et al. [23]. This combined approach enables the surgeon to expose the ventral area from C3 down to T4/T5 [23, 24].

Sternal Splitting (Transsternal) Approach

The general setup is similar to modified anterior approach in terms of positioning and anesthesia considerations. The surgeon can access lesions down to T3 level. The incision starts at the anterior border of SCM and extends obliquely down to the suprasternal notch and then vertically over the sternum to the xiphoid process. After exposing the cervical portion as an ACDF approach, the retrosternal space is dissected bluntly and then the sternum is cut midline down to the xiphoid process with a Gigli or an oscillating saw. Sternal retractors are placed, and, after retraction of vascular structures, the retropleural fascia is identified and dissected meticulously to expose the CTJ.

Posterior Approach

The posterior approach to CTJ is more popular than the anterior approaches, because of the surgeon's familiarity to both the anatomy and the surgical technique. When combined with costotransversectomy, it has the added advantage to address ventral pathologies, as well as accomplish transpedicular corpectomy in experienced hands. Similarly, pedicle subtraction osteotomy makes correcting severe kyphotic deformities feasible. Fin addition fixation can be applied to as many segments as needed.

The patient is positioned prone on the operating table, and the Mayfield skull clamp is applied. All pressure points are safely padded. The shoulders are tucked down with adhesive tape to maximize radiographic visualization. Anatomical localization is confirmed by the lateral view. After preparing and draping, a midline skin incision is made, subcutaneous dissection is done, and paravertebral fascia is opened bilaterally with electrocautery. Subperiosteal dissection proceeds to expose cervical lateral masses and thoracic facet joints, bilaterally. The exposure of the upper thoracic spine might go beyond the facet joints, if ventral access is planned via costotransversectomy. Instrumentation is usually achieved by inserting pedicular screws at C7 and upper thoracic vertebrae. We prefer to choose the entry points in line with subaxial cervical lateral mass screws to avoid an offset connecting construct. A small laminotomy at each level helps to keep a safe trajectory by palpating the medial, upper, and lower borders of the corresponding pedicle. Laminectomy is usually done in a standard fashion to address the pathology at the affected level. If the aim is to reverse a kyphotic deformity, an attempt should be made after doing laminectomy and possible osteotomy by maneuvering the head within the three-point-fixation skull clamp. After putting the rod connectors and finalizing the construct, posterolateral decortication and bone graft material are placed. The wound is irrigated with copious antibiotic saline, and posterolateral arthrodesis is made by a suitable bone graft. Hemostasis is achieved, a Hemovac drain is put subfascially, muscular layers are reapproximated at the laminectomy site, and sequential closure of the fascia, subcutaneous tissue, and skin is done. We prefer to use supplemental posterior fusion constructs extending from two levels up to two levels down at the laminectomy site at the CTJ.

Illustrative Case

A 57-year-old male patient presented with neck pain and head falling forward. On neurological examination, he appeared to have mild gait ataxia, intact sensation, and full strength in four limbs. MRI of the cervical spine revealed homogenously contrast-enhancing epidural soft tissue mass with cord compression at T1–T2 with the involvement of T1 and T2 vertebral bodies (Fig. 14.1). The collapse of T1 and T2 vertebral bodies resulted in a local cervicothoracic kyphosis and spinal cord stretching at the CVJ. The patient underwent C7 and T1 corpectomy plus C6–C7 to T1–T2 discectomy via the modified anterior cervical approach. A strut graft without an anterior cervical plate was placed at the corpectomy site to restore the segmental height and to reverse the kyphotic deformity (Fig. 14.2).This was supplemented by posterior cervicothoracic fusion (Fig. 14.2). Histopathology confirmed the diagnosis to be multiple melanoma. The patient was referred to the oncology colleagues for adjuvant therapies. At 5 years follow-up, the patient is neurologically intact and has no neck pain or tumor recurrence.

Technical Pearls

- Regardless of the type of anterior approach chosen to CTJ, the lowest surgically accessible vertebrae remains T4.
- Access to the lower cervical vertebra is limited with transthoracic approach, and it is best suited for pathologies affecting T1 to T4 vertebra. Because of the lateral nature of the approach, the risk of injury to the sympathetic chain is higher than other anterior approaches. Often, insertion of a chest tube is necessary at the end of procedure.
- Because of the morbidities of transsternal approach and no more visualization than other sternal sparing approaches, it is rarely used to approach CTJ anteriorly.
- During a left anterior approach, working medial to carotid sheath will save the thoracic duct from injury. Most often, the thoracic duct is hidden from the surgeon's view, and it can only be seen after the injury occurs. If diagnosed intraoperatively, primary repair should be attempted even on friable tissue.
- Injury to the recurrent laryngeal nerve is avoided partly by choosing a left-side anterior

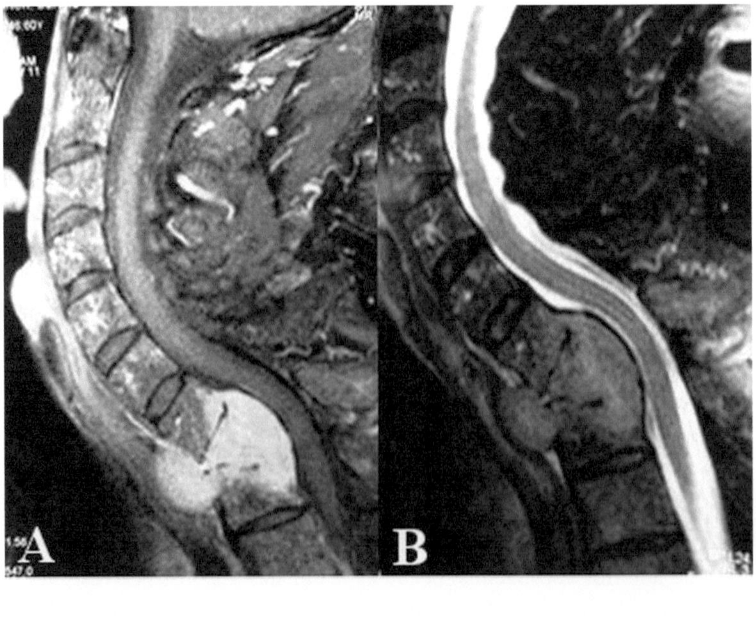

Fig. 14.1 (**a**) Post-contrast T1 sagittal MRI reveals a homogenously enhancing tumor affecting C7, T1, and T2 vertebral bodies with extension into the epidural space. Stretching of the spinal cord and segmental kyphosis due to the collapse of the vertebral bodies are also evident at the CTJ. (**b**) T2 sagittal MRI illustrates a hypersignal mass originating from the vertebral bodies at the CTJ with apparent cord compression but no associated myelopathy

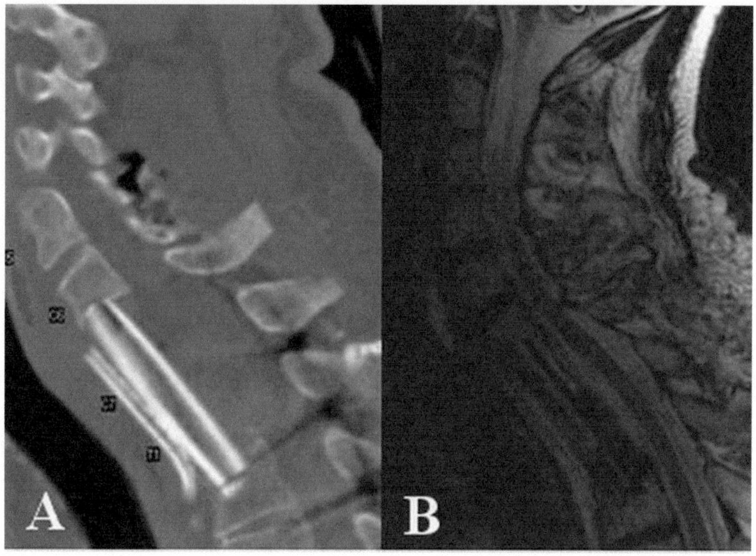

Fig. 14.2 (**a**) Postoperative reconstructed sagittal CT scan of the same patient shows appropriate placement of a strut graft at the corpectomy site. (**b**) Sagittal T2WI confirms spinal cord decompression. The restoration of the height and the reversal of the segmental kyphosis were achieved through a modified anterior cervical approach

approach. A carefully placed medial retractor under the esophagus (and not within the tracheoesophageal groove) also helps to prevent injury to the nerve.

- Longus colli muscles have surgical importance in an anterior approach. Working medial to these muscles prevents injury to the sympathetic chain. They are also regarded as surgical landmarks for the midline and correct level.
- External and internal jugular veins and inferior thyroid vessels may hinder anterior access to the CTJ in some patients and may need to be ligated and cut.
- Anterior reconstruction with autograft bone is superior to allograft or synthetic cages in multilevel anterior corpectomies.
- When closing a pedicle subtraction osteotomy during a posterior approach, care should be taken to prevent spinal cord buckling by removing two-thirds of the rostral and caudal lamina.
- Because of the convexity of vertebral bodies at the anterior border and the risk of injury to vital structures, ventral pedicle screw penetration should not exceed beyond 80% of the vertebral body on a lateral radiograph.
- In comparison to conventional AP view, a slightly oblique AP is better for identifying the entry point at the midpoint of the pedicle.
- A posterior fusion may skip C7 for better alignment of the connecting rods between lower cervical and upper thoracic vertebrae.

Complications and Strategies for Avoidance

The complications can be of a systemic or a direct operative cause. Systemic complications include deep venous thrombosis, pulmonary embolism, and cardiovascular problems in elderly patients or prolonged surgeries. Direct operative complications include early or late complications. Early complications are dysphagia, temporary hoarseness, vocal cord paresis, Horner's syndrome, postoperative hematoma or emphysema (tracheal injury), esophageal rupture, lung injury, vascular injury, exaggerated preexisting myelopathy, and infection. Late complications include pseudoarthrosis, device failure, muscular atrophy, and late infection.

Recommended strategies for prevention are as follows:

Intraoperative pneumatic compression stockings and early initiation of IV anticoagulants (after 24 h) should be used in high risk patients. Awake intubation and intraoperative neuromonitoring reduce the risk of postoperative aggravated myelopathy. Any vascular injury should be repaired primarily. During a left anterior approach, the plane of dissection should always stay medial to the carotid sheath to avoid thoracic duct injury. In a right anterior approach, the retractors should be placed deep to esophagus and not within the tracheoesophageal groove to prevent an injury to recurrent laryngeal artery. The surgeon should be very meticulous about esophageal injury and the possibility of occult ruptures should be excluded at the end of surgery by the instillation of Indigo carmine via a retracted nasogastric tube. If leakage happens, primary esophageal repair is mandatory to avoid acute mediastinitis. A Hemovac drain should be kept under the fascia (posterior approach) or platysma (anterior approach) for 12–24 h postoperatively to prevent the formation of postoperative hematoma. To decrease the risk of pseudoarthrosis, the patient should be encouraged to stop smoking. Because the risk of pseudoarthrosis grows up with the number of anteriorly operated segments, the use of autografts is advocated for these patients.

Conclusion

The cervicothoracic junction is a tricky area to the spine surgeons in terms of the complex ventral anatomy and biomechanical concerns. A spectrum of different pathologies seen elsewhere throughout the spinal column may necessitate an anterior, posterior, or circumferential approach with instrumentation at this area. Anterior surgical access is limited by the sternum and crowding of neurovascular structures which may pose significant postoperative morbidity, while the posterior approach is complexed by the anatomy of the pedicles and intraoperative X-ray drawbacks. Two main postoperative concerns are adjacent segment disease and treatment failure/pseudarthrosis, which usually mandate supplemental posterior instrumentation and fusion crossing the cervicothoracic junction.

References

1. Kretzer RM, Hsu W, Hu N, Umekoji H, Jallo GI, McAfee PC, et al. Adjacent-level range of motion and intradiscal pressure after posterior cervical decompression and fixation: an in vitro human cadaveric model. Spine. 2012;37:E778–85.
2. Vasavada AN, Li S, Delp SL. Influence of muscle morphometry and moment arms on the moment-generating capacity of human neck muscles. Spine. 1998;23:412–22.
3. Iizuka H, Shimizu T, Tateno K, Toda N, Edakuni H, Shimada H, et al. Extensor musculature of the cervical spine after laminoplasty: morphologic evaluation by coronal view of the magnetic resonance image. Spine. 2001;26:2220–6.
4. Kreshak JL, Kim DH, Lindsey DP, Kam AC, Panjabi MM, Yerby SA. Posterior stabilization at the cervicothoracic junction. A biomechanical study. Spine. 2002;27:2763–70.
5. Prybis BG, Tortolani PJ, Hu N, Zorn CM, McAfee PC, Cunningham BW. A comparative biomechanical analysis of spinal instability and instrumentation of the cervicothoracic junction: an in vitro human cadaveric model. J Spinal Disord Tech. 2007;20(3):233–8.
6. Wang VY, Chou D. The cervicothoracic junction. Neurosurg Clin N Am. 2007;18(2):365–71.
7. Vaccaro AR, Rizzolo SJ, Allardyce TJ, Ramsey M, Salvo J, Balderston RA, et al. Placement of pedicle screws in the thoracic spine. Part I: morphometric analysis of the thoracic vertebrae. J Bone Joint Surg Am. 1995;77:1193–9.
8. Cinotti G, Gumina S, Ripani M, Postacchini F. Pedicle instrumentation in the thoracic spine. A morphometric and cadaveric study for placement of screws. Spine. 1999;24:114–9.
9. Panjabi MM, O'Holleran JD, Crisco JJ 3rd, Kothe R. Complexity of the thoracic spine pedicle anatomy. Eur Spine J. 1997;6:19–24.
10. Singh K, Berta SC, Albert TJ. Anterior Cervicothoracic junction approach. Tech Orthop. 2003;17(3):365–73.
11. Amin A, Saifuddin A. Fractures and dislocations of the cervicothoracic junction. J Spinal Disord Tech. 2005;18:499–505.
12. Chapman JR, Anderson PA, Pepin C, Toomey S, Newell DW, Grady MS. Posterior instrumentation of the unstable cervicothoracic spine. J Neurosurg. 1996;84:552–8.
13. Mazel C, Hoffmann E, Antonietti P, Grunenwald D, Henry M, Williams J. Posterior cervicothoracic instrumentation in spine tumors. Spine. 2004;29:1246–53.
14. Ulmar B, Cakir B, Huch K, Puhl W, Richter M. Posterior stabilisation of a malignant cervico-thoracic vertebral bone defect. Acta Orthop Belg. 2005;71:349–52.
15. Le H, Balabhadra R, Park J, Kim D. Surgical treatment of tumors involving the cervicothoracic junction. Neurosurg Focus. 2003;15:E3.

16. Mihir B, Vinod L, Umesh M, Chaudhary K. Anterior instrumentation of the cervicothoracic vertebrae: approach based on clinical and radiologic criteria. Spine. 2006;31:E244–9.
17. Mummaneni PV, Mummaneni VP, Haid RW Jr, Rodts GE Jr, Sasso RC. Cervical osteotomy for the correction of chin-on-chest deformity in ankylosing spondylitis. Technical note Neurosurg Focus. 2003;14:E9.
18. Steinmetz MP, Miller J, Warbel A, Krishnaney AA, Bingaman W, Benzel EC. Regional instability following cervicothoracic junction surgery. J Neurosurg Spine. 2006;4:278–84.
19. Boockvar JA, Philips MF, Telefeian AE, O'Rourke DM, Marcotte PJ. Results and risk factors for anterior cervicothoracic junction surgery. J Neurosurg. 2001;94(1 Suppl):12–7.
20. An HS, Vaccaro A, Cotler JM, Lin S. Spinal disorders at the cervicothoracic junction. Spine. 1994;19:2557–64.
21. Fielding JW, Stillwell WT. Anterior cervical approach to the upper thoracic spine. Spine. 1976;1: 158–61.
22. Kurz L, Stewart P, Herkowitz H. Modified anterior approach to cervicothoracic junction. Spine. 1995;16(suppl):542–7.
23. Nazzaro JM, Arbit E, Burt M. "trap door" exposure of the cervicothoracic junction. Technical note J Neurosurg. 1994;80:338–41.
24. Gokaslan ZL, York JE, Walsh GL, et al. Transthoracic vertebrectomy for metastatic spinal tumors. J Neurosurg. 1998;89:599–609.

15 Open Anterior and Lateral Thoracic Interbody Approaches and Techniques

Hesham Mostafa Zakaria and Victor Chang

Introduction

The first reported case of a thoracic herniated disc causing spinal cord compression was published in 1838 [1], with the next reported case 73 years later [2]. The original surgical treatment for herniated discs was laminectomy, which was introduced in 1922 [3]. Unfortunately the procedure was morbid, rendering many patients paraplegic [4]. The first lateral approach to the thoracic spine was via costotransversectomy in 1900 [5], which was subsequently modified for Pott's disease [6]. A modernized approach of costotransversectomy for thoracic herniated disc was implemented in 1960 [7], and it was soon observed to be more effective and safer than laminectomy [8]. The first transthoracic procedure for herniated disc was described in 1958 [9] and was soon deemed as a viable alternative to costotransversectomy [10, 11]. The original description of an open anterior approach to the thoracic spine is from 1928 [12], which was subsequently modified in 1969 for scoliosis [13]. All of these approaches have evolved with time, and current iterations include microsurgical techniques, video-assisted thoracoscopic surgery, and minimally invasive surgery [8, 14–21]. This chapter will focus on open anterior and lateral approaches to the thoracic spine for the purpose of interbody placement.

H.M. Zakaria, MD (✉) • V. Chang, MD
Department of Neurosurgery, Henry Ford Hospital, 2799 W Grand Blvd, Detroit, MI 48202, USA
e-mail: Hzakari1@hfhs.org; Vicchang@gmail.com

Specific Pathologies

The main rationale for an anterolateral approach to the thoracic spine is to gain direct access to pathology of the thoracic vertebral body and/or disc space. For the purpose of interbody placement, these approaches provide the largest access corridor for placement of a strut graft and subsequent arthrodesis. Operative indications and approaches for interbody placement depend on patient symptoms and the specific diagnosis seen on imaging, as well as the specific anatomical location of any pathology. Pathologies to be treated include five broad categories: degenerative, neoplastic, infectious, spinal deformity, and trauma. Degenerative pathologies can include but are not limited to thoracic disc herniation and ossification of the posterior longitudinal ligament (OPLL). Neoplastic lesions include most commonly metastatic tumors to the spinal column as well as primary bone tumors. Infectious etiologies include the spectrum from discitis to osteomyelitis and, rare today, tuberculous lesions. Deformity can include adolescent idiopathic scoliosis and Scheuermann's kyphosis, as well as adult degenerative deformities. Trauma includes a variety of fractures or ligamentous injuries that can involve the thoracic spine.

L.T. Holly, P.A. Anderson (eds.), *Essentials of Spinal Stabilization*,
DOI 10.1007/978-3-319-59713-3_15

Indications for Surgery

In general, surgery should be offered for (1) symptomatic lesions that have failed conservative therapy, (2) lesions compromising spinal stability, and (3) lesions that cause progressive neurological symptoms (i.e., myelopathy, extremity weakness, paralysis, bowel or bladder dysfunction, imbalance, ataxia, and debilitating pain refractory to nonoperative treatments). A simplified guideline is that surgery is indicated for lesions that cause any neurological deficit and lesions that compromise the stability of the spinal column in such a manner that normal physiological load-bearing activity can lead to neurological injury. Stable asymptomatic lesions can be monitored with serial imaging, especially if the surgery has potential morbidities. Specific considerations for different classes of pathology are discussed below. It is important to keep in mind that symptoms of thoracic spinal cord compression have been described as variable and nonspecific [3, 22, 23]. The typical chronologic progression of symptoms is that of band-like thoracic pain, followed by sensory disturbances, and ultimately bowel/bladder dysfunction [24–26]. Therefore, all other sources of myelopathy should be ruled out before proceeding to surgery in pursuit of thoracic spine pathology.

Degenerative Disc Disease

Asymptomatic thoracic disc pathology is common, with 73% of patients having abnormalities on magnetic resonance imaging (MRI), including spinal cord deformation in 29% [27]. Asymptomatic disc herniations warrant surgery only if there is concern that they may progress and become symptomatic; however, most asymptomatic discs do not become symptomatic. Progression of disc degeneration over time has been reported [25, 28]. The location, size, or laterality of asymptomatic disc herniations does not indicate that it is benign, as lateral discs can cause severe deficits if they compress a feeding vessel, [29] and a small asymptomatic herniation has the potential to suddenly enlarge and become symptomatic, with severe and sudden neurological deficits [30, 31]. Symptomatic herniated discs can cause thoracic myelopathy and are most commonly found in the lower thoracic region between T8 and T11 (Fig. 15.1) [32]. Herniated thoracic discs are often central (77–94%) as well

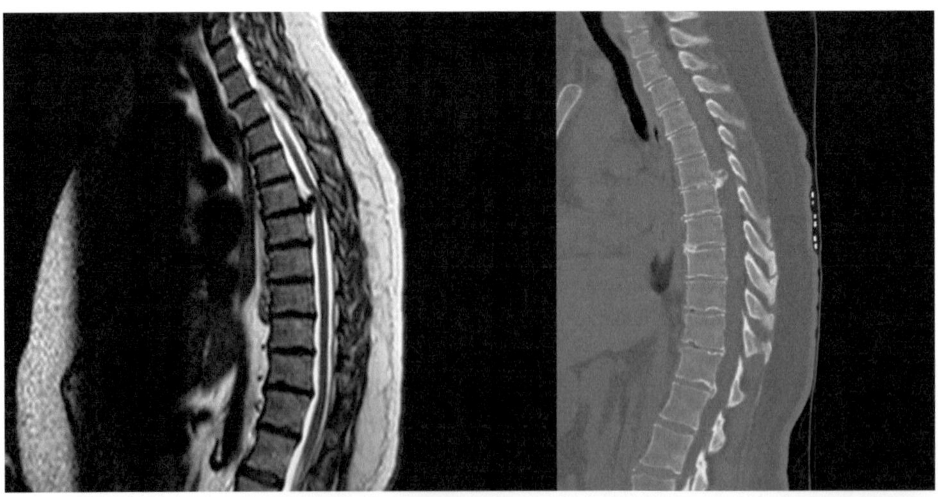

Fig. 15.1 Example of a calcified herniated disc causing spinal cord compression. The patient had clear signs of myelopathy on physical examination, including hyperreflexia and weakness of his lower extremities. Lesion requires an anterolateral approach to best access the disc space for safe removal of the calcified disc material

as calcified (22–65%). A small number of these discs are intradural (~6%) [26] and can only be treated safely using an anterior/lateral approach.

While occurring predominantly in the cervical region, OPLL can occur at any level of the spine [33–35]. Long-term longitudinal studies of OPLL have shown myelopathy-free survival at 30-year follow-up to be 71% [36]. Despite these results, there are reports of rapid progression of symptoms [37, 38]. Further studies have shown that spinal canal stenosis of over 60% and lateral calcification are radiographic risk factors for the development of myelopathy [39–41]. Anterior decompression and reconstruction within the cervical spine for OPLL have been shown to be safe and effective [42–44]. Surgery on thoracic OPLL is potentially morbid, with recent studies showing a 14.7–34.6% rate of postoperative neurological deterioration [45–47]. Therefore, for the young asymptomatic patient, deferring surgery while closely following the physical exam with imaging correlates is appropriate [44].

Neoplastic

Surgery for malignancy is indicated for tissue diagnosis, neurological decompression, and spinal stabilization (Fig. 15.2). Operative intervention is also appropriate when neoplasms are resistant to radiation therapy and for removal of isolated recurrences. Surgery has been shown to improve quality of life for metastases [48–51], but the improvements may be compromised if there are postoperative complications [52, 53]. Preoperative considerations about whether patients are surgical candidates include preoperative functional status, medical comorbidities, life expectancy, and need for tissue diagnosis [54–56], while new evidence suggests that age is not an absolute contraindication [57].

Trauma

Thoracic spinal fractures occur most frequently at the thoracolumbar junction, with 50–80% between T10 and L2 [58, 59]. This area is more susceptible to injury because the thoracic spine has additional mechanical stability via the rib cage, while the more caudal junctional levels undergo transitioning from kyphosis to lordosis in conjunction to a change in orientation of the facet joints [60, 61]. The most common fracture types are compression and burst [61, 62], with the traditional teaching being that surgery is considered for patients with more than 40% height loss, 50% compromise of the spinal canal without

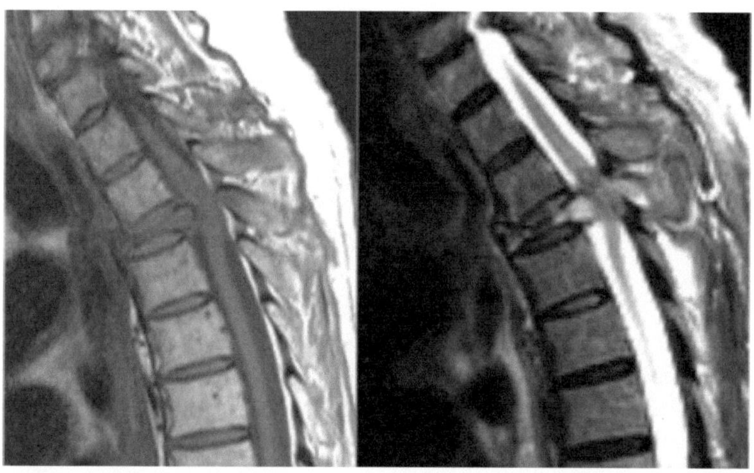

Fig. 15.2 Example of a metastatic lesion to the T3/T4 disc space causing spondylolisthesis and spinal column instability. Surgery only for tissue sampling and decompression would be inappropriate, as there is risk for spinal cord injury with worsening spondylolisthesis. Placement of an interbody with fusion would restore spinal alignment and provide stability for arthrodesis

neurological deficits, or a kyphotic deformity greater than 300 degrees [63–65].

Deformity

Thoracic spine deformity may be congenital, idiopathic, degenerative, and as a sequelae of previous trauma, infection, neoplasm, or surgery. Again, it is appropriate to perform surgery on symptomatic deformity, including intractable axial or radicular pain and progressive neurological deficits. Often, surgery is deferred until kyphosis is greater than 30 degrees or if there is progression of deformity on serial imaging.

Infectious

With the advent of modern antibiotics, vertebral osteomyelitis and discitis without mechanical instability or a neurological deficit can be primarily treated nonsurgically [66–69]. Surgery is warranted to identify the causative organism, for neurological progression, or osseous deformity causing pain. Recent evidence has shown that spinal instrumentation within an infected locus, including from an anterior approach and with tuberculosis, is safe and warranted to confer additional stability [70–75].

Imaging

Adequate imaging is vital before surgery on the thoracic spine. Plain radiographs are a versatile and fairly inexpensive imaging modality. They are sensitive enough to identify vertebral body alignment/deformity, fractures, evidence of discitis or spondylosis, osteolytic/blastic lesions (malignancy), and calcifications within the spinal canal that are indicative of posterior osteophytes and calcified discs. They can be used preoperatively to count the number of ribs and vertebral bodies for correlation with intraoperative fluoroscopy and can be helpful for accurate intraoperative localization to minimize the risk of surgery at an incorrect level. Plain radiographs are also useful to assess pulmonary function and to identify possible risk factors for complications, including COPD/emphysema, heart failure, and pulmonary metastasis. In addition, 36″ standing radiographs can be used to assess for alignment under physiological loads as well as with bending to illustrate whether a deformity is fixed or mobile. One caveat with plain radiographs is that it may be ineffectual in patients with a large body habitus, as bony anatomy may be obscured.

MRI functions as the mainstay imaging modality, with sufficient sensitivity and specificity to differentiate disc disease from infectious, neoplastic, traumatic, or demyelinating pathologies [76–78]. CT can also be useful and in some cases is superior to MRI when imaging bony anatomy, calcified discs, and OPLL. It may also be used to define bony architecture for surgical approaches and instrumentation [23, 79, 80]. CT myelography is useful to assess bone anatomy in relation to neural structures.

It is important to note that both CT myelography and MRI have a relatively high false-positive rate when it comes to identifying symptomatic disc disease, about 14% for both [23, 81, 82]. In rare cases where the pain generator cannot be identified, or if there are multiple sites of disc disease, or no clear pathology at all, provocative discography has been useful in localizing the specific site of axial back pain [83–85]. This procedure should not be used when there is large disc prolapse with cord deformity, as the saline injection may cause further disc herniation and increase the risk of spinal cord injury.

Medical Optimization

Patients should be medically optimized before any open anterior or lateral approach to the spine. These procedures are potentially morbid with a risk for major blood loss and can place considerable physiological stress on the patient in the perioperative period. Plain chest AP and lateral radiographs are part of routine screening for any patient undergoing elective surgery and are a useful screening modality for COPD/

emphysema, heart failure, and pulmonary metastasis. Echocardiography is indicated for those patients who may have elements of heart failure. Pulmonary function testing is useful to quantify pulmonary disease and identify patients whose lung capacities may be insufficient to tolerate surgery; this is especially important if the operative plan is to deflate a lung and to ventilate with only one lung. Marginal surgical candidates should undergo these additional tests and excluded if there is clinical indication that they may not tolerate the procedures. These approaches are known to produce severe pain from rib resection, soft tissue retraction, and chest tube placement, which is necessary when entering the thoracic cavity. Many of these approaches require preoperative coordination with an access surgeon, who will provide spinal exposure. However, in the case of acute neurological deficit, such considerations are not feasible, and therefore it is imperative that the treating surgeon weigh the potential risks of a morbid approach with the potential benefits. It is also critical that the surgeon discusses these considerations with the patient, if possible, prior to undergoing surgery.

Neuromonitoring

Intraoperative neuromonitoring has efficacy to detect spinal cord injury, but its ability to prevent injury remains controversial [86–91]. There are specific reports of poor sensitivity and specificity of neuromonitoring for thoracic spine surgery [92, 93]. Neuromonitoring may be used to identify and avoid potential ischemic injury to the spinal cord, which may occur during ligation of radicular arteries [94]. Recent literature has shown that three levels of bilateral arterial sacrifice are safe without evidence of cord ischemia or compromise [95], although there are case reports where just a single artery ligation caused spinal cord ischemia [96]. The number of segmental vessels ligated is proportional to the risk of cord ischemia and should therefore be minimized if possible [97]. This may be more pronounced if the artery of Adamkiewicz (great anterior radiculomedullary artery) is targeted. Localization of this vessel, which normally arises from the left side from T9–L2, may be achieved using modern imaging modalities [98–100].

Ultimately, the specific monitoring modality used, whether SSEP, MEP, or EMG, is contentious, as currently there is no universal standard of care [101, 102]. It may be able to provide real-time feedback about injury to the spinal cord, but its utility to prevent injury is still uncertain. A baseline reading should be obtained before initiation of surgery, which is used for intraoperative comparisons. Changes from this baseline indicate injury, and the surgeon should correlate these changes with intraoperative findings. Some aberrations from baseline may be caused by physiologic changes, anesthetic parameters, or technical problems, which are outside the scope of this chapter [103–105].

The exact approaches utilized will be dictated by the location of pathology. As a general rule, T1 to T3 requires an anterior transmanubrial approach, T4 to T10 a lateral transthoracic approach, and T10 to T12 a lateral thoracoabdominal approach, which may be used for upper lumbar pathology as well.

T1–T3: Transmanubrial (Possibly with Clavicular Resection)

As compared to the remainder of the thoracic spine, surgical pathology in this area is uncommon. In patients with long and thin necks, the C7/T1 and T1/T2 discs are potentially approachable via the standard anterior cervical discectomy approach. However, in most patients, a transmanubrial approach is necessary and will allow access up to the T3/T4 disc space. The transmanubrial corridor requires dissection and manipulation of the superior mediastinum, including the left brachiocephalic vein, subclavian veins, aortic arch, and great vessels, putting these structures at risk. Other structures at risk include the carotid sheath and contents, trachea, esophagus, recurrent laryngeal nerves, sympathetic trunk and stellate ganglion, and pleural apices. There are several variations to this approach [106–108], but this section will cover the most commonly used technique.

The patient is positioned supine with a towel roll or bolster between the scapulae to allow for head and shoulder extension. Additional extension can be achieved by lowering the head of the operating table. The shoulders are pulled down using adhesive tape to allow for lateral fluoroscopy, but placing too much tension on the shoulders puts the patient at risk for brachial plexus injury. Trendelenburg positioning may allow for enhanced venous drainage from the operative site. An orogastric tube should be placed to help identify the esophagus intraoperatively.

An incision through the skin and subcutaneous layer is performed along the medial border of the right sternocleidomastoid (SCM) muscle or along the superior border of the clavicle if a clavicular resection is planned. The incision should extend caudally to the sternal notch and then down the midline of the manubrium to the sternal angle. Platysmal flaps are then elevated while ensuring the safety of the anterior jugular vein underneath; however, this vessel may be ligated if necessary to aid in exposure. The strap muscles and the SCM are dissected, and their insertions onto the clavicle and manubrium are identified and elevated subperiosteally proximally and laterally. Subperiosteal exposure of both the clavicle and the manubrium is performed, which requires elevation of the pectoralis major muscle. Subperiosteal exposure should also be accomplished along the posterior aspect of the manubrium with finger dissection. At this point, if necessary, the clavicle may be sectioned with care, as the subclavian vein is in close proximity underneath. Up to the middle of the clavicle may be taken, with greater removal improving exposure. After sectioning, it is disarticulated from the manubrium and stored for reimplantation during closure.

The manubrium is split longitudinally along its midline while being careful not to injure the mediastinal structures. Sternal retractors are placed to help exposure, and the major vessels, the pericardium, and the thymus are identified. The inferior thyroid artery and vein may be ligated to assist in exposure. The thymus and surrounding fat are reflected to the right, and the trachea, esophagus, and carotid sheath are identified. The left innominate vein may be sacrificed to enhance the exposure. The approach to the spine is between the left common carotid and the right innominate (brachiocephalic) artery, trachea/esophagus, and thyroid (Fig. 15.3). The recurrent laryngeal nerve lies posterior to the trachea and anterior to the esophagus, and so to avoid injury, care should be taken to avoid dissection or manipulation of this area, including during placement of the retractor. The brachio-

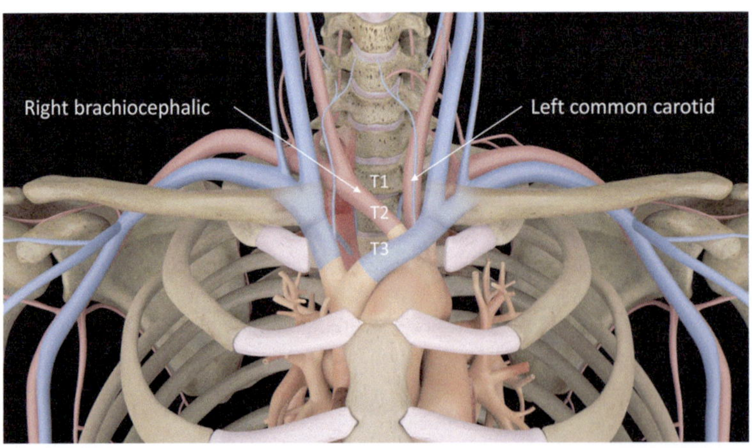

Fig. 15.3 The vascular anatomy encountered during the transmanubrial approach to the spine. The final corridor to the vertebrae during this approach is between the left common carotid artery and the right innominate (brachiocephalic) artery. This pathway yields a relatively avascular plane, which upon careful and blunt dissection will yield the vertebral column

cephalic and subclavian veins can be displaced inferolaterally to approach the prevertebral fascia, which can be thinned by using a Kitner to visualize the longus colli muscles [106, 109]. The thoracic duct lives in close proximity and to the left of the esophagus from around T4 to where it joins with the internal jugular or subclavian vein, and care must be taken to not injure it.

The remainder of the procedure should be performed in a similar fashion as a cervical spine anterior cervical discectomy. Briefly, osteophytes that narrow the access to the disc space should be cleaned away using rongeurs or a high-speed drill. A sharp knife is used to incise the anterior longitudinal ligament and the annulus fibrosis, allowing access into the interbody space. The bulk of the disc should be removed with pituitary forceps. The superior and inferior aspects of the end plates should be prepared by cleaning away any residual disc material: an osteotome or various curettes are excellent tools for this task. Once all the residual disc material has been cleared away, the desired interbody device can be placed. Additional instrumentation and fusion are often required to ensure stability of the interbody device (Fig. 15.4). Hemostasis is achieved with bipolar cautery and hemostatic agents.

Closure is performed in layers. The sternum and manubrium should be wired to approximate the split halves. If the clavicle was disarticulated and removed, it should be fixed back into place. The strap muscles and SCM are reattached to their insertion sites and repaired. A drain is placed, and the platysma and skin are closed in the usual fashion.

T4–T12: Transthoracic (Possibly with Scapula Mobilization)

The transthoracic approach to the spine allows for straightforward access from T6 to T12. Access to T4 and T5 is possible but requires elevation of the scapula to reach this height.

The patient is intubated with a double lumen endotracheal tube to allow for deflation of the lung and is subsequently placed in a lateral decubitus position. An axillary roll is often necessary to prevent pressure on the brachial plexus. The laterality of the surgery should be ipsilateral to the pathology. However, the left-sided approach avoids potential injury to the thoracic duct as well as the fragile azygos vein and vena cava, and the view is not obstructed by

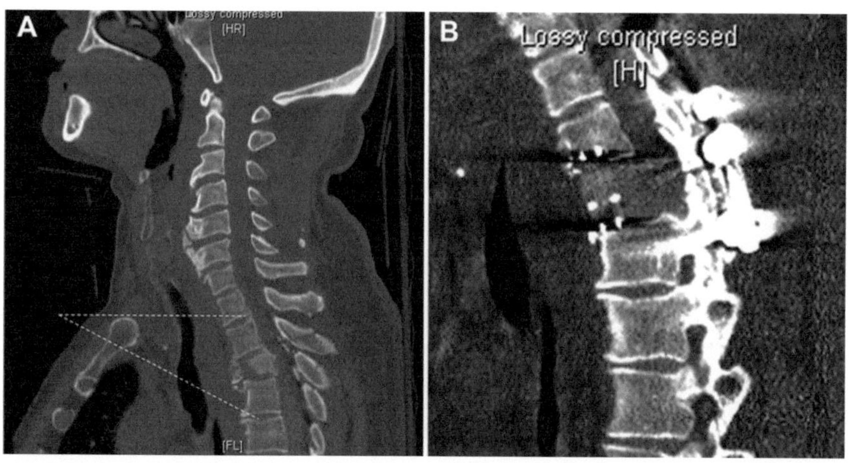

Fig. 15.4 (**a**) Computed tomographic scan of the cervicothoracic junction illustrating a T3 vertebral body fracture with retropulsion into the spinal canal. The *dotted lines* show the rostral and caudal limits to a transmanubrial approach to the spinal column. (**b**) Postoperative imaging after a T3 corpectomy with instrumentation and fusion was performed on this lesion (Reprinted with permission from Lam and Groff [109])

the dome of the liver in the lower thoracic spine. For the upper thoracic spine, a right-sided approach avoids the heart, carotid, and subclavian vessels. Scoliosis may prompt an approach from the convexity, instead of being confined within the concavity. A final consideration is if the patient has had previous surgery or pulmonary disease which would make access to a specific thoracic cavity preferable. The patient should be placed at the break of the table such that a mild convex curve is created, which assists in opening of the rib interspaces.

The location of the incision is determined with fluoroscopy; it should be located two rib levels cranial to the pathology, and the incision itself is oblique along the superior aspect of the rib and should reach past the anterior axillary line for adequate exposure. The skin is incised, and there are often several layers of musculature that need to be divided in a layered fashion and overlying the rib, including the trapezius, latissimus dorsi, rhomboid major, rhomboid minor, serratus anterior, and serratus posterior. At the rib, a subperiosteal plane is used to dissect away the neurovascular bundle from the inferior aspect of the rib using an Alexander-Farabeuf periosteotome and a Doyen elevator. The rib is then cut at the costal junction anteriorly and the costotransverse junction posteriorly; it should be harvested and used as autograft to enhance arthrodesis.

Within the upper thoracic spine, the scapula limits exposure, and so additional rib resections may be necessary. Alternatively, the scapula may be mobilized. If this is the plan, then the incision should start from the T1 spinous process and travel along the medial/inferior border of the scapula. At the most inferior aspect of the scapula, the incision should curve anteriorly along the sixth or seventh rib to end at the costal cartilage of the third rib. Dissection is performed in a layered fashion through the musculature (i.e., trapezius, latissimus dorsi, rhomboids, serratus posterior), which mobilizes the scapula and allows it to be retracted proximally and away from the operative site. The removal of the rib is similar to the procedure described previously, with a subperiosteal dissection and harvesting at the desired rib being performed while sparing the neurovascular bundle.

The lung is then deflated, and the parietal pleura incised, allowing access to the thoracic cavity. It is possible to dissect the pleura away from the chest wall after rib removal, which allows for an extrapleural approach to the spine and thus no need for a chest tube [110]. Extrapleural dissection also has a theoretically decreased risk of perioperative morbidity. A rib spreader provides rib retraction and eases entry into the thoracic cavity, and the lung may be protected with a malleable retractor covered with a sponge.

At this time, it is prudent to again use fluoroscopy to identify the correct interspace. Alternatively, the surgeon may count the ribs by palpation within the thoracic cavity. The neurovascular structures should also be identified, including the aorta, parietal pleura, azygos veins, vena cava, and sympathetic plexus, and avoided if possible. The parietal pleura is dissected to expose the subperiosteal plane on the interspace, with care taken to avoid the segmental vessels if possible; these vessels may be ligated but should be tied or clipped away from the aorta to avoid bleeding. The vertebral bodies and disc space are exposed subperiosteally to enhance visualization (Fig. 15.5). If necessary, the sympathetic chain can be displaced dorsally. The intercostal neurovascular bundle can be used to localize the neural foramen. The rib head is removed with a rongeur or a drill, allowing full exposure and access to the disc space. Additional rib resections may be performed if greater exposure is needed to approach multiple levels. The surgeon should be able to see clearly the disc margins, the intervertebral foramen, and the pedicle above and below the operative site.

The pedicle below the disc space may require removal using a burr and Kerrison rongeurs to enhance exposure of the exiting nerve root and the thecal sac, as well as osteophytes which may crowd the disc space. The disc annulus is incised sharply, and the disc material can be removed with a pituitary rongeur, a Kerrison rongeur, or a drill. The goal at this stage should be decompression and preparation of the inter-

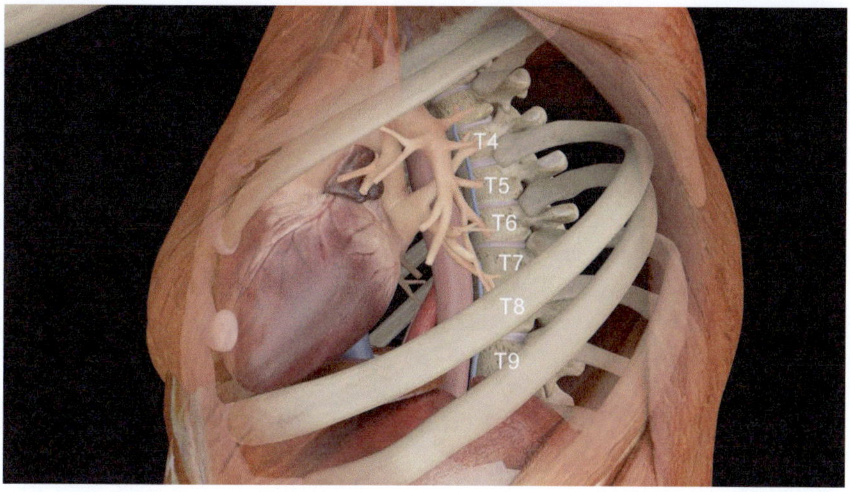

Fig. 15.5 This illustration shows the operative view of the bony and vascular anatomy after exposure of a left-sided transthoracic approach to the spinal column. The descending aorta partially obscures the view, but this vessel may be mobilized with relative ease if necessary. The sympathetic chain and ganglia lay just lateral to the vertebral bodies, and, if necessary, subperiosteal elevation is possible

space for arthrodesis, which requires removal of as much of the disc as possible. For calcified central discs, decompression is ensured if the entirety of the thecal sac is visualized and the contralateral pedicle can be palpated with a blunt instrument. After removal of the disc, bleeding of the epidural veins can be treated with hemostatic agents or careful bipolar cautery at a low setting. An interbody is placed, and the vertebral bodies are instrumented to allow for fusion.

Calcified discs with dural adhesions are at the highest risk for CSF leak [26, 111]. If a CSF leak is encountered, primary approximation for watertight closure is always the most ideal treatment choice. However, this is often not possible due to the narrow working space, or the tear may be so large that it is better classified as a dural defect. Subsequently, other standard methods of dural closures should be attempted, including the muscle, fat, or fascia onlay to plug the hole. The use of fibrin glue sealants is common in these situations. For large CSF leaks or inadequate repairs, a subarachnoid drain for CSF diversion should be placed as cranial to the dural defect as possible. Drains should undergo attempted wean by POD5-7, and patients who have a persistent CSF leak through the incision despite prolonged drainage perhaps need permanent shunting.

At the time of closure, irrigation of the thoracic cavity allows for removal of bone fragments and dust as well as identification of air leaks within the visceral pleura. A chest tube is placed along the posterior aspect of the thoracic cavity via a separate incision. The parietal pleura should be closed, with visual confirmation of lung reinflation afterward. The ribs are reapproximated with nonabsorbable suture or wire, with the assistance of a rib reapproximator. The overlying musculature should be closed in layers and the skin closed in the usual fashion. The chest tube should be set to water suction and monitored for air leakage.

T10–L2: Thoracoabdominal Approach

This versatile approach allows for spinal access from T10 to L2 by partial mobilization of the diaphragm to give access to the thorax and retroperitoneum. It is important to note that extending the incision to the iliac crest does allow for exposure of the lower lumbar disc spaces. This approach does carry with it unique risks, including injury to the abdominal viscera, splanchnic nerves, sympathetic trunk, thoracic duct, and great vessels, as well as postoperative ileus. It should not be performed on patients with respiratory compromise or those with adhesions from previous retroperitoneal surgery.

The patient is intubated with a double-lumen endotracheal tube. A nasogastric tube should be placed to assist with intraoperative identification of the esophagus. The patient is placed in a lateral decubitus position. The approach may be from the left or right side, but a left-sided approach is advantageous because the liver will not obscure the view and the thin-walled vena cava does not need to be mobilized. The table should be broken to spread out the operative field, with the center of break positioned over the site of the incision. Fluoroscopy is used to confirm the operative level, and an incision is made along the 9th, 10th, or 11th rib, depending on the location of the pathology. Its course starts from the posterior angle of the rib and continues anteriorly along the rib past the costal cartilage, and once at the anterior surface of the abdomen and before the rectus abdominus, it should curve inferiorly to end at the level of the pathology. The muscles and fascia are divided in a layered fashion to reach the surface of the rib, which is exposed to the costal cartilage. The rib is raised subperiosteally, avoiding damage to the neurovascular bundle, and cut at the costal junction and the costotransverse junction. It may be used as autograft to enhance fusion.

The lung is deflated and the pleura is identified. The retropleural space is entered by blunt dissection through the cartilaginous portion of the rib. The peritoneum is then swept off the rectus abdominus and the diaphragm with the use of fingertip or a sponge stick. The internal oblique, external oblique, and transversus abdominis muscles are cut in a layered fashion. Further exposure and dissection allow visualization of the psoas muscle, and the peritoneum should again be swept off of it carefully. The peritoneum often covers the diaphragm posteriorly, and after sweeping it off it can be clearly visualized. Entry into the thoracic cavity is performed by opening the rib bed, and the collapsed lung may be further retracted with a malleable covered with a sponge. At this time, the diaphragm may be sectioned and released circumferentially from within the chest cavity, being sure to maintain at least 1 cm to allow for reattachment of this muscle. If access to L1 and L2 is necessary, then the diaphragmatic crus may also need to be incised. Suture may be placed in the diaphragm remnant to aid closure at the end of procedure.

Access to the disc space and placement of an interbody is performed as described previously, making sure to respect the great vessels and sympathetic plexus. If mobilization of the great vessels is required to access the vertebral body, then the intercostal vessels may need to be ligated safely and away from their origin. If the psoas muscle needs to be mobilized, a subperiosteal dissection should be performed to avoid injury of the lumbar plexus.

At the time of closure, a chest tube is placed using a different entry site. Closure of the wound should be performed in layers, including the diaphragm, the pleura, and the intra-abdominal muscles. Careful closure of this area is crucial, as any defect may allow for the development of a hernia. Visual confirmation of lung reinflation should be performed before closing the superficial muscular layer. The skin is closed in the usual fashion.

Choice of Interbody Device

Depending on whether a discectomy or discectomy with corpectomy is necessary, a variety of instrumentation and grafting options are available (Fig. 15.6). Iliac crest graft either as autograft from the patient or as an allograft from cadaveric donor bone is viable. One consideration with iliac crest graft is the potential harvest site morbidity. Other structural allografts such as a fibular strut or femoral ring allografts can be used. As technology has evolved, a variety of other synthetic strut grafts have been developed, ranging from static titanium cages to expandable cages with modular end caps made either out of titanium or polyether ether ketone (PEEK). Traditionally, these strut grafts were used in conjunction with an anterior plate secured by screws.

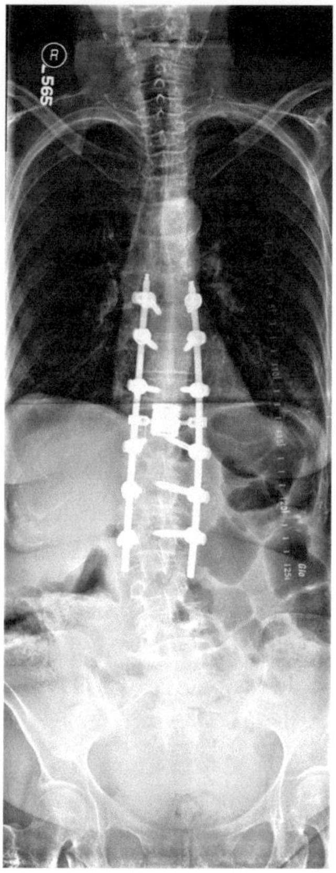

Fig. 15.6 This AP radiograph is an example of instrumentation options. The patient has a T8–L2 pedicle fixation with a T12 corpectomy and placement of an expandable cage

Newer implants have emerged with integrated plating systems that allow for securing of the cage to the bone without the use of a plate. Bone grafting options range from locally harvested and morselized autografts to a variety of allograft products that are available on the market. Other biologic extenders such as recombinant human bone morphogenetic protein and silicone-based bioglasses are also available to help facilitate arthrodesis. More recently, a number of allograft preparations enriched with mesenchymal stem cells have also emerged as grafting options. A detailed discussion of all these options is outside the scope of this chapter, but numerous options exist to promote arthrodesis, and surgeons must familiarize themselves with the potential risks and benefits of each [112].

Minimally Invasive Anterior Thoracic Approaches

More recently minimally invasive approaches, which were initially developed for the lumbar spine, have been also adapted for the thoracic spine. These techniques most often utilize a modular expandable retractor which can be used in conjunction with a fiber optic light source to allow for visualization through a relatively small opening. However, these approaches are outside the scope of this chapter.

Illustrative Case

A 59-year-old man with diabetes mellitus and hypertension presented to clinic with a 2-month history of "pins and needles" in his feet. He reported that the sensation traveled up his legs and ended in his lower back. He reported axial mid-back pain, which was made worse with movement. He denied any bowel or bladder incontinence, weakness, or numbness. He was able to perform his normal activities of daily living without difficulty. On examination, his strength was intact in both his upper and lower extremities, and rectal tone was intact. He had diminished light touch in a stocking distribution in his bilateral lower extremities. His reflexes were 1+ in his upper extremities and 3+ in his patellar and Achilles tendons with cross adduction. A test of pathological reflexes revealed three beats of clonus in his bilateral lower extremities, as well as positive Babinski's sign bilaterally. MRI of the thoracic spine revealed a large gadolinium-enhancing mass that was centered at the right T10 pedicle; the mass encroached into the vertebral body of T10 and caused impingement of the spinal cord at that level (Fig. 15.7).

Due to need for tissue sampling for pathology, the clear myelopathy on physical exam, and the potential for spinal column destabilization due to erosion of the vertebral body, the decision for operative intervention was made. The operative plan was to perform a two-stage surgery. The first stage was a posterior approach T9–T11 laminectomy and right facetectomy with resection, followed by T9–T11 pedicle screw instrumentation and fixation. The second stage of the surgery was

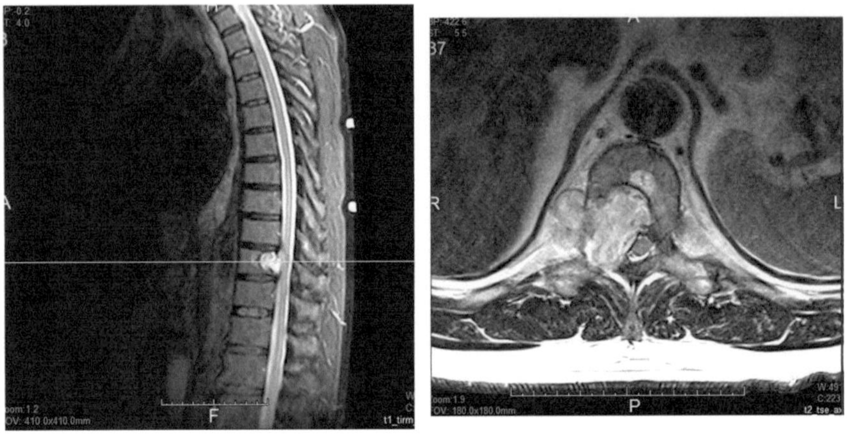

Fig. 15.7 Preoperative MRI of a 59-year-old man who presented to the clinic with signs of myelopathy. The lesion is centered at the right pedicle and is causing erosion of the vertebral body. There is significant stenosis of the spinal canal with impingement on the spinal cord

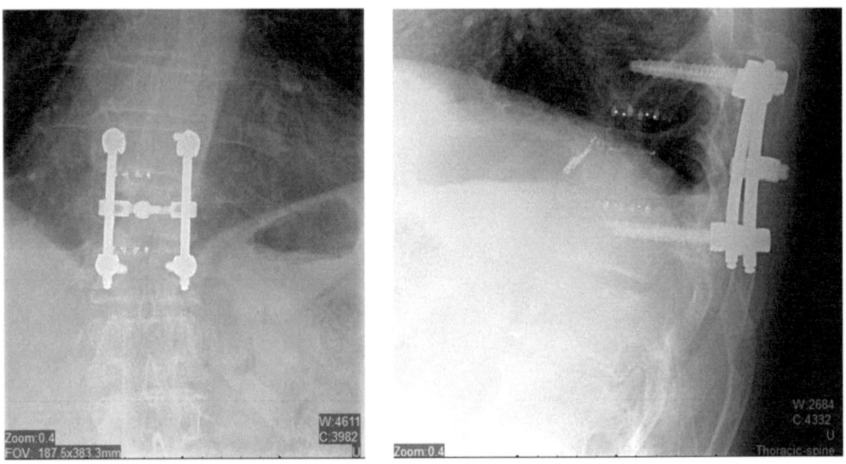

Fig. 15.8 Postoperative imaging for the patient in Fig. 15.7. The patient underwent a two-stage operation. The first stage was a T9–T11 laminectomy, right facetectomy, and pedicle screw fixation. The second stage was a right transthoracic T10 corpectomy and placement of an expandable PEEK cage. The patient continued to do well 1 year postoperatively

a right lateral transthoracic approach for T10 corpectomy and resection of tumor. The vertebral body defect was repaired with an expandable PEEK cage with T9–T11 anterior fusion.

The patient tolerated surgery without any intraoperative complications. His postoperative course was benign; his chest tube was removed on postoperative day 3, and he was discharged to inpatient rehabilitation on postoperative day 5. Postoperative anterior/posterior and lateral x-rays showed good placement of hardware and stable construct (Fig. 15.8). Final pathology revealed the tumor to be a schwannoma. Imaging performed at 1-year follow-up showed gross total resection of the lesion.

Technical Pearls

- A double-lumen ET tube should be used to facilitate lung collapse.
- An access often surgeon is recommended to safely reach the desired spinal cord level.

- For the lateral decubitus position, a beanbag or foam bolster may be used to assist in placement, with an axillary roll used to prevent brachial plexus injury.
- Placing the incision over the break in the table helps to improve exposure by spreading out the operative field.
- If the table is broken during surgery, then it should be returned to flat position before instrumentation to prevent iatrogenic scoliosis.
- Flexion of the patient's hips and knees helps relax the abdominal musculature.
- For approaching the cervicothoracic junction, the recurrent laryngeal nerve has a more reliable course on the left, and a left-sided approach may be favored.
- For patients with extreme kyphosis, the transmanubrial approach may not be successful to allow for access to the disc space, and there are radiological methods to predict whether patients are amenable to this approach [108].
- Preoperative recognition of a calcified disc is important for planning of the surgical approach and techniques and can be identified with plain radiographs or CT myelogram.
- The transthoracic approach is best for treatment of calcified disc, and partial corpectomies may be needed to ensure safe exposure of the disc.
- The best way to avoid a durotomy is to limit manipulation of the thecal sac if possible.
- For the transabdominal approach, a gauze-covered finger or a Kitner may be used to dissect out the peritoneum as well as the parietal pleura without violating the peritoneum.
- When splitting muscles, their ends should be tagged to allow for anatomic approximation during repair, especially for the diaphragm.
- Psoas muscle should be mobilized subperiosteally to avoid injury to the lumbar plexus.
- Due to the potential for blood loss, an intraoperative blood salvage device may be useful in patients without a history of malignancy or infection.
- When it is necessary to ligate segmental arteries, they should be sectioned away from the aorta, but ligation should be avoided in general to prevent spinal cord ischemia.
- If vessels are taken, prevent hypotension to ensure perfusion, especially in the setting of severe cord compression, where the cord may already have compromised blood flow.
- An intraoperative test occlusion can also be performed to assess whether a segmental artery is safe to ligate; the vessel can be temporarily clamped for a few minutes to see if any signal changes develop on either SSEP or MEPs. If no changes are observed, then the vessel can be ligated safely and divided.

Complications and Strategies for Avoidance

These procedures are potentially morbid, medically as well as surgically. The best way to avoid a medical complication after surgery is to ensure preoperative optimization as well as the appropriate level of postoperative care. Patients should be screened to see if they can tolerate the procedure, including potentially major blood loss as well as lung collapse. Adequate pain management postoperatively is essential to promote ventilation and inflation of the lung, especially with a chest tube in place. Thoracic rib blocks by anesthesia can provide excellent localized pain control and may be safely repeated as necessary. Pulmonary toilet using cough, deep breathing exercises, and incentive spirometry is important to prevent atelectasis and pneumonia. For the patient with multiple medical comorbidities, ICU monitoring is appropriate.

Accurate and precise localization of a thoracic spine lesion is important to prevent surgery at the incorrect level. Intraoperative fluoroscopy is used to count ribs or vertebral body pedicles superiorly until the correct level is reached. However, in a small but clinically relevant number of patients, variations from normal anatomy in the number of ribs and vertebral bodies may potentially lead a surgeon to localize at the wrong level if unnoticed preoperatively. Preoperative anterior/posterior and lateral radiographs may be used to establish a baseline and correlate with intraoperative fluoroscopy. Consultation prior to surgery with the radiologist who will be aiding in determination of disc level can aid identification of correct level. Preoperative marking of the correct level with a radiopaque dye by interventional radiology is also another option. When palpating ribs to check the operative level, the second rib is often the most caudal rib that can be easily palpated. The first rib lies inside the second rib and may not be easily felt. Fluoroscopy should be used to confirm the correct operative level.

Dural openings causing CSF leaks have the potential of becoming CSF fistulas, which are difficult to treat. Primary, tension-free, and watertight repair of any dural opening is ideal, but this may be technically difficult to achieve, especially with ventral tears. When this is not possible, a muscle graft or a pleural flap may be used. Processed allograft or xenograft is another option. Fibrin glue is useful as an adjunct to reinforce the suture line [113, 114]. If these techniques are not successful, then the use of a lumbar drain for CSF diversion until the dural tear heals may be required to prevent a CSF-pleural fistula. If there is concern regarding a CSF leak, then the chest tube should be removed early before discontinuation of the lumbar drain.

Conclusion

Surgery for thoracic spine disease should be offered for symptomatic lesions that have failed conservative therapy, compromise spinal stability, and/or cause progressive neurological symptoms. Preoperative assessment of the specific pathology, with evaluation of calcified discs, is essential to minimize morbidity. Patients should be critically assessed for fitness for surgery and medically optimized preoperatively. Approaches to the T1–T4 disc spaces frequently require an anterior transmanubrial approach, to T4–T10 a lateral transthoracic approach, and T10–T12 and below a lateral thoracoabdominal approach. An access surgeon is often necessary to reach the desired level. Postoperative mobilization and pain control are needed to minimize morbidity.

References

1. Key C. On paraplegia depending on disease of the ligaments of the spine. Guys Hosp Rep. 1838;3:17–34.
2. Middleton GS, Teacher JH. Injury of the spinal cord due to rupture of an intervertebral disk during muscular effort. Glascow Medical Journal. 1911;76(1):1.
3. Love JG, Schorn VG. Thoracic-disk protrusions. JAMA. 1965;191:627–31.
4. Mixter WJ, Barr JS. Rupture of the intervertebral disc with involvement of the Spinal Canal. N Engl J Med. 1934;211(5):210–5.
5. Menard V. Etude Pratique sur le Mal de Pott. Paris: Masson et Cie; 1900.
6. Hodgson AR, Stock FE. Anterior spinal fusion a preliminary communication on the radical treatment of Pott's disease and Pott's paraplegia. Br J Surg. 1956;44(185):266–75.
7. Hulme A. The surgical approach to thoracic intervertebral disc protrusions. J Neurol Neurosurg Psychiatry. 1960;23:133–7.
8. Arce CA, Dohrmann GJ. Herniated thoracic disks. Neurol Clin. 1985;3(2):383–92.
9. Crafoord C, Hiertonn T, Lindblom K, Olsson SE. Spinal cord compression caused by a protruded thoracic disc; report of a case treated with antero-lateral fenestration of the disc. Acta Orthop Scand. 1958;28(2):103–7.
10. Perot PL Jr, Munro DD. Transthoracic removal of midline thoracic disc protrusions causing spinal cord compression. J Neurosurg. 1969;31(4):452–8.
11. Ransohoff J, Spencer F, Siew F, Gage L Jr. Transthoracic removal of thoracic disc. Report of three cases. J Neurosurg. 1969;31(4):459–61.
12. Royle ND. The operative removal of an accessory vertebra. Med J Aust. 1928;1(467–468):387–91.
13. Dwyer AF, Newton NC, Sherwood AA. An anterior approach to scoliosis. A preliminary report. Clin Orthop Relat Res. 1969;62:192–202.
14. Snyder LA, Smith ZA, Dahdaleh NS, Fessler RG. Minimally invasive treatment of thoracic disc herniations. Neurosurg Clin N Am. 2014;25(2):271–7.
15. Anand N, Regan JJ. Video-assisted thoracoscopic surgery for thoracic disc disease: classification and outcome study of 100 consecutive cases with a 2-year minimum follow-up period. Spine (Phila Pa 1976). 2002;27(8):871–9.
16. Yoshihara H. Surgical treatment for thoracic disc herniation: an update. Spine (Phila Pa 1976). 2014; 39(6):E406–12.
17. Falavigna A, Piccoli CL. Minimally invasive approaches for thoracic decompression from discectomy to corpectomy. J Neurosurg Sci. 2013;57(3): 175–92.
18. Deviren V, Kuelling FA, Poulter G, Pekmezci M. Minimal invasive anterolateral transthoracic transpleural approach: a novel technique for thoracic disc herniation. A review of the literature, description of a new surgical technique and experience with first 12 consecutive patients. J Spinal Disord Tech. 2011;24(5):E40–8.
19. Vollmer DG, Simmons NE. Transthoracic approaches to thoracic disc herniations. Neurosurg Focus. 2000;9(4):e8.
20. McCormick WE, Will SF, Benzel EC. Surgery for thoracic disc disease. Complication avoidance: overview and management. Neurosurg Focus. 2000;9(4):e13.

21. Burke TG, Caputy AJ. Treatment of thoracic disc herniation: evolution toward the minimally invasive thoracoscopic technique. Neurosurg Focus. 2000;9(4):e9.
22. Hou X, Sun C, Liu X, Liu Z, Qi Q, Guo Z, et al. Clinical features of thoracic spinal stenosis-associated myelopathy: a retrospective analysis of 427 cases. Clin Spine Surg. 2016;29(2):86–9.
23. Awwad EE, Martin DS, Smith KR Jr, Baker BK. Asymptomatic versus symptomatic herniated thoracic discs: their frequency and characteristics as detected by computed tomography after myelography. Neurosurgery. 1991;28(2):180–6.
24. Tovi D, Strang RR. Thoracic intervertebral disk protrusions. Acta Chir Scand Suppl. 1960;Suppl 267:1–41.
25. Brown CW, Deffer PA Jr, Akmakjian J, Donaldson DH, Brugman JL. The natural history of thoracic disc herniation. Spine (Phila Pa 1976). 1992;17(6 Suppl):S97–102.
26. Stillerman CB, Chen TC, Couldwell WT, Zhang W, Weiss MH. Experience in the surgical management of 82 symptomatic herniated thoracic discs and review of the literature. J Neurosurg. 1998;88(4):623–33.
27. Wood KB, Garvey TA, Gundry C, Heithoff KB. Magnetic resonance imaging of the thoracic spine. Evaluation of asymptomatic individuals. J Bone Joint Surg Am. 1995;77(11):1631–8.
28. Wood KB, Blair JM, Aepple DM, Schendel MJ, Garvey TA, Gundry CR, et al. The natural history of asymptomatic thoracic disc herniations. Spine (Phila Pa 1976). 1997;22(5):525–9. discussion 9-30
29. Mansour H, Hammoud F, Vlahovitch B. Brown-Sequard syndrome caused by foramen and calcified disk herniation, responsible for direct compression of Adamkiewicz's artery. Neurochirurgie. 1987; 33(6):478–81.
30. Campbell E, Kite WC Jr, Whitfield RD. The thoracic herniated intervertebral disc syndrome. J Neurosurg. 1957;14(1):61–7.
31. Lesoin F, Rousseaux M, Autricque A, Reesaul Y, Villette L, Clarisse J, et al. Thoracic disc herniations: evolution in the approach and indications. Acta Neurochir. 1986;80(1–2):30–4.
32. Debnath UK, McConnell JR, Sengupta DK, Mehdian SM, Webb JK. Results of hemivertebrectomy and fusion for symptomatic thoracic disc herniation. Eur Spine J. 2003;12(3):292–9.
33. Tsuyama N. Ossification of the posterior longitudinal ligament of the spine. Clin Orthop Relat Res. 1984;184:71–84.
34. Kawaguchi Y, Nakano M, Yasuda T, Seki S, Hori T, Kimura T. Ossification of the posterior longitudinal ligament in not only the cervical spine, but also other spinal regions: analysis using multidetector computed tomography of the whole spine. Spine (Phila Pa 1976). 2013;38(23):E1477–82.
35. Fujimori T, Watabe T, Iwamoto Y, Hamada S, Iwasaki M, Oda T. Prevalence, concomitance, and distribution of ossification of the spinal ligaments: results of whole spine CT scans in 1500 Japanese patients. Spine (Phila Pa 1976). 2016;41(21):1668–76.
36. Matsunaga S, Nakamura K, Seichi A, Yokoyama T, Toh S, Ichimura S, et al. Radiographic predictors for the development of myelopathy in patients with ossification of the posterior longitudinal ligament: a multicenter cohort study. Spine (Phila Pa 1976). 2008;33(24):2648–50.
37. Chiba K, Yamamoto I, Hirabayashi H, Iwasaki M, Goto H, Yonenobu K, et al. Multicenter study investigating the postoperative progression of ossification of the posterior longitudinal ligament in the cervical spine: a new computer-assisted measurement. J Neurosurg Spine. 2005;3(1):17–23.
38. Hori T, Kawaguchi Y, Kimura T. How does the ossification area of the posterior longitudinal ligament progress after cervical laminoplasty? Spine (Phila Pa 1976). 2006;31(24):2807–12.
39. Matsunaga S, Sakou T, Taketomi E, Yamaguchi M, Okano T. The natural course of myelopathy caused by ossification of the posterior longitudinal ligament in the cervical spine. Clin Orthop Relat Res. 1994;305:168–77.
40. Matsunaga S, Kukita M, Hayashi K, Shinkura R, Koriyama C, Sakou T, et al. Pathogenesis of myelopathy in patients with ossification of the posterior longitudinal ligament. J Neurosurg. 2002;96(2 Suppl):168–72.
41. Hori T, Kawaguchi Y, Kimura T. How does the ossification area of the posterior longitudinal ligament thicken following cervical laminoplasty? Spine (Phila Pa 1976). 2007;32(19):E551–6.
42. Sugrue PA, McClendon J Jr, Halpin RJ, Liu JC, Koski TR, Ganju A. Surgical management of cervical ossification of the posterior longitudinal ligament: natural history and the role of surgical decompression and stabilization. Neurosurg Focus. 2011;30(3):E3.
43. Saetia K, Cho D, Lee S, Kim DH, Kim SD. Ossification of the posterior longitudinal ligament: a review. Neurosurg Focus. 2011;30(3):E1.
44. Smith ZA, Buchanan CC, Raphael D, Khoo LT. Ossification of the posterior longitudinal ligament: pathogenesis, management, and current surgical approaches. A review. Neurosurg Focus. 2011;30(3):E10.
45. Ito Z, Matsuyama Y, Ando M, Kawabata S, Kanchiku T, Kida K, et al. Postoperative paralysis from thoracic ossification of posterior longitudinal ligament (OPLL) surgery-risk factor of neurologic injury: Nationwide multi-institution survey. Spine (Phila Pa 1976). 2016;41:E1159–63.
46. Hu P, Yu M, Liu X, Liu Z, Jiang L. A circumferential decompression-based surgical strategy for multilevel ossification of thoracic posterior longitudinal ligament. Spine J. 2015;15(12):2484–92.
47. Matsumoto M, Toyama Y, Chikuda H, Takeshita K, Kato T, Shindo S, et al. Outcomes of fusion surgery for ossification of the posterior longitudinal ligament of the thoracic spine: a multicenter

retrospective survey: clinical article. J Neurosurg Spine. 2011;15(4):380–5.
48. Choi D, Fox Z, Albert T, Arts M, Balabaud L, Bunger C, et al. Rapid improvements in pain and quality of life are sustained after surgery for spinal metastases in a large prospective cohort. Br J Neurosurg. 2016;30(3):337–44.
49. Choi D, Crockard A, Bunger C, Harms J, Kawahara N, Mazel C, et al. Review of metastatic spine tumour classification and indications for surgery: the consensus statement of the global spine tumour study group. Eur Spine J. 2010;19(2):215–22.
50. Tang Y, Qu J, Wu J, Liu H, Chu T, Xiao J, et al. Effect of surgery on quality of life of patients with spinal metastasis from non-small-cell lung cancer. J Bone Joint Surg Am. 2016;98(5):396–402.
51. Park SJ, Lee CS, Chung SS. Surgical results of metastatic spinal cord compression (MSCC) from non-small cell lung cancer (NSCLC): analysis of functional outcome, survival time, and complication. Spine J. 2016;16(3):322–8.
52. Dea N, Versteeg A, Fisher C, Kelly A, Hartig D, Boyd M, et al. Adverse events in emergency oncological spine surgery: a prospective analysis. J Neurosurg Spine. 2014;21(5):698–703.
53. Zairi F, Karnoub MA, Vieillard MH, Bouras A, Marinho P, Allaoui M, et al. Evaluation of the relevance of surgery in a retrospective case series of patients who underwent the surgical treatment of a symptomatic spine metastasis from lung cancer. Eur Spine J. 2016;25:4052–9.
54. Ghori AK, Leonard DA, Schoenfeld AJ, Saadat E, Scott N, Ferrone ML, et al. Modeling 1-year survival after surgery on the metastatic spine. Spine J. 2015;15(11):2345–50.
55. Schoenfeld AJ, Le HV, Marjoua Y, Leonard DA, Belmont PJ Jr, Bono CM, et al. Assessing the utility of a clinical prediction score regarding 30-day morbidity and mortality following metastatic spinal surgery: the New England spinal metastasis score (NESMS). Spine J. 2016;16(4):482–90.
56. Tokuhashi Y, Matsuzaki H, Oda H, Oshima M, Ryu J. A revised scoring system for preoperative evaluation of metastatic spine tumor prognosis. Spine (Phila Pa 1976). 2005;30(19):2186–91.
57. Amelot A, Balabaud L, Choi D, Fox Z, Crockard HA, Albert T, et al. Surgery for metastatic spine tumors in the elderly. Advanced age is not a contraindication to surgery! Spine J. 2015;17(6): 759–67.
58. Keene JS. Radiographic evaluation of thoracolumbar fractures. Clin Orthop Relat Res. 1984;189:58–64.
59. Mumford J, Weinstein JN, Spratt KF, Goel VK. Thoracolumbar burst fractures. The clinical efficacy and outcome of nonoperative management. Spine (Phila Pa 1976). 1993;18(8):955–70.
60. Berg EE. The sternal-rib complex. A possible fourth column in thoracic spine fractures. Spine (Phila Pa 1976). 1993;18(13):1916–9.
61. Denis F. The three column spine and its significance in the classification of acute thoracolumbar spinal injuries. Spine (Phila Pa 1976). 1983;8(8):817–31.
62. Hanley EN Jr, Eskay ML. Thoracic spine fractures. Orthopedics. 1989;12(5):689–96.
63. Wood KB, Li W, Lebl DR, Ploumis A. Management of thoracolumbar spine fractures. Spine J. 2014;14(1):145–64.
64. Bohlman HH. Treatment of fractures and dislocations of the thoracic and lumbar spine. J Bone Joint Surg Am. 1985;67(1):165–9.
65. Devilee R, Sanders R, de Lange S. Treatment of fractures and dislocations of the thoracic and lumbar spine by fusion and Harrington instrumentation. Arch Orthop Trauma Surg. 1995;114(2):100–2.
66. Cahill DW, Love LC, Rechtine GR. Pyogenic osteomyelitis of the spine in the elderly. J Neurosurg. 1991;74(6):878–86.
67. Lehovsky J. Pyogenic vertebral osteomyelitis/disc infection. Baillieres Best Pract Res Clin Rheumatol. 1999;13(1):59–75.
68. Pola E, Logroscino CA, Gentiempo M, Colangelo D, Mazzotta V, Di Meco E, et al. Medical and surgical treatment of pyogenic spondylodiscitis. Eur Rev Med Pharmacol Sci. 2012;16(Suppl 2):35–49.
69. Boody BS, Jenkins TJ, Maslak J, Hsu WK, Patel AA. Vertebral osteomyelitis and spinal epidural abscess: an evidence-based review. J Spinal Disord Tech. 2015;28(6):E316–27.
70. Baker AS, Ojemann RG, Swartz MN, Richardson EP Jr. Spinal epidural abscess. N Engl J Med. 1975;293(10):463–8.
71. Kostuik JP. Anterior spinal cord decompression for lesions of the thoracic and lumbar spine, techniques, new methods of internal fixation results. Spine (Phila Pa 1976). 1983;8(5):512–31.
72. Oga M, Arizono T, Takasita M, Sugioka Y. Evaluation of the risk of instrumentation as a foreign body in spinal tuberculosis. Clinical and biologic study. Spine (Phila Pa 1976). 1993;18(13):1890–4.
73. Gorensek M, Kosak R, Travnik L, Vengust R. Posterior instrumentation, anterior column reconstruction with single posterior approach for treatment of pyogenic osteomyelitis of thoracic and lumbar spine. Eur Spine J. 2013;22(3):633–41.
74. Dai LY, Chen WH, Jiang LS. Anterior instrumentation for the treatment of pyogenic vertebral osteomyelitis of thoracic and lumbar spine. Eur Spine J. 2008;17(8):1027–34.
75. Jin D, Qu D, Chen J, Zhang H. One-stage anterior interbody autografting and instrumentation in primary surgical management of thoracolumbar spinal tuberculosis. Eur Spine J. 2004;13(2):114–21.
76. Blumenkopf B. Thoracic intervertebral disc herniations: diagnostic value of magnetic resonance imaging. Neurosurgery. 1988;23(1):36–40.
77. Francavilla TL, Powers A, Dina T, Rizzoli HV. MR imaging of thoracic disk herniations. J Comput Assist Tomogr. 1987;11(6):1062–5.

78. Videman T, Battie MC, Gill K, Manninen H, Gibbons LE, Fisher LD. Magnetic resonance imaging findings and their relationships in the thoracic and lumbar spine. Insights into the etiopathogenesis of spinal degeneration. Spine (Phila Pa 1976). 1995;20(8):928–35.
79. Arce CA, Dohrmann GJ. Thoracic disc herniation. Improved diagnosis with computed tomographic scanning and a review of the literature. Surg Neurol. 1985;23(4):356–61.
80. Ryan RW, Lally JF, Kozic Z. Asymptomatic calcified herniated thoracic disks: CT recognition. AJNR Am J Neuroradiol. 1988;9(2):363–6.
81. Williams MP, Cherryman GR. Thoracic disk herniation: MR imaging. Radiology. 1988;167(3):874–5.
82. Williams MP, Cherryman GR, Husband JE. Significance of thoracic disc herniation demonstrated by MR imaging. J Comput Assist Tomogr. 1989;13(2):211–4.
83. Wood KB, Schellhas KP, Garvey TA, Aeppli D. Thoracic discography in healthy individuals. A controlled prospective study of magnetic resonance imaging and discography in asymptomatic and symptomatic individuals. Spine (Phila Pa 1976). 1999;24(15):1548–55.
84. Schellhas KP, Pollei SR, Dorwart RH. Thoracic discography. A safe and reliable technique. Spine (Phila Pa 1976). 1994;19(18):2103–9.
85. Shah RV, Everett CR, McKenzie-Brown AM, Sehgal N. Discography as a diagnostic test for spinal pain: a systematic and narrative review. Pain Physician. 2005;8(2):187–209.
86. Nuwer MR, Dawson EG, Carlson LG, Kanim LE, Sherman JE. Somatosensory evoked potential spinal cord monitoring reduces neurologic deficits after scoliosis surgery: results of a large multicenter survey. Electroencephalogr Clin Neurophysiol. 1995;96(1):6–11.
87. Lall RR, Lall RR, Hauptman JS, Munoz C, Cybulski GR, Koski T, et al. Intraoperative neurophysiological monitoring in spine surgery: indications, efficacy, and role of the preoperative checklist. Neurosurg Focus. 2012;33(5):E10.
88. Fehlings MG, Brodke DS, Norvell DC, Dettori JR. The evidence for intraoperative neurophysiological monitoring in spine surgery: does it make a difference? Spine (Phila Pa 1976). 2010;35(9 Suppl):S37–46.
89. Gonzalez AA, Jeyanandarajan D, Hansen C, Zada G, Hsieh PC. Intraoperative neurophysiological monitoring during spine surgery: a review. Neurosurg Focus. 2009;27(4):E6.
90. Malhotra NR, Shaffrey CI. Intraoperative electrophysiological monitoring in spine surgery. Spine (Phila Pa 1976). 2010;35(25):2167–79.
91. Raynor BL, Padberg AM, Lenke LG, Bridwell KH, Riew KD, Buchowski JM, et al. Failure of intraoperative monitoring to detect postoperative neurologic deficits: a 25-year experience in 12,375 spinal surgeries. Spine. 2016;41(17):1387–93.
92. Deutsch H, Arginteanu M, Manhart K, Perin N, Camins M, Moore F, et al. Somatosensory evoked potential monitoring in anterior thoracic vertebrectomy. J Neurosurg. 2000;92(2 Suppl):155–61.
93. Eggspuehler A, Sutter MA, Grob D, Porchet F, Jeszenszky D, Dvorak J. Multimodal intraoperative monitoring (MIOM) during surgical decompression of thoracic spinal stenosis in 36 patients. Eur Spine J. 2007;16(Suppl 2):S216–20.
94. Eleraky MA, Setzer M, Papanastassiou ID, Baaj AA, Tran ND, Katsares KM, et al. Role of motor-evoked potential monitoring in conjunction with temporary clipping of spinal nerve roots in posterior thoracic spine tumor surgery. Spine J. 2010;10(5):396–403.
95. Murakami H, Kawahara N, Demura S, Kato S, Yoshioka K, Tomita K. Neurological function after total en bloc spondylectomy for thoracic spinal tumors. J Neurosurg Spine. 2010;12(3):253–6.
96. Ikard RW. Methods and complications of anterior exposure of the thoracic and lumbar spine. Arch Surg. 2006;141(10):1025–34.
97. Yuan L, Ni GX, Luk KK, Cheung KM, Lu DS, Hu Y, et al. Effect of segmental artery ligation on the blood supply of the thoracic spinal cord during anterior spinal surgery: a quantitative histomorphological fresh cadaver study. Spine (Phila Pa 1976). 2005;30(5):483–6.
98. Murthy NS, Maus TP, Behrns CL. Intraforaminal location of the great anterior radiculomedullary artery (artery of Adamkiewicz): a retrospective review. Pain Med. 2010;11(12):1756–64.
99. Yoshioka K, Niinuma H, Ehara S, Nakajima T, Nakamura M, Kawazoe K. MR angiography and CT angiography of the artery of Adamkiewicz: state of the art. Radiographics. 2006;26(Suppl 1):S63–73.
100. Melissano G, Bertoglio L, Rinaldi E, Leopardi M, Chiesa R. An anatomical review of spinal cord blood supply. J Cardiovasc Surg. 2015;56(5):699–706.
101. Dormans JP. Establishing a standard of care for neuromonitoring during spinal deformity surgery. Spine (Phila Pa 1976). 2010;35(25):2180–5.
102. Halpin RJ, Sugrue PA, Gould RW, Kallas PG, Schafer MF, Ondra SL, et al. Standardizing care for high-risk patients in spine surgery: the northwestern high-risk spine protocol. Spine (Phila Pa 1976). 2010;35(25):2232–8.
103. Sutter M, Eggspuehler A, Grob D, Jeszenszky D, Benini A, Porchet F, et al. The diagnostic value of multimodal intraoperative monitoring (MIOM) during spine surgery: a prospective study of 1,017 patients. Eur Spine J. 2007;16(Suppl 2):S162–70.
104. Sutter M, Eggspuehler A, Muller A, Dvorak J. Multimodal intraoperative monitoring: an overview and proposal of methodology based on 1,017 cases. Eur Spine J. 2007;16(Suppl 2):S153–61.
105. Deletis V. Basic methodological principles of multimodal intraoperative monitoring during spine surgeries. Eur Spine J. 2007;16(Suppl 2):S147–52.

106. Liu YL, Hao YJ, Li T, Song YM, Wang LM. Trans-upper-sternal approach to the cervicothoracic junction. Clin Orthop Relat Res. 2009;467(8): 2018–24.
107. Pointillart V, Aurouer N, Gangnet N, Vital JM. Anterior approach to the cervicothoracic junction without sternotomy: a report of 37 cases. Spine (Phila Pa 1976). 2007;32(25):2875–9.
108. Teng H, Hsiang J, Wu C, Wang M, Wei H, Yang X, et al. Surgery in the cervicothoracic junction with an anterior low suprasternal approach alone or combined with manubriotomy and sternotomy: an approach selection method based on the cervicothoracic angle. J Neurosurg Spine. 2009;10(6):531–42.
109. Lam FC, Groff MW. An anterior approach to spinal pathology of the upper thoracic spine through a partial manubriotomy. J Neurosurg Spine. 2011;15(5):467–71.
110. McCormick PC. Retropleural approach to the thoracic and thoracolumbar spine. Neurosurgery. 1995;37(5):908–14.
111. Stillerman CB, Weiss MH. Management of thoracic disc disease. Clin Neurosurg. 1992;38:325–52.
112. Oppenheimer JH, DeCastro I, McDonnell DE. Minimally invasive spine technology and minimally invasive spine surgery: a historical review. Neurosurg Focus. 2009;27(3):E9.
113. Jankowitz BT, Atteberry DS, Gerszten PC, Karausky P, Cheng BC, Faught R, et al. Effect of fibrin glue on the prevention of persistent cerebral spinal fluid leakage after incidental durotomy during lumbar spinal surgery. Eur Spine J. 2009;18(8):1169–74.
114. Shaffrey CI, Spotnitz WD, Shaffrey ME, Jane JA. Neurosurgical applications of fibrin glue: augmentation of dural closure in 134 patients. Neurosurgery. 1990;26(2):207–10.

16 Thoracic Lateral Extracavitary Decompression and Fusion

Christopher D. Witiw and Richard G. Fessler

Introduction

The lateral extracavitary approach (LECA) was first described by Capener in 1954 and then modified by Larson et al. in 1976 [1, 2]. The approach affords access to all three columns of the spine, and the primary indication of this posterolateral intervention is resection of ventral compressive pathology on the spinal cord [3]. Anterior decompression and circumferential reconstruction of the integrity of the spinal column may be performed all through a single incision, and all steps of the operation can be accomplished without the need for any substantial manipulation of patient positioning. Moreover, efforts to minimize the invasiveness of the operation and reduce the likelihood of complications have led to advances in minimally invasive techniques. Now, similar decompression and reconstruction may be accomplished with limited muscular disruption [4].

The LECA is one of the numerous options to address ventral compressive pathology in the thoracic spine, leaving the spinal surgeon with numerous considerations. With this chapter, we will describe appropriate indications for the LECA to assist with decision-making. This will be followed by essential preoperative considerations, a detailed review of the surgical steps for the classic open LECA, and more recent modifications to make the operation minimally invasive. This is supplemented by a discussion of the essential details of the costotransversectomy and transpedicular approaches to the vertebral body. These allow for ventral decompression with less invasive access, albeit at the expense of a decrease in ventral visualization. Following this, we will outline the modifications needed for a posterolateral approach to the upper thoracic vertebrae (T1–T4) through the lateral parascapular extrapleural approach. The chapter concludes with technical pearls, a case illustration and a discussion of potential complications along with strategies for avoidance.

Indications and Patient Selection

The LECA may be employed for posterolateral access to compressive thoracic pathology from T5 to T12. Lesions from the cervicothoracic

C.D. Witiw, MD
Department of Neurological Surgery, Rush University Medical Center, 1725 W. Harrison St., Suite 855, Chicago, IL 60612, USA

Division of Neurosurgery, Department of Surgery, University of Toronto, Toronto, ON, Canada
e-mail: christopher.witiw@mail.utoronto.ca

R.G. Fessler, MD, PhD (✉)
Department of Neurological Surgery, Rush University Medical Center, 1725 W. Harrison St., Suite 855, Chicago, IL 60612, USA
e-mail: rfessler@rush.edu

L.T. Holly, P.A. Anderson (eds.), *Essentials of Spinal Stabilization*,
DOI 10.1007/978-3-319-59713-3_16

junction down to T4 may be approached by the lateral parascapular extrapleural approach (LPEA) which will also be described within this chapter [5]. The LECA or LPEA is certainly not the sole option, and spine surgeons are often challenged to decide which of the myriad of techniques for decompression of ventral spinal pathology is optimal. Broadly these may be divided into anterior intracavitary, anterolateral, and posterolateral.

The anterior thoracotomy based and modifications for the upper thoracic spine such as trans-sternal, trans-manubrial, and trans-clavicular exposure approaches allow a direct visualization of the anterior and middle columns of the spine for decompression and reconstruction [6]. However, visualization often comes at the cost of approach-specific complications such as pulmonary contusions, pleural effusions, atelectasis, and hemothoracies [7]. Less invasive, thoracoscopic technologies hold some promise to reduce complications, but these techniques are less familiar to spine surgeons, and the steep learning curve reduces its practicality for surgeons who do not perform them routinely [8]. An alternative to the intracavitary approach is the retropleural approach [9, 10]. This affords the benefit of avoiding entrance into the thoracic cavity and provides excellent exposure to the anterior spinal column. However, challenges include an ongoing risk of pleural breach along with obtaining appropriate angulation to sufficiently decompress the spinal cord and a risk to the segmental arteries. For these reasons and more, this approach has yet to garner widespread acceptance.

The posterolateral approaches offer more familiarity and are the preferred method for many surgeons. These include the transpedicular approach, the costotransversectomy, or the LECA. Of these three, the LECA affords greater exposure and allows for excellent visualization [11]. The only anatomical structures of the spinal column falling outside of surgeon visualization are the contralateral edge of the vertebral body and contralateral pedicle, and, if needed, these may often be approached from the contralateral side [12].

The specific pathological indications for a posterolateral approach are quite broad. Most conditions of the thoracic spinal column that result in ventrally oriented compressive forces on the spinal cord are amenable to this approach. A recent systematic review of the literature conducted by Foreman et al. identified multiple series describing the approach to address numerous pathological conditions and include trauma, intervertebral disc herniation, tumor, and infection [3]. A summary of the typical indications for LECA may be found in Table 16.1. We strongly advocate for the consideration of a LECA where a thoracic corpectomy is mandated to achieve sufficient decompression and/or resection of pathological tissue. We also suggest a LECA for cases of calcified, central intervertebral disc herniations. Soft laterally oriented thoracic disc herniations are most often amenable to treatment by a posterolateral microendoscopic thoracic discectomy [13]. In cases where ventral decompression is required but patient comorbidities may limit LECA as an option, then a transpedicular or costotransversectomy approach may be considered; however, more recent modifications to the traditional LECA to make it less invasive generally make it appropriate even in these scenarios.

Table 16.1 Indications for lateral extracavitary approach for thoracic spinal decompression and fusion

Trauma
Vertebral body fracture
Spinal cord compression
Painful progressive deformity
Intervertebral disc herniation
Calcified centralized disc herniations
Tumor
Extradural
Vertebral body metastases
Primary osseous lesions of the spinal column
Intradural extramedullary
Meningioma
Peripheral nerve sheath tumors
Infection
Osteomyelitis
Epidural abscess
Spinal tuberculosis

Preoperative Considerations

Accurate intraoperative localization of the correct surgical level is of paramount importance for any surgical intervention involving the thoracic spine. While the ultimate localization occurs in the operating room, the preoperative steps ensure success. It is thus imperative that the presurgical imaging includes sufficient anatomical features to allow the surgeon to determine that correct level of the thoracic pathology. Imaging should include the second cervical vertebra to allow for a downward count of the vertebral levels or the sacrum to allow for an upward count. An upward count from the sacrum is preferred because intraoperatively, it is easier to count in a cranial direction from the sacrum or from the lowest rib because the anatomical relation of the musculoskeletal structures of the pectoral girdle can obstruct radiographic visualization of the lower cervical and upper thoracic spine. All patients must also have a preoperative chest radiograph to account for the possibility of an additional rib as well as a lateral lumbosacral radiograph to assess for the presence of a lumbosacral transitional vertebra. Further consideration may be given to implementation of an institution level protocol to ensure availability of radiology expertise during surgical intervention to confirm interpretation of level localization. Taking these steps prior to surgical intervention will serve greatly to mitigate the risk of operating at an incorrect thoracic level. We also suggest that somatosensory evoked potentials and motor evoked potentials should be arranged preoperatively to ensure they are available at the time of surgery. These should be initiated once the patient is positioned and then monitored throughout the operation to detect any changes during the intervention.

Surgical Technique

There have been numerous modifications to the LECA since its early description, but these can be generally classified as traditional open approaches and minimally invasive approaches. The senior author exclusively uses the minimally invasive approach; however, both will be described as many surgeons prefer the open approach. This will be followed by a discussion of the essential technical surgical considerations for the costotransversectomy and transpedicular approaches. This section will conclude with a description of the LEPA which may be used to address upper thoracic (T1–T4) pathology and afford similar access to this region as the LECA does for the more caudal thoracic levels.

Open Lateral Extracavitary Approach

Surgical Exposure

The patient is positioned prone on a Wilson frame or a Jackson table. The side of approach should be dictated by side of pathology. The skin incision may be oriented in a number of ways but two often predominate. The first is a long midline "hockey-stick" incision with the apex of the curvature located at the level of the pathology (Fig. 16.1a) [14]. The other is a curvilinear incision beginning at the midline three levels above the pathology and ending at the midline three levels below with the apex of the arc 7.5 cm off the midline on the ipsilateral side of the approach (Fig. 16.1b) [3]. Both afford access to the posterior aspect of the contralateral side if posterior instrumentation is needed. With the

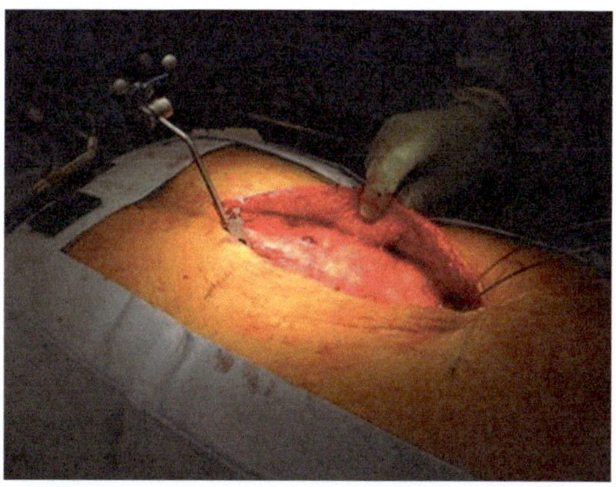

Fig. 16.1 Options for cutaneous incision. (**a**) "Hockey-stick" incision with apex of the curve at the level of pathology; (**b**) curved incision with apex of the curve approximately 7.5 cm lateral to the level of pathology

curvilinear incision, the initial dissection is carried down to the thoracodorsal fascia, and the cutaneous flap is mobilized across midline. Then the spinous processes and lamina are exposed through midline subperiosteal dissection at the level of the pathology and a level above and below. Then dissection is carried laterally at the affected level to identify the angle of the ipsilateral rib. Following this, the latissimus dorsi muscle is identified at the lateral edge of the cutaneous incision, and a vertical incision is carried down to the ribs. The muscle is dissected to free the muscle from the rib cage which facilitates mobilization of the ipsilateral latissimus muscle. With the "hockey-stick" incision, the skin flap is raised with the plane of dissection immediately above the thoracodorsal fascia, and the fascia is opened in a linear fashion over the spinous processes. The fascial incision is then carried out laterally at the level of interest, exposing the erector spinae muscles. The erector spinae muscles are elevated from lateral to medial and then retracted medially. This may necessitate splitting all or part of the erector spinae muscle to achieve sufficient exposure. Surgeon preference and familiarity will generally dictate the technique selected.

The rib resection is initiated by opening the posterior periosteum with monopolar electrocautery. A periosteal elevator is used to strip the periosteum from the posterior aspect of the rib and then carried further to elevate the periosteum from the cranial and caudal aspects of the rib. The cranial rib edge is easiest to strip from medial to lateral, and the inferior edge is easiest to strip from lateral to medial. Caution is needed to preserve the neurovascular bundle when dissecting the caudal aspect of the rib. A curved periosteal elevator such as a Doyen rib raspatory should be employed to complete the circumferential periosteal dissection. A guillotine-type rib cutter should be used to transect the rib 5–10 cm from the costovertebral joint. Remove the transverse process with a Leksell rongeur back toward the pedicle and lamina. Incise the costotransverse and costovertebral ligaments with a scalpel. Elevate the rib and disarticulate it at the costotransverse and costovertebral joints using a Kerrison rongeur. If properly dissected, the periosteum, endothoracic fascia, and retropleural fat should provide protection against a breach of the pleura. Then the rib is transected 5–10 cm from the costovertebral joint and removed. The neurovascular bundle is identified, and the intercostal nerve is followed to the neural foramen. The thoracic nerve root and vasculature may be ligated with silk ties followed by sharp division if it is felt that additional exposure is needed at this stage. The laminofacet on the ipsilateral side should be removed with an osteotome, and this will be followed by removal of the ipsilateral pedicle using a high-speed burr. An inside-out method for the pediculectomy will help prevent injury to the exiting nerve root by leaving a thin rim of cortical bone. This can be carefully resected using a Kerrison punch. At this stage, there is excellent visualization of the intervertebral disc, lateral spinal canal, and vertebral body at the pathological level, and attention may be turned to the ventral decompression (Fig. 16.2). The segmental artery should be identifiable at the caudal limit of the concavity corresponding to the vertebral body. If it is felt that the intercostal vessel cannot be spared, then intraoperative neuromonitoring should be used to monitor for potential disruption of a major supply to the spinal cord. A temporary vascular clip should be applied and then somatosensory evoked potentials monitored for a few minutes. If there is no significant change, then this suggests the vessel can be ligated; otherwise, the vessel should be spared. The sympathetic chain, located on the lateral vertebral surface, should be identified and the rami communicantes transected.

Ventral Decompression

If the nature of the pathology requires corpectomy, the intervertebral discs above and below the involved vertebral body are identified and resected with sharp dissection. Disc material is cleared with curettes and pituitary rongeurs. The adjacent endplates should be completely free of disc or cartilaginous material to optimize bony fusion. A high-speed burr should be used to decompress the center of the vertebral body with the inside-out method. A thin cortical shell should be maintained at the ventral, dorsal, and

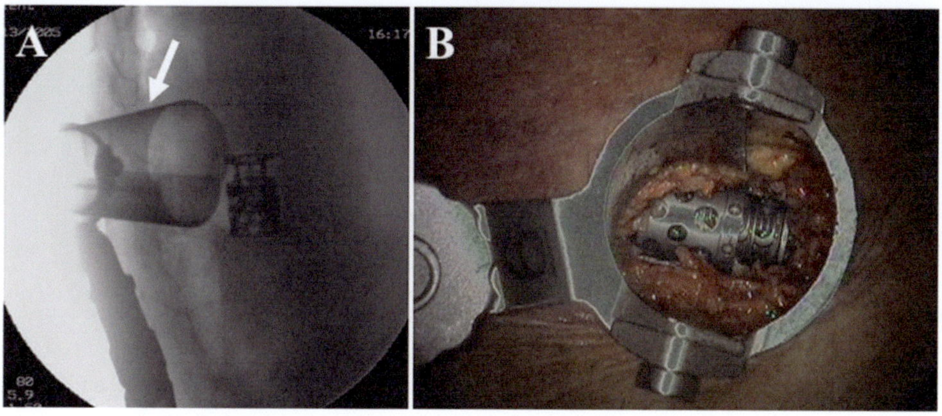

Fig. 16.2 View following removal of the rib (Adapted from Rice et al. [15])

contralateral edges. Once all pathological tissue has been removed, the posterior cortical rim can be carefully removed by dissecting between the posterior longitudinal ligament with a curette. Once the cortical bone is removed, the posterior longitudinal ligament should be removed to expose the dura mater with careful inspection to identify any remaining ventral compression on the spinal cord. Any pathology identified should be removed, avoiding any manipulation of the spinal cord. If necessary, the resection of an additional adjacent rib may improve exposure and allow for adjacent vertebral body decompression in a similar manner.

Treatment of calcified central intervertebral disc herniations generally does not require a full corpectomy. Instead, a working cavity should be created around the pathological disc space. Beforehand, the lateral edge of the posterior longitudinal ligament should be identified to ensure identification of the spinal canal. Once this important anatomical landmark is confirmed, the inferior endplate of the cranial vertebral level and the superior endplate of the caudal vertebral level can be drilled away. A thin rim of cortical bone should be maintained along the posterior aspect of the vertebral bodies. Then a curette may be used to create a dissection plane between the posterior longitudinal ligament and the remaining cortex. This can then be pushed into the superior and inferior resection cavities above and below the disc. Then the remaining calcified disc can be pushed inferiorly and removed to relieve the compressive forces on the spinal cord without requiring undue manipulation.

Spinal Reconstruction

Generally, in all cases where the decompressive steps involved all three columns of the spinal column, internal fusion and fixation will be needed to ensure the maintenance of biomechanical stability. Allograft, autograft, or synthetic structural cages are all options for reconstruction of the defect (Fig. 16.3). The choice of graft material is typically dictated by the nature of the pathology. The anterior graft should be supported with posterior pedicle screw instrumentation. This is typically done with bilateral pedicle screws inserted into at least two levels above and two levels below the level of decompression with joining posterior rods. If there is concern for instability and progressive development of deformity during the decompressive stages of the operation, the pedicle screws may be placed following the initial stages of boney exposure and the contralateral rod placed to maintain alignment. The ipsilateral rod will then be placed following the decompression and ventral reconstruction. If there is a preexisting deformity requiring reduction to attain normal alignment, a rod may be placed through the contralateral pedicle screws to maintain temporary positioning. Then following decompression and ventral reconstruction, the ipsilateral rod may be placed and held loosely in place by blocker caps. The blocker caps on the contralateral rod may then be loosened, and the

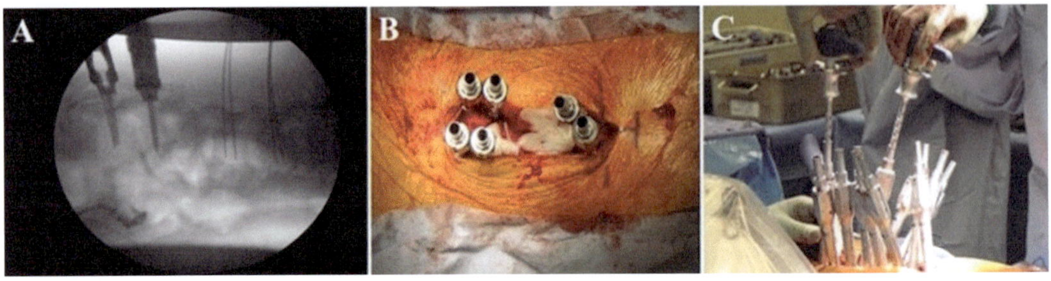

Fig. 16.3 Ventral reconstruction following decompression (Adapted from Scheer et al. [16])

deformity may be corrected using sequential reduction maneuvers and blocker fixation until appropriate alignment is achieved. Final blocker tightening is then used to maintain the alignment.

Minimally Invasive Lateral Extracavitary Approach

Substantial tissue dissection is required for the traditional open LECA, and this has compelled efforts to reduce the invasiveness of the approach. The initial description of a minimally invasive lateral extracavitary approach (MI-LECA) was presented by Kim et al. in 2009 [12]. The steps involved with the decompression are quite similar to the traditional approach; however, there are important differences in the surgical exposure and spinal reconstruction.

Initial exposure may be accomplished by either a small paramedian cutaneous incision to accommodate the tubular dilator or one longer midline cutaneous incision to the level of the thoracodorsal fascia (Fig. 16.4). Our preference is for the longer midline incision. This obviates the need for multiple stab incisions for insertion of the percutaneous posterior instrumentation, and we have found that the larger cutaneous incision has minimal impact on postoperative pain and recovery. After cutaneous exposure, an initial dilator is docked on the lateral facet of the pathological level. Sequential tubular dilators are inserted, and once sufficient nontraumatic muscular dilatation is achieved, an expandable tubular retractor is inserted and fixed in place by a table-mounted adjustable arm. The lamina, facet, transverse process, costovertebral and costotransverse joints, and the rib head are exposed with subperiosteal dissection through the tubular retractor using electrocautery in a similar manner to the traditional open approach.

The removal of the rib head and proximal segment of the rib allows for improved ventromedial visualization. During rib removal, blunt dissection of the ventral and inferior aspect of the rib can be performed with a Penfield #1 which helps avoid injury to the underlying pleura and neurovascular bundle. The rib is then resected distally with a Leksell rongeur. This is followed by the pediculectomy as previously described which affords visualization of the spinal canal and identification of the posterior longitudinal ligament before the stages of ventral decompression are performed. The remaining steps of spinal cord decompression are similar to the traditional open approach, and the spinal column reconstruction may be performed by inserting the anterior graft through the expandable tubular retractor into position (Fig. 16.5a, b).

Following anterior decompression and reconstruction, posterior pedicle screw instrumentation is inserted percutaneously. Intraoperative fluoroscopy is used to dock a Jamshidi needle at the junction of the lateral margin of the superior facet and midpoint of the transverse process. Next, a Kirschner wire (K-wire) is drilled in 2 cm, and the Jamshidi needle is removed. The K-wire is then advanced into the vertebral body using lateral fluoroscopy to visualize depth (Fig. 16.6a), and sequential tubular dilators (Fig. 16.6b) are used to create a nontraumatic pathway through overlying muscle to tap the pedicle and insert the pedicle screw (Fig. 16.6c), and

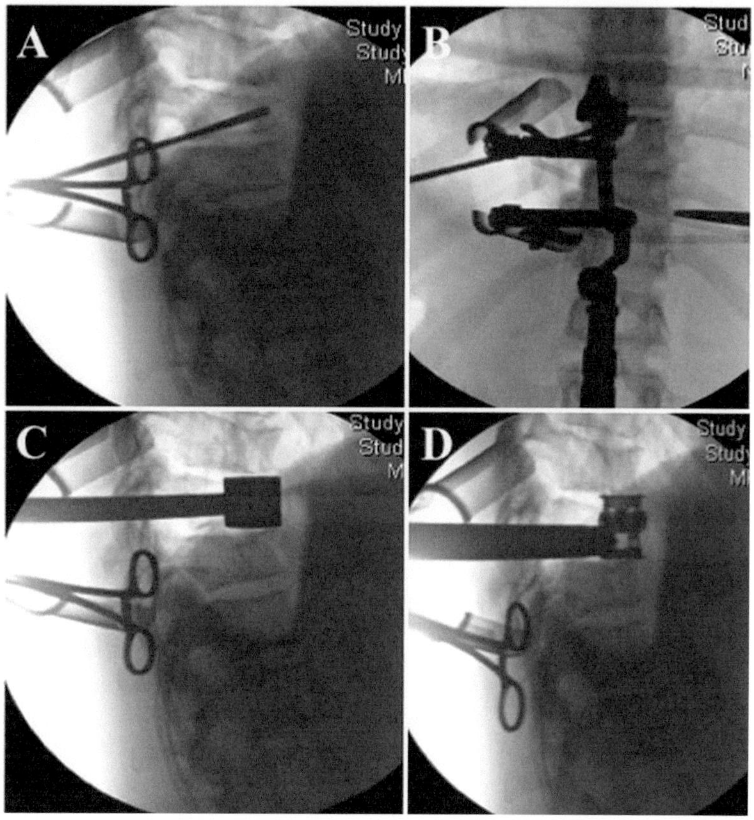

Fig. 16.4 Cutaneous exposure with the thoracodorsal fascia intact for a minimally invasive lateral extracavitary approach. This affords sufficient exposure for muscular dilatation for ventral decompression and fusion, as well as insertion of posterior instrumentation without requiring multiple cutaneous incisions

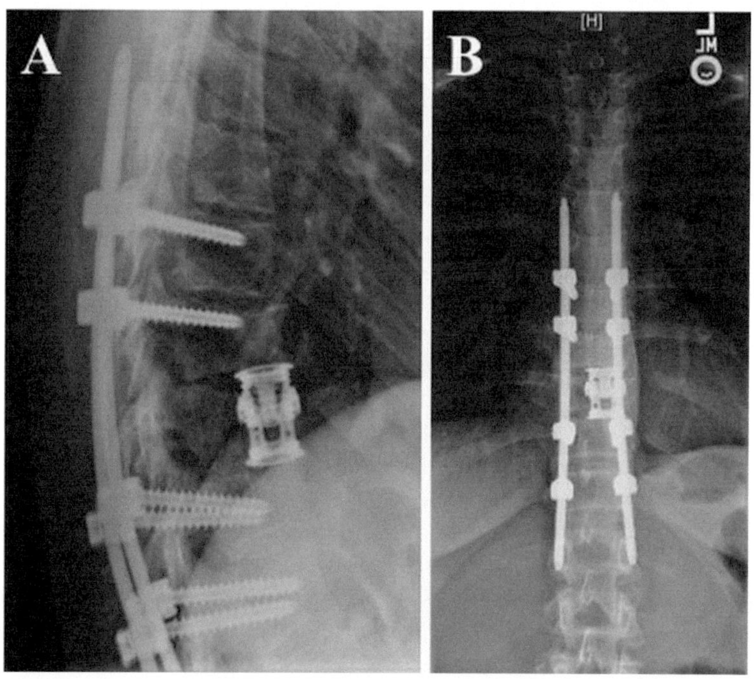

Fig. 16.5 Minimally invasive insertion of an expandable titanium cage for reconstruction of the thoracic spinal column after single level corpectomy. (**a**) Lateral fluoroscopic image showing the positioning of the expandable tubular retractor (*white arrow*) and the expandable titanium cage. (**b**) Intraoperative photograph following insertion of the cage from the surgeon's perspective looking down the expandable tubular retractor

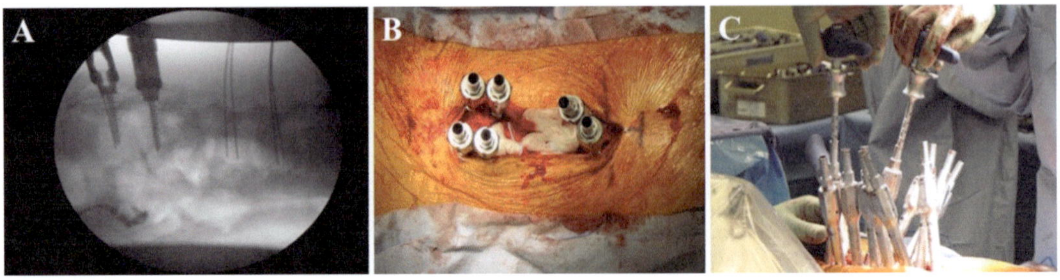

Fig. 16.6 Posterior percutaneous pedicle screw instrumentation. (**a**) Lateral intraoperative fluoroscopic image of the K-wires inserted into the thoracic vertebral bodies cranial to the lesion; (**b**) tubular dilatators; (**c**) insertion of the pedicle screws through the tubular dilators

this step of the operation is completed with the insertion of the posterior rods.

Transpedicular or Costotransversectomy Approaches

In cases where the patient may not require or tolerate the lateral exposure afforded by the LECA, then a transpedicular approach or costotransversectomy may be considered (Fig. 16.7). The primary difference between the LECA and the costotransversectomy is the lateral extent of rib resection. The surgeon should be aware that the costotransversectomy will afford less ventromedial visualization, thus making ventral decompression and spinal column resection more challenging. With the transpedicular approach, the costovertebral articulation complex is left intact. This affords much less ventromedial visualization and will make insertion of a graft for ventral spinal column reconstruction a challenge and often not possible; however, a bilateral transpedicular approach will often be sufficient to relieve ventral compression on the thoracic spinal cord and is particularly useful in metastatic tumor cases when separation of the tumor margin and dura mater is desired prior to radiotherapy.

Maintain artist signiture. A midline cutaneous incision is sufficient to provide exposure for both the costotransversectomy and transpedicular approach. Paraspinal musculature should be dissected from the posterior osseous elements along a subperiosteal plane and then retracted in bulk laterally using a self-retaining retractor. Visualization of the transverse processes is sufficient for a transpedicular approach; however, if a costotransversectomy is planned, then the dissection should be carried further laterally to identify the angle of the rib and the costotransverse joint. When performing a costotransversectomy, the steps of resecting the transverse process, costovertebral articulation complex, laminofacet, and ipsilateral pedicle will proceed in a manner similar to that of the LECA. When performing a transpedicular approach, the transverse process should be removed with a Leksell rongeur, and a laminectomy should be performed to permit palpation of the medial wall of the pedicle. The ipsilateral laminofacet can then be removed with an osteotome, and a high-speed burr can be used to perform the pediculectomy using an inside-out method as previously described which will afford access to the ventrally located compressive pathology.

Lateral Parascapular Extrapleural Approach

The upper thoracic vertebrae are difficult to approach surgically because of the parascapular shoulder musculature and the narrowing of the thoracic cage to reach the thoracic inlet. The lateral parascapular extrapleural approach provides a similar ventral exposure as the traditional LECA but should be used for neural decompression and vertebral reconstruction at T1–T4. The following description outlines the technical details of this exposure as it differs from the traditional open LECA performed at the lower

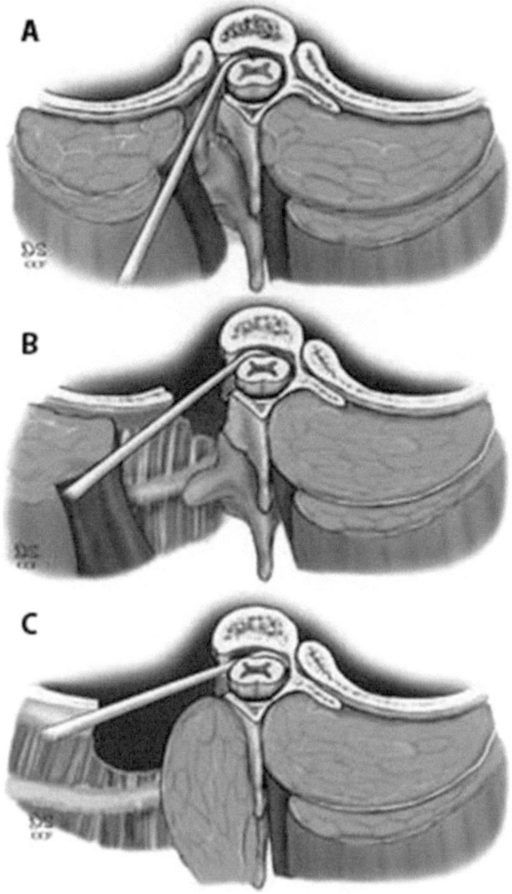

Fig. 16.7 Artist rendition of the exposure afforded by each of the three posterolateral approaches to the thoracic spine: (**a**) transpedicular approach, (**b**) costotransversectomy, and (**c**) lateral extracavitary approach (Adapted from Steinmetz et al. [17])

thoracic levels; however, the decompression and vertebral column reconstruction are largely similar to the open LECA.

A midline incision down to the deep facial plane is made extending from three spinous processes above and below the level of the level of the lesion. This should be curved lateral to the scapular line on the side of approach. The incision is extended down to the spinous processes, and the trapezius and rhomboid muscles are dissected free in the subperiosteal plane. Blunt finger dissection is used to free the muscle layers. A myocutaneous flap that incorporates the skin, rhomboid, and trapezius muscles is then reflected laterally toward the medial boarder of the scapula (Fig. 16.8a). This muscular mobilization will induce lateral movement of the scapula and increase the lateral exposure to the spinal column. Next, the splenius cervicis and erector spinae muscles are dissected from the spinous processes, and this muscular mass is retracted medially toward the contralateral side (Fig. 16.8b).

Sufficient exposure to the level of the lesion is generally provided by removing the rib at the level of interest along with the rib below. This is accomplished using the technique outlined in the section describing the open LECA. The rib should be sectioned laterally at the angle of the rib and then disarticulated from the costotransverse and costovertebral joints after subperiosteal dissection and careful protection of the neurovascular bundle running along the underside of the rib (Fig. 16.8c). The sympathetic chain, located on the lateral vertebral surface, should be identified and the rami communicantes transected.

The stages of lateral and ventral decompression and vertebral column reconstruction proceed in a manner similar to that described previously in the section on open LECA (Fig. 16.8d). Wound closure should proceed systematically to ensure appropriate layered re-approximation. The splenius cervicis and erector spinae muscles are returned from their retracted positioning on the contralateral side, and the trapezius and rhomboid muscles are returned from their lateral positioning. The deep and superficial facial layers are re-approximated to ensure obliteration of any potential dead space.

Illustrative Case

While the primary indication of the LECA is for ventral decompression of the spinal cord, it also may be used to provide spinal column reconstruction in instances of trauma where the primary issue is painful deformity rather than spinal cord compression. In this instance, a 29-year-old female presented with a 2-year history of progressively worsening mid-thoracic back pain that began after a motor vehicle collision where she

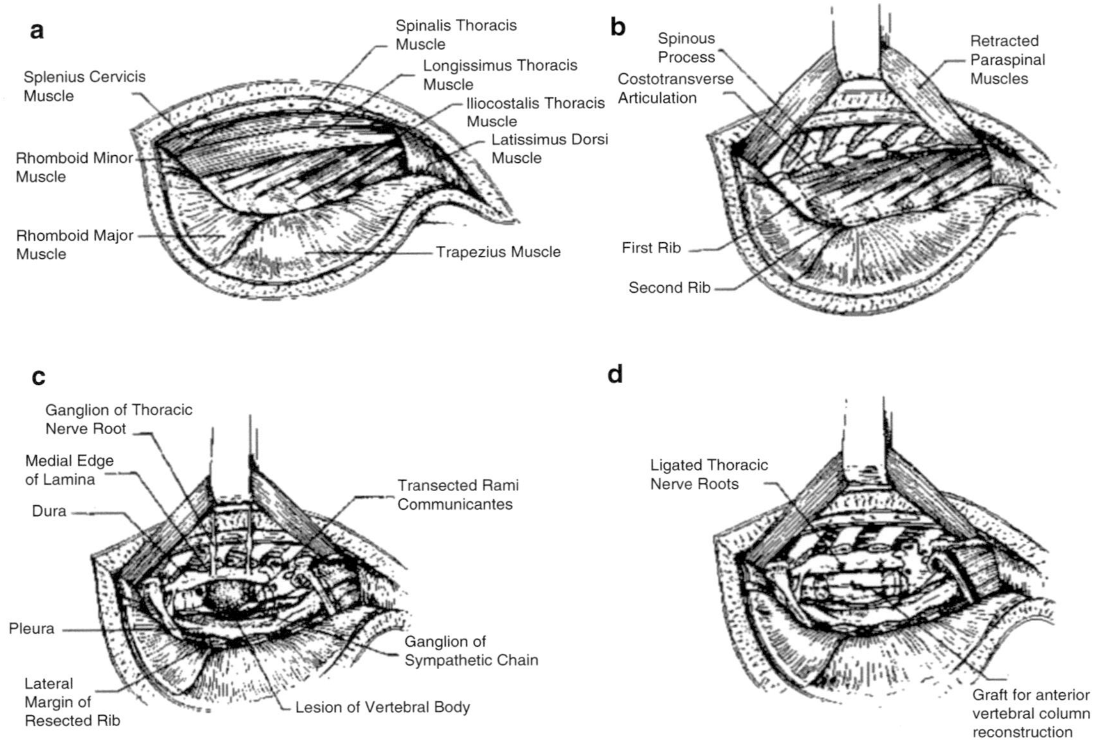

Fig. 16.8 Surgical stages of the lateral parascapular extrapleural approach to the upper thoracic spine. (**a**) Lateral reflection of the myocutaneous flap incorporating the trapezius and rhomboid muscles; (**b**) medial reflection of the paraspinal muscles; (**c**) view following the removal of the ribs; (**d**) view following vertebral column reconstruction (Adapted from Fessler et al. [5])

sustained a T10 compression fracture with subsequent progressive kyphotic deformity (Fig. 16.9a).

Surgical intervention was planned to restore alignment at the affected segment. An MI-LECA as previously described was used. A partial anterior corpectomy at T10 was performed through the tubular retractor (Fig. 16.9b). After bony resection, a trial cage was inserted to determine the appropriate size (Fig. 16.9c), and this was followed by inserting an expandable titanium cage to correct the segmental deformity (Fig. 16.9d) which was followed by posterior instrumentation at the final stage. Postoperative standing radiographs demonstrated restoration of spinal alignment (Fig. 16.10a, b), and the patient's debilitating pain symptomatology was relieved.

Technical Pearls

Several important technical surgical considerations were described during the technical descriptions of the preceding section; however, there are some additional factors that all surgeons performing posterolateral access to the thoracic spine should be aware of. We have outlined these by each stage of the operation.

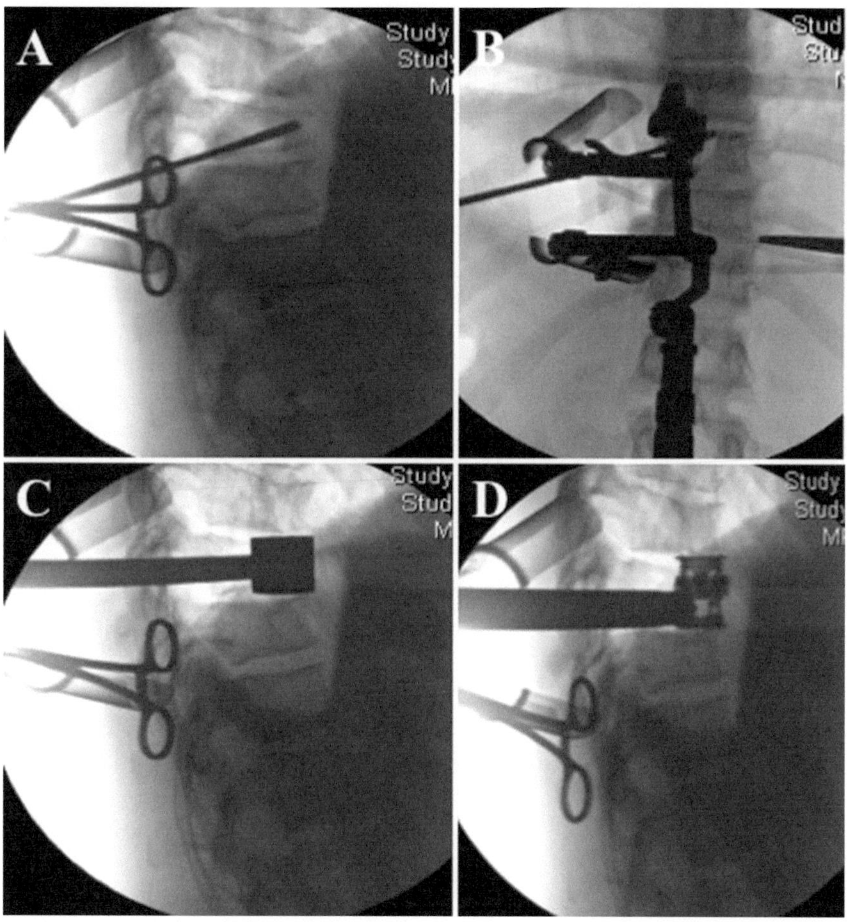

Fig. 16.9 Intraoperative fluoroscopic images. (**a**) Lateral view demonstrating positioning of the tubular retractor and segmental kyphotic deformity at T10 from a chronic traumatic compression fracture: (**b**) Anteroposterior view demonstrating the positioning of the tubular retractor lateral to the affected level; (**c**) Lateral view with insertion of the trial spacer following partial anterior corpectomy at T10; (**d**) Lateral view with insertion to the expandable titanium cage

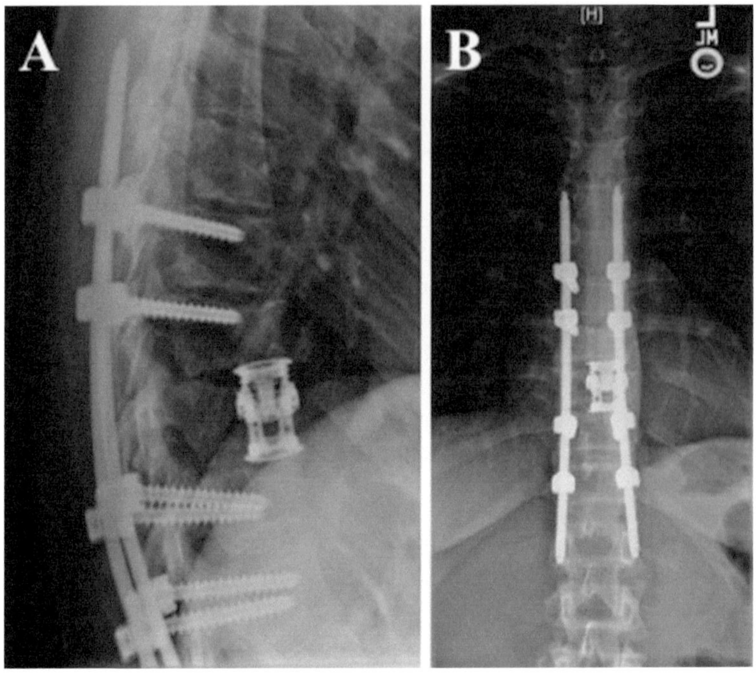

Fig. 16.10 Postoperative standing plain film radiographs. (**a**) Lateral view demonstrating restoration of segmental alignment with an interbody expandable cage at T10 and pedicle screw instrumentation two levels above and below providing posterior support; (**b**) Anteroposterior view demonstrating the same construct

Exposure Stage

- During intraoperative localization, the anatomic relationship between the vertebral body and intervertebral disc space is important. The rib belongs to the inferior level of the disc space of interest. For example, the seventh rib articulates with the transverse process and vertebral body of T7 and overlies the T6/T7 disc space. This recognition is critical to ensure appropriate exposure.
- Similarly, it is necessary to accurately identify where the transverse process articulates with the proximal rib. Aggressive dissection with electrocautery in this area may cause an unintended pleural breach or an injury to the neurovascular bundle running along the underside of the rib.

Ventral Decompression Stage

- To protect the thoracic vascular structures, the anterior cortex of the vertebral body should be left intact whenever possible. The only exception to this is cases where the surgery is being performed for tumor resection.
- When decompression is required for a calcified central intervertebral disc herniation, we have found it helpful to drill away 2 or 3 mm of the pedicle at the caudal level to improve medial visualization and enhance surgical access to the herniation without requiring undue manipulation of the spinal cord.

Ventral Instrumentation Stage

- It is necessary to ensure that the vertebral body endplates adjacent to the site of decompression are sufficiently exposed to allow for optimal fusion.
- Care should be taken to remove the anterior and posterior lips of the endplates to avoid a central separation between the endplates and the graft.
- Conversely, excessive iatrogenic destruction of the vertebral body endplates should be

avoided to mitigate the risk of graft subsidence into the cancellous bone.

Posterior Instrumentation Stage

- An appreciation of the changing anatomical orientation of the thoracic pedicles moving caudally in the thoracic spine is important to avoid misplaced instrumentation. The thoracic pedicles are angled most medially in the upper thoracic spine and then become increasingly more anteriorly oriented moving caudally down to T12.
- When placing percutaneous pedicle screws, unintended anterior migration of the K-wire through the vertebral body represents a potential source of complications. An assistant should fix the wire with an instrument, particularly when tapping the pedicle.
- K-wire fracture is another risk during percutaneous pedicle screw insertion. It is important to maintain a consistent parallel trajectory of the K-wire with the pedicle as a loss of alignment may lead to a fracture of the K-wire.

Complications and Strategies for Avoidance

The LECA is technically challenging, often the interventions are prolonged, and there is a notable potential for adverse events. Resnick et al. reported a 55% incidence of morbidity from a series of 33 patients undergoing a traditional open LECA for thoracic trauma in the acute setting. Their mean surgical time was approximately 7.5 h and a mean blood loss of just over 3 l. The most common complications were pleural fluid collections, pneumonia, and surgical wound infections. Moreover, with any large exposure to the spine, the potential for cutaneous cerebrospinal fluid leaks is ever present. A number of strategies may be employed to mitigate these risks, and these are reviewed in this section.

Pulmonary Complications

While one of the primary advantages of the LECA is the theoretical avoidance of the pulmonary complications associated with an intracavitary anterior approach, there is still a notable risk of pulmonary-related adverse events [18]. The best approach for avoidance is to stay extrapleural. Meticulous dissection of the pleura from the rib and rib head, as well as gentle retraction of the lung, will serve to help avoid an unintentional breach of the pleural membrane. Prior to wound closure, the operative field should be filled with saline irrigation and observed for the presence of an air leak. Identified pleural breaches may be repaired primarily with nonabsorbable interrupted sutures. If the pleural breach cannot be identified or repaired and the air leak persists intraoperatively, then a 24-French thoracostomy tube should be placed and tunneled to a percutaneous exit site inferior to the incision. In the instance of a significant pleural fluid collection diagnosed postoperatively, it is best to treat this with tube thoracostomy because initial thoracentesis has been found frequently to be ineffective in preventing recurrence [14].

Excessive Bleeding

The LECA is often employed when substantial decompression is needed. As such, there is a notable risk of blood loss, and it is critical to ensure that the abdomen is decompressed when the patient is placed in the prone position to reduce venous stasis and avoidable intraoperative bleeding.

When the approach is used for extradural tumors of the spinal column, a preoperative tissue diagnosis will allow for the recognition of highly vascularized pathological lesion types. In such cases, preoperative angiographic embolization may be undertaken to reduce the risk of intraoperative blood loss. Even with preoperative embolization, however, tumor bleeding can still be quite significant. Most often the source of hemorrhage is from the tumor bed, and this is best managed with complete removal of all visible tumors whenever possible. Bleeding should not be treated with bone wax, as this may limit osteogenesis and predispose to pseudarthrosis [18]. Vigilance for sites of epidural bleeding is important, and hemostasis should be attained with bipolar coagulation. Identified epidural vessels may be coagulated and then sharply dissected when needed during the stages of decompression. Hemostatic gelatin or other packing agents may also be employed as needed while being careful not to apply any force on the spinal cord.

Wound Infections

With large, traditional open exposures, the risk for postoperative wound infection is high. This is further exacerbated by the presence of hardware and, in cases of malignancy, wound breakdown from postoperative radiation therapy. For these reasons, meticulous multilayer wound closure is critical, and the surgical field should always be copiously irrigated. A substantial body of evidence has now emerged to support the use of vancomycin powder as an adjunct to reduce infection, and we support its use [19, 20]. Furthermore, the use of minimally invasive technique may represent an opportunity to lower the incidence of infection [21, 22].

Cutaneous Cerebrospinal Fluid Leaks

An incidental durotomy may occur during decompression along the thecal sac. At other times, tumor erosion may lead to sections of absent dura mater. In instances of a discrete dural breach, primary repair should be attempted with a nonabsorbable 4-0 suture. However, in certain cases, this may not be possible. We suggest these should be managed with a synthetic dural patch onlay and supplemented with fibrin glue. The patient should be maintained on strict fully supine bedrest for 24 h following the surgery for small breaches in the dura; however, at times, larger durotomies may necessitate cerebrospinal fluid (CSF) diversion with the use of a percutaneously inserted lumbar intrathecal catheter. As with wound infections, minimally invasive techniques may also represent a means of lowering the incidence of postoperative cutaneous CSF leaks [23].

Conclusion

The LECA represents a well-accepted surgical technique to address ventral compressive pathology in the thoracic spine. The primary advantages are the ability to address the ventral pathology while supplementing the spinal column reconstruction with posterior instrumentation, all through a single incision without the need for patient repositioning. Modifications to the technique such as the LEPA for the upper thoracic spine as well as selection of a costotransversectomy or transpedicular approach may be employed as appropriate. However, these procedures are technically challenging and should generally be reserved for those with substantial familiarity with spinal interventions. There is a notable risk of surgical complications with any of these approaches, but the techniques outlined within this chapter should serve to reduce the risk. Advancements made in minimally invasive techniques and technologies have lowered the soft tissue destruction required, and it is likely that the posterolateral approach to the thoracic spine will continue to serve as a mainstay in the spinal surgeon's armamentarium.

References

1. Larson SJ, Holst RA, Hemmy DC, Sances A Jr. Lateral extracavitary approach to traumatic lesions of the thoracic and lumbar spine. J Neurosurg. 1976;45(6):628–37.
2. Capener N. The evolution of lateral rhachotomy. J Bone Joint Surg Br. 1954;36-b(2):173–9.
3. Foreman PM, Naftel RP, Moore TA 2nd, Hadley MN. The lateral extracavitary approach to the thoracolumbar spine: a case series and systematic review. J Neurosurg Spine. 2016;24(4):570–9.
4. Lall RR, Smith ZA, Wong AP, Miller D, Fessler RG. Minimally invasive thoracic corpectomy: sur-

gical strategies for malignancy, trauma, and complex spinal pathologies. Minim Invasive Surg. 2012;2012:213791.
5. Fessler RG, Dietze DD Jr, Millan MM, Peace D. Lateral parascapular extrapleural approach to the upper thoracic spine. J Neurosurg. 1991;75(3):349–55.
6. Kaya RA, Turkmenoglu ON, Koc ON, Genc HA, Cavusoglu H, Ziyal IM, et al. A perspective for the selection of surgical approaches in patients with upper thoracic and cervicothoracic junction instabilities. Surg Neurol. 2006;65(5):454–63. discussion 63
7. Faciszewski T, Winter RB, Lonstein JE, Denis F, Johnson L. The surgical and medical perioperative complications of anterior spinal fusion surgery in the thoracic and lumbar spine in adults. A review of 1223 procedures. Spine (Phila Pa 1976). 1995;20(14):1592–9.
8. Khoo LT, Beisse R, Potulski M. Thoracoscopic-assisted treatment of thoracic and lumbar fractures: a series of 371 consecutive cases. Neurosurgery. 2002;51(5 Suppl):S104–17.
9. Moskovich R, Benson D, Zhang ZH, Kabins M. Extracoelomic approach to the spine. J Bone Joint Surg Br. 1993;75(6):886–93.
10. McCormick PC. Retropleural approach to the thoracic and thoracolumbar spine. Neurosurgery. 1995;37(5):908–14.
11. Graham AW 3rd, Mac Millan M, Fessler RG. Lateral extracavitary approach to the thoracic and thoracolumbar spine. Orthopedics. 1997;20(7):605–10.
12. Kim DH, O'Toole JE, Ogden AT, Eichholz KM, Song J, Christie SD, et al. Minimally invasive posterolateral thoracic corpectomy: cadaveric feasibility study and report of four clinical cases. Neurosurgery. 2009;64(4):746–52. discussion 52-3
13. Perez-Cruet MJ, Kim BS, Sandhu F, Samartzis D, Fessler RG. Thoracic microendoscopic discectomy. J Neurosurg Spine. 2004;1(1):58–63.
14. Resnick DK, Benzel EC. Lateral extracavitary approach for thoracic and thoracolumbar spine trauma: operative complications. Neurosurgery. 1998;43(4):796–802. discussion -3
15. Rice RA, Daniel F, Voyadzis JM. Open costotransversectomy. In: Fessler RG, Sekhar LN, editors. Atlas of neurosurgical techniques: spine and peripheral nerves. Second ed. New York: Thieme; 2016.
16. Scheer JK, Dahdaleh NS, Smith ZA. MIS Costotransversectomy. In: Fessler RG, Sekhar LN, editors. Atlas of neurosurgical techniques: spine and peripheral nerves. Second ed. New York: Thieme; 2016.
17. Steinmetz MP, Mekhail A, Benzel EC. Management of metastatic tumors of the spine: strategies and operative indications. Neurosurg Focus. 2001 Dec 15;11(6):e2.
18. Lubelski D, Abdullah KG, Steinmetz MP, Masters F, Benzel EC, Mroz TE, et al. Lateral extracavitary, costotransversectomy, and transthoracic thoracotomy approaches to the thoracic spine: review of techniques and complications. J Spinal Disord Tech. 2013;26(4):222–32.
19. Khan NR, Thompson CJ, DeCuypere M, Angotti JM, Kalobwe E, Muhlbauer MS, et al. A meta-analysis of spinal surgical site infection and vancomycin powder. J Neurosurg Spine. 2014;21(6):974–83.
20. Dennis HH, Wei DT, Darren KZ, Shantakumar JT, Kumar N, Lau LL, et al. Is intraoperative local Vancomycin powder the answer to surgical site infections in spine surgery? Spine (Phila pa 1976). 2016.
21. Ee WW, Lau WL, Yeo W, Von Bing Y, Yue WM. Does minimally invasive surgery have a lower risk of surgical site infections compared with open spinal surgery? Clin Orthop Relat Res. 2014;472(6):1718–24.
22. O'Toole JE, Eichholz KM, Fessler RG. Surgical site infection rates after minimally invasive spinal surgery. J Neurosurg Spine. 2009;11(4):471–6.
23. Wong AP, Shih P, Smith TR, Slimack NP, Dahdaleh NS, Aoun SG, et al. Comparison of symptomatic cerebral spinal fluid leak between patients undergoing minimally invasive versus open lumbar foraminotomy, discectomy, or laminectomy. World Neurosurg. 2014;81(3–4):634–40.

Posterior Thoracic Spinal Fixation

17

Stephen K. Mendenhall and Saad A. Khairi

Introduction

Spinal stability is defined as the ability to protect the neural structures from damage and to prevent neurologic deficit/deformity under normal physiologic loads [1]. Posterior thoracic spinal instrumentation is used to restore spinal stability when its mechanical functions are disrupted by trauma, tumor, infection, degenerative disease, deformity, or surgical management of these disorders. The particular indications for each disease process may be different, but the goal is the same – increasing stability, prevention of deformity, maintenance of load bearing, and promotion of bone fusion.

Posterior thoracolumbar instrumentation is divided into rigid and nonrigid constructs. The earliest constructs involved wiring the spinous process or other posterior elements alone or with autograft. These early wiring techniques were then replaced with wire-rod techniques. The most common technique, Luque wiring, involved sublaminar wires wrapped around rods to form a segmental nonrigid spine construct. These techniques were considered nonrigid because they allowed movement of the spine in the craniocaudal direction. Wire-rod techniques were replaced with simple hook-based distraction devices that were used to correct scoliosis. Early hook-based constructs allowed lordosis to be contoured into the rod and anchored at multiple points. These constructs were significantly more rigid, greatly improving fusion rates and greatly decreasing the amount of time needed for postoperative bracing or cast immobilization.

Posterior thoracic pedicle screw instrumentation has succeeded posterior hook-rod fixation and wiring techniques because it has been proven to be biomechanically advantageous, i.e., pedicle screw fixation requires fixation to fewer levels, allows for laminectomy to be performed at the levels to be fused, decreases operative time, and reduces construct motion [2–6]. Additionally, pedicle screw constructs employ three-column spine fixation, whereas hooks anchor to the posterior elements alone and therefore have weaker reduction power [7]. In a comparison of pullout strength, thoracic pedicle screws were found to be significantly stronger than hooks and are recommended for rigid curves [8]. Although mostly supplanted by pedicle screw fixation, hooks are still used for salvage procedures, deformity, and backup in osteoporotic cases.

Pedicle screw instrumentation of the thoracic spine is challenging due to large anatomic variability and the intimate relationships between the bony, neural, vascular, and visceral elements that compose and surround the thoracic spine [9–14].

S.K. Mendenhall, MD • S.A. Khairi, MD (✉)
Indiana University Health Neuroscience Center, 355 W. 16th Street, Suite 5100, Indianapolis, IN 46202, USA
e-mail: skmenden@iupui.edu; skhairi@goodmancampbell.com

L.T. Holly, P.A. Anderson (eds.), *Essentials of Spinal Stabilization*, DOI 10.1007/978-3-319-59713-3_17

Therefore, the surgeon must have a thorough understanding of thoracic spinal anatomy, in addition to individual patient anatomy and pathology via proper clinical and radiographic evaluation to achieve an excellent outcome. The purpose of this chapter is to review the indications, anatomy, biomechanics, and surgical techniques for posterior thoracic spinal fixation.

Indications and Patient Selection

The main pathologic processes of the thoracic spine that require instrumentation are deformity, trauma, tumor, and infection. Patients are selected for surgery for the following reasons:

1. Pain that is not improved with nonoperative management
2. Functional limitations not improved with nonoperative management
3. Deformity progression
4. Neurologic deficit

Patients who require osteotomies and destabilization of the spine will require posterior thoracic pedicle screw and rod instrumentation due to the creation of instability by release of the facet joints to correct coronal imbalance.

The most common indication for posterior thoracic fusion is trauma. There are many different types of spine fractures which are destabilizing to the spine, either creating initial neurologic injury or having the potential to cause neurologic injury without spinal fixation. Operative decision-making in thoracolumbar trauma is based on the thoracolumbar injury classification and severity score (TLICS). Injury is graded based on the morphology of the fracture, integrity of the posterior longitudinal ligament, and neurologic status [15].

Patients with tumor or infections of the spine often require extensive decompression of the vertebral column to treat the underlying pathology. When decompression creates spinal instability, it is typically stabilized with posterior instrumentation across the unstable vertebral levels.

Exclusion criteria for patients undergoing posterior thoracic instrumentation include severe osteoporosis, morbid obesity, and multisystem trauma. Patients with osteoporosis are generally poor spine surgery candidates because reduced bone mineral density is associated with higher rates of hardware failure. Morbidly obese patients have much higher rates of all complication types including cardiac, renal, pulmonary, and wound complications [16]. Lastly, patients with severe multisystem trauma who meet criteria for thoracic spinal instrumentation may not be candidates for surgery in general due to coagulopathy and risk of death from other immediate injuries. The spine surgeon must be able to weigh the benefits of posterior thoracic instrumentation with the risks of the procedure for each individual patient. Only when the benefits outweigh the risks of surgery is spinal instrumentation justified.

Preoperative Considerations

Anatomy

The thoracic spine consists of 12 vertebral bodies. The vertebral bodies decrease in size from T1 to T3 and then increase in size to T12 [17]. The spinous processes of the thoracic spine are angulated posteroinferiorly and are palpable in most individuals. In the midline, a layer of fat separates the skin from the thoracic fascia and supraspinous ligaments. The muscles of the thoracic spine are lateral and deep to this fatty layer.

There are three groups of muscles in the thoracic spine: superficial, intermediate, and deep. The superficial layer contains the trapezius and latissimus dorsi muscles. Deep to these are the rhomboid major and minor muscles [18]. The intermediate muscle layer contains the serratus superior and inferior muscle groups. The deep layer contains the erector spinae muscles, which consist of the semispinalis, multifidus, and rotator muscles. The thoracolumbar fascia originates from the dorsal layer of investing fascia from the deep muscle layer and is continuous with the transverse abdominis aponeurosis [19].

Surgical exposure of the posterior thoracic spine is performed midline, over the spinous processes. Midline dissection minimizes risk to nerves innervating the thoracic musculature. The superficial muscles are innervated by the spinal accessory, thoracodorsal, and C5 nerve root. The intermediate muscles are innervated by the anterior rami of thoracic nerves. The deep muscle layer is innervated by the posterior rami of the thoracic nerves.

The ligaments and joint capsules of the spine are responsible for maintaining spinal motion in a restricted manner. From superficial to deep, they include the supraspinous ligament, interspinous ligament, ligamentum flavum, facet capsule, posterior longitudinal ligament, and anterior longitudinal ligament. The supraspinous ligament attaches to the tips of the spinous processes. The interspinous ligament extends from the root to the apex of each spinous process and connects adjacent spinous processes. The interspinous ligament blends with the ligamentum flavum near the base of the spinous process and joins the supraspinous ligament at the apex or each spinous process. The ligamentum flavum inserts on the undersurface of the lamina above and attaches to the top of the inferior lamina. The posterior longitudinal ligament (PLL) is a thick band that runs midline along the dorsal aspect of the vertebral bodies and intervertebral discs. The PLL has been shown to be biomechanically important for posterior instrumentation when attempting to perform indirect reduction of fractures by means of ligamentotaxis [20]. The anterior longitudinal ligament (ALL) is a similar structure traversing the ventral aspect of the vertebral bodies and intervertebral discs. The ALL is important for prevention of hyperextension and overdistraction [21].

In the thoracic spine, the pedicle width is smallest at T4. In general, the pedicle width decreases from T1 to T4 and then increases from T4 to T12. The pedicle height increases from T1 to T12 in most patients. For T1 and T2, the pedicles have a medial projection of 30–40°; at T3–T11, this angle decreases to 20–25°; at T12, the angle is around 10° (Fig. 17.1). In the sagittal plane, the thoracic angulation is constant between 10 and 20° downward (Fig. 17.2) [10, 12–14, 22].

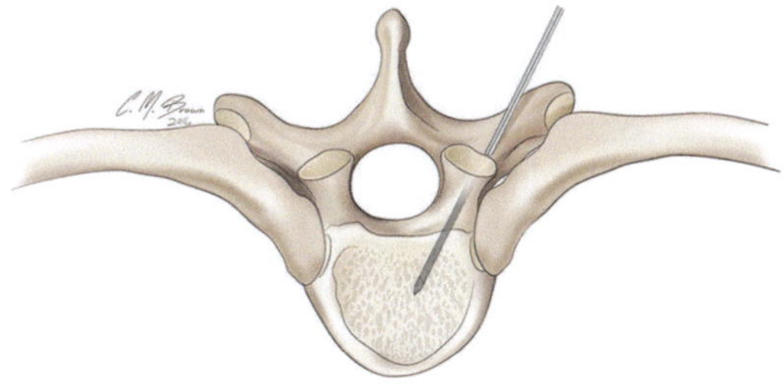

Fig. 17.1 Axial view. Medial angulation of the pedicle and trajectory of pedicle screw placement. T1–T2, 30–40°; T3–T11, 20–25°; T12, 10°

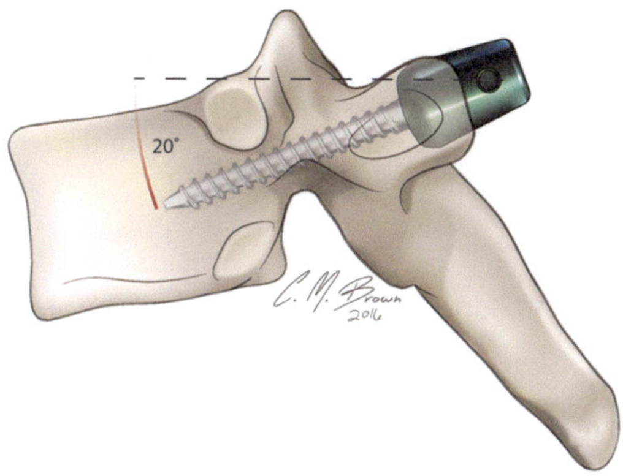

Fig. 17.2 Sagittal view after pedicle screw placement. Thoracic pedicles maintain a downward 10–20° angulation throughout the length of the thoracic spine

The relationships of the nerve roots and thecal sac to the pedicle have been well described. The thecal sac typically rests against the medial wall of the pedicle. The nerve root exits underneath the same numbered pedicle at that level. In general, the distance from the pedicle to the inferior root and superior root increases from T1 to T12 [10]. Special care should be taken to avoid superior and inferior breaches in the upper thoracic vertebral segments. Additionally, it has been shown that the distance from the medial pedicle to the thecal sac is shortest in the middle thoracic segments [10]. Therefore, medial pedicle breach at these levels should be avoided. It is important to stress that there exists a wide variety of three-dimensional pedicle anatomy mandating thorough preoperative CT pedicle anatomic evaluation.

The thoracic aorta is located anterior and/or lateral to the thoracic vertebral bodies. Hell et al. examined the distance from the aortic wall to the thoracic vertebral body and found that in normal patients, this distance is approximately 2.5 mm. In addition, the aorta is positioned more laterally and posteriorly from T5 to T12 [23]. Care must be taken when placing thoracic pedicle screws in this region to prevent inadvertent, catastrophic injury to the aorta. The dominant supply to the anterior spinal cord is the anterior spinal artery. In the thoracic and upper lumbar region, the anterior spinal artery is mainly supplied by segmental radicular arteries. The dominant artery at the thoracolumbar region is the artery of Adamkiewicz, which is always located between T8 and L3, at T9 or T10 in 50% of cases, and coming from the left side in 75% of cases [24].

Biomechanics

Instrumentation of the thoracic spine requires a thorough understanding of its biomechanical properties. Relative to the cervical and lumbar regions, the thoracic spine is relatively less mobile except at the cervicothoracic and thoracolumbar regions. The transition areas at either end of the thoracic spine are more susceptible to destabilization through traumatic injury.

In the thoracic spine, the vertebral bodies support the axial loading forces and the intervertebral discs stabilize the axial loading forces. The vertical orientation of the thoracic facets limits sagittal motion. The rib cage and sternum provide a significant amount of stability to the thoracic spine in flexion/extension, lateral bending, and axial rotation [25]. This has been proven in canine models, where unilateral resection of a rib head after partial discectomy in a spinal model caused a significant decrease in thoracic spinal stability [26].

The point of posterior thoracic spinal fixation is to preserve neurologic function, maintain alignment, correct deformity, and/or provide support until bony fusion occurs. Before spine surgeons can accurately address a specific pathology, they must fully understand several key points listed below: [27]

1. What forces are acting on the spine?
2. In what plane(s) is the spine unstable?
3. How will instrumentation counteract the forces applied to the spine?
4. What are the destabilizing effects of the operative procedure itself?
5. How will the instrumentation affect the forces that are passing through the structural grafts?
6. What is the extent of postoperative muscular force?
7. What is the time course needed for bone healing?

In general, the surgeon will evaluate the degree of anatomic disruption seen on MRI/CT scan or envision the destabilization that will be caused by treatment of pathology and use his knowledge of the forces applied by instrumentation to counteract the anatomic disruption. To do this effectively, the surgeon must understand the different planes in which forces are acting on the spine and how well the construct will hold when subjected to these forces. Failure to understand the forces acting on the spine can lead to overly large or inappropriately small fusion constructs. The better the surgeon understands the key points listed above, the more able he/she will be to choose the optimum construct for the treatment of a specific surgical pathology.

Surgical Technique

The posterior approach to the thoracic spine is well established and is the workhorse for many spine surgeons. Its versatility allows access to the osseoligamentous regions of the posterior thoracic spine for treatment of trauma, neoplasms, deformity, and infection.

Prior to starting the case, all preoperative images should be reviewed in detail and made available for viewing throughout the procedure. The patient is evaluated by an anesthesiologist, whose selection of general anesthetic is made based on the patient's comorbidities and the preference of the spine surgeon.

After induction with general anesthesia, the patient is positioned in the prone position on a radiolucent table with chest, thigh, and hip pads. The exception to this positioning is patients with ankylosing spondylitis. These patients are positioned using the Jackson table with Wilson Frame in order to recreate the normal curvature of the thoracic spine before instrumentation. The arms can either be tucked at the patient's side or overhead on arm boards (Fig. 17.3). It is important to ensure that the abdomen is not under tension. Abdominal wall tension is transmitted to the inferior vena cava, causing increased caval pressure. Increase caval pressure is transmitted to the vertebral venous plexus and can contribute to a significant increase in blood loss [28]. Additionally, high venous pressures can result in decreased spinal cord perfusion, putting the patient at risk for neurologic injury [29].

The patient is positioned in a manner that approximates normal thoracic kyphosis. This step is important to prevent abnormal thoracic kyphosis or deformity under-correction after instrumentation. The thoracic levels to be addressed are then identified using intraoperative fluoroscopy, and the incision is planned. A longitudinal line is drawn directly over midline, using palpation of the spinous processes at the desired level. Typically, the incision is extended one level proximal and distal to obtain adequate exposure. The patient is then prepped and draped in the normal sterile fashion.

Surgical localization in the thoracic spine is achieved by counting ribs on an AP radiograph intraoperatively. Confusion can arise when the patient has more ribs than normal, fewer ribs than

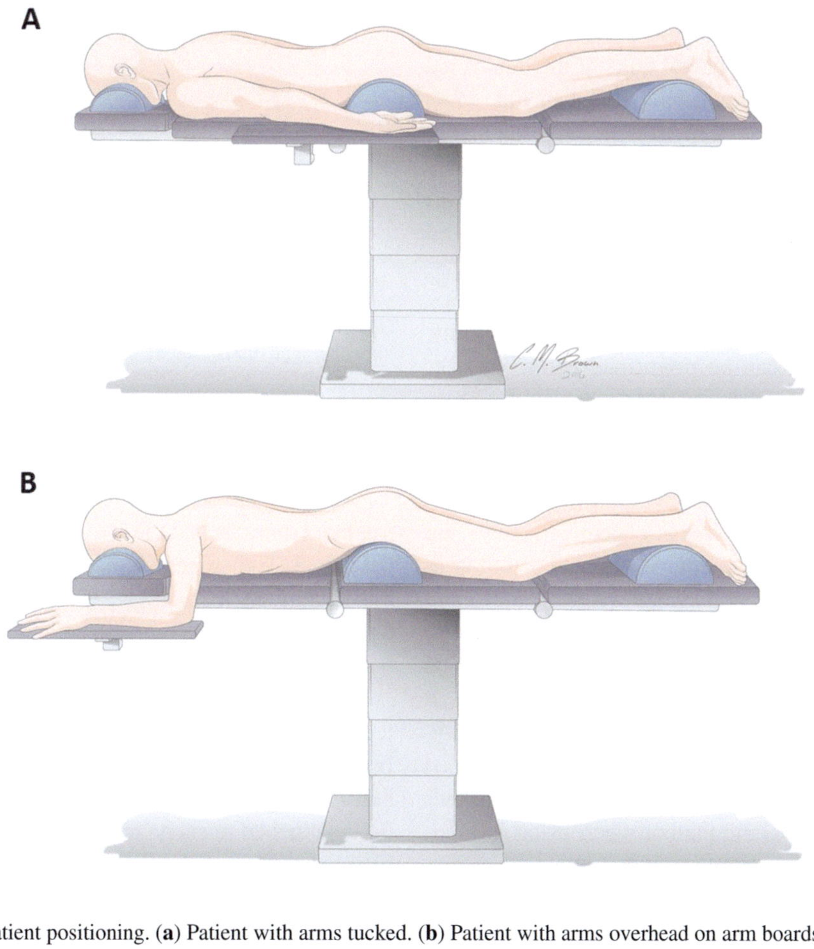

Fig. 17.3 Patient positioning. (**a**) Patient with arms tucked. (**b**) Patient with arms overhead on arm boards

normal, or elongated transverse processes that are counted as ribs. The prevalence of cervical ribs is 0.05–6% [30]. The prevalence of thoracic rib aplasia is approximately 6% [30]. The prevalence of a lumbar rib is approximately 1% [30]. Elongated transverse processes have a prevalence of 2.2% [31]. The overall prevalence of rib number abnormalities has been estimated to be 8% [31]. It is imperative to evaluate preoperative imaging to identify rib abnormalities to prevent wrong level surgery.

The initial skin incision is made with a No. 10 blade. Electrocautery is used to deepen the incision through the subcutaneous tissues. Any bleeding is coagulated with care so that the skin is not devascularized. After the subcutaneous tissue dissection, the muscles of the back are encountered. They are dissected subperiosteally from the spinous processes and laminae bilaterally to minimize muscular bleeding. In preparation for pedicle screw placement, the dissection is carried out to the lateral edge of the transverse processes bilaterally, as illustrated in Fig. 17.4. Dissection of the deep muscle layer from the lamina out over the lateral transverse process edge can be facilitated using Cobb elevators and electrocautery. Self-retaining Gelpi retractors are then placed, and hemostasis is obtained.

At this point, surgical correction of pathology occurs, sometimes involving laminectomy. Laminectomy can be performed before or after pedicle screw placement. It is our practice to perform pedicle screw placement before decompression, utilizing the lamina as a safe guard in case of pedicle screw instrumentation slippage.

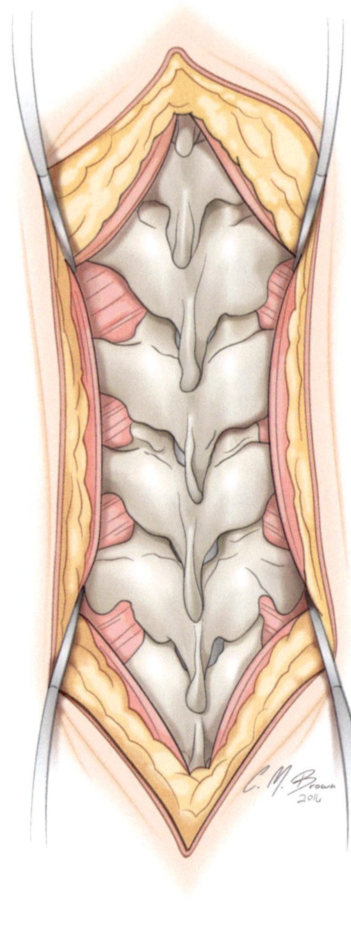

Fig. 17.4 Posterior thoracic exposure of T7–T10. Subperiosteal dissection of the muscle layers, showing exposure of the mid-thoracic spine using two Gelpi retractors. The exposure is carried out to the lateral edge of the transverse processes bilaterally

In our practice, thoracic pedicle screws are placed using intraoperative computed tomography (CT) reference-based navigation tools and instruments. Image-guided spinal instrumentation is relatively new and has been shown to be highly safe, accurate, and effective [32–35]. It should be noted that with the use of intraoperative navigation, patients should be positioned with the arms tucked at the sides. This allows easier access to the patient when using intraoperative CT. The authors feel that an extensive discussion of CT-navigated pedicle screws is not warranted in this book chapter. Instead, the freehand thoracic pedicle screw technique will be described. The spine surgeon should understand this technique to facilitate a three-dimensional understanding of the thoracic pedicle and its relationship to the nerve roots and thecal sac.

The authors use the freehand pedicle screw technique described by Kim et al. [36]. Instrumentation is started at the most distal vertebra. A Leksell rongeur is used to remove the soft tissue attached to each facet joint associated with instrumentation (Fig. 17.5). In the lower thoracic region (T11–T12), the pedicle screw entry points are located at the junction of the bisected

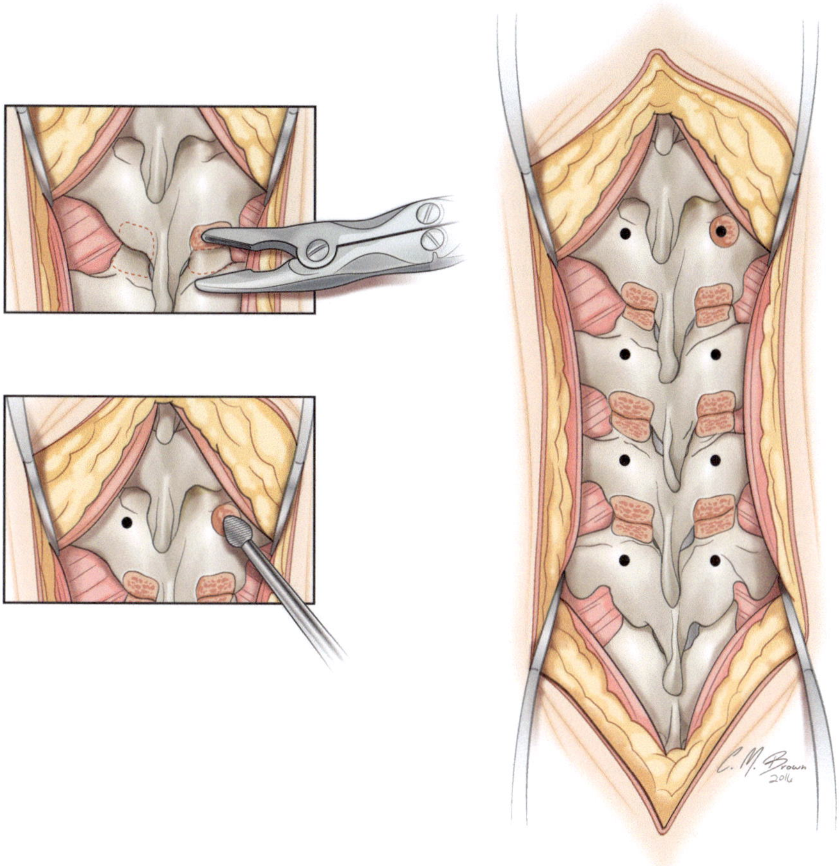

Fig. 17.5 Posterior thoracic exposure of T7–T10. A Leksell rongeur is used to remove the facet joint capsule and soft tissue. A high-speed burr was used to create the pedicle screw entry point at the junction of the proximal edge of the transverse process and lamina

transverse process and lamina, directly medial to the lateral aspect of the pars. As one progresses to the apical mid-thoracic region, the entry point is more medial and cephalad. At the mid-thoracic region (T7–T9), the entry point is the most medial and located at the junction of the proximal edge of the transverse process and lamina, just lateral to the midportion of the base of the superior articular process. Above the mid-thoracic region, the entry point moves slightly caudally and laterally with each successive level. At the proximal thoracic region (T1–T2), the entry point is at the junction of the bisected transverse process and lamina at the lateral pars. As one places each successive pedicle screw cranially, these trends should be noted and used to make slight adjustments to each successive pedicle screw based on the previous level. Once the entry points are delineated, a high-speed burr is used to decorticate the entry points (Fig. 17.5).

After decortication, the thoracic gearshift probe is placed into the entry point in search of a "soft" spot, which indicates entry into the cancellous bone of the pedicle. Initially, the gearshift should point laterally for safety and advance 15–20 mm. It is then directed medially and advanced down the path of the pedicle to its final depth. Preoperative imaging should be used to measure the approximate lengths of the instrumented pedicles in preparation for this step. It should be noted that most spine surgeons use intraoperative fluoroscopy to guide gearshift probing. Anterior-posterior (AP) fluoroscopy views "looking" down the pedicle are used to guide the gearshift probe along the length of the pedicle using the exact same steps as mentioned above. After probing, a ball-tip probe is placed into the pedicle and used to feel for medial/lateral wall breach. This is a critical portion of the procedure. A missed pedicle breach could potentially lead to pedicle screw-induced neurologic injury postoperatively. If any breach is found, the pedicle probe is used to redirect the path for the pedicle screw. Once an adequate path is created, the ball-tip probe is placed to the base of the tract, and the length marked with a hemostat to measure pedicle screw length.

The pedicle tract is then tapped with a smaller diameter screw tract. The tract is palpated for breach. If no breach is found, the pedicle screw is placed into the pedicle following the same trajectory as the tapping device (Fig. 17.6). The screw placement is then confirmed with intraoperative fluoroscopy and is tested with electromyography (EMG) stimulations utilizing real-time thoracic nerve root recordings from the rectus abdominis musculature. EMG assesses screws placed from T6 to T12. It has been shown that an EMG threshold less than 6.0 mA, with values 65% or less from the "average" of all other screws at T6–T12, is indicative of a potential medial pedicle screw breach [37].

As the life expectancy of the general population increases, more patients with advanced age and osteoporosis are undergoing spine surgery. In this population, surgery typically involves instrumented stabilization and reconstruction. Rigid instrumentation is associated with high mechanical demand at the implant-bone interface, and as bone quality decreases, the risk of mechanical degradation at the implant-bone interface increases. Several studies have demonstrated that screw pullout strength is directly related to bone mineral density and that pedicle screws fail by stripping the cancellous bone within the pedicle tract [38–40]. Longer screws have been shown to achieve significantly better fixation, especially screws that are placed bicortically [38, 40]. In addition, augmentation of the screw tract with cement has been shown to increase fixation in the

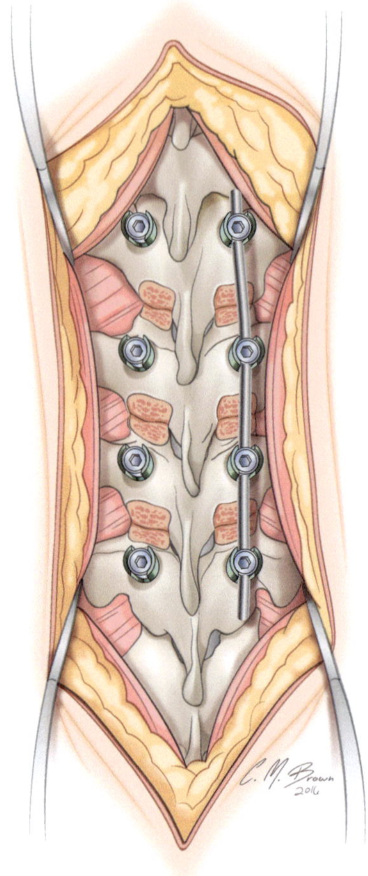

Fig. 17.6 Posterior thoracic exposure of T7–T10. Pedicle screws have been placed and unilateral rod fixation completed

osteoporotic bone. Injecting polymethyl methacrylate into the screw tract prior to screw placement has been shown to significantly increase pullout resistance [41, 42]. 1–3 mL of cement is generally recommended for injection since larger volumes of cement have not shown benefit in regard to pullout strength [43].

After pedicle screw placement is complete, laminectomy and/or deformity correction for the operative pathology is performed. Rods are cut to an appropriate length and bent to maintain proper thoracic curvature. They are placed in the screw heads bilaterally and finally tightened (Fig. 17.6). Depending on the degree of spine instability and motion segments instrumented, placement of transverse rod cross-links is recommended. Cross-links have been proven to increase rotational and bending stiffness significantly [44–47]. If two cross-links are used, one is placed as proximal as possible and the second as distal as possible. If the instrumentation exceeds 30 cm in length, a third transverse cross-link connector should be considered. A high-speed drill is then used to decorticate the lateral aspects of the transverse processes, and bone graft material is laid along the lateral aspect of the instrumentation construct.

Closure of the wound is performed in a sequential fashion. The surgeon meticulously obtains hemostasis and carefully inspects for cerebral spinal fluid (CSF) leak. Bleeding is controlled with electrocautery, and CSF leak is primarily repaired using a 4-0 Nurolon suture and is covered with fibrin glue sealant. The wound is copiously irrigated with antibiotic irrigation. Two grams of vancomycin powder is rubbed into the muscle, fascia, and subcutaneous tissues in order to reduce postoperative infection rate [48, 49]. Typically, an epidural drain is left postoperatively to limit the buildup of epidural fluid. The aponeurosis of the paraspinal muscles is reapproximated with Vicryl suture. The skin is reapproximated with staples or a running Monocryl suture. A sterile dressing is applied. The patient is awoken from anesthesia and checked postoperatively for neurologic deficit.

Illustrative Case

History

A 66-year-old previously healthy male presented to the emergency department by ambulance after a skydiving accident. While approaching the ground after deploying his parachute, it malfunctioned around 20–30 feet in the air. He plummeted, landed on his feet, and collapsed to the ground. There was no loss of consciousness. He had back pain immediately after the fall. He was able to move his legs after the accident, but they were mildly weak. On his way to the hospital, he began feeling burning pain down both of his legs into the toes. He denied any bowel or bladder incontinence.

Physical Exam

Neurologic examination revealed point tenderness to his mid- and lower thoracic spine. He had 4+/5 strength in his lower extremities. He had 3+ patellar and Achilles reflexes without clonus. He had normal sensation. Lastly, he was noted to have urinary retention and needed intermittent catheterization.

Imaging

CT of the head and cervical, thoracic, and lumbar spine were ordered. CT of the thoracic spine was remarkable for T7 compression fracture and T12 burst fracture with retropulsion into the spinal canal (Fig. 17.7). MRI was performed to evaluate for spinal cord injury and ligamentous injury to the vertebral column. Short T1 inversion recovery (STIR) MRI revealed high signal intensity within the T7 and T12 vertebral bodies, posterior ligamentous injury at T12, and spinal cord injury at T12 from compression and ischemia caused by the burst fracture (Fig. 17.7). There were no other injuries found on clinical exam or radiographic analysis.

Treatment

Operative decision-making in thoracolumbar trauma is based off the thoracolumbar injury classification and severity core (TLICS). Injury is graded based on the morphology of the fracture, integrity of the posterior longitudinal ligament, and neurologic status. The following are the scores and management decision: 0–3 = nonoperative management, 4 = management based on surgeon choice, and greater than 4 = operative management [15]. The TLICS score for this patient is 7, indicating operative management.

The patient was selected to undergo a T5–L2 posterior thoracolumbar fusion with laminectomy at T12 (Fig. 17.8). The surgical correction was

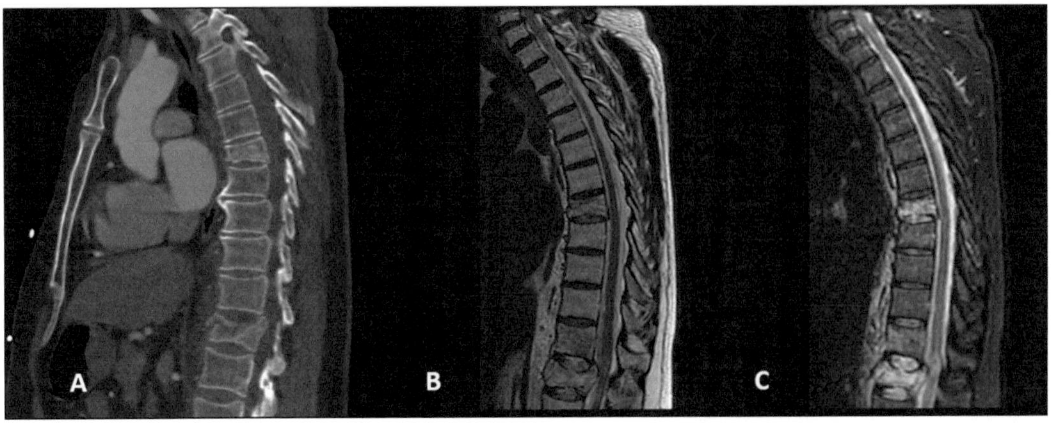

Fig. 17.7 Preoperative imaging. (**a**) Sagittal CT. (**b**) Sagittal T2 MRI. (**c**) Sagittal STIR MRI

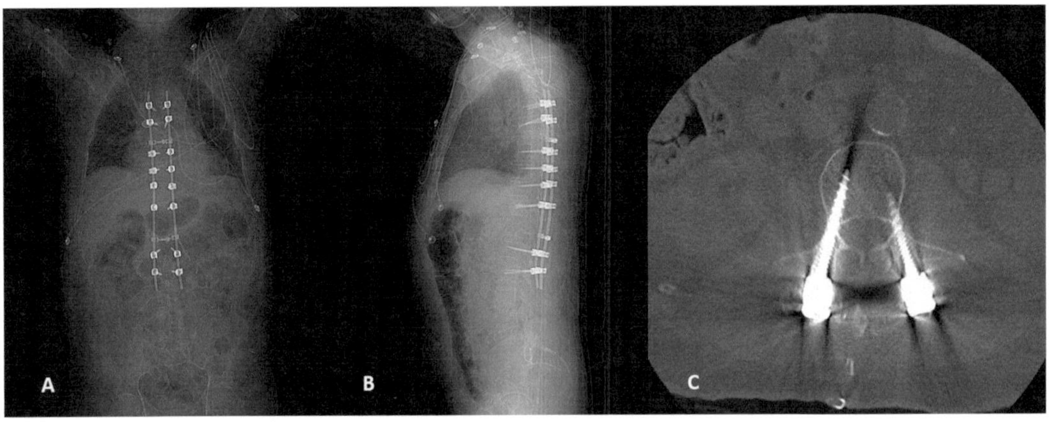

Fig. 17.8 Postoperative films. (**a**) AP standing X-ray. (**b**) Lateral standing X-ray. (**c**) Axial CT

based on the biomechanical considerations discussed previously. This patient suffered an axial loading injury causing a compression fracture at T7 and a burst fracture at T12. These injuries lead to axial loading instability in the sagittal plane. Posterior thoracic instrumentation with pedicle screws and rods counteract the axial loading instability by providing strength and rigidity to the posterior elements. In this case, the most unstable portion of the thoracic spine is at T12. Laminectomy was performed at this level to decompress the spinal cord from the retropulsed burst fracture fragments. At the thoracolumbar junction, there is greater motion than the other thoracic segments, and therefore instrumentation was carried down two levels to L2. The construct was extended past T7 because the patient has low-density bone for a male. Extending the instrumentation to T5 will help prevent further degeneration of the T7 compression fracture over time.

Outcome

The patient underwent surgical decompression and fusion without complication. He was followed up in a clinic at 1 month, 3 months, 6 months, and 1 year postoperatively. By his 6-month follow-up, his neurologic exam had returned to baseline, and he was ambulating well. By 1 year postoperatively, he had evidence of radiographic bony fusion from T5 to L2.

Technical Pearls

- Patient positioning that prevents abdominal tension greatly reduces blood loss during spinal surgery.
- The use of intraoperative fluoroscopy should be routinely used to confirm the spinal level before decompression and instrumentation.
- Careful preoperative measurement of the pedicle width and length should be performed prior to each posterior spinal fusion to help prevent nerve root, thecal sac, and aortic injury.
- The distance from the medial wall of the pedicle to the thecal sac is closest in the mid-thoracic region. Special care should be taken at these levels to prevent medial pedicle breach.
- Placement of pedicle screws before laminectomy utilizes the lamina as a safe guard for the possibility of pedicle screw instrumentation slippage.
- Understanding the biomechanics of the spine will help build solid fusion constructs that counteract destabilizing forces acting on the spine.
- Fusion should be considered across the cervical thoracic junction in cases of C7–T1 instability.
- Long segment fixation of the thoracic spine should incorporate the thoracolumbar junction through L5 or the sacrum to prevent adjacent segment kyphosis.
- Bracing after spine surgery is controversial. Patients with poor bone quality and factors that may affect bone fusion should have careful consideration for external orthosis postoperatively.
- Smoking cessation prior to spinal instrumentation improves arthrodesis rates.
- Preoperative antibiotics 30 min to 1 h prior to surgery are effective at reducing the incidence of surgical site infection.
- 1–2 grams of vancomycin powder applied before closure is helpful in reducing surgical site infection.

Complications and Strategies for Avoidance

Complications associated with posterior thoracic spinal instrumentation can be broken down into several main categories: (1) patient positioning, (2) thoracic spine exposure, (3) instrumentation, and (4) postoperative.

The surgical and anesthesia teams are responsible for proper and safe positioning of the patient prior to thoracic instrumentation. Detailed attention is paid to positioning of the neck and limbs in the prone position. The neck must be in a neutral position and the limbs properly padded to avoid injury to peripheral nerves. There are case reports of excessive neck rotation causing carotid artery occlusion and resultant stroke [50]. The shoulders need to be padded and placed in a neutral position to avoid brachial plexus injury. Padding must be placed under the arms at the elbow, iliac crests, and knees to prevent skin breakdown and pressure ulcer development.

Prone positioning has the risk of ocular complications. Postoperative visual deficits have been reported with an incidence as high as 0.1–0.2% [51]. The most common cause of postoperative visual deficit is ischemic optic neuropathy (ION). The major risk factors include prolonged intraoperative hypotension, postoperative anemia, and facial swelling. Avoiding or immediately correcting these risk factors greatly reduces the incidence of ION [52]. Visual deficit can also result from central retinal artery occlusion, isolated stroke, or embolic phenomenon. While ocular complications are rare, prevention of such complications in high-risk patients (e.g., patients with diabetes, hypertension, history of prior stroke or cases with long operative time) is achieved by reducing the central venous pressure [53, 54].

Safe thoracic exposure entails a comprehensive knowledge of the local anatomy and neurovascular structures within the region of dissection. During posterior thoracic exposure, the neural elements are at risk once the spinal canal is entered. Care must be taken to avoid plunging instruments into the spinal canal during exposure. This becomes especially true when the spine is flexed on the Wilson Frame, revision spine surgery, and trauma. Additionally, the correct level must be identified prior to exposure. In one study, 50% of spine surgeons admitted to performing a wrong-level surgery at least once during their career [55]. Wrong-level spine surgery can be avoided with careful preoperative planning and intraoperative localization utilizing fluoroscopy.

Pedicle screw placement places the nerve roots, thecal sac, spinal cord, and aorta at risk for injury. Preoperative imaging should be reviewed for any anatomic abnormalities that would increase the chance for neurologic injury and plans made to circumvent the abnormal anatomy. Intraoperatively, anatomic landmarks and image guidance, when available, should be used to ensure proper screw placement. Pedicle diameter and length are measured preoperatively to ensure correct screw diameter and length intraoperatively. Screws that are "long" and placed on the left side of the spine have the potential to injure the aorta because of its close proximity to the ventral vertebral body. Additionally, screws placed on the right side of the body have the potential to injure the superior intercostal vessels at T4–T5, esophagus at T4–T9, azygous vein at T5–T11, inferior vena cava at T11–T12, and thoracic duct at T4–T12. Techniques that check for medial and lateral breach during pedicle cannulation are essential. Medial and lateral pedicle screw breaches have the potential to injure the thecal sac and nerve root, respectively.

Many complications associated with instrumentation occur due to disruption of the interface between the bony tissue and pedicle screws. Wound infection rates have been shown to be higher in instrumented spine procedures compared to ones that are non-instrumented and lead to erosion of the bone around the pedicle screws [56]. Patients with osteoporosis often experience early fixation failure or pedicle screw pullout. Other conditions associated with hardware failure include steroid use, smoking, cancer, radiation therapy, and poor nutrition. Poor nutritional status in spinal instrumentation candidates should be reversed to improve surgical outcome [57]. Smoking cessation improves fusion outcomes [58].

The most common complication after spine surgery is postoperative wound infection. The incidence reported in the literature is quite variable and ranges from 0.5% to 15% [59–61]. This is likely due to variation in case complexity across the different studies examining spine infection rates. Infection can be prevented by use of prophylactic antibiotics [62]. The most effective prophylactic antibiotic agents are those that have action against the most common bacteria present in tissues adjacent to the surgical site. Cefazolin is commonly used at our institution. It is currently recommended that perioperative antibiotics be administered 30 min to 1 h preoperatively to ensure adequate levels at the surgical site at the time of skin incision [63, 64]. In addition to preoperative antibiotics, irrigation solutions are commonly used intraoperatively. Common irrigants include bacitracin, iodine, chlorhexidine, neomycin, and polymyxin. There is no clinical evidence that these irrigants reduce infection rates in spine surgery, but in vitro studies show a significant reduction in bacterial counts [65]. More recently, vancomycin powder has gained popularity for reducing surgical site infections. Typically 1–2 g is added generously to the wound upon closure. This is the typical practice at our institution. There is no class 1 evidence proving vancomycin powder effectiveness, but there are many retrospective and prospective studies that validate its everyday use in spinal instrumentation surgery [66–72].

Conclusion

Posterior thoracic spinal fixation is used to restore spinal stability when its mechanical functions are disrupted by trauma, tumor, infection, degenerative disease, deformity, or surgical management of these disorders. Achieving safe and optimal results requires a thorough knowledge of the anatomy and the biomechanical properties of the thoracic spine. Pedicle screw fixation has supplanted previous techniques because of its advantageous biomechanical properties and greater reduction power. Familiarity with the instrumentation techniques discussed in this chapter will help the surgeon minimize complications while enabling the treatment of a wide variety of spinal pathologies.

References

1. Whitesides TE Jr. Traumatic kyphosis of the thoracolumbar spine. Clin Orthop Relat Res. 1977;128:78–92.
2. An HS, Singh K, Vaccaro AR, Wang G, Yoshida H, Eck J, et al. Biomechanical evaluation of contemporary posterior spinal internal fixation configurations in an unstable burst-fracture calf spine model: special references of hook configurations and pedicle screws. Spine (Phila Pa 1976). 2004;29(3):257–62.
3. Hitchon PW, Brenton MD, Black AG, From A, Harrod JS, Barry C, et al. In vitro biomechanical comparison of pedicle screws, sublaminar hooks, and sublaminar cables. J Neurosurg. 2003;99(1 Suppl):104–9.
4. Karatoprak O, Unay K, Tezer M, Ozturk C, Aydogan M, Mirzanli C. Comparative analysis of pedicle screw versus hybrid instrumentation in adolescent idiopathic scoliosis surgery. Int Orthop. 2008;32(4):523–8. discussion 9
5. Gurr KR, McAfee PC, Shih CM. Biomechanical analysis of anterior and posterior instrumentation systems after corpectomy. A calf-spine model. J Bone Joint Surg Am. 1988;70(8):1182–91.
6. Gurr KR, McAfee PC, Shih CM. Biomechanical analysis of posterior instrumentation systems after decompressive laminectomy. An unstable calf-spine model. J Bone Joint Surg Am. 1988;70(5):680–91.
7. Lee SM, Suk SI, Chung ER. Direct vertebral rotation: a new technique of three-dimensional deformity correction with segmental pedicle screw fixation in adolescent idiopathic scoliosis. Spine (Phila Pa 1976). 2004;29(3):343–9.
8. Liljenqvist U, Hackenberg L, Link T, Halm H. Pullout strength of pedicle screws versus pedicle and laminar hooks in the thoracic spine. Acta Orthop Belg. 2001;67(2):157–63.
9. Rampersaud YR, Simon DA, Foley KT. Accuracy requirements for image-guided spinal pedicle screw placement. Spine (Phila Pa 1976). 2001;26(4):352–9.
10. Ebraheim NA, Jabaly G, Xu R, Yeasting RA. Anatomic relations of the thoracic pedicle to the adjacent neural structures. Spine (Phila Pa 1976). 1997;22(14):1553–6. discussion 7
11. Liljenqvist U, Hackenberg L. Morphometric analysis of thoracic and lumbar vertebrae in idiopathic scoliosis. Stud Health Technol Inform. 2002;88:382–6.
12. Vaccaro AR, Rizzolo SJ, Allardyce TJ, Ramsey M, Salvo J, Balderston RA, et al. Placement of pedicle screws in the thoracic spine. Part I: morphometric analysis of the thoracic vertebrae. J Bone Joint Surg Am. 1995;77(8):1193–9.
13. Vaccaro AR, Rizzolo SJ, Balderston RA, Allardyce TJ, Garfin SR, Dolinskas C, et al. Placement of pedicle screws in the thoracic spine. Part II: an anatomical and radiographic assessment. J Bone Joint Surg Am. 1995;77(8):1200–6.
14. Ebraheim NA, Xu R, Ahmad M, Yeasting RA. Projection of the thoracic pedicle and its morphometric analysis. Spine (Phila Pa 1976). 1997;22(3):233–8.
15. Vaccaro AR, Lehman RA Jr, Hurlbert RJ, Anderson PA, Harris M, Hedlund R, et al. A new classification of thoracolumbar injuries: the importance of injury morphology, the integrity of the posterior ligamentous complex, and neurologic status. Spine (Phila Pa 1976). 2005;30(20):2325–33.
16. Kalanithi PA, Arrigo R, Boakye M. Morbid obesity increases cost and complication rates in spinal arthrodesis. Spine (Phila Pa 1976). 2012;37(11):982–8.
17. Magee DJ. Orthopedic physical assessment. Philadelphia: Saunders; 2002.
18. Hoppenfeld SDP, Hutton R. Surgical exposures in Orthopaedics: the anatomic approach. 2nd ed. Philadelphia: JB Lippincott; 1994.
19. Kim DH. Surgical anatomy and techniques to the spine. Philadelphia: WB Saunders; 2006.
20. Whang PG, Vaccaro AR. Thoracolumbar fracture: posterior instrumentation using distraction and ligamentotaxis reduction. J Am Acad Orthop Surg. 2007;15(11):695–701.
21. White AAPM. Clinical biomechanics of the spine. 3rd ed. Philadelphia: JB Lippincott; 1990.
22. Xu R, Ebraheim NA, Shepherd ME, Yeasting RA. Thoracic pedicle screw placement guided by computed tomographic measurements. J Spinal Disord. 1999;12(3):222–6.
23. Sucato DJ, Duchene C. The position of the aorta relative to the spine: a comparison of patients with and without idiopathic scoliosis. J Bone Joint Surg Am. 2003;85-A(8):1461–9.
24. Charles YP, Barbe B, Beaujeux R, Boujan F, Steib JP. Relevance of the anatomical location of the Adamkiewicz artery in spine surgery. Surg Radiol Anat. 2011;33(1):3–9.
25. Watkins R, Watkins R 3rd, Williams L, Ahlbrand S, Garcia R, Karamanian A, et al. Stability provided by the sternum and rib cage in the thoracic spine. Spine (Phila Pa 1976). 2005;30(11):1283–6.
26. Takeuchi T, Abumi K, Shono Y, Oda I, Kaneda K. Biomechanical role of the intervertebral disc and costovertebral joint in stability of the thoracic spine. A canine model study. Spine (Phila Pa 1976). 1999;24(14):1414–20.
27. Orndorff DGZT. Rothman-Simeone the spine. 6th ed. Philadelphia: Elsevier; 2011.
28. Schonauer C, Bocchetti A, Barbagallo G, Albanese V, Moraci A. Positioning on surgical table. Eur Spine J. 2004;13(Suppl 1):S50–5.
29. Palmon SC, Kirsch JR, Depper JA, Toung TJ. The effect of the prone position on pulmonary mechanics is frame-dependent. Anesth Analg. 1998;87(5):1175–80.

30. Brewin J, Hill M, Ellis H. The prevalence of cervical ribs in a London population. Clin Anat. 2009;22(3):331–6.
31. Merks JH, Smets AM, Van Rijn RR, Kobes J, Caron HN, Maas M, et al. Prevalence of rib anomalies in normal Caucasian children and childhood cancer patients. Eur J Med Genet. 2005;48(2):113–29.
32. Scheufler KM, Franke J, Eckardt A, Dohmen H. Accuracy of image-guided pedicle screw placement using intraoperative computed tomography-based navigation with automated referencing, part I: cervicothoracic spine. Neurosurgery. 2011;69(4):782–95. discussion 95
33. Scheufler KM, Franke J, Eckardt A, Dohmen H. Accuracy of image-guided pedicle screw placement using intraoperative computed tomography-based navigation with automated referencing. Part II: thoracolumbar spine. Neurosurgery. 2011;69(6):1307–16.
34. Dinesh SK, Tiruchelvarayan R, Ng I. A prospective study on the use of intraoperative computed tomography (iCT) for image-guided placement of thoracic pedicle screws. Br J Neurosurg. 2012;26(6):838–44.
35. Lee CY, Wu MH, Li YY, Cheng CC, Hsu CH, Huang TJ, et al. Intraoperative computed tomography navigation for transpedicular screw fixation to treat unstable thoracic and lumbar spine fractures: clinical analysis of a case series (CARE-compliant). Medicine (Baltimore). 2015;94(20):e757.
36. Kim YJ, Lenke LG, Bridwell KH, Cho YS, Riew KD. Free hand pedicle screw placement in the thoracic spine: is it safe? Spine (Phila Pa 1976). 2004;29(3):333–42. discussion 42
37. Raynor BL, Lenke LG, Kim Y, Hanson DS, Wilson-Holden TJ, Bridwell KH, et al. Can triggered electromyograph thresholds predict safe thoracic pedicle screw placement? Spine (Phila Pa 1976). 2002;27(18):2030–5.
38. Hackenberg L, Link T, Liljenqvist U. Axial and tangential fixation strength of pedicle screws versus hooks in the thoracic spine in relation to bone mineral density. Spine (Phila Pa 1976). 2002;27(9):937–42.
39. Halvorson TL, Kelley LA, Thomas KA, Whitecloud TS 3rd, Cook SD. Effects of bone mineral density on pedicle screw fixation. Spine (Phila Pa 1976). 1994;19(21):2415–20.
40. Soshi S, Shiba R, Kondo H, Murota K. An experimental study on transpedicular screw fixation in relation to osteoporosis of the lumbar spine. Spine (Phila Pa 1976). 1991;16(11):1335–41.
41. Zindrick MR, Wiltse LL, Widell EH, Thomas JC, Holland WR, Field BT, et al. A biomechanical study of intrapeduncular screw fixation in the lumbosacral spine. Clin Orthop Relat Res. 1986;203:99–112.
42. Sarzier JS, Evans AJ, Cahill DW. Increased pedicle screw pullout strength with vertebroplasty augmentation in osteoporotic spines. J Neurosurg. 2002;96(3 Suppl):309–12.
43. Frankel BM, D'Agostino S, Wang C. A biomechanical cadaveric analysis of polymethylmethacrylate-augmented pedicle screw fixation. J Neurosurg Spine. 2007;7(1):47–53.
44. Dick JC, Zdeblick TA, Bartel BD, Kunz DN. Mechanical evaluation of cross-link designs in rigid pedicle screw systems. Spine (Phila Pa 1976). 1997;22(4):370–5.
45. Dick JC, Jones MP, Zdeblick TA, Kunz DN, Horton WC. A biomechanical comparison evaluating the use of intermediate screws and cross-linkage in lumbar pedicle fixation. J Spinal Disord. 1994;7(5):402–7.
46. Johnston CE 2nd, Ashman RB, Baird AM, Allard RN. Effect of spinal construct stiffness on early fusion mass incorporation. Experimental study Spine (Phila Pa 1976). 1990;15(9):908–12.
47. Lynn G, Mukherjee DP, Kruse RN, Sadasivan KK, Albright JA. Mechanical stability of thoracolumbar pedicle screw fixation. The effect of crosslinks. Spine (Phila Pa 1976). 1997;22(14):1568–72. discussion 73
48. Schroeder JE, Girardi FP, Sandhu H, Weinstein J, Cammisa FP, Sama A. The use of local vancomycin powder in degenerative spine surgery. Eur Spine J. 2016;25(4):1029–33.
49. Bakhsheshian J, Dahdaleh NS, Lam SK, Savage JW, Smith ZA. The use of vancomycin powder in modern spine surgery: systematic review and meta-analysis of the clinical evidence. World Neurosurg. 2015;83(5):816–23.
50. Wang LC, Liou JT, Liu FC, Hsu JC, Lui PW. Fatal ischemia stroke in a patient with an asymptomatic carotid artery occlusion after lumbar spine surgery--a case report. Acta Anaesthesiol Taiwanica. 2004;42(3):179–82.
51. Chang SH, Miller NR. The incidence of vision loss due to perioperative ischemic optic neuropathy associated with spine surgery: the Johns Hopkins Hospital experience. Spine (Phila Pa 1976). 2005;30(11):1299–302.
52. Dunker S, Hsu HY, Sebag J, Sadun AA. Perioperative risk factors for posterior ischemic optic neuropathy. J Am Coll Surg. 2002;194(6):705–10.
53. American Society of Anesthesiologists Task Force on Perioperative B. Practice advisory for perioperative visual loss associated with spine surgery: a report by the American Society of Anesthesiologists Task Force on perioperative blindness. Anesthesiology. 2006;104(6):1319–28.
54. American Society of Anesthesiologists Task Force on Perioperative Visual L. Practice advisory for perioperative visual loss associated with spine surgery: an updated report by the American Society of Anesthesiologists Task Force on perioperative visual loss. Anesthesiology. 2012;116(2):274–85.
55. Upadhyaya CD, Wu JC, Chin CT, Balamurali G, Mummaneni PV. Avoidance of wrong-level thoracic spine surgery: intraoperative localization with preoperative percutaneous fiducial screw placement. J Neurosurg Spine. 2012;16(3):280–4.
56. Weinstein MA, McCabe JP, Cammisa FP Jr. Postoperative spinal wound infection: a review of

2,391 consecutive index procedures. J Spinal Disord. 2000;13(5):422–6.
57. Klein JD, Hey LA, Yu CS, Klein BB, Coufal FJ, Young EP, et al. Perioperative nutrition and postoperative complications in patients undergoing spinal surgery. Spine (Phila Pa 1976). 1996;21(22):2676–82.
58. Glassman SD, Anagnost SC, Parker A, Burke D, Johnson JR, Dimar JR. The effect of cigarette smoking and smoking cessation on spinal fusion. Spine (Phila Pa 1976). 2000;25(20):2608–15.
59. El-Gindi S, Aref S, Salama M, Andrew J. Infection of intervertebral discs after operation. J Bone Joint Surg Br. 1976;58(1):114–6.
60. Rechtine GR, Bono PL, Cahill D, Bolesta MJ, Chrin AM. Postoperative wound infection after instrumentation of thoracic and lumbar fractures. J Orthop Trauma. 2001;15(8):566–9.
61. Fernandez-Sousa JM, Gavilanes JG, Municio AM, Paredes JA, Perez-Aranda A, Rodriguez R. Primary structure of cytochrome c from the insect *Ceratitis capitata*. Biochim Biophys Acta. 1975;393(2):358–67.
62. Savitz MH, Malis LI, Savitz SI. Efficacy of prophylactic antibiotic therapy in spinal surgery: a meta-analysis. Neurosurgery. 2003;53(1):243–4. author reply 4-5
63. Swoboda SM, Merz C, Kostuik J, Trentler B, Lipsett PA. Does intraoperative blood loss affect antibiotic serum and tissue concentrations? Arch Surg. 1996;131(11):1165–71. discussion 71-2
64. Polly DW Jr, Meter JJ, Brueckner R, Asplund L, van Dam BE. The effect of intraoperative blood loss on serum cefazolin level in patients undergoing instrumented spinal fusion. A prospective, controlled study. Spine (Phila Pa 1976). 1996;21(20):2363–7.
65. Rosenstein BD, Wilson FC, Funderburk CH. The use of bacitracin irrigation to prevent infection in postoperative skeletal wounds. An experimental study. J Bone Joint Surg Am. 1989;71(3):427–30.
66. Caroom C, Tullar JM, Benton EG Jr, Jones JR, Chaput CD. Intrawound vancomycin powder reduces surgical site infections in posterior cervical fusion. Spine (Phila Pa 1976). 2013;38(14):1183–7.
67. Heller A, McIff TE, Lai SM, Burton DC. Intrawound Vancomycin powder decreases staphylococcal surgical site infections after posterior instrumented spinal arthrodesis. J Spinal Disord Tech. 2015;28(10):E584–9.
68. Martin JR, Adogwa O, Brown CR, Bagley CA, Richardson WJ, Lad SP, et al. Experience with intrawound vancomycin powder for spinal deformity surgery. Spine (Phila Pa 1976). 2014;39(2):177–84.
69. O'Neill KR, Smith JG, Abtahi AM, Archer KR, Spengler DM, McGirt MJ, et al. Reduced surgical site infections in patients undergoing posterior spinal stabilization of traumatic injuries using vancomycin powder. Spine J. 2011;11(7):641–6.
70. Strom RG, Pacione D, Kalhorn SP, Frempong-Boadu AK. Lumbar laminectomy and fusion with routine local application of vancomycin powder: decreased infection rate in instrumented and non-instrumented cases. Clin Neurol Neurosurg. 2013;115(9):1766–9.
71. Strom RG, Pacione D, Kalhorn SP, Frempong-Boadu AK. Decreased risk of wound infection after posterior cervical fusion with routine local application of vancomycin powder. Spine (Phila Pa 1976). 2013;38(12):991–4.
72. Evaniew N, Khan M, Drew B, Peterson D, Bhandari M, Ghert M. Intrawound vancomycin to prevent infections after spine surgery: a systematic review and meta-analysis. Eur Spine J. 2015;24(3):533–42.

Anterior Spinal Column Augmentation Techniques

18

Ian K. White, Eric Potts, and Jean-Pierre Mobasser

Introduction

Vertebral fractures are a major source of morbidity in the United States in terms of pain, work days lost to patients and families, and dollars spent on medical treatment. Osteoporosis accounts for the majority of these fractures (85%), with high-impact trauma (12%) and pathologic fractures (3%) accounting for a much lower cohort [1]. The incidence of osteoporotic-related spine fracture in the United States is 117 per 100,000 life years with the number approaching 2.1 million in 2016. This is not surprising with the aging population and 10 million Americans (8 million women/2 million men) meeting the criteria for osteoporosis.

Vertebral compression fractures (VCF) are the most common fragility fractures followed by the hip, wrist, and ankle. Although commonly thought to have a benign course, osteoporotic fractures are associated with significant morbidity and increased mortality and costs. Once an individual suffers a compression fracture, it increases the patient's risk of sustaining a second fracture by 5–10 times [2].

Traditionally, nonoperative medical management including lifestyle changes (smoking cessation, diet, supplements), medications (anti-resorptive and anabolic), pain control, and bracing has served as the standard of care. Despite treatment, many patients have debilitating residual pain, functional limitations, and decreased independence. Open surgery is associated with high rates of adverse events in this population due to poor fixation and further fracture especially at adjacent segments and from medical comorbidities.

Neoplasm commonly affects the spine in more than one-third of cancer patients and is the presenting symptom in 10–15%. Metastatic disease from breast, lung, and prostate cancer accounts for 60–65% of these cases. In addition, multiple myeloma commonly presents with severe osteoporosis and spinal fracture. The mechanism of bone loss is due to osteoclastic activation and resorption of bone architecture that predisposes patients to fractures resulting in pain, neurologic deficits, and progressive spinal deformity that have a severe impact on their quality of life.

Limitations in effective management of VCFs in these patients have led to the development of percutaneous vertebral augmentation. These techniques include vertebroplasty and kyphoplasty.

I.K. White, MD (✉) • E. Potts, MD
J.-P. Mobasser, MD
Goodman Campbell Brain and Spine, Department of Neurological Surgery, Indiana University School of Medicine, 355 W. 16th Street, Suite 5100, Indianapolis, IN 46202, USA
e-mail: ian.k.white33@gmail.com; epotts@goodmancampbell.com; jmobasser@goodmancampbell.com

L.T. Holly, P.A. Anderson (eds.), *Essentials of Spinal Stabilization*,
DOI 10.1007/978-3-319-59713-3_18

In both techniques, polymethylmethacrylate (PMMA) is placed percutaneously into the vertebral body, although other materials are being investigated. Vertebral augmentation provides rapid improvement in pain with some restoration in vertebral body height and prevention of progressive deformity. In addition, surgeons have begun to use cement augmentation to improve pedicle screw fixation. In this chapter, we explore the indications and techniques for vertebroplasty and kyphoplasty along with the growing use of PMMA in open surgery.

History

Galibert performed the first vertebroplasty in France in 1984 where PMMA was used to treat a painful hemangioma of the C2 vertebra [3, 4]. One year later, vertebroplasty was used to treat a compression fracture in an osteoporotic patient, and, subsequently, the first North American vertebroplasty was performed at the University of Virginia in 1993. Balloon assistance to create a cavity and expand the vertebral body, termed kyphoplasty, was first reported in 1998, and its use became widespread [5–10]. In 2003, in a randomized controlled trial, Diamond et al. demonstrated the efficacy of vertebroplasty in providing rapid and effective pain control after osteoporotic compression fractures [11]. Since then, there have been many uses for PMMA that are reviewed later in this chapter.

Patient Evaluation and Indications

Patient Selection

The majority of patients sustaining a compression fracture from trauma or osteoporotic/pathologic etiologies benefit from a trial of nonoperative treatment. However, a detailed neurological examination must first occur to guide the patient's post-injury course. Most often, compression fractures are first identified on plain radiographs or CT. If not already available, three-dimensional imaging is used to evaluate the posterior body wall and estimate stability. CT may also be used to estimate bone mineral density using x-ray attenuation, Hounsfield units (HU). Schreiber has shown that patients having spinal HU greater than 140 have normal bone mineral density (BMD), those between 100 and 130 are osteopenic, and those less than 100 are likely osteoporotic [12]. Patients with neurologic deficits require MRI for a more thorough evaluation of the soft tissue and neuro-elements. MRI is useful to determine the age of a fracture, and it is always indicated when it is believed that spinal metastasis is the etiology of the fracture. If the fracture has occurred with low-energy mechanism, a dual-energy x-ray absorptiometry (DEXA) scan should also be considered to evaluate patient's future risk of fracture.

Most patients with vertebral compression fractures should initially be treated nonoperatively. Patients who have intractable pain and are unable to mobilize should be considered for operative intervention. Pain is poorly controlled in 20–30% of osteoporotic and metastatic fractures [13, 14]. Radiotherapy oftentimes can help the lytic pain due to spinal metastasis-related fractures, but can take 1 month to have any pain-related benefits and 2–6 months to show any bony reinforcement, subjecting patients to high risk of further instability during this time period.

The ideal candidate for vertebral augmentation is a patient with intractable pain localized to an acute fracture level that has an intact posterior cortex, who is neurologically intact after the fracture, and who has failed conservative management. Relative contraindications to treatment include vertebra plana, comminuted burst fracture, spinal canal compromise greater than 20%, epidural tumor extension, myelopathy, and coagulopathy.

Tumor and Metastatic Disease

Spinal metastasis is involved in over two-thirds of patients who die of metastatic disease. These bone lesions are in themselves very painful and oftentimes result in vertebral body fractures in 10–20% of cases. The most common sites of disease are the thoracic vertebrae (60–80%), followed by the lumbar (20%) and cervical (10%) spine [15].

Spinal metastasis is a painful process involving intrinsic pain to the vertebra through bony erosion and propensity toward fracture. Many of these patients have multiple metastases and will need to undergo chemotherapy and radiation which would be delayed from open surgery due to wound healing issues. Still, these patients live with substantial pain, oftentimes for the remainder of their lives. Vertebral column augmentation has been shown to provide quick relief in these patients without delaying their primary cancer treatments [16]. It can provide palliative relief in a variety of tumor and fracture patterns. The mechanism of pain relief is believed to be from stabilization of the fractures and through thermochemical ablation of pain fibers in the bone through the exothermic chemical reaction of PMMA.

Classically, vertebroplasty was indicated for neoplastic disease in patients having single-level compression fractures, without posterior wall compromise and without [1]epidural compression. These indications have recently been challenged. Liu and colleagues described 104 spinal levels in 28 patients all treated with VP and all in single operations. Patient pain levels were decreased prior to pre-op and maintained these levels as well as vertebral body height for 12 months [15]. Cianfoni treated patients with posterior wall erosion and epidural invasion, showing low clinically significant, perioperative adverse events with good pain relief scores [17]. They did recommend that the technique requires careful attention to detail in these high-risk patients. Although less common, cervical cement augmentation has been shown to be an option if no open procedure is available [18]. These procedures can also be performed in the setting of multiple myeloma-related fractures. Due to the diversity of cancer-related pain and expanding indications for these procedures, vertebral augmentation is an essential part of the spine surgeon's armamentarium.

An Adjunct to Open Surgery

Recently PMMA along with other biologics cements such as calcium phosphate and calcium sulfate has been used to augment fixation in open surgery [33, 34]. In addition, screw modifications to improve fixation have been developed including expandable and hydroxyapatite-coated screws. In biomechanical models of osteoporosis, both expandable and hydroxyapatite-coated screws show greater pullout resistance when further augmented with PMMA [19, 20]. Pullout strength was noted to be 1.5 times that of equivalent segments in one study [21]. Screw pullout strength was the only parameter tested, and more complex torsional and directional forces still need to be evaluated. Some studies suggest a greater amount of bone cement to a point of increasing screw pullout strength, and it has been suggested that pretreating with kyphoplasty provides the best pullout strength with reduced toggle [21]. The differing screw augmentation techniques are shown in Fig. 18.1. Interestingly, augmented pedicle screws can be removed if revision is necessary without catastrophic damage to the vertebral body or pedicle.

One strategy for providing screw PMMA augmentation is the cannulated and fenestrated pedicle screw. A number of modifications of the fenestrated screw are available, but no known differences in efficacy have been established. This screw allows pedicle screw placement and then vertebroplasty to be performed through the screw fenestrations using a fitted cannulated plungerFenestrated pedicle screw technique (Fig. 18.2). The PMMA is injected into the body as the fenestrations are near the tip, and this can be performed minimally invasively or through an open incision. All screws should be tapped. Prefilling the tapped holes may provide an additional benefit in resistance to toggle and pullout strength [19, 20, 22]. This technique appears safe as Klingler reported 157 cannulated and fenestrated pedicle screws placed in this manner had no cement- or vascular-related complications [19, 20, 22].

Another indication for vertebral augmentation is the treatment of burst fractures in a combined

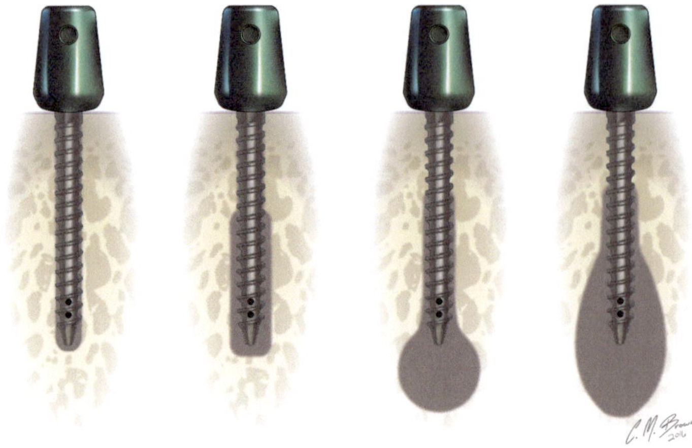

Fig. 18.1 Elder and colleagues described the pullout strength using different strategies for cement augmentation in fenestrated screws [21]. From *left* to *right*: no augmentation, cement down the pedicle track, cement through the screw fenestrations, vertebroplasty with cement down the pedicle and in the vertebral body, and kyphoplasty augmentation with cement down the pedicle and in the vertebral body

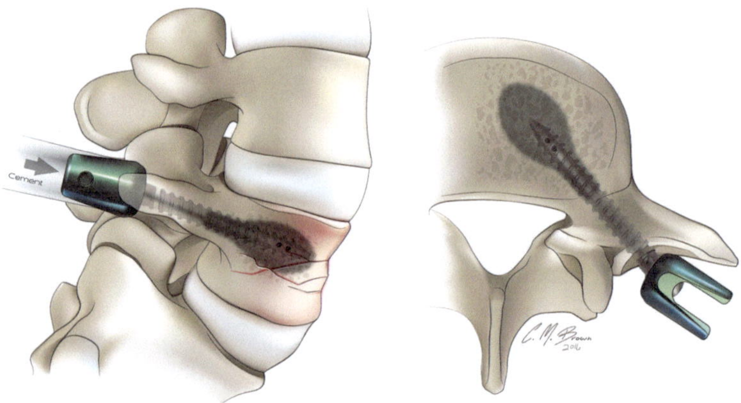

Fig. 18.2 Fenestrated pedicle screw technique with fenestrations at the tip of the screw similar to that seen in Fig. 18.1. Once the screw is inserted in the standard technique, a cannula is inserted through the screw to the end, and a plunger pushes the cement out the fenestrations into the anterior aspect of the vertebral body

open procedure. Posterior fixation with pedicle screws can improve lordosis and sometimes indirectly reduce the retropulsed fragment but often will not correct the vertebral collapse and wedging. Balloon-assisted end plate reduction restores vertebral body height and provides for better anterior column support. Oner and colleagues reported 20 consecutive patients treated by posterior pedicle screw fixation and balloon-assisted reduction of the vertebral body and PMMA augmentation. Reduction of kyphosis from 11 degrees to 1.6 and an average vertebral body height restoration from 66% to 81% occurred. This correction was maintained over a 17-month period. No patients experienced clinically related extravasation complications [23].

Timing

The timing of vertebral augmentation is controversial. The majority of compression fractures improve with time, thus making the role of immediate intervention contraindicated in most patients [32]. Some authors advocate time periods ranging from 6 weeks to 1 year [24–26].

There does seem to be a trend toward early intervention showing that patients treated less than 7 weeks after their fracture event do better from a pain standpoint than those treated later [27]. Patients who are hospitalized for pain control do benefit from early vertebral augmentation. This results in shortened hospitalization, fewer readmissions, and lower overall costs [28].

Preoperative Considerations

When planning the procedure, the following factors must be taken into account: the size of the vertebral body, the size of the pedicle, if transpedicular or parapedicular approaches will be used, if KP or VP is desired, and if unilateral or bilateral needle placement is the chosen technique. A wide vertebral body with a severe compression deformity and wide pedicles may dictate a bilateral approach to restore height and ensure there is enough volume of PMMA to reach both sides equally. However, in the smaller vertebral body where fracture height restoration is of less interest, a unilateral approach may be sufficient.

Two pedicle approaches are used. Transpedicular is used whenever possible dictated by pedicle diameter. In patients with diameters <4 mm, a parapedicular approach may be used. In this technique, the cannula enters the bone, exits along the lateral edge of the pedicle, and reenters the vertebral body. This is possible in the thoracic spine where the rib shields any neurovascular structure. Pedicles in the high to mid-thoracic spine may be small and severely angled making the parapedicular approach the more viable option. The differing trajectories for transpedicular and parapedicular are shown in Fig. 18.3. Vertebroplasty at our institution is almost always performed from a unilateral approach. Preoperative trajectories should avoid the neuroforamina starting high on the pedicle with a slightly inferior and medial trajectory, planning length, and angles of approach.

Due to longer procedural time, at our institution, kyphoplasty is reserved to single-level deformity or disease in younger patients where the level of deformity is believed to cause progression of deformity in the future and where fracture reduction is believed to have a reasonable chance of being accomplished. Vertebroplasty is done over multiple levels due to its speed in older patients where the goal is pain control and maintaining fracture stability without reduction.

Surgical Technique

Vertebroplasty

This procedure is performed under conscious sedation or general anesthesia and should be done in a facility with spine surgery capabilities. Biplanar fluoroscopy is essential and can be done either in the interventional suite or the operating room. It can be done with single C-arm alternating between lateral and AP pictures or by using

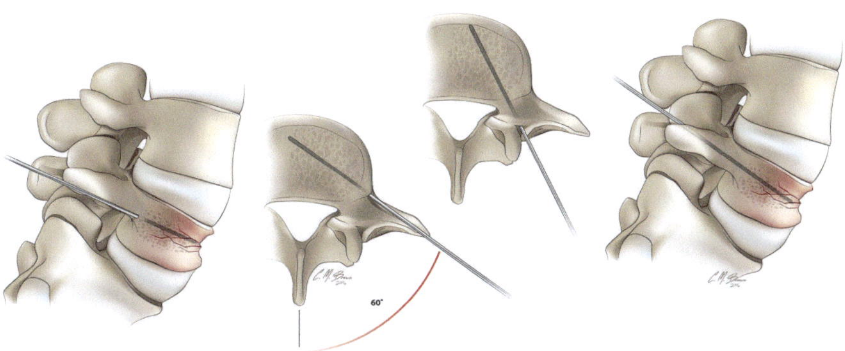

Fig. 18.3 Trajectories showing parapedicular and transpedicular approaches

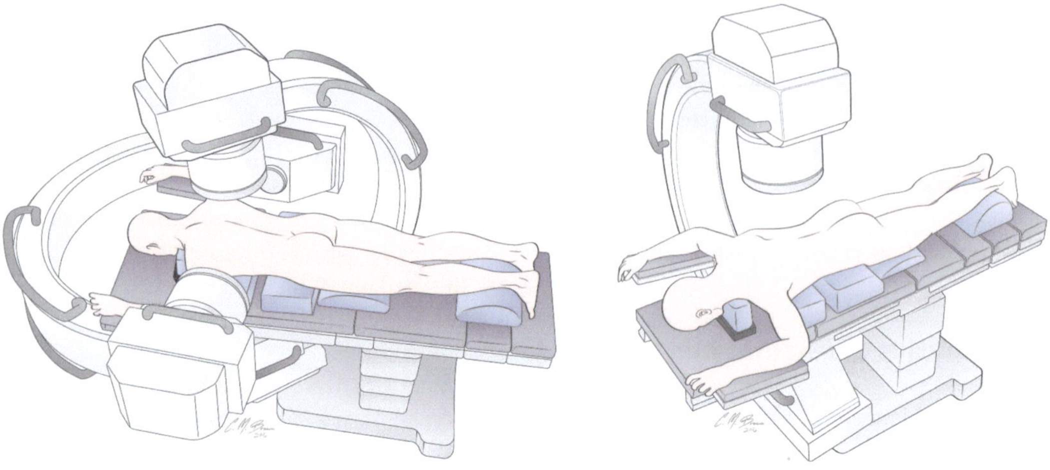

Fig. 18.4 Showing patient positioning with standard C-arm positioning and two C-arms allowing for biplanar fluoroscopy. This same setup can be done in the interventional suite

dual arms which speed the procedure, especially when treating multiple levels.

The patient is positioned prone on a radiolucent operating table, and the face and pressure points are padded as well as the elbows and axilla to prevent brachial plexus and ulnar injuries (Fig. 18.4). We have not found a Foley catheter necessary. Although general anesthesia is not necessary, trained personnel should administer the conscious sedation, and vital signs should be continually monitored. The patient is then prepped and draped sterilely.

Based on preoperative images, the parapedicular or transpedicular approach is selected. The level of interest is then localized using fluoroscopy, placing the initial mark on the skin just lateral to the superior lateral border of the pedicle of interest on the AP image when using transpedicular trajectory (Fig. 18.5). When using the parapedicular trajectory, the skin incision should be made 7–11 cm off of midline to allow for a more medial trajectory. The cranial/caudal trajectory should be the same as transpedicular. The skin is injected with 1% lidocaine with 1:200,000 epinephrine or 0.5% Marcaine with 1:200,000 epinephrine down to the pedicle making sure to inject the periosteum. A 2 mm incision is then made either with an 11 blade or 15 blade knife and a No. 11 Jamshidi biopsy needle with trocar in place. Fluoroscopy can be used to plan the ideal trajectory. If using the transpedicular approach, the needle is advanced to the bone and located at the superior lateral aspect of the pedicle. Alternating between AP and lateral views, the course of the needle should follow the trajectory of the pedicle with slight triangulation ending up in the anterior half of the vertebral body. The needle should be advanced in 1–2 mm increments. When using the transpedicular approach, this is usually done bilaterally as the PMMA has difficulty reaching the contralateral aspect of the body.

When using the parapedicular approach, the cannula is initially located on the transverse process. The junction of the transverse process and the facet is felt, and the Jamshidi needle is walked inferiorly until it falls off the inferior edge of the transverse process. The entry point is at the lateral vertebral body, immediately caudal to the transverse process, and at the lateral junction of the pedicle on the AP fluoroscopy. From this entry point, the goal is to reach the middle of the body on the AP while reaching the anterior half of the vertebral body. It should be noted that the parapedicular approach theoretically increases the patient's risk for pneumothorax in thoracic cases. The location of the needle for unilateral approaches is important as the amount of cement able to be infused into the body is proportional up to a point in pain reduction, and poor needle

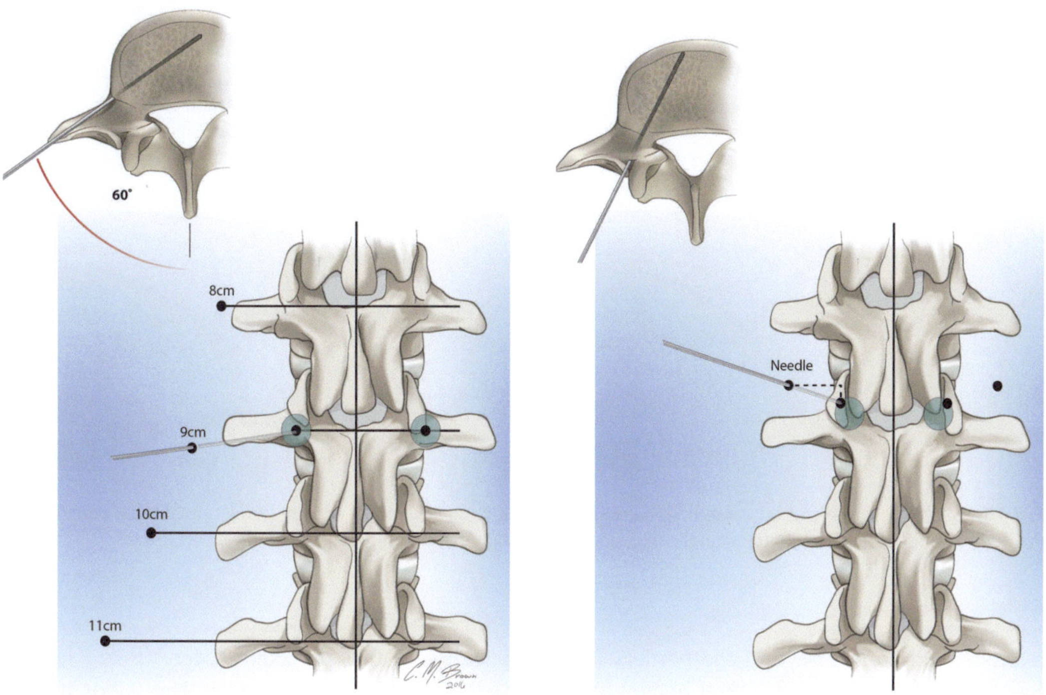

Fig. 18.5 Choosing entry point on transpedicular and parapedicular trajectories on the AP radiograph. Notice the lateral starting point approximately 7–11 cm off of midline at the level of the pedicle for the parapedicular, whereas the transpedicular is 1 cm off the superolateral border of the pedicle of interest

placement can reduce the amount of cement that is able to be symmetrically injected [27].

The surgeon should practice safety from excessive radiation by using a clamp or lead gloves to shield their hands. If multiple levels are going to be done, it is preferred to place all needles before cement injections. It used to be common practice before cement injection to inject a small amount of contrast to visualize the venous channels present; however, this practice has not been proven to have clinical utility [29]. Before injecting the bone cement, the operator should check the needle to make sure it is deemed to be in a suitable position. If the needle position is deemed to be non-ideal, there is the option of either replacing the needle or a curved inner cannula can be used to deliver bone cement throughout the entirety of the vertebral body.

There are several cement products on the market with differing properties; however, for the majority of cases, PMMA is the bone cement of choice. In commercial kits, it comes as two parts (a methyl-methacrylate polymer powder and a liquid monomer), and, once mixing occurs, the components begin polymerization. A radio-dense material such as barium is added to aid visualization. The PMMA is mixed for 3–5 min until it is the consistency of hair conditioner and loaded into a 10 cc syringe. The cement for vertebroplasty is slightly less thick than that for kyphoplasty, which is more similar to the consistency of toothpaste. During the hardening process, PMMA undergoes an exothermic reaction which may be responsible for some of the pain relief experienced from the procedure. After the cement is deemed to be at the appropriate consistency, the injection tool is connected to the needle. There are a number of devices now available, but generally they are threaded through the needle and have an attachment at the base for the needle and for the syringe. The cement is then injected under steady pressure. In the lumbar spine, usually 5–10 cc can be injected safely with decreasing amounts for severe fracture patterns and fractures higher in the thoracic spine. During injection, care must be taken not to let cement

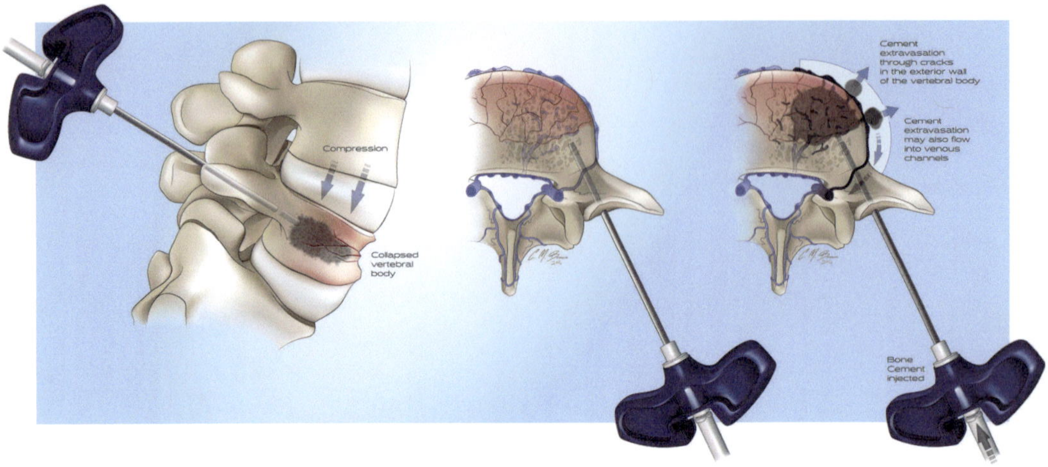

Fig. 18.6 After needle is placed, complications can arise with extravasation of cement into large draining veins, along the body into the foramen, into the spinal canal, and out the fracture site into the paravertebral soft tissues

extravasation course beyond the borders of the body. Anteroposterior and lateral images should be taken to assess that the cement remains within the borders of the body. The spinal canal should be critically evaluated as cement extrusion into the spinal canals should be avoided. Complications related to extravasation are shown in Fig. 18.6.

After the cement is injected and the surgeon satisfied with the amount injected and the fluoroscopic picture, the injection device is removed, and the inner cannula of the Jamshidi needle replaced. This needs to be maintained until the cement has completely hardened as polymerization causes volume expansion of the PMMA which can back up into the needle. After the PMMA is hardened, the Jamshidi needle is removed by twisting motion, and each incision can be closed with a monofilament suture. The patient should be kept supine for 1–2 h post-op and then discharged home after meeting discharge criteria. Neurological examination should be performed before discharge.

Kyphoplasty

Kyphoplasty is a procedure similar to vertebroplasty with the exception that an inflatable balloon tamp is inserted into the vertebral body. The benefits of this procedure over VP are largely radiographic and theoretical. The major benefit is some height restoration to acute fractures and decreased extravasation of cement due to lower injection pressures and compacted bone around the cavity which was created [30, 31]. Kyphoplasty has been shown to have greater volumes of cement injected per level, better short-term pain relief, and better short- and long-term kyphosis angles. Long-term clinical outcomes in terms of pain at 1 year are similar [30, 31]. The downside of kyphoplasty is the longer operative times often necessitating general anesthesia. Recently, the Kyphon device has come “off patent” making the procedure more affordable since generic devices have entered the market reducing costs. Kyphoplasty is often performed bilaterally as this allows for maximal height restoration. In our experience, end plate restoration is more likely to occur in the acute period before fractures organize into the chronic phase.

In kyphoplasty, docking of the needle tends to be done in a similar fashion to vertebroplasty done by the bipedicular approach (Fig. 18.7). The kyphoplasty needle should have a mildly triangulated trajectory and lie in the posterior half of the vertebral body. The stylet is moved, and a hand drill is used to create a pathway for the balloon. The drill should be stopped 3–6 mm from the

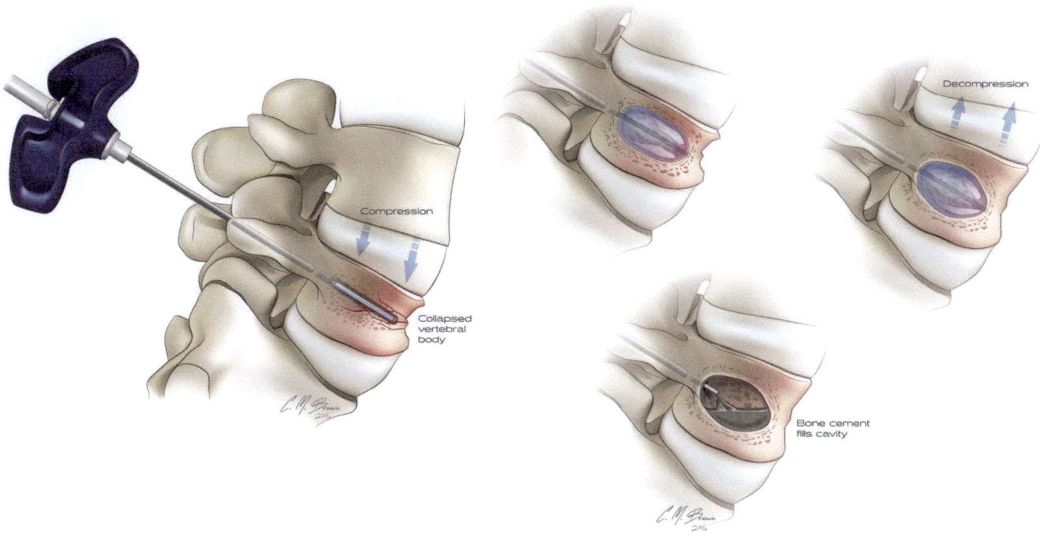

Fig. 18.7 Balloon-assisted kyphoplasty showing restoration of vertebral body height with packing out of cancellous bone to create cavity and filling with cement under low pressure

most posterior aspect of the anterior cortex of the body, and, at this point, the drill tip should approximate the midline. The drill is then removed, and the balloon tamp is inserted. The markings on the balloon tamp are on the posterior aspect of the balloon, and these markings should be at least 5 mm from the tip of the cannula. The tip of the tamp should not be less than 5 mm from the anterior aspect of the vertebral body to assure that inflation will not be inside the cortical bone.

Once the operator is satisfied with the balloon position, balloons are inflated with contrast under fluoroscopy and with continuous pressure monitoring. It is important to make sure that balloon tamps do not violate the cortical bone on any surface as this will increase the risk of cement extravasation. The balloons should not be inflated to more than 220 psi, which is the maximum recommended pressure. From our experience, staggering the balloon inflation helps delineate the level of inflation of each balloon as the contrast can obscure visualization if one is fully inflated on the lateral imaging. This also aids in symmetric fracture reduction. Once satisfactory inflation is achieved, balloons are deflated and removed. In the event that the fracture displaces after the balloons are deflated, there is the option to keep one inflated for the injection of the cement. Small cannulas containing PMMA at the consistency of toothpaste are inserted. It should be noted that this is thicker than the consistency of PMMA used for vertebroplasty. These are injected by hand, taking care to watch for extravasation. Typically cement is injected in small increments bilaterally to allow for better visualization and less fluoroscopy time. Once the surgeon is satisfied with the final images and cement has hardened, the trocars are removed, and the incisions can be closed with monofilament suture. Postoperative imaging can be left to the surgeon's discretion, but oftentimes the patient can be discharged the same day.

Kiva

The Kiva implant is a polyetheretherketone (PEEK-Optima) coil deployment system that allows fracture reduction in a controlled manner over a removable Nitinol Osteo guidewire. As the implant is deployed, the coil stacks upon itself adding substance to the body while reducing the fractured end plate. Once the coil is completely deployed, it forms a hollow cylinder ideally with its borders from end plate to end plate. PMMA is injected after the device is deployed to fill the

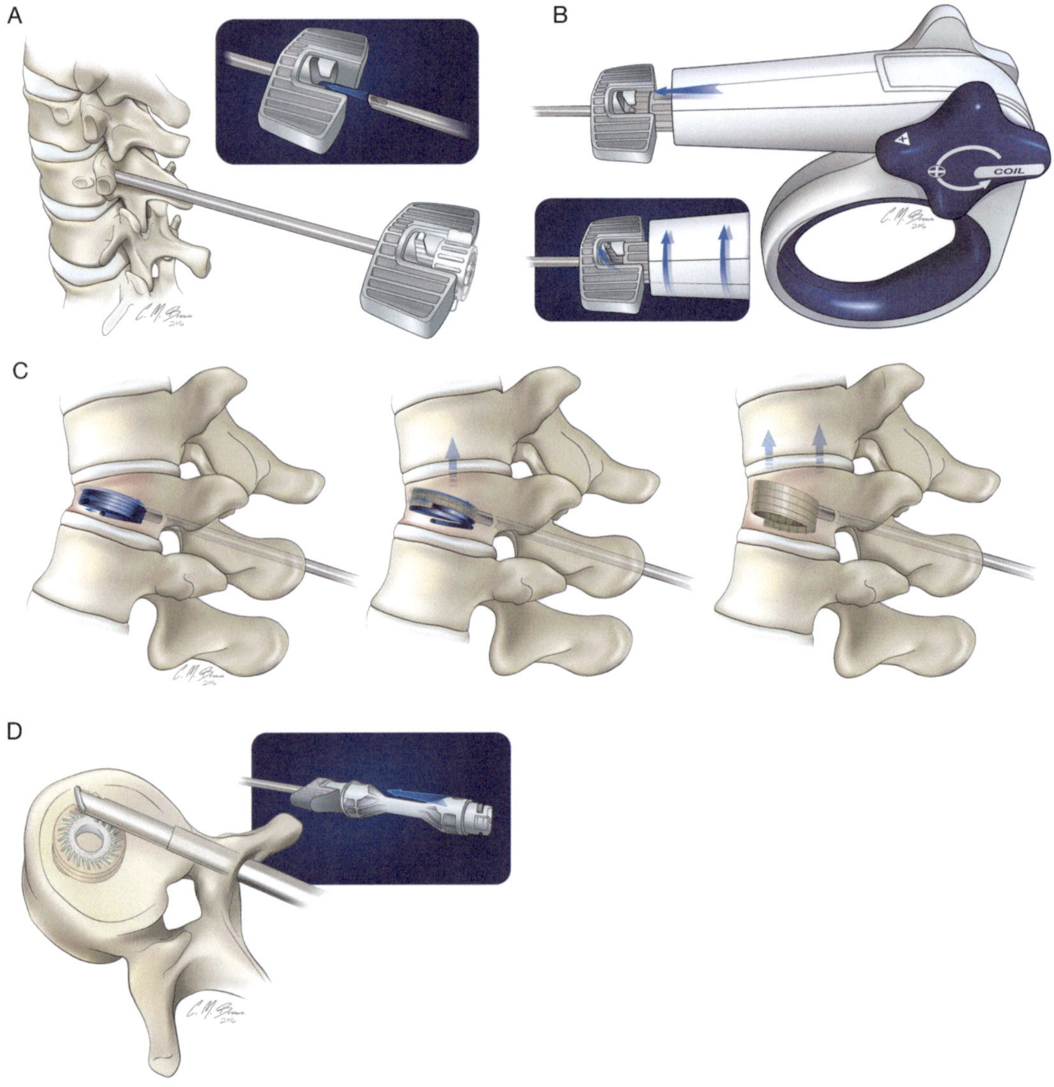

Fig. 18.8 (**a**) KIVA device docking needle is placed in a transpedicular trajectory with inner trocar in place. (**b**) Trocar is removed, and KIVA deployment device is attached. (**c**) The coil knob is turned to deploy the coil completely. The KIVA device is then deployed over the coil using the knob on the other side. The coil is then retracted and the device detached, and (**d**) a polymethylmethacrylate-filled plunger fills the center of the device through holes in the center of the device in a controlled fashion similar to kyphoplasty. The device both restores height and decreases radiographic cement extravasation

center, containing the PMMA within the walls of the cylinder as shown in Fig. 18.8a–d.

The Kiva implant is deployed through a unilateral transpedicular approach. The setup is the same for both vertebroplasty and kyphoplasty, and the procedure can be done under local or general anesthesia. The initial needle is placed in a similar fashion in the anterior half of the vertebral body. It does not have to reach the midline as with other unilateral approaches. At this point, the stylet for the needle is removed, and the head of the device is inserted near the most anterior part of the vertebral body. The device is then turned medially with the top of the device deploying the coil. Once the coil is deployed, the implant is deployed over the coil slowly increasing the anterior vertebral body height. Once the graft is deployed, PMMA is injected through the deploying device through the graft into the center of the cylinder that the graft created. The graft is then detached from the deploying device, and the wound is closed.

The Kiva device was recently compared to kyphoplasty in the KAST trial. The major finding was the Kiva device showed significantly less cement extravasation. This can be explained by the device's ability to keep the PMMA central. This finding did not result in any difference in clinical outcomes. There was also a decrease in adjacent level fractures but this failed to meet significance. Overall the trial showed that the Kiva implant is a safe alternative to kyphoplasty.

Using Navigation

In a very select set of instances, visualization of the vertebral column may be obscured in the severely osteoporotic, severely obese, or when vertebral levels are near the diaphragm. In these patients where the landmarks are obscured, placing the needle can be very dangerous. Spinal navigation in these patients should be considered.

A reference arc should be attached to the spinous process rostral to the most superior level that needs to be addressed with the camera at the head of the bed. The areas of fracture can be localized with C-arm. The patient is then prepped and draped, and the O-arm is also draped so as to use the biplanar fluoroscopy function of the O-arm. Once acquisition is taken, the O-arm is moved rostral, and the navigated pedicle access needle can be used using three-dimensional navigation for either parapedicular or transpedicular trajectories. A Kirschner wire is then placed down the needle into the vertebral body, and the access needle is removed leaving the K-wire in place. If multiple levels are to be done, K-wires should be placed at every level that needs to be addressed. Vertebral augmentation cannulas are then placed over the K-wires, and vertebroplasty is performed under the fluoroscopy function of the O-arm, and, after all levels are completed, a three-dimensional scan can be taken to confirm the location of the cement within the body.

Although this technique is substantially more time consuming, it provides a greater level of safety in those patients with anatomy that one is unable to visualize on plain fluoroscopy.

Illustrative Case

History of Present Illness

This is a case of an 82-year-old female who has a history of osteoporosis confirmed by DEXA scan (T scores <-2.5) on calcium supplementation and teriparatide, who sustained an osteoporotic compression fracture at T10 3 years prior to vertebroplasty treatment due to intractable pain. She did well after the procedure and returned to her prior functional status until 6 weeks later when, while mopping her floor, the patient felt a pop in her back causing her to lose her breath and fall to the floor in pain. She did not note any numbness, tingling, weakness, or loss of continence.

Physical Examination

Upon initial presentation, she was at her neurologic baseline without deficits. She was alert and conversational, oriented x3. She was very tender to palpation over her mid to lower back. All extremities were moving with 5/5 movement with good sensation in all and she did not have any perigenital/anal anesthesia.

Radiographic Evaluation

Her preoperative radiographs are shown in Fig. 18.9a, b showing acute compression fractures at T11 and T12.

Initial Management

She was treated with bracing and pain control, and, although she was able to return home, her activity level decreased secondary to pain at her 2- and 6-week appointments. Her standing

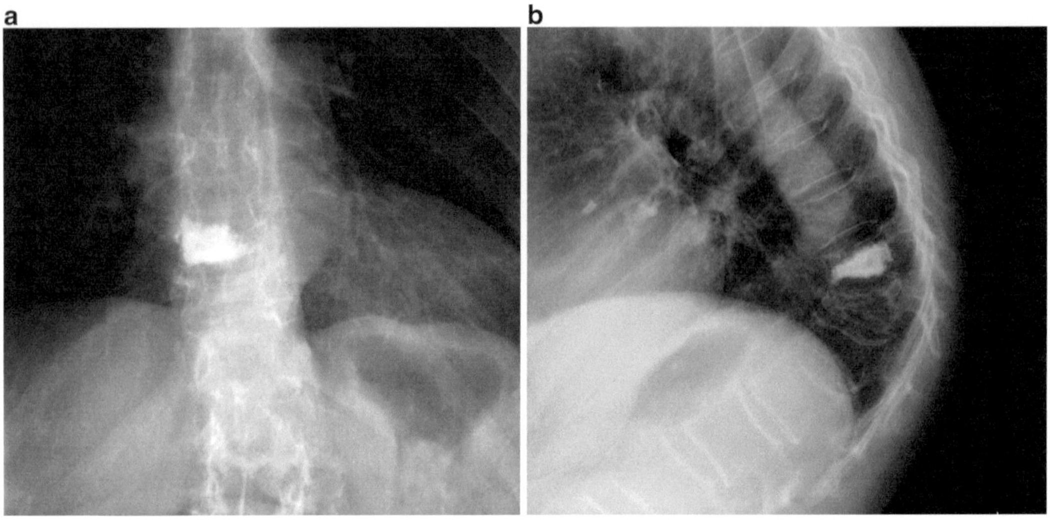

Fig. 18.9 (**a**) AP preoperative radiographs demonstrating compression fractures at T11 and T12. (**b**) Sagittal radiographs demonstrating the same pathology

radiographs looked grossly similar at this appointment showing an intact posterior cortex, but her son reported that she mainly was sitting in her wheelchair without much activity over this time period. It was at this point they decided she would like to undergo vertebroplasty.

Procedure and Outcome

The unilateral parapedicular vertebroplasty was performed under conscious sedation. Fourteen milliliters of PMMA was injected at each level without complication. Trajectories are shown in Fig. 18.10a and b. In recovery, she felt immediate pain relief. Postoperative radiographs show excellent cement fill without extravasation (Fig. 18.11a, b). At 3 months post-surgery, she has returned to her baseline functional status.

Technical Pearls

- When performing these procedures and especially when doing multiple levels, biplanar fluoroscopy can be used. This can be done in an interventional suite or positioning two C-arms.
- It is always imperative to obtain true AP and lateral images of the targeted vertebrae.
- When doing multiple vertebrae, it should be noted that a single batch of cement should be kept at cool temperatures to slow polymerization. One batch typically can do three vertebrae, and, at our institution, no more than three levels are ever done at one time due to PMMA toxicity and a higher risk of adverse events. A larger amount of PMMA should be used in kyphoplasty as there should be enough bone cement to fill the cavity created and the surrounding trabecular bone.
- When treating a significantly collapsed vertebra with kyphoplasty, there are two techniques that have been shown to keep the fracture reduced. If there is unilateral collapse, the cavity contralateral to the collapse can be filled first, allowing some cement to pack the trabecular bone providing a structural buttress. The second balloon can then be withdrawn.
- The second technique can be used in the setting of vertebra plana which re-collapses after balloon withdrawal. One milliliter of PMMA can be injected into the body, and the balloon can be reinserted and inflated allowing cement

a b

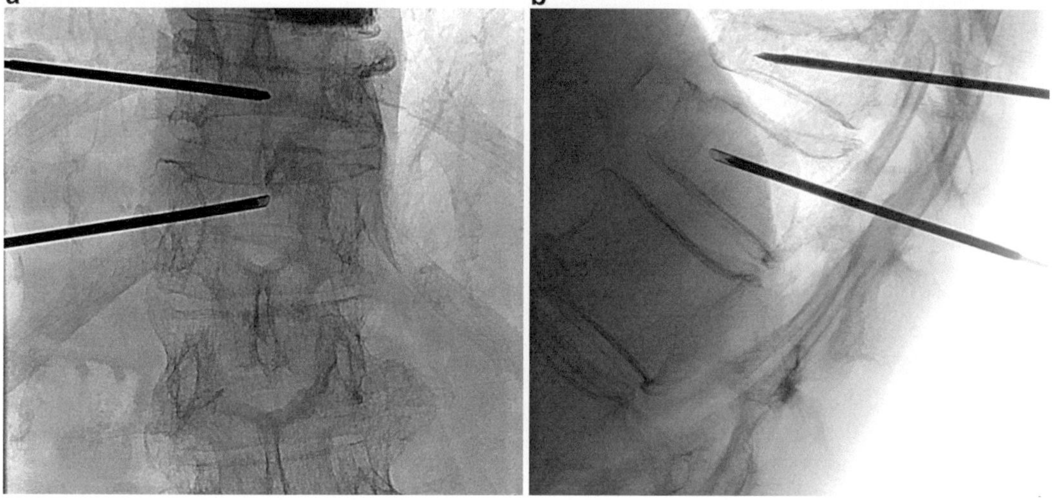

Fig. 18.10 (**a**) Showing intraoperative parapedicular trajectory in the AP plane reaching the midline. (**b**) Showing the same in the sagittal plane

a b

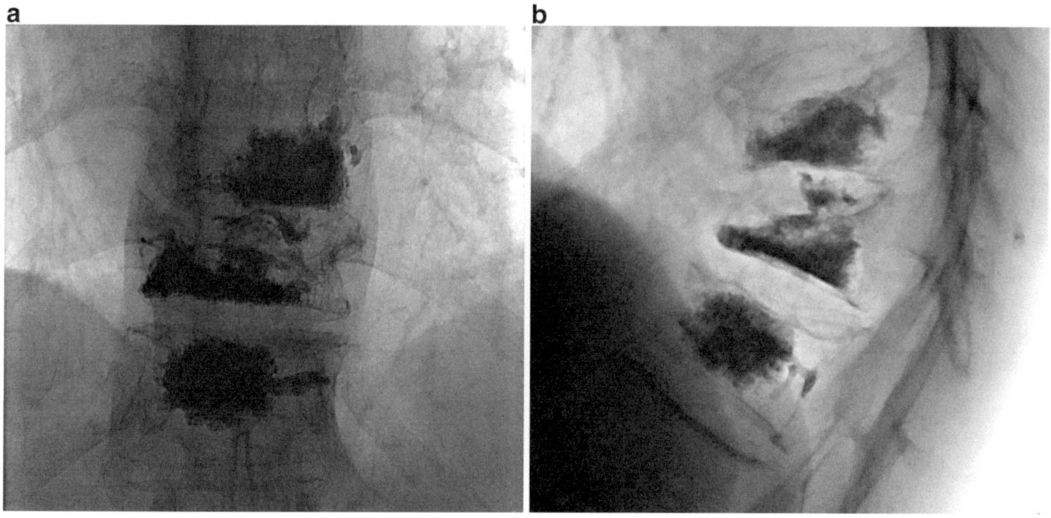

Fig. 18.11 (**a**) Showing postoperative AP radiographs and (**b**) sagittal radiographs post-augmentation. It should be noted that with vertebroplasty, end plate reduction and deformity correction are no different than preoperative imaging

to harden forming a thin shell of cement. The balloon can then be withdrawn and the rest of the cavity filled with cement.

Complications and Avoidance

Preoperative planning must always focus on the goals of the surgery while preventing complications. The two complications that can arise from this procedure involve the initial placement of the trocars and extravasation of bone cement. Placing Jamshidi needles through the neuro-elements can be avoided by obtaining true AP and lateral radiographs, lining up the end plates, pedicles, and facet joints. If the image needs to be improved in the osteoporotic patient, magnification on the C-arm may be increased, the tube may be brought closer to the patient, and the respirations may be held until the Jamshidi needle is placed. As stated before, the transpedicular approach should start on the superolateral aspect of the pedicle to avoid damage to the nerve roots. The parapedicular approach can be started lateral to the pedicle and medial to the costovertebral joint. It should be noted that the needle on this approach should not be medial to the medial aspect of the pedicle until it reaches the posterior aspect of the vertebral body to once again avoid nerve root injury and damage to the spinal cord. The parapedicular approach is usually done in mid to high thoracic fractures with transpedicular being reserved for low thoracic and lumbar fractures. With these precautions taken, the operator can be certain that the needle is in good position and has not damaged any of the neural elements.

The most common complication occurring in both vertebroplasty (VP) and kyphoplasty (KP) is PMMA extravasation that occurs in 11–75% of VP patients and 5–38% of KP patients. These are radiographic leaks and are rarely symptomatic. Symptomatic leaks were reported in 1.48% of VP patients and 0.06% of the KP patients [30]. This higher leak rate is thought to be caused by the higher pressures that VP cement is injected under, the lower viscosity of the cement, and the ability of kyphoplasty to pack out the bone around the cavity that it creates. The majority of these leaks go into the paravertebral soft tissue, but extravasation into the spinal canal can be catastrophic, and having a spine surgeon at the institution available to perform emergent decompression is imperative. In order to avoid this, it is advisable to do this under live fluoroscopy and to confirm an intact posterior cortex when starting out.

Cement extravasation can be minimized first by patient selection, choosing patients with an intact posterior cortex if possible. The needle should be placed in the anterior two-thirds of the vertebral body to allow some room to fill the body without reaching the posterior cortex too early. It is essential to make sure the PMMA is at a consistency thick enough to maintain its integrity. When doing a kyphoplasty, the balloon should not be inflated to the point where there is any outpouching through any of the cortical bone so as not to create any breaches. When deploying the PMMA, it should be done in small increments 0.2–0.5 ml at one time with frequent fluoroscopy. When using the bilateral approach, small amounts of PMMA should be placed alternating each side one at a time as on the lateral image large amounts of PMMA on one side can obscure visualization of the contralateral PMMA as it is being deployed. If there is any evidence of breaches in the contrast, the procedure should be stopped immediately. If vertebroplasty is being performed and it is felt that a less than adequate amount of contrast has been deployed, the cannula can be repositioned. Although most cement leaks are clinically inconsequential, if there is a significant leak, the patient must be examined before leaving the operating room, and, in the face of a neurologic deficit, if a deficit is appreciated, emergent decompression should be considered.

Conclusion

Vertebral augmentation is a minimally invasive technique with expanding indications in the fields of oncology, trauma, and metabolic dysfunction providing pain relief, deformity correction, and spinal stability with minimal surgical morbidity and, if careful, low complication rates. Surgeon familiarity with these techniques have led to utilization of these materials in hybrid models both in the augmentation of pedicle screw pullout strength and providing anterior stiffness to an unstable spine allowing fewer segments to be fixated. Newer devices are currently being developed that may provide greater deformity correction with less chance of cement extravasation.

References

1. Cooper C, Atkinson EJ, O'Fallon WM, Melton LJ 3rd. Incidence of clinically diagnosed vertebral fractures: a population-based study in Rochester, Minnesota, 1985–1989. J Bone Miner Res. 1992;7(2):221–7.
2. Lindsay R, Silverman SL, Cooper C, et al. Risk of new vertebral fracture in the year following a fracture. JAMA. 2001;285(3):320–3.

3. Galibert P, Deramond H. Percutaneous acrylic vertebroplasty as a treatment of vertebral angioma as well as painful and debilitating diseases. Chirurgie. 1990;116(3):326–34. discussion 335
4. Galibert P, Deramond H, Rosat P, Le Gars D. Preliminary note on the treatment of vertebral angioma by percutaneous acrylic vertebroplasty. Neuro-Chirurgie. 1987;33(2):166–8.
5. Allen RT, Kum JB, Weidner N, Hulst JB, Garfin SR. Biopsy of osteoporotic vertebral compression fractures during kyphoplasty: unsuspected histologic findings of chronic osteitis without clinical evidence of osteomyelitis. Spine. 2009;34(14):1486–91.
6. Garfin SR, Buckley RA, Ledlie J. Balloon Kyphoplasty outcomes G. Balloon kyphoplasty for symptomatic vertebral body compression fractures results in rapid, significant, and sustained improvements in back pain, function, and quality of life for elderly patients. Spine. 2006;31(19):2213–20.
7. Garfin SR, Yuan HA, Reiley MA. New technologies in spine: kyphoplasty and vertebroplasty for the treatment of painful osteoporotic compression fractures. Spine. 2001;26(14):1511–5.
8. Ghofrani H, Nunn T, Robertson C, Mahar A, Lee Y, Garfin S. An evaluation of fracture stabilization comparing kyphoplasty and titanium mesh repair techniques for vertebral compression fractures: is bone cement necessary? Spine. 2010;35(16):E768–73.
9. Perry A, Mahar A, Massie J, Arrieta N, Garfin S, Kim C. Biomechanical evaluation of kyphoplasty with calcium sulfate cement in a cadaveric osteoporotic vertebral compression fracture model. Spine J. 2005;5(5):489–93.
10. Theodorou DJ, Theodorou SJ, Duncan TD, Garfin SR, Wong WH. Percutaneous balloon kyphoplasty for the correction of spinal deformity in painful vertebral body compression fractures. Clin Imaging. 2002;26(1):1–5.
11. Diamond TH, Champion B, Clark WA. Management of acute osteoporotic vertebral fractures: a nonrandomized trial comparing percutaneous vertebroplasty with conservative therapy. Am J Med. 2003;114(4):257–65.
12. Schreiber JJ, Anderson PA, Hsu WK. Use of computed tomography for assessing bone mineral density. Neurosurg Focus. 2014;37(1):E4.
13. Weninger P, Schultz A, Hertz H. Conservative management of thoracolumbar and lumbar spine compression and burst fractures: functional and radiographic outcomes in 136 cases treated by closed reduction and casting. Arch Orthop Trauma Surg. 2009;129(2):207–19.
14. Gertzen H, Hallberg O, Laage-Hellman JE, Lundblad L, Odelberg-Johansson O, Widstrom A. Radiotherapy of differentiated thyroid neoplasms. Lakartidningen. 1978;75(34):2857.
15. Liu W, Zhou S, Wang S. Application of percutaneous vertebroplasty in the treatment of multiple thoracic metastases. Oncol Lett. 2015;9(6):2775–80.
16. Berenson J, et al. Balloon kyphoplasty versus nonsurgical fracture management for treatment of painful vertebral body compression fractures in patients with cancer: a multicentre, randomised controlled trial. Lancet Oncol. 2011;12(3):225–35.
17. Cianfoni A, Raz E, Mauri S, et al. Vertebral augmentation for neoplastic lesions with posterior wall erosion and epidural mass. AJNR Am J Neuroradiol. 2015;36(1):210–8.
18. De la Garza-Ramos R, Benvenutti-Regato M, Caro-Osorio E. Vertebroplasty and kyphoplasty for cervical spine metastases: a systematic review and meta-analysis. Int J Spine Surg. 2016;10:7.
19. Costa F, Ortolina A, Galbusera F, et al. Pedicle screw cement augmentation. A mechanical pullout study on different cement augmentation techniques. Med Eng Phys. 2016;38(2):181–6.
20. Tan QC, Wu JW, Peng F, et al. Augmented PMMA distribution: improvement of mechanical property and reduction of leakage rate of a fenestrated pedicle screw with diameter-tapered perforations. J Neurosurg Spine. 2016;24:971–7.
21. Elder BD, Lo SF, Holmes C, et al. The biomechanics of pedicle screw augmentation with cement. Spine J. 2015;15(6):1432–45.
22. Klingler JH, Scholz C, Kogias E, et al. Minimally invasive technique for PMMA augmentation of fenestrated screws. ScientificWorldJournal. 2015;2015:979186.
23. Oner FC, Verlaan JJ, Verbout AJ, Dhert WJ. Cement augmentation techniques in traumatic thoracolumbar spine fractures. Spine. 2006;31(11 Suppl):S89–95. discussion S104
24. McGraw JK, Cardella J, Barr JD, et al. Society of Interventional Radiology quality improvement guidelines for percutaneous vertebroplasty. J Vasc Interv Radiol. 2003;14(7):827–31.
25. McGraw JK, Cardella J, Barr JD, et al. Society of Interventional Radiology quality improvement guidelines for percutaneous vertebroplasty. J Vasc Interv Radiol. 2003;14(9 Pt 2):S311–5.
26. Stallmeyer MJ, Zoarski GH, Obuchowski AM. Optimizing patient selection in percutaneous vertebroplasty. J Vasc Interv Radiol. 2003;14(6):683–96.
27. Papanastassiou ID, Filis A, Aghayev K, Kokkalis ZT, Gerochristou MA, Vrionis FD. Adverse prognostic factors and optimal intervention time for kyphoplasty/vertebroplasty in osteoporotic fractures. Biomed Res Int. 2014;2014:925683.
28. Svedbom A, et al. Balloon kyphoplasty compared to vertebroplasty and nonsurgical management in patients hospitalised with acute osteoporotic vertebral compression fracture: a UK cost-effectiveness analysis. Osteoporos Int. 2013;24(1):355–67.
29. Wong W, Mathis J. Is intraosseous venography a significant safety measure in performance of vertebroplasty? J Vasc Interv Radiol. 2002;13(2 Pt 1):137–8.
30. Zaryanov AV, Park DK, Khalil JG, Baker KC, Fischgrund JS. Cement augmentation in vertebral burst fractures. Neurosurg Focus. 2014;37(1):E5.
31. Bae JW, Gwak HS, Kim S, Joo J, et al. Percutaneous vertebroplasty for patients with metastatic compression

fractures of the thoracolumbar spine: clinical and radiological factors affecting functional outcomes. Spine J. 2016;16(3):355–64.
32. Tezer M, Erturer RE, Ozturk C, Ozturk I, Kuzgun U. Conservative treatment of fractures of the thoracolumbar spine. Int Orthop. 2005;29(2):78–82.
33. Lu WW, Cheung KM, Li YW, et al. Bioactive bone cement as a principal fixture for spinal burst fracture: an in vitro biomechanical and morphologic study. Spine 2001;26(24):2684–2690; discussion 2690–81.
34. Mermelstein LE, McLain RF, Yerby SA. Reinforcement of thoracolumbar burst fractures with calcium phosphate cement. A biomechanical study. Spine 1998;23(6):664–670; discussion 670–61.

19 Anterior Lumbar Interbody Fusion of the Lumbosacral Spine: L3 Through the Sacrum

J. Kenneth Burkus

Introduction

Degenerative disc disease in the lumbar spine is a specific pain syndrome that originates from changes and instability patterns within the intervertebral disc. This syndrome is diagnosed by a history of clinical complaints, physical findings, and neuroradiographic studies. Identifying patients with a symptomatic degenerative disc who will benefit from interventional treatment is challenging. The selection of appropriate treatment modalities depends on the patient's symptoms, physical findings, and diagnostic testing.

Discogenic pain syndromes are a continuum of diagnostic categories that involve degenerative conditions of the intervertebral disc [1]. These clinical syndromes are commonly referred to as *internal disc disruption* (IDD) and *degenerative disc disease* (DDD). These degenerative processes occur in the majority of people as the result of aging. However, in addition to the degenerative patterns seen with aging, certain biologic and biomechanical factors predispose some people to painful degenerative changes within the spinal motion segment. Clinically painful discs have been shown to have specific patterns of altered stresses in the annulus and vertebral end plates. These heightened stresses reflect abnormal biomechanical loading patterns across the disc space.

The first clinical report on the treatment of symptomatic degenerative lumbar disc disease by anterior lumbar interbody fusion (ALIF) was published in 1948 [2]. Crock later introduced the term internal disc disruption (IDD) based upon a retrospective analysis of patients who had continued to complain of disabling back and leg pain after operations for lumbar disc prolapse [3]. Contemporary reports of large clinical series of anterior lumbar interbody fusion (ALIF) results have shown varying rates of fusion and differing clinical outcomes [4–7]. Loguidice et al. [8] found ALIF had an 80% rate of successful fusion and an 80% rate of clinical success. Blumenthal et al. [9] found a 73% successful fusion rate and 74% clinical success rate. Newman et al. [10] found that 86% of their patients with internal disc derangement had successful clinical results following an ALIF procedure. A successful fusion alone does not guarantee an improved clinical outcome [11–14].

Interbody fusion devices have been introduced recently that have been used to improve rates of fusion, reestablish disc space height, and restore normal sagittal contours [15–17]. The design characteristics of these implants provide significant advantages and benefits over traditional

J.K. Burkus, MD (✉)
Attending Physician, Spine Service, The Hughston Clinic, 6262 Veterans Parkway, Columbus, GA 31908, USA
e-mail: jkb66@knology.net

L.T. Holly, P.A. Anderson (eds.), *Essentials of Spinal Stabilization*,
DOI 10.1007/978-3-319-59713-3_19

interbody fusion techniques including intersegmental distraction, immediate stabilization, and facilitation of fusion. The intradiscal fusion devices provide mechanical support that promotes fusion and prevents subsidence and disc space collapse. Restoration of anatomic disc space height and the reduction of any frontal or sagittal plane deformities are important in reducing disabling complaints and enhancing clinical outcomes [18–20].

A failed posterior spinal fusion can also be salvaged with an ALIF procedure. A posterolateral or intertransverse process fusion provides stability in the presence of rotational, translational, and iatrogenic instability patterns when the disc is intact or is not the source of pain. However, a posterior or posterolateral fusion does not always restore the structural integrity of a painful degenerative or unstable lumbar disc. During the traditional posterior approach, the paraspinal muscles are detached from the posterior spinal elements and transverse processes. The loss of their normal anatomic attachment sites, formation of scar tissue, and loss of independent muscle function compromise the paravertebral muscles. Lumbar spine stabilization procedures that do not interfere with the posterior spinal muscles or that limit posterolateral dissection offer some significant advantages.

Indications and Patient Selection

Anterior lumbar interbody fusion (ALIF) is an effective treatment for patients with symptomatic degenerative discogenic conditions that include lumbar spondylosis, instability, and radiculopathy from L3 through the sacrum. One- or two-level degenerative lumbar disc disease can be treated with stand-alone anterior lumbar interbody fusion procedures; however, three-level lumbar disc disease can rarely be treated by anterior interbody fusion alone. This condition usually requires additional posterior segmental spinal stabilization.

These treatable degenerative conditions of the lumbosacral spine are manifested by persistent back pain and referred leg pain that are recalcitrant to nonoperative treatment modalities. Patients often exhibit restricted range of motion of the lumbar spine, tenderness to palpation over the affected lumbar motion segments, and paravertebral muscle spasm. They commonly describe pain that is exacerbated by activities and that is relieved with rest. Sitting can be uncomfortable, and patients frequently complain of difficulty finding a comfortable position. Pain is commonly referred to the buttock and posterior aspect of the thigh. This referred leg pain pattern rarely extends below the knees and radiates in a nondermatomal distribution into the lower extremities. Objective neurologic deficits, such as diminished or altered sensation and depressed reflexes, can be demonstrated; however, significant motor weakness, such as a foot drop, is rarely seen in patients suffering from these degenerative conditions. These patients do not commonly have positive sciatic tension signs. Straight-leg raising usually causes low back pain and referred buttock and posterior thigh pain.

Degenerative disc disease can be readily identified in symptomatic patients with plain radiographic findings. Degenerative changes within the lumbar motion segment are evidenced on plain radiographs by disc space collapse, radial osteophyte formation, and vertebral end plate sclerosis. Plain radiographs can also identify specific patterns of segmental instability by demonstrating excessive translational or rotational segmental motion at the intervertebral disc space. Painful instability patterns include spondylolisthesis, retrolisthesis, lateral listhesis, rotatory subluxation, and scoliosis. These abnormal motion patterns may require dynamic stress radiographs to be seen. Radiographic criteria for sagittal or rotational instability have been established and involve angular displacement on a flexion-extension lateral radiograph or translational shift to be considered in this diagnostic group. Segmental imbalance and loss of normal sagittal contours can also cause painful symptoms from the overloading of the facet joint and muscle fatigue.

Sagittal plane deformities with more than 20% subluxation cannot be treated reliably and predictably with a stand-alone anterior interbody fusion. Similarly, patients with severe segmental instability, as evidenced by more than 5 mm of sagittal plane translation on dynamic flexion-extension lateral radiographs, are not candidates for anterior interbody fusion alone. These patients would require additional posterior stabilization.

Imaging studies, such as magnetic resonance imaging (MRI), are helpful in identifying degenerative disc disease. MRI scans confirm desiccation of the disc and often Modic changes in the adjacent vertebral end plates [21]. However, disc desiccation, radial annular tears, and high-intensity zones documented on MRI are not, by themselves, indications for surgery. Correlative discography may be helpful in identifying the painful disc levels. Importantly, discography cannot be used alone to identify painful disc levels. Discography is often not effective in reproducing concordant pain stimulation at the affected level. The annulus of the disc can be incompetent, and distension of the annular pain fibers is not the primary source of pain. Discography may be helpful in the diagnostic evaluation by assessing adjacent spinal segments.

The level of bifurcation of the great vessel is highly variable. Most commonly, it occurs over the L5 vertebral body. The bifurcation of the vessels should be identified on preoperative neuroradiographic studies; evaluation of the axial cuts of preoperative MRI images or CT scans can help to identify the level of the bifurcation. These studies are essential when anterior instrumentation is being considered to stabilize the intradiscal implant. In addition, occult calcification of the great vessel can be seen on these studies.

Preoperative Considerations

Identifying patients with symptomatic degenerative disc disease who will benefit from surgical treatment is challenging for the physician. Approximately 30% of asymptomatic subjects have degenerative changes on plain radiographic studies. The selection of appropriate treatment modalities depends on the patient's symptoms, physical findings, and diagnostic testing. Only one-third of those patients who have pain for more than 3 months develop significant disabling symptoms that warrant further diagnostic evaluation.

Before surgery is considered, patients should be treated with vigorous aerobic lumbar conditioning programs that include isometric trunk-strengthening exercises and flexibility exercises. Nonimpact aerobic exercise, such as swimming or warm-water hydrotherapy, is well tolerated by these patients. In addition, isometric trunk-stabilization strengthening exercises consisting of a series of rigorous abdominal and paraspinal isometric exercises performed without much trunk mobilization have proven beneficial.

Chiropractic manipulation has been found to be effective in the treatment of short-duration low back pain. Similarly, the use of a nonnarcotic anti-inflammatory medication and the use of muscle relaxants are indicated for short-term relief of pain. The use of narcotic pain medication for the control of chronic pain is not efficacious. Neither bracing nor the use of acupuncture offers any substantial advantage in the treatment of discogenic pain syndromes.

Patients with previous disc space infection, metabolic bone disease, or osteoporosis also cannot be effectively treated with stand-alone anterior lumbar interbody fusion. The interbody fusion cages rest on the bony end plates of the intervertebral disc space. In patients with osteoporosis, the host trabecular and cortical bone cannot sustain the stresses from the cages. Microstress fractures occur, and the cages subside through the end plates and into the trabecular bone of the vertebral body. Subsidence leads to loss of soft tissue tensioning and instability at the disc space. Subsidence of the implants is also associated with loss of lordosis and loss of foraminal height. The micromotion associated with subsidence can lead to a delayed union or fibrous nonunion.

The overriding concern for the treating physician is proper patient selection. The majority of patients with discogenic pain do not require surgical treatment. Fusion surgery, or arthrodesis, should be reserved for patients who are highly motivated, carefully selected, and without psychological magnification of their symptoms.

Surgical Technique

Patient Positioning

The patient is placed in the supine position on the operating room table. The table must accommodate fluoroscopy in both the anteroposterior and lateral dimensions. The patient's arms may be tucked to the sides or suspended laterally from the table. Importantly, the arm position should not interfere with the fluoroscopic visualization of the spine. A radiolucent roll is placed under the lumbar spine and directly underneath the affected lumbar motion segment. The lumbar roll increases lumbar lordosis and frequently opens the collapsed disc space. This maneuver facilitates intraoperative distraction of the disc space and often partially reduces any sagittal plane deformity.

The lumbar spine is visualized in both the anteroposterior and lateral dimensions. The spine is checked for rotation. The posterior spinous process should be able to be well visualized between the pedicles. After a radiographic marker is placed on the skin, fluoroscopy is used to confirm its optimal position over the disc space. The entire abdomen and pelvis are prepared and draped in the surgical field in the usual and sterile fashion.

Open Retroperitoneal Exposure of the Lumbosacral Spine

A vertical or transverse skin incision is made over the appropriate disc space. The incision is sharply carried down through subcutaneous tissues. The ventral portion of the rectus abdominus muscle sheath is exposed. The muscle sheath is divided vertically approximately 2 cm from the midline. The medial border of the rectus abdominus muscle is bluntly dissected free from the muscle fascial sheath, and the rectus abdominus muscle is mobilized with blunt dissection and retracted laterally.

The arcuate line and posterior rectus sheath is visualized. The posterior rectus sheath is often a very thin layer overlying the peritoneal sac. First, the posterior rectus sheath bluntly separates from the peritoneal sac starting inferiorly and working superiorly and laterally. The posterior rectus sheath can be sharply incised and blunt dissection continued. A fatty plane is encountered directly overlying the psoas muscle. The entire peritoneal sac is then easily reflected past the midline. The ureter can be seen within the peritoneal sac crossing the iliac vessels. Care is taken to ensure that the left ureter is retracted along with the peritoneal contents. The genitofemoral nerve is seen lying directly on top of the psoas muscle. This nerve should not be mobilized.

The bifurcation of the great vessels occurs most commonly over the L5 vertebral body and should be identified on preoperative imaging studies. The L5–S1 disc space is most often located directly inferior to the bifurcation of the iliac vein, and the L4–L5 disc space is usually found directly lateral to the bifurcation of the iliac artery. The L4–L5 disc can be palpated at the junction between the bifurcation of the iliac artery and the psoas muscle. The sacral promontory and the L5–S1 disc can be palpated directly below the iliac vein bifurcation.

Exposure of the L3–L4 and L4–L5 Disc Spaces

The L4–L5 disc space is initially identified with gentle palpation along the medial border of the psoas muscle adjacent to the bifurcation of the iliac artery. The rounded soft annulus is readily identified. The L3–L4 disc space can be localized in the same plane, approximately 4 cm cephalad to the iliac bifurcation.

Direct dissection is carried down on top of the disc space through an avascular plane. Once the anterior surface of the annulus has been exposed, soft tissues can be swept off the disc space medially and laterally. Segmental vessels tether the aorta, vena cava, and iliac vessels. The segmental vessels lie in the midportion of the vertebral bodies of L3 and L4.

In exposing the L3–L4 disc space, the segmental vessels above and below the disc space must be identified, ligated, and divided. After this maneuver, blunt dissection allows the surgeon to mobilize the great vessels well past the midline of the disc space.

Exposure of the L4–L5 interspace requires the surgeon to mobilize the left iliac artery and vein. Once the disc space has been identified, dissection is bluntly carried cephalad, and segmental vessels crossing the midportion of the L4 vertebral body are identified, ligated, and divided. With blunt dissection, the iliac artery and aorta can be gently reflected past the midline. Directly under the artery is the left iliac vein. Before the vein is mobilized, blunt dissection must be carried out inferiorly along the lateral border of the left iliac vein. The recurrent iliolumbar vein should be identified. This lateral branch of the left iliac vein often needs to be securely ligated and divided to adequately mobilize the vein. The iliac artery and vein can then be reflected past the midline, exposing the L4–L5 disc space.

Exposure of the L5–S1 Disc Space

The L5–S1 disc space can be palpated gently within the bifurcation of the great vessels. Blunt dissection is carried down directly on top of the left iliac artery. Underneath the artery is the left iliac vein. Soft tissues should be separated from the vein and bluntly mobilized past the midline of the disc. Dissection is carried out superiorly to the bifurcation of the iliac vein. All soft tissues are then bluntly swept from left to right. The middle sacral artery and vein are exposed after this maneuver. These vessels are sequentially identified, ligated, and divided; they should not be cauterized. The disc space is further exposed with blunt dissection. Quite frequently, the left iliac vein must be retracted laterally and superiorly.

Superior Hypogastric Plexus and Retrograde Ejaculation

In male patients, retrograde ejaculation (RE) is a potential complication of anterior lumbar interbody fusion. The reported incidence of retrograde ejaculation after anterior lumbar interbody fusion varies widely in the literature. Plausible causes include direct injury to nerve and inflammation. Proposed various factors related to an increased risk of RE include the use of rhBMP-2, the interbody implant used, surgical approach, surgical technique (use of monopolar electrocautery), and surgeon experience.

The pelvic preaortic sympathetic plexus travels down from the thoracolumbar sympathetic chain in the retroperitoneal space. The superior hypogastric plexus is the terminal extension of this plexus. It lies anterior to the aorta and vertebra and covers the iliac bifurcation. The plexus has a variable structure. The nerve fibers are most commonly found arching over the left iliac artery crossing the L51 disc space. The hypogastric plexus can be injured by removing prevertebral tissue from the front of the L5–S1 disc space or by liberal use of electrocautery in the bifurcation.

Blunt dissection of presacral tissues, lateral retraction of these tissues, and avoidance of electrocautery in the bifurcation preserve the sympathetic plexus. No transverse incisions across the disc interspace are made until the annulus is clearly exposed and isolated from all soft tissues. For transperitoneal midline approaches, the posterior peritoneum must be careful opened. A sharp incision should be made over the level of the bifurcation and extended inferiorly over the L5S1 disc space. Electrocautery should not be used. Blunt dissection should begin on the right side of the disc space, and soft tissues should be swept from right to left across the disc space.

The Bulldog Discectomy

A complete anterior discectomy is carried out. The entire anterior portion of the vertebral body should be readily visualized. The rounded anterior surface and anterior longitudinal ligament and lateral borders of the annulus should be exposed. A radiographic marker is placed in the midportion of the disc space. Its position is confirmed with fluoroscopy in both the anteroposterior and lateral dimensions. The cartilaginous end plates are separated from the bony end plate. Great care is taken to preserve the bony end plates. Dissection is carried out lateral and posterior with the disc space. The lateral portions of the annulus must also be preserved. The posterior annulus and posterior radial osteophytes may be removed under direct visualization. Contained disc protrusions and disc herniations can be removed through this approach.

Following the thorough discectomy, the disc space can be mobilized. Distraction can be achieved with the use of serial impacted dilators. Expansion of the collapsed disc space re-tensions the soft tissues and ligamentous structures surrounding it. Anterior distraction maneuvers often reduce sagittal plane deformity (spondylolisthesis, retrolisthesis), reduce lateral plane deformity (scoliosis, lateral listhesis), and increase lumbar lordosis by tensioning the surrounding soft tissue elements. Establishing normal disc space height indirectly decompresses the neuroforamina and enlarges the neuroforaminal opening. Distraction of the disc space tensions the annulus fibrosus and compresses the interbody implant.

Disc space distraction should be limited to the anatomic restoration of disc space height assessed on preoperative standing plain lateral radiographs. Anterior intradiscal distraction instruments are powerful and can easily overcome the stabilizing soft tissue elements of the disc space. Overdistraction should be avoided. Similarly, segmental hyperlordosis of the disc space should be avoided. Templates are available that enable the surgeon to accurately measure the disc space height of adjacent normal discs. Having an understanding of anatomic disc space height, the surgeon can anticipate the amount of disc space distraction necessary to achieve uniform tensioning of the soft tissue elements across the disc space in the operating room. Fluoroscopy and tactile feedback is used to assess disc space expansion and reduction and any sagittal deformity during the impaction of the disc space distracters.

Interbody Implants

Structural autografts and allograft impacted intradiscal spacers have been a popular graft source and have a long and well-documented record of clinical safely and efficacy. Advanced biomaterial options, such as titanium, resorbable polymers, carbon fiber, and PEEK (polyetheretherketone) materials, are also available. These materials have proven biocompatibility, excellent chemical stability, and good mechanical properties. The implants differ in their modulus of elasticity. The PEEK material is comparable to bone, which minimizes stress shielding following implantation and is radiographically transparent. Synthetic polymers are increasingly used as alternatives to titanium not only because of their mechanical properties but also because of their properties in terms of molding, processing, and in vivo radiographic imaging. In assessing postoperative fusion, these implants have no imaging interference—osteoinduction and bone graft maturation can be demonstrated on radiographs without artifact.

Porous metal implants and PEEK implants with porous or rough metal coatings have found their way into clinical use. Both titanium and PEEK materials are currently being enhanced with several physical and chemical surface treatments which have been shown to improve osseointegration into the host bone. Implant surface treatments alter the micrometer- or nanometer-scale surface roughness with a high degree of precision. These surface treatments promote osteoblastic differentiation and foster a specific cellular environment that enhances bone formation. The long-term clinical and radiographic outcomes from the use of the advanced materials have not been established.

The shape of the vertebral body is important in planning the depth of insertion of the spinal implants. The implants should be recessed within the confines of the intervertebral disc space. The implants should contact the vertebral apophysis but remain well seated within the intervertebral disc space. Axial sections of preoperative MRI and CT scan will help to document the size of the implants to be used.

Cage Choices

Stand-alone anterior interbody implants can be impacted or threaded. The impacted implants are driven into the disc space. Preoperative evaluation of plane radiographs and axial images of the spinal motion segments are important in planning and establishing the goals of an anterior interbody fusion. Preoperative templating helps to ensure that the appropriate interbody fusion cage is selected for each interspace. It also aids the surgeon in planning the extent of intraoperative distraction necessary to tension the annulus fibrosus adequately and to reestablish the normal anatomic relationship of the intervertebral motion segment. The intradiscal implant should be placed parallel to the end plates of the adjacent vertebra. The anterior head wall of the device should be seated along the anterior margins of the vertebral bodies. The device should not penetrate the posterior or posterolateral corner of the disc space. The shape of the vertebral body must be evaluated on axial scans to determine how deeply the cages can be inserted in the disc space without risks of posterolateral perforation.

Depending upon the bone quality, the intradiscal implant can be used as a stand-alone device or supplemental fixation can be used. An anterior plate can be fixed to the vertebral bodies. The plate must be placed away from contact with adjacent vascular structures and therefore is most commonly used at the L5S1 disc level. The intradiscal device itself can incorporate screws or fins that insert into the adjacent vertebral bodies. Expandable devices within the disc space can be used. Hyperlordotic implants should be avoided. The implant should match the geometry of the disc space following appropriate distraction. The implant should not establish segmental hyperlordosis.

Bone Graft/Substitute

The standard for bone grafting in spinal fusion procedures has long been autogenous cancellous bone harvested from the iliac crest. Autologous bone grafts provide osteoinductive and osteoconductive elements that are not immunogenic and are usually well incorporated into the transplantation site. Harvesting autogenous bone grafts for spinal surgery has been associated with many complications; recent publications have also documented the long-term incidence of donor site pain to occur in 22–45% of the patients.

Contemporary bone grafting options eliminate the high rates of complications associated with autogenous bone harvesting. The biologic activity and structural composition of these grafting materials determine whether these materials are used as bone graft extenders or bone graft replacements. Human cadaver allograft bone products have an osteoconductive scaffold; however, they have minimal osteoinductive factors.

Demineralized bone matrices (DBMs) are the product formed by the acid treatment of allograft bone. DBMs do not have structural strength but possess osteoconductivity and the osteoinductive growth factors. The osteoinductive ability in DBMs to stimulate bone regeneration is dependent upon the activity of the bone morphogenic proteins (BMPs). DBM does not function as a replacement for autograft; it expands the volume and enhances the inductivity of autograft but does not replace it.

Ceramic scaffolds are not osteoinductive or osteogenic. They do not enhance the ability of the graft material to form new bone; they have not been demonstrated to perform comparable to iliac crest autograft in lumbar fusions. They cannot be used alone in spinal fusions; ceramics are not bone graft substitutes.

Platelet gels contain multiple growth factors but do not contain any BMPs; they are not regarded as osteoinductive. They encourage local cellular proliferation but are unable to induce bone formation alone and are not capable of mediating the process of bone formation. These gels have little clinical evidence of their efficacy and also cannot be used alone as a bone graft substitute.

Only bone morphogenetic proteins are capable of inducing the entire bone formation cascade. It is this unique property that allows these proteins with a suitable carrier to be used as a bone graft replacement. Recombinant human bone morphogenetic protein-2 (rhBMP-2) is an osteoinductive protein that when combined with the proper carrier (absorbable college sponge ACS) at an appropriate concentration has the potential to obviate the need for autogenous bone grafting. The use of rhBMP-2/ACS was shown to be an effective treatment in inducing fusion as well as improving pain and function in subjects with single-level lumbar degenerative disc disease. The fusion rate in those patients treated with rhBMP-2/ACS was significantly higher than those patients treated with autogenous bone grafts. Recent studies using pooled data have confirmed that patients with radiographically confirmed fusion had significantly better improvements in clinical outcomes than those of patients with radiographic nonunion. Additional studies have reported decreased reoperation rates are caused by the improved fusion with the use of rhBMP-2/ACS. Appropriately dosed rhBMP-2/ACS can be used in patients who are at risk for developing a pseudarthrosis following lumbar intradiscal fusion surgery.

Supplemental Fixation

Supplemental posterior stabilization should be considered if there is any residual sagittal or frontal plane deformity following the interbody fusion. Patients with osteoporosis, patients at risk of pseudarthrosis, patients who have undergone a posterior decompression, and those patients desiring aggressive postoperative mobilization can befit from posterior stabilization.

Closure

The great vessels are inspected to ensure that there have been no injuries. The ureter and retroperitoneal structures are also inspected. The wounds are then closed, along with any inadvertent perforations in the peritoneum. No attempts are made to suture the posterior rectus sheath. The anterior rectus sheath is approximated with divided absorbable sutures and the wound margins are approximated with a subcuticular stitch.

Oblique Lumbar Approach

A minimally invasive retroperitoneal oblique lumbar interbody fusion (OLIF) has been developed [10]. The minimally invasive OLIF technique is feasible for exposure from L3 through the sacrum. This approach to the lower lumbar spine for arthrodesis may be associated with a higher incidence of complications than open techniques [22, 23].

Illustrative Case

A 51-year-old white male had incapacitating low back pain and referred bilateral leg pain into his buttocks and posterior thighs. He had undergone an L5–S1 discectomy in the remote past. He had no complaints of pain radiating below his knees. His symptoms were exacerbated with activities and partially relieved with rest. His symptoms were recalcitrant to a 6-month course of physical therapy, anti-inflammatory medications, and antispasmodic medications.

An anteroposterior lumbar radiograph shows bilateral laminotomy defects at L5 (Fig. 19.1). A standing lateral radiograph shows 3 mm of retrolisthesis at L5–S1 (Fig. 19.2). There is significant narrowing of the neural foramina at L5–S1 secondary to the retrolisthesis and disc space narrowing (arrow). Figures 19.3 and 19.4 demonstrate the disc space narrowing, anterior osteophyte formation (arrow), and retrolisthesis at L5–S1 and normal motion patterns at discs above that level.

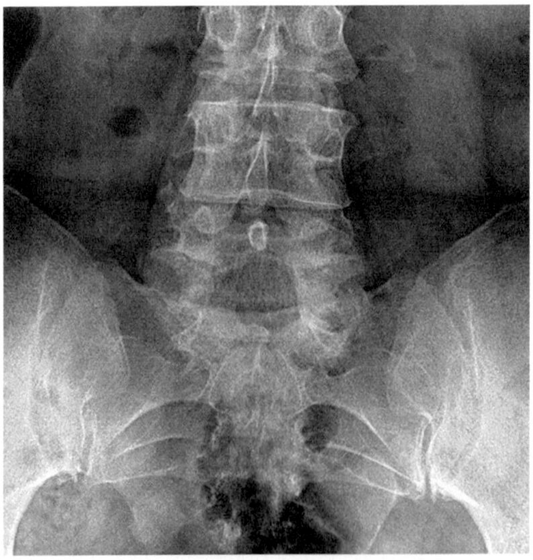

Fig. 19.1 Anteroposterior lumbar radiograph

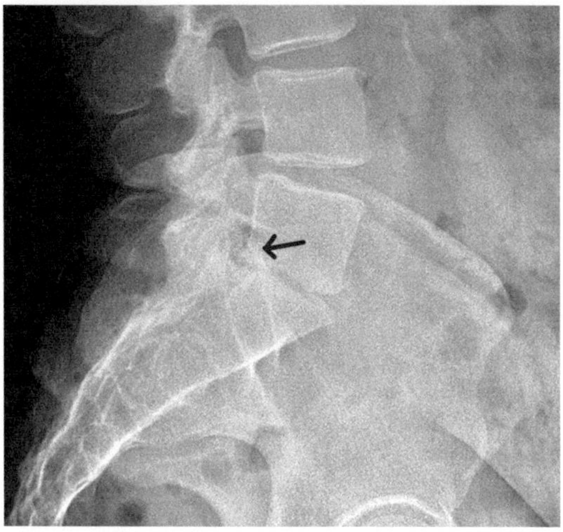

Fig. 19.2 Standing lateral radiograph shows 3 mm of retrolisthesis at L5–S1 (*arrow*)

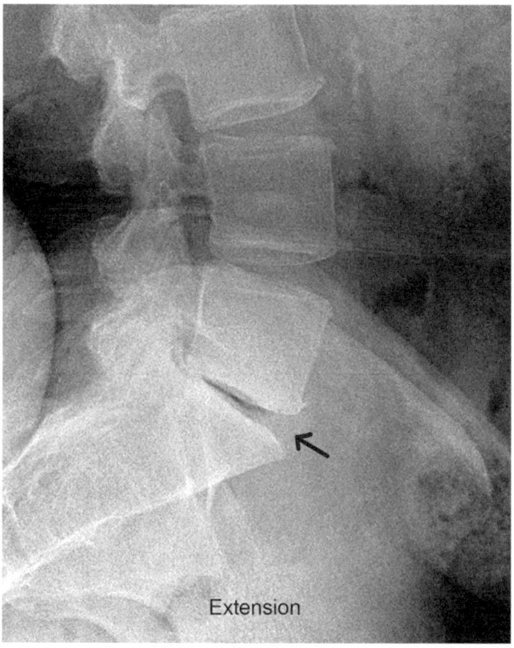

Fig. 19.3 Extension radiograph demonstrates the disc space narrowing, anterior osteophyte formation (*arrow*)

Postoperative anteroposterior (Fig. 19.5) and lateral (Fig. 19.6) radiographs show central positioning of the interbody cage, expansion of disc space height, enlargement of the neural foramina, and segmental fixation of the interbody fusion device.

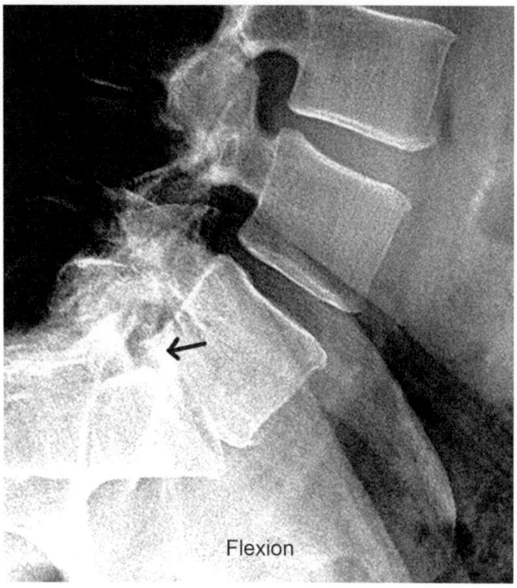

Fig. 19.4 Flexion radiograph shows retrolisthesis at L5–S1 and normal motion patterns at discs above that level

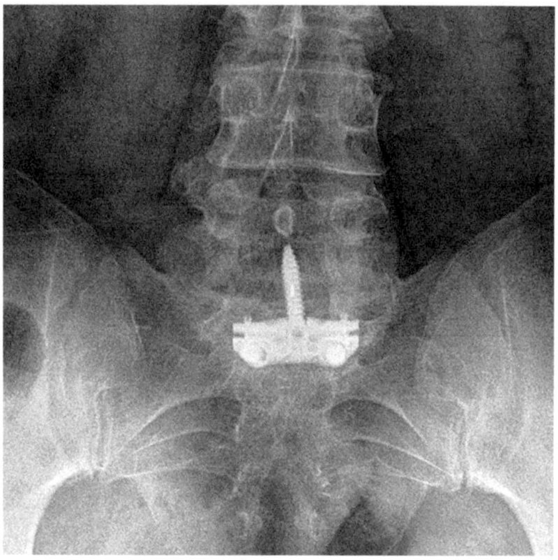

Fig. 19.5 Postoperative anteroposterior radiograph shows interbody cage device

Technical Pearls

- Axial cuts of the MRI or computerized axial tomography scan are helpful in documenting the dimensions of the intervertebral disc space and the size of implants to be used. The shape of the vertebral body is important in planning the depth of insertion of the spinal implants.

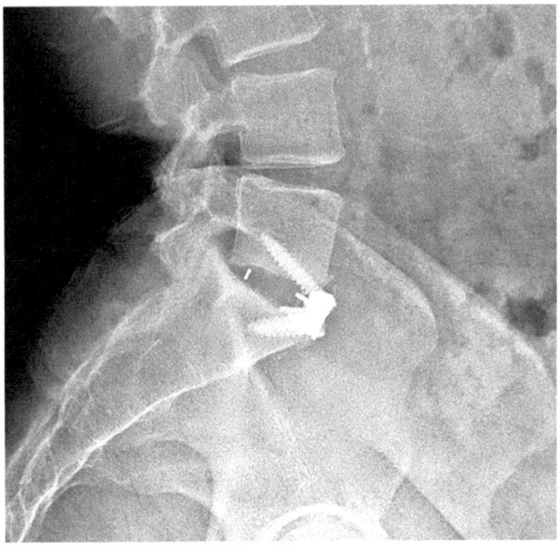

Fig. 19.6 Postoperative lateral radiograph

The implants should be recessed within the confines of the intervertebral disc space. The implants should contact the vertebral apophysis but remain well seated within the intervertebral disc space.

- Position the patient with a roll under the affected lumbar motion segment to increase lumbar lordosis and facilitate disc space distraction.
- Critically assess the vascular structures on preoperative MRI. Knowledge of anomalies and the location of bifurcation are important to avoid iatrogenic injury.
- Perform a complete discectomy under direct visualization. This will prevent retropulsion of any disc fragments, ensure an adequate fusion bed for the intervertebral body grafts, and allow for appropriated mobilization of the disc for restoration of an anatomic configuration of the disc.
- Adequately distract the disc space to the height of the adjacent vertebral motion segment. Avoid overdistraction and underdistraction.

Complications and Strategies for Avoidance

Intraoperative problems usually involve mobilization of the great vessels. The left iliac vein is generally the anatomic structure the surgeon has the most trouble adequately mobilizing [24]. Inadvertent tears in the vein should be promptly repaired using fine sutures. ALIF is a safe procedure when performed by a combined surgical team of vascular surgeon and spine surgeon with acceptably low complication rates [23]. The team approach results in short operative times and length of stay, with rapid control of intraoperative vessel injury and low overall blood loss.

Patients with previous abdominal surgery or calcified vascular disease involving the aorta and iliac vessel are not candidates for stand-alone anterior interbody fusion. These patients are better treated by posterior posterolateral approaches to the lumbosacral spine.

Retrograde ejaculation can occur in men after this procedure [25]. This problem can be avoided by careful blunt dissection, bifurcation of the great vessels, and ligation along the lateral border of the iliac. Avoiding electrocautery during the initial dissection of disc spaces will also limit the occurrence of this problem.

Multilevel lumbar fusions (more than two disc space levels) are associated with high rates of pseudarthrosis. Long lumbar fusions are also associated with restricted lumbar motion and stress transfer to the sacroiliac joints.

Conclusion

Anterior lumbar interbody fusions have clinical advantages over posterior lumbar approaches. Interbody fusion procedures place bone grafts within the disc space at the center of rotation of the vertebral motion segment. The intervertebral area is highly vascular, and the grafts have a wide contact area and are inserted in the weight-bearing axis of the spinal motion segment. An anterior interbody fusion allows the surgeon to directly manipulate the spinal motion segment through the collapsed disc space. Intersegmental distraction enables the surgeon to restore the normal sagittal plane contours of the spine, achieve immediate stabilization of the spinal motion segment, and facilitate the fusion process without damaging the posterolateral soft tissues or mobilizing and retracting neural tissues.

References

1. Wilder DG, Pope MH, Frymoyer JW. The biomechanics of lumbar disc herniation and the effect of overload and instability. J Spinal Disord. 1988;1(1):16–32.
2. Lane JD, Moore ES. Transperitoneal approach to the intervertebral disc in the lumbar area. Ann Surg. 1948;127:537–51.
3. Crock HV. Anterior lumbar interbody fusion. Clin Orthop. 1982;165:157–63.
4. Chow SP, Leong JCY, Ma A, Yau ACMC. Anterior spinal fusion for deranged lumbar intervertebral disc. Spine. 1980;5:452–8.
5. Goldner JL, Urbaniak JR, McCollom DE. Anterior excision and interbody spinal fusion for chronic low back pain. Orthop Clin North Am. 1971;2:543–68.
6. Harmon DH. Anterior excision and vertebral body fusion operation for intervertebral disc syndromes of the lower spine: three to five year results in 244 cases. Clin Orthop. 1963;26:107–27.
7. Sacks S. Anterior interbody fusion of the lumbar spine. J Bone Joint Surg Br. 1965;47:211–23.
8. Loguidice VA, Johnson RG, Guyer RD, Stith WJ, Ohnmeiss DD, Hochschuler SH, Rashbaum RF. Anterior lumbar interbody fusion. Spine. 1988;13:366–9.
9. Blumenthal SL, Baker J, Dossett A, Selby DK. The role of anterior lumbar fusion for internal disc disruption. Spine. 1988;13:566–9.
10. Newman MH, Grinstead GL. Anterior lumbar interbody fusion for internal disc disruption. Spine. 1992;17:831–3.
11. Kumar A, Kozak JA, Doherty BJ, Dickson JH. Interspace distraction and graft subsidence after anterior lumbar fusion with femoral strut allograft. Spine. 1993;18:2393–400.
12. Leong JCY, Chun SY, Grange WJ, Fang D. Long-term results of lumbar intervertebral disc prolapse. Spine. 1983;8:793–9.
13. Schroeder GD, Kepler CK, Millhouse PW, Fleischman AN, Maltenfort MG, Bateman DK, Vaccaro AR. L5/S1 fusion rates in degenerative spine surgery: a systematic review comparing ALIF, TLIF, and axial interbody arthrodesis. Clin Spine Surg. 2016;29(4):150–5.
14. Verbruggen D, Tampere T, Uyttendaele D, Sys G, Poffyn B. Long-term follow-up of the anterior lumbar interbody fusion procedure. Acta Orthop Belg. 2015;81(3):546–52.
15. Burkus JK, Gornet MF, Dickman C, Zdeblick TA. Anterior lumbar interbody fusion using rhBMP-2 with tapered interbody cages. J Spinal Disord. 2002;15:337–49.
16. Kuslich SD, Ulstrom CL, Griffith SL, Ahern JW, Dowdle JD. The Bagby and Kuslich method of lumbar interbody fusion: history, techniques, and 2-year follow-up results of a United States prospective, multicenter trial. Spine. 1998;21:1267–79.
17. Li J, Dumonski ML, Liu Q, Lipman A, Hong J, Yang N, Jin Z, Ren Y, Limthongkul W, Bessey JT, Thalgott J, Gebauer G, Albert TJ, Vaccaro AR. A multicenter study to evaluate the safety and efficacy of a stand-alone anterior carbon I/F cage for anterior lumbar interbody fusion: two-year results from a Food and Drug Administration investigational device exemption clinical trial. Spine. 2010;35(26):E1564–70.
18. Dennis S, Watkins R, Landaker S, Dillin W, Springer D. Comparison of disc space heights after anterior lumbar interbody fusion. Spine. 1989;14:876–8.
19. Schuler TC, Burkus JK, Gornet MF, Subach BR, Zdeblick TA. The correlation between preoperative disc space height and clinical outcomes after anterior lumbar interbody fusion. J Spinal Disord Tech. 2005 Oct;18(5):396–401.
20. Burkus JK, Gornet MF, Schuler TC, Kleeman TJ, Zdeblick TA. Six-year outcomes of anterior lumbar interbody arthrodesis with use of interbody fusion cages and recombinant human bone morphogenetic protein-2. J Bone Joint Surg Am. 2009;91:1181–9.
21. Modic MT, Steinberg PM, Ross JS, Masaryk TJ, Carter JR. Degenerative disc disease: assessment of changes in vertebral body marrow with MR imaging. Radiology. 1988;166:193–9.
22. Escobar E, Transfeldt E, Garvey T, Ogilvie J, Graber J, Schultz L. Video-assisted versus open anterior lumbar spine fusion surgery: a comparison of four techniques and complications in 135 patients. Spine. 2003;28(7):729–32.
23. Mobbs RJ, Phan K, Daly D, Rao PJ, Lennox A. Approach-related complications of anterior lumbar interbody fusion: results of a combined spine and vascular surgical team. Global Spine J. 2016;6(2):147–54.
24. Sasso RC, Best NM, Mummaneni PV, Reilly TM, Hussain SM. Analysis of operative complications in a series of 471 anterior lumbar interbody fusion procedures. Spine. 2005;30:670–4.
25. Sasso RC, Burkus JK, LeHuec JC. Retrograde ejaculation after anterior lumbar interbody fusion: transperitoneal versus retroperitoneal exposure. Spine. 2003;28:1023–6.

Transformational Lumbar Interbody Fusion

20

Robert F. Heary and John C. Quinn

Introduction

Lumbar spinal fusion has evolved as a treatment option for symptomatic spinal instability, spinal stenosis, spondylolisthesis, and degenerative scoliosis [1, 2]. Lumbar spinal fusion is often performed after a posterior decompressive procedure when there is evidence of preoperative lumbar spinal deformity or instability that could worsen after laminectomy alone [3]. When performing a lumbar spine fusion, attaining a solid interbody arthrodesis through the intravertebral disc space has distinct biomechanical advantages when compared to intertransverse or posterolateral fusions [4]. The advantages of interbody fusions include increased surface area for fusion to occur, the ability to restore and/or maintain foraminal height, and the ability to restore segmental lordosis across the fused segment [4]. Restoration of disc space height through placement of structural interbody grafts increases foraminal size which allows for indirect neural decompression [5, 6]. The posterior lumbar interbody fusion (PLIF) and transforaminal lumbar interbody fusion (TLIF) are effective techniques for lumbar interbody fusion via a posterior-only approach, and each technique has distinct advantages and disadvantages [3, 4, 7]. The purpose of this chapter will be to describe our technique for performing a transforaminal lumbar interbody fusion in a step-by-step fashion. We will discuss important technical considerations as well as specific techniques for complication avoidance.

First described by Cloward in 1953, the posterior lumbar interbody fusion (PLIF) involves placing two grafts on either side of the interbody space after a wide laminectomy and partial facetectomy [8]. The pars interarticularis is preserved in the traditional PLIF operation, and graft placement is carried out through a direct posterior approach which is limited by the amount the thecal sac can be retracted to either side. A traditional PLIF requires retraction of the thecal sac and nerve roots to gain sufficient access to the posterior disc space through the spinal canal which increases the risks of incidental durotomy and/or injury to the traversing nerve roots [3].

The transforaminal lumbar interbody fusion (TLIF) is a modification of the PLIF that approaches the disc space from a more lateral-to-medial transforaminal corridor [9] (Fig. 20.1). This lateral trajectory is created by a more extensive facetectomy including an osteotomy with complete removal of the pars interarticularis and its subjacent inferior articular facet. The lateral-to-medial trajectory with TLIF has several

R.F. Heary, MD (✉) • J.C. Quinn, MD
Department of Neurological Surgery, New Jersey Medical School, Rutgers, The State University of New Jersey, 90 Bergen Street – Suite 8100, Newark, NJ 07103, USA
e-mail: heary@njms.rutgers.edu; quinnj1719@gmail.com

L.T. Holly, P.A. Anderson (eds.), *Essentials of Spinal Stabilization*,
DOI 10.1007/978-3-319-59713-3_20

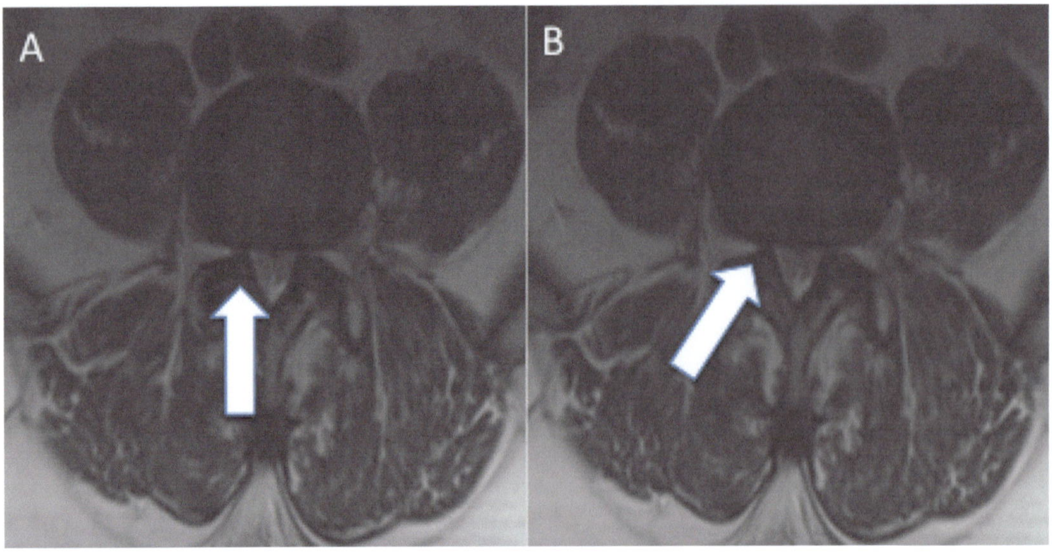

Fig. 20.1 Operative corridor PLIF versus TLIF. An axial T2-weighted MR at the L4–L5 disc space demonstrating the operative corridor for intervertebral disc space access during PLIF and TLIF. (**a**) The operative corridor during PLIF is more medial due to the intact facet joints and requires retraction of the thecal sac and traversing nerve root to gain access to the disc space. (**b**) TLIF allows for a more lateral-to-medial access to the disc space through removal of the inferior facet and pars interarticularis

advantages over the more direct, medial trajectory with PLIF. These advantages include less retraction of the thecal sac and the traversing nerve roots, a decreased in the risk of an incidental durotomy or nerve root injury, and the ability to fit a larger interbody graft compared with the PLIF technique [5, 10]. In the setting of a reoperation following prior posterior decompression (laminectomy or laminotomy), epidural scar tissue may limit the ability to mobilize and retract the neural elements. In these cases a transforaminal approach may be advantageous as the lateral-to-medial approach allows for avoidance of midline epidural scar tissue. The original description of the TLIF procedure involved a unilateral facetectomy for unilateral interspace access for discectomy and unilateral graft placement. The contralateral facet was preserved and can be decorticated and used as a fusion surface. Further modifications of the original TLIF to include bilateral medial facetectomies with removal of the pars interarticularis bilaterally or the posterior column osteotomy (chevron or Smith-Petersen osteotomy) have been described. The benefit of the complete posterior column osteotomy is that it allows for a generous bilateral neural decompression and facilitates realignment in both the coronal and sagittal planes. With a complete posterior column release, segmental distraction across the interspace can be applied across the pedicle screws. Distraction across the interspace facilitates an aggressive discectomy and also allows for placement of large lordotic-shaped interbody cages into the anterior half of the disc space. After placement of the interbody cages, posterior compression is applied utilizing the pedicle screws, with the cages acting as fulcrums, allowing for restoration of segmental lordosis [5]. The combination of a posterior column osteotomy with bilateral discectomy and bilateral interbody cage placements has been described and has the advantage of being able to perform a more complete discectomy compared to the unilateral approach [11].

Indications and Patient Selection

Surgical intervention may be indicated for patients with degenerative disc disease that is refractory to conservative management. Previous studies have demonstrated that lumbar fusion surgery is superior to nonoperative treatment in patients with debilitating low back pain and/or radiculopathy that have failed conservative treatment [1]. Fusion is also indicated in patients with lumbar instability and for correction of spinal deformity including symptomatic spondylolisthesis, degenerative scoliosis, and spinal stenosis associated with instability [1, 2, 12]. Circumferential fusions with interbody graft placement have several advantages over posterolateral or intertransverse fusions. These advantages include greater surface area for fusion, restoration of disc space height for additional indirect decompression, and restoration of and/or preservation of segmental lordosis. Recent evidence from the spine deformity literature demonstrates the importance of global and regional alignment on patient outcomes. Inadequate restoration of lordosis or loss of lordosis through these segments can have a dramatic effect on the overall lumbar lordosis, which can impact sagittal alignment, patient outcomes, and need for revision surgery. Not restoring adequate lumbar lordosis during lumbar fusion may result in mechanical low back pain, sagittal malalignment, and increased risk of adjacent segment degeneration. Several short-term studies comparing posterolateral fusions to interbody techniques including TLIF have not reported a dramatic difference in short term outcomes. The ability to restore segmental lordosis with TLIF is a distinct advantage over PLF and may result in more durable long-term outcomes.

When an interbody fusion is considered, it is mandatory that an extensive trial of nonoperative treatment has been attempted. At a minimum, we encourage a trial of physical therapy as well as the use of epidural injections. The great majority of patients can benefit from optimizing their body weight (which frequently involves an attempt at dieting) as well as attempting to strengthen midsections using core strengthening exercise programs. In addition, alternative approaches, which may include chiropractic treatment, acupuncture, and biofeedback, can be attempted. Only after failure of nonoperative treatment attempts for a minimum period of 6 months should an interbody fusion surgery be considered or offered to the patient. It is noteworthy that the majority of patients can avoid surgical intervention with a comprehensive conservative treatment regimen. Advanced radiographic imaging studies are reserved for those patients who have failed conservative treatments. If the imaging studies concur with the clinical scenario, then an interbody fusion surgery may be considered.

Preoperative Considerations

Preoperative planning should include preoperative anteroposterior (AP) and lateral standing 36-in. radiographs and flexion/extension lateral radiographs of the lumbosacral spine. A magnetic resonance imaging (MRI) or a computed tomography (CT) myelogram is routinely obtained to assist with understanding, complementing, and comparing the anatomy reflected on the radiographs and to assess the severity and anatomic location of stenosis. These studies will serve to better plan the surgical approach regarding side, pedicle size and orientation, nerve root location, and disc space height. If unilateral facetectomy is planned, this should always be performed on the most symptomatic side unless contraindicated. In very specific cases of discogenic pain, discography may be useful in determining the level of the pain generator; the clinician ordering this study must follow very selective criteria due to its controversial utility.

Relative contraindications include severe osteoporosis and active infections. Anatomic variations encountered during surgery including conjoined nerve roots or the presence of a high takeoff of the traversing nerve root may limit access to the disc space from the transforaminal approach. If a safe corridor cannot be created with mobilization of the neural elements, a contralateral approach should be considered.

Surgical Technique

Patient Positioning

Under general anesthesia, the patient is placed on a radiolucent Jackson table in the prone position. It is essential to extend the hips fully to allow the lumbar spine to achieve maximum lordosis [13]. Any hip flexion can be associated with kyphotic angulation of the lumbar spine and may predispose to the development of flat-back syndrome and adjacent segment disease [14]. Care is taken to position the arms in a 90° extension–90° flexion orientation to prevent any stretch or compression injuries to the peripheral nerves, which can occur during prolonged surgery in the prone position. It is essential to pad all osseous prominences and take precautions to protect the eyes. Placing a soft foam cushion around the periphery of the face avoids any direct pressure on the eyes, and a 10° reverse Trendelenburg position can reduce the risk of postoperative blindness, a rare but debilitating complication. A radiolucent table is used to aid in intraoperative fluoroscopic imaging in both the coronal and sagittal planes.

Incision and Exposure

Before the initial skin incision, the operative site, including both the lumbar spine and the iliac crest regions, is prepared and draped. A preoperative dose of 2 g of cefazolin is administered intravenously, and repeat antibiotic dosing of 1 g every 2 h is given over the course of the surgery. Vancomycin is used in patients with hypersensitivity to penicillin or cephalosporins or those known to be carriers of methicillin-resistant *Staphylococcus aureus*. A standard midline approach is used. After radiographic confirmation of the correct operative level, the deep lumbodorsal fascia is identified and a subperiosteal dissection of the posterior elements is performed. Care is taken to avoid cauterization of the facet joint capsules of the adjacent levels, which will not be included in the fusion procedure. The lateral extent of the exposure includes the transverse processes at each operative level and the sacral alae in cases that extend to the sacrum. When fusing to the sacrum, adequate exposure of the sacral alae is essential as the L5–S1 space is the most difficult level to achieve successful arthrodesis in the lumbar spine. This exposure may require significant retraction of the paraspinal muscles in larger patients. Large Gelpi self-retaining retractors are placed to limit compressive forces on the paraspinal muscles. In addition, these Gelpi retractors work well to allow correct placement of pedicle screws by permitting proper medial and cranial-caudal orientation of instruments during screw placement owing to their smaller footprint within the operative field relative to other retractors commonly used in the posterior lumbar surgery. On an hourly basis, the retractors are released for 90 s; during which time the wound is irrigated with a pulse lavage irrigation system. The retractors are then replaced and the procedure is continued. This maneuver of releasing the retractors and irrigating hourly prevents excessive ischemia of the paraspinal musculature and removes any mechanical debris during prolonged operative procedures.

Decompression

Decompression is undertaken with bilateral removal of the spinous processes, laminae, pars interarticularis, and the inferior facets of the operative levels. In addition, resection of the medial and superior portions of the subjacent superior facets is helpful in limiting neural retraction later in the operation when intervertebral struts are placed. Importantly, a wide foraminotomy is also accomplished by this maneuver. All resected bones are cleaned of soft tissue and morselized and saved for use later in the operation as autologous local bone graft. This aggressive bony decompression provides a generous amount of bone graft material. The exposed ligamentum flavum is completely resected. After decompression, the thecal sac and the exiting and traversing nerve roots are well visualized and widely exposed.

Instrumentation

After decompression, pedicle screws are placed. The superior, medial, and inferior margins of the pedicles are readily palpable at this point which makes placement of the screws easier. Lateral fluoroscopy can be used if any concern exists regarding the optimal entry site or trajectory for the screw placement. The technique for screw placement involves use of a high-speed burr to decorticate the entry site. A pedicle probe or a drill is then placed to help localize the pedicle. After localization of the pedicle, a small tap is used to access the pedicle. A ball-tipped probe is used to confirm that the tapped track has not deviated out of the pedicle or that it has not violated the far vertebral cortex. Based on the preoperative imaging studies, sequentially larger diameter taps can be inserted with a ball-tipped probe used to confirm the adequacy of each tapped track after the larger tap is utilized. Routinely, the largest tap used is one size, or approximately 0.5–1.0 mm, smaller than the screw to be placed. In so doing, the screw purchase and insertional torque are improved [15].

Discectomy

In order to facilitate the discectomy and interbody placement, a temporary rod is placed opposite the side of the planned discectomy and distraction is applied. Use of an offset distraction device on the ipsilateral side may improve access to the disc space while maintaining distraction. With the disc space under distraction, the thecal sac and exiting nerve roots are identified and protected, the disc space is identified, and discectomy is performed. First, the outer annulus fibrosis of the intervertebral disc is incised lateral to the traversing nerve root. If the medial aspect of the subjacent superior facet has been adequately resected, the discectomy can be accomplished with minimal or no retraction of the exiting or the traversing nerve roots. Pituitary rongeurs and bone rasps are used to remove the great majority of disc material from the interspace. Care is taken to preserve the ventral and lateral margins of the annulus to allow the graft material, both structural and morselized, to be contained.

Interbody Graft Placement

In all cases, we use generous amounts of autologous bone graft for both the intervertebral space and the posterolateral gutters. Autogenous iliac crest graft is combined with the previously prepared local autograft bone. Corticocancellous iliac crest autograft may be obtained, through either the same incision or a separate incision, using bone gouges. Recently, we have modified our technique and have started using bone marrow aspirates from the iliac crest. Using a large bore trocar, the bone marrow is aspirated and no incision is necessary. A total of 20 mL of combined blood/bone marrow is removed for processing. This technology allows for concentration of the osteogenic precursor cells which are isolated from the bone marrow. These cells are combined with the previously obtained local bone graft to produce a generous amount of fusion substrate bone for later grafting. The fusion substrate bone is packed within radiolucent, carbon-fiber reinforced PEEK cages (CFRP cages; DePuy Synthes Spine). In our current technique, after a thorough discectomy, autologous morselized graft is packed into the ventral aspect of the disc space.

A custom-made funnel is positioned through the discectomy defect into the ventral disc space. The morselized graft material is then introduced through this funnel into the ventral disc space. After this is completed, two carbon fiber cages are packed with the morselized graft material. These cages are radiolucent except for tantalum beads which are embedded in the extremes of the cage and allow fluoroscopic confirmation of cage placement. The cages have a lordotic sagittal contour with the anterior surface at least 2 mm taller than the posterior surface. These cages are designed to be inserted straight or in a slight oblique manner to allow for lordosis restoration when posterior compression is applied. A variety of cage heights, lengths, and widths are available, and the appropriate sizing is based on the preoperative neuroimaging studies and the intraoperative clinical impression. The cages are impacted bilaterally so that the dorsal most aspect of each cage is countersunk 2 mm ventral to the dorsal

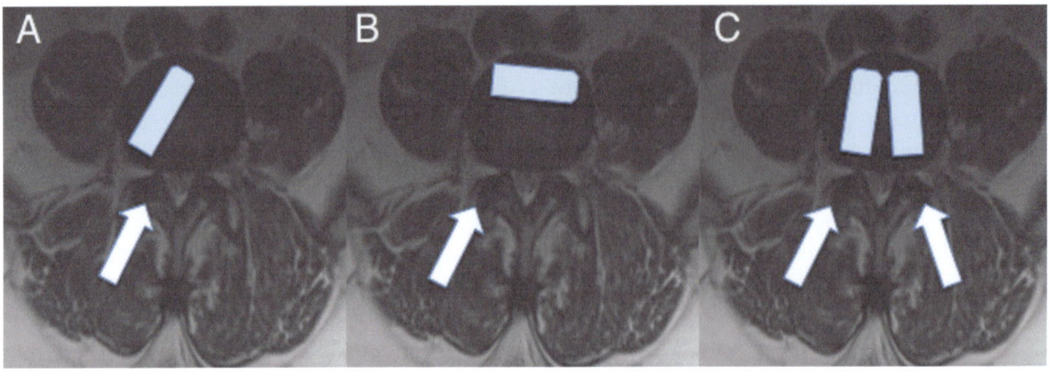

Fig. 20.2 Techniques for graft placement during TLIF. An axial T2-weighted MR at the L4–L5 disc space demonstrating different approaches for placement of intervertebral cages when performing a TLIF. Straight cages may be placed in a diagonal fashion across the disc space to maximize disc space height restoration (**a**). Alternatively cages may be placed horizontally across the anterior 1/3 of the disc space which when combined with segmental compression acts as a fulcrum for restoration of segmental lordosis (**b**). Bilateral TLIF cages may be placed after bilateral facetectomies (**c**)

margin of the vertebral bodies above and below (Fig. 20.2). In cases of spondylolisthesis, a cage of shorter depth is used. Additional morselized graft is placed between the cages if there is space available. By resecting the medial aspects of the subjacent superior facets, manipulation of the thecal sac and nerve roots is kept to a minimum. A nerve root retractor may be used to protect the thecal sac, though, often, there is no need to retract neural structures. Throughout the cage impaction process, all neural structures are directly visualized and gently protected.

After placement of the interbody struts has been completed, the epidural space is inspected to assure that no bone fragments have been deposited into the spinal canal inadvertently. At this point, we copiously irrigate the wound with 3 L of warm normal saline to remove mechanical debris and assist with hemostasis.

Posterolateral Fusion

Attention is now directed to the lateral gutters. Generous amounts of morselized autograft are placed over the decorticated transverse processes and sacral alae. This is performed before connecting the pedicle screws together to allow for the bone to be in direct apposition to the exposed donor sites.

Rod Placement

After placement of the lateral fusion bone, the screws are connected to each other with either plates or rods. When possible, plates are preferentially used for shorter constructs. The plates or rods are contoured in the sagittal plane to achieve a lumbar lordosis. When rods are used, cross-connectors may be attached to each rod to aid in achieving rotational stability. If necessary for alignment and if the bone is of adequate density, compression of the screws posteriorly can be performed to improve the extent of lordosis able to be obtained. Following placement of the instrumentation, biplanar radiographs are obtained using fluoroscopy.

Closure

At this point, care is taken to achieve meticulous hemostasis. Particular attention is directed to the epidural venous structures to confirm control of any bleeding sites. Depending on surgeon preference, suction drains may be placed at this time. For single-level fusions, closure is most often performed without drain placement; in multilevel cases, drains are used routinely. When used, the drains are routinely brought out through two separate stab wounds in the skin. Drains remain in place until output decreases to less than 50 mL over a 24-h period. Vancomycin powder (1 gm or 2 gms) can be placed into the lateral gutters covering the graft material and the metallic instrumentation in an attempt to limit the likelihood of developing a postoperative wound infection. Standard wound closure is performed in layers.

Illustrative Case

History

A 59-year-old male with a history of progressive mechanical back pain, lumbar stenosis with neurogenic claudication, and bilateral L5 radiculopathies. Extensive conservative management had been attempted without improvement. These therapies included multiple epidural steroid injections and several courses of both land-based physical therapy and aquatic physical therapy.

Physical Examination

On physical examination the patient demonstrated normal posture and gait. He was able to toe and heel walk without difficulty. His lower extremity motor strength exam was symmetric; 5/5 in hip flexion, knee extension, ankle dorsiflexion, and plantar flexion; and 4+/5 in extensor hallucis longus. His sensory exam was notable for paresthesias in an L5 distribution bilaterally, and his lower extremity reflexes were diminished +1 and symmetric.

Imaging

Plain radiographs and magnetic resonance (MR) imaging showed significant disc degeneration which was greatest at the L4–L5 and L5–S1 levels with loss of disc height and severe L4–L5 and L5–S1 lateral recess and foraminal stenoses as well as a low-grade degenerative spondylolisthesis at L4–L5.

Treatment

Given the significant disc height loss causing severe foraminal stenosis, as well as the degenerative spondylolisthesis at L4–L5, a two-level TLIF was offered to decompress the nerve roots, stabilize the L4–L5 and L5–S1 interspaces, restore the disc space heights, and attempt to restore the segmental lordosis across the L4–S1 segments (Figs. 20.3 and 20.4).

Outcome

The patient tolerated the procedure well with an immediate improvement in his radicular leg pain. At 6-month follow-up, the patient reported a dramatic improvement in his back and leg pain and was able to ambulate over a mile pain free. His motor strength improved to 5/5 in all muscle groups with mild residual paresthesias in the right L5 distribution.

Technical Pearls

- TLIF can be a powerful tool for restoration of segmental lordosis. This can be achieved by performing a posterior column osteotomy (chevron or Smith-Petersen osteotomy) followed by compression across the segment. This is facilitated by anterior placement of the interbody cages which acts as a fulcrum when compression is applied across the segment.
- Cages with lordotic shapes are used to maintain or restore sagittal plane alignment. In addition, the large degree of bony decompression allows the application of compressive, lordotic forces if needed to correct or maintain sagittal plane alignment.
- The placement of large bilateral, lordotic interbody grafts is both structurally robust and biomechanically advantageous for posterior column compression and the subsequent restoration of sagittal plane alignment. In addition, utilizing large quantities of autograft bone in the disc spaces, in and between the

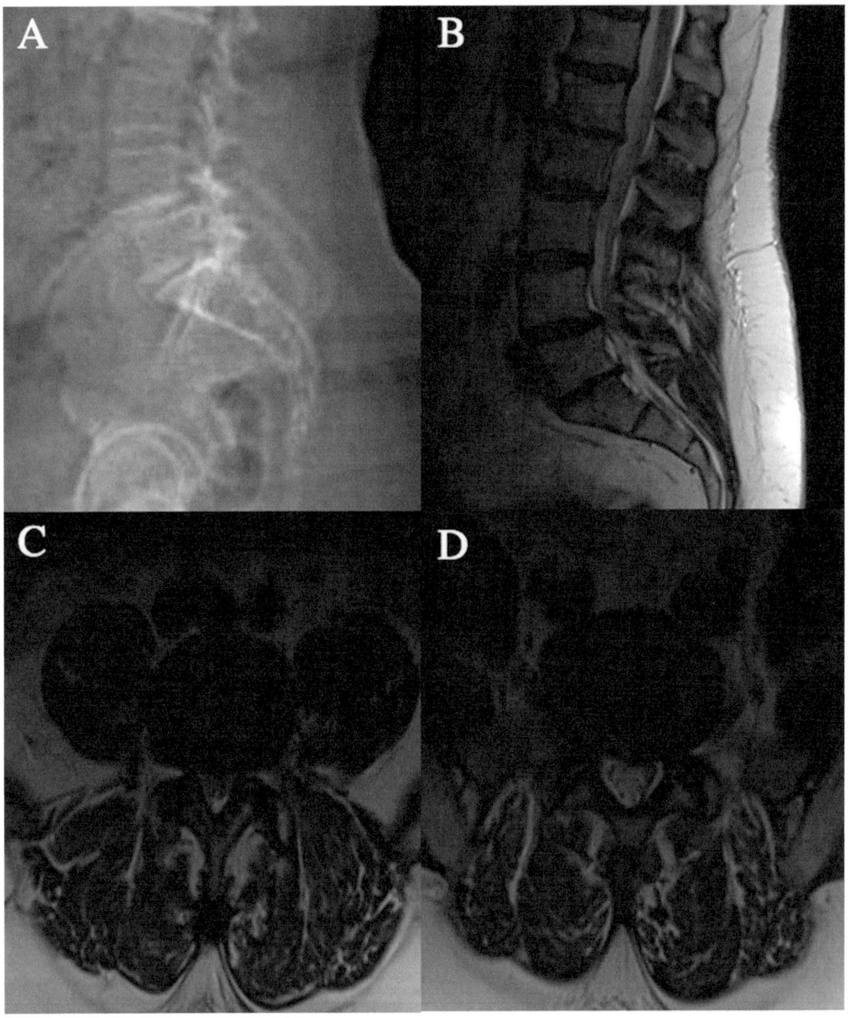

Fig. 20.3 Case example preoperative imaging. A lateral radiograph (**a**) and sagittal (**b**) and axial MR of the L4–L5 (**c**) and L5–S1 (**d**) disc space demonstrate an L4–L5 degenerative spondylolisthesis with significant bilateral foraminal stenosis at L4–L5 and L5–S1

cages, and in the lateral gutters is ideal for achieving stable arthrodesis.

- A variety of interbody cages of different design made of different materials have been developed. Some options include titanium mesh cages, wedged structural allograft, threaded cylindrical cages, banana-shaped cages, and straight cages.
- Straight cages are typically inserted in an oblique fashion. Lordosis restoration using straight cages relies the anterior height of the cage being larger than the posterior height. Use of banana cages with a rotatable inserter allows for the ability to "steer" the implant into a horizontal position along the anterior portion of the disc space. With posterior compression the cage acts as a fulcrum and allows for a greater degree of segmental lordosis.
- Careful, meticulous end plate preparation is critical to achieve interspace fusion. Avoid violation of end plate during discectomy to prevent graft subsidence which may lead to loss of indirect decompression.

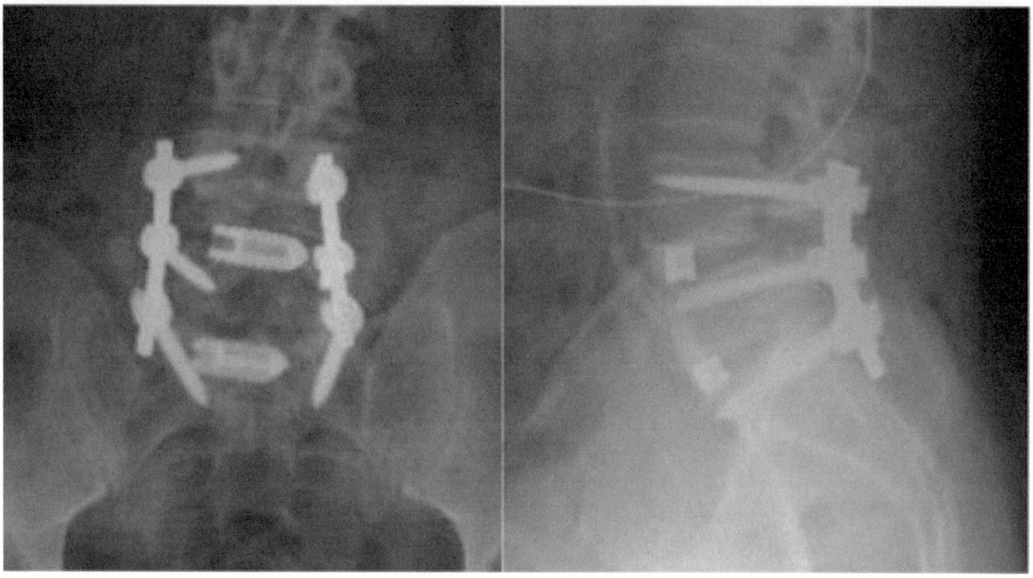

Fig. 20.4 Case example postoperative imaging. Postoperative AP (**a**) and lateral (**b**) radiographs following L4–L5 and L5–S1 TLIFs. Complete posterior column osteotomies were performed at each level; discectomy and cage placement were performed from the right side at both levels. Titanium cages were placed into the anterior third of the disc spaces at each level followed by compression across these segments allowing for a restoration of segmental lordosis across the L4–S1 segments

Complications and Strategies for Avoidance

TLIF has been shown to be a safe and effective technique for lumbar spine fusion. Complication rates for single-level TLIF are relatively low with fusion rates of greater than 90% for single-level procedures. Rates of transient neurological deficit in the range of 2–7% have been reported [16–18]. Care should be taken to identify and protect all neural structures during discectomy and interbody placement to avoid inadvertent injury. Following interbody grafting the neural foramen should be palpated with blunt probe to ensure there is no residual compression of the exiting nerve. There have been reports of the development of contralateral radicular pain symptoms following unilateral TLIF. It is hypothesized that with compression and lordosis correction, there is risk for increased foraminal stenosis when a facetectomy is not completed. Care must be taken to evaluate both foramen on the preoperative MRI regardless of which side the symptoms are on.

Hardware complications from misplaced pedicle screws are relatively rare with an incidence of less than 5% in most studies. Cage migration rates have been reported as high as 8% without posterior instrumentation. This is a rare complication with the additional stabilization afforded by segmental pedicle screw instrumentation, which allows for compression across the interspace after graft placement. Appropriate sizing of interbody graft, preservation of the anterior annulus, and proper placement within the anterior 1/3 of the interspace graft migration are important in limiting the rates of graft migration. Graft subsidence may occur and result in loss of correction, loss of indirect decompression, and hardware failure. Factors predisposing to subsidence include inadequate graft technique, sizing, end plate violation during discectomy, and patient factors such as osteoporosis. Biomechanical load-sharing properties of the interbody graft are predicated on the bony stability of intact end plates. Fracture or violation of the end plate during the procedure may result in subsidence. To minimize this risk, particular care must be taken to appreciate the sagittal orientation of the end plates with intraoperative imaging and to maintain the trajectory of the instruments parallel to this orientation.

Vascular injury during TLIF, though rare, is a potentially catastrophic complication that all surgeons must be aware of. Violation of the anterior annulus may result in inadvertent entry into the retroperitoneum with either an instrument or an implant, which may lead to catastrophe because of the nearby location of the large vessels. During preparation of the disc space, implant placement, the surgeon must maintain direct visualization of the working space. Intraoperative fluoroscopy may be used to confirm location of instruments during discectomy and during placement of the interbody grafts to ensure the anterior annulus is not violated. If there is a decline in hemodynamics stability at any point after beginning the discectomy, the potential of a vascular injury must be considered.

Conclusion

The transforaminal lumbar interbody fusion (TLIF) is a safe and versatile procedure and can be used to treat a number of degenerative conditions in the lumbar spine. The transforaminal corridor has advantages over other direct posterior approaches in that it provides direct access to the disc space and lateral recess with minimal retraction of neural elements through a lateral-to-medial trajectory. TLIF allows for excellent fusion rates, the ability to provide indirect decompression and restore segmental lordosis with relatively low complication rates.

References

1. Madigan L, Vaccaro AR, Spector LR, Milam RA. Management of symptomatic lumbar degenerative disk disease. J Am Acad Orthop Surg. 2009;17(2):102–11.
2. Eismont FJ, Norton RP, Hirsch BP. Surgical management of lumbar degenerative spondylolisthesis. J Am Acad Orthop Surg. 2014;22(4):203–13.
3. Humphreys SC, Hodges SD, Patwardhan AG, Eck JC, Murphy RB, Covington LA. Comparison of posterior and transforaminal approaches to lumbar interbody fusion. Spine (Phila Pa 1976). 2001;26(5):567–71.
4. Ames CP, Acosta FL Jr, Chi J, Iyengar J, Muiru W, Acaroglu E, et al. Biomechanical comparison of posterior lumbar interbody fusion and transforaminal lumbar interbody fusion performed at 1 and 2 levels. Spine (Phila Pa 1976). 2005;30(19):E562–6.
5. Jagannathan J, Sansur CA, Oskouian RJ Jr, Fu KM, Shaffrey CI. Radiographic restoration of lumbar alignment after transforaminal lumbar interbody fusion. Neurosurgery. 2009;64(5):955–63. discussion 63–4
6. Harris BM, Hilibrand AS, Savas PE, Pellegrino A, Vaccaro AR, Siegler S, et al. Transforaminal lumbar interbody fusion: the effect of various instrumentation techniques on the flexibility of the lumbar spine. Spine (Phila Pa 1976). 2004;29(4):E65–70.
7. Heary RF, Bono CM. Circumferential fusion for spondylolisthesis in the lumbar spine. Neurosurg Focus. 2002;13(1):E3.
8. Cloward RB. The treatment of ruptured lumbar intervertebral discs; criteria for spinal fusion. Am J Surg. 1953;86(2):145–51.
9. Harms J, Rolinger H. A one-stager procedure in operative treatment of spondylolistheses: dorsal traction-reposition and anterior fusion (author's transl). Z Orthop Ihre Grenzgeb. 1982;120(3):343–7.
10. Hackenberg L, Halm H, Bullmann V, Vieth V, Schneider M, Liljenqvist U. Transforaminal lumbar interbody fusion: a safe technique with satisfactory three to five year results. Eur Spine J. 2005;14(6):551–8.
11. Heary RF, Kumar S, Karimi RJ. Dorsal lumbar interbody fusion for chronic axial, mechanical low back pain: a modification of two established techniques. Neurosurgery. 2008;63(1 Suppl 1):ONS102–6. discussion ONS6–7
12. Awad JN, Moskovich R. Lumbar disc herniations: surgical versus nonsurgical treatment. Clin Orthop Relat Res. 2006;443:183–97.
13. Peterson MD, Nelson LM, McManus AC, Jackson RP. The effect of operative position on lumbar lordosis. A radiographic study of patients under anesthesia in the prone and 90–90 positions. Spine (Phila Pa 1976). 1995;20(12):1419–24.
14. Potter BK, Lenke LG, Kuklo TR. Prevention and management of iatrogenic flatback deformity. J Bone Joint Surg Am. 2004;86-A(8):1793–808.
15. Kuklo TR, Lehman RA Jr. Effect of various tapping diameters on insertion of thoracic pedicle screws: a biomechanical analysis. Spine (Phila Pa 1976). 2003;28(18):2066–71.
16. Hee HT, Castro FP Jr, Majd ME, Holt RT, Myers L. Anterior/posterior lumbar fusion versus transforaminal lumbar interbody fusion: analysis of complications and predictive factors. J Spinal Disord. 2001;14(6):533–40.

17. Villavicencio AT, Burneikiene S, Bulsara KR, Thramann JJ. Perioperative complications in transforaminal lumbar interbody fusion versus anterior-posterior reconstruction for lumbar disc degeneration and instability. J Spinal Disord Tech. 2006;19(2):92–7.

18. Potter BK, Freedman BA, Verwiebe EG, Hall JM, Polly DW Jr, Kuklo TR. Transforaminal lumbar interbody fusion: clinical and radiographic results and complications in 100 consecutive patients. J Spinal Disord Tech. 2005;18(4):337–46.

21 Percutaneous Spinal Fixation

Ken Hsuan-kan Chang, David McCarthy, and Michael Y. Wang

Introduction

Pedicle screw fixation has been utilized for the surgical management of thoracolumbar spinal deformities, degenerative disease, and trauma since the middle 1980s [1]. Pedicle screw fixation creates a rigid construct, establishing a stable spine among destabilizing spinal pathologies, and further facilitates the process of bone fusion after fixation. Initially, pedicle screw fixation was performed as an open procedure; however, as surgical techniques evolved, a minimally invasive percutaneous screw fixation approach has developed in the last two decades.

Overall, both open screw fixation and percutaneous screw fixation approaches result in similar radiographic and clinical outcomes [2, 3]. In the twenty-first century, there has been increased interest in percutaneous spinal fixation due to its less invasive nature, technological advances in devices and imaging, less radiation exposure, and shorter procedure time. Many physicians that were initially trained in the open screw fixation approach are starting to embrace percutaneous screw fixation nowadays. As surgical techniques and devices continue to advance, percutaneous screw fixation is also being adapted for spine deformity and robotic surgery and has demonstrated the ability to achieve an equivalent outcome.

In this chapter, percutaneous pedicle screw (PPS), facet screw, and iliac screw fixation protocol are described. This chapter will detail the indications/contraindications, preoperative considerations, surgical technique, outcomes, complications, and new technology for these procedure.

Two-Dimensional Image Considerations (C-arm)

The major breakthrough for the development of the percutaneous technique was the recognition and utilization of image guidance when it comes to pedicle screw fixation. Fluoroscopy-guided method is by far the most common technique adopted by spine surgeons in regard to percutaneous screw placement. Unlike open surgery, the bony landmarks and relative anatomy cannot be identified through direct visualization in the percutaneous technique. Thus, the entire percutaneous screw placement process relies heavily on a series of intraoperative fluoroscopic images. Satisfactory intraoperative fluoroscopic imaging

K.H.-k. Chang, MD • D. McCarthy, BS
M.Y. Wang, MD, FACS (✉)
Department of Neurological Surgery and Rehabilitation Medicine, University of Miami Miller School of Medicine, Lois Pope Life Center, 1095 Northwest 14th Terrace, Miami, FL 33136, USA
e-mail: mwang2@med.miami.edu

L.T. Holly, P.A. Anderson (eds.), *Essentials of Spinal Stabilization*,
DOI 10.1007/978-3-319-59713-3_21

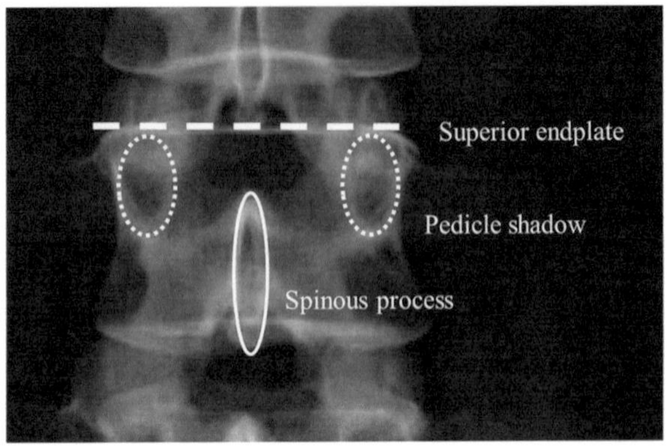

Fig. 21.1 Illustration of the critical anatomic landmarks on a true AP image

is imperative for successful percutaneous screw placement in minimally invasive (MIS) spine surgery. A radiological technician is the main person that operates the C-arm during a surgery, although the spine surgeon is responsible for training the technicians and collaborating with them during percutaneous screw placement. Therefore, a surgeon must have the capability to recognize the adequate two-dimensional images acquired by C-arm fluoroscopy.

The primary obstacle for intraoperative fluoroscopy is obtaining a clear image with properly aligned bony structures. A distorted image is usually caused by malalignment of the bone structure, in this case, the target vertebrae. Image distortion can easily mislead the surgeon, resulting in misplacement of the percutaneous screw in surgery. To avoid image distortion, the fluoroscope should be manipulated to a certain position and angle in which the X-ray beam from the source lies perpendicular to the vertebrae of interest. The optimal image may be difficult to capture under certain circumstances, such as deformity, osteoporosis, obesity, abnormal anatomy, or revision surgery, etc.

A true anteroposterior (AP) fluoroscopic image is the first step and might be the most useful image when performing K-wire cannulation for PPS (Fig. 21.1). Lateral fluoroscopic image is usually the second step and allows the surgeon to examine if the guidewire and Jamshidi needle are in an appropriate place inside the pedicle and vertebral body. The optimal image can be achieved with several aids. First, the target vertebrae should be placed in the center of the image. Peripherally placed vertebrae will generate a parallax phenomenon. In a true AP image, the C-arm needs to be adjusted to an angle that makes the superior endplate of the target vertebrae parallel to the central X-ray beam. Therefore, the superior endplate can appear as one single superimposed line. The pedicle should appear as two oval shadows just caudal and lateral to the single superimposed line of superior endplate (Fig. 21.1). The spinous process has to be in the true midline of the rectangle image of vertebrae to complete a true AP image (Fig. 21.2). In a lateral view, the superior endplate as well as the anterior and posterior border of the target vertebrae should appear as single superimposed lines to avoid malrotation of the fluoroscopic image. The superior and inferior borders of the pedicle shadow need to be superimposed while performing lateral fluoroscopy.

The pivotal pearl of the percutaneous technique is to always perform the whole procedure under well-aligned fluoroscopic images. The interpretation and knowledge of the fluoroscopic images are essential for minimally invasive spine surgery.

Indications and Contraindications

Percutaneous screw fixation is indicated in minimally invasive surgery for cases of instability in degenerative disease, thoracolumbar trauma, infection, and neoplasia [4]. The cannulation technique can also be applied for vertebroplasty/kyphoplasty and vertebral body biopsy. PPS may be advantageous in comparison to open procedures for obese patients since the approach and soft tissue dissection are often more significant in such cases. In theory, percutaneous techniques avoid

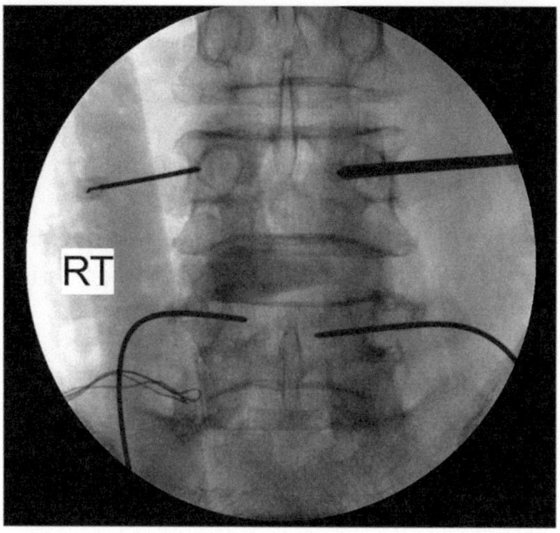

Fig. 21.2 An adequate anteroposterior (AP) fluoroscopic image for L4, undergoing Jamshidi needle cannulation. L5 is already cannulated with a K-wire. The shadow of superior endplate of L4 is superimposed. The pedicle shadow is clear and just caudal to the superior endplate. The spinous process is centered at the midline

the extensive dissection of an open procedure, in return reducing the rate of wound infection, intraoperative blood loss, total operative time, and postoperative pain [5].

A contraindication of PPS placement is the absence of high-quality intraoperative fluoroscopic images. It is unsafe to perform the percutaneous procedure if anatomic landmarks are unable to be identified on fluoroscopic imaging. The situation may be encountered in patients with obesity, osteoporosis, spine deformity, and congenital abnormality or with inexperienced surgeons and C-arm technicians. In these situations, navigated image guidance or robotic screw placement is another option.

Surgical Technique

Percutaneous Pedicle Screw

The patient is almost always positioned prone for percutaneous pedicle screw (PPS) placement, although lateral position is sometimes adopted if PPS procedure follows a lateral lumbar interbody fusion. A radiolucent table, like the Jackson table or Allen table, is mandatory for PPS placement because intraoperative AP fluoroscopic images

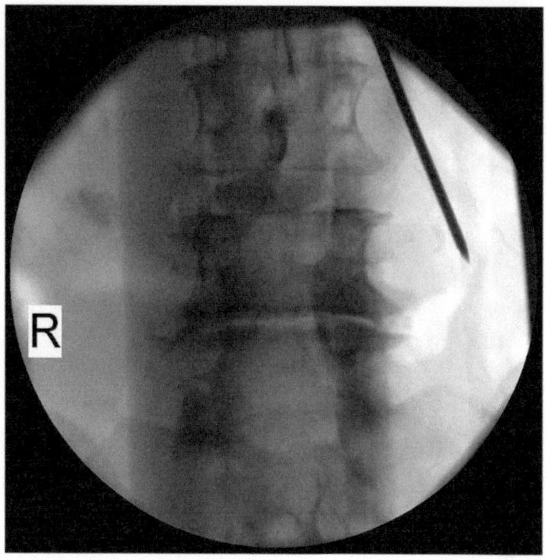

Fig. 21.3 The tip of the needle is placed laterally to the lateral border of the pedicle shadow to estimate the appropriate entry point for the Jamshidi needle on the skin

are required. The true AP image technique is most commonly used for cannulation of the K-wire in a PPS procedure.

A well-centered AP image for target vertebrae is checked and is the first and most important step for PPS placement. Marking the midline can help the X-ray technician to properly center the X-ray beam repeatably. Jamshidi needles are often used for cannulation of the K-wire. The tip of the needle can be placed laterally to the lateral border of the pedicle shadow before skin incision (Fig. 21.3). This allows estimation of appropriate entry point for Jamshidi needles on the skin under fluoroscopy. The distance between the needle tip and the lateral border of pedicle is approximately 1 centimeter (cm), but may vary depending on individual patient conditions such as obesity, muscularity, body habitus, etc. A 1.5 cm incision through the skin and fascia is sufficient for Jamshidi needle and screw insertion. Finger palpation of surface bony landmarks may also facilitate or enhance recognition of the vertebral body anatomy. Simultaneous placement of the Jamshidi needle on both sides can save time and reduce radiation dose.

Jamshidi needles should dock on the junction between the transverse process and the lateral border of the facet joint. On AP image, the needle tip would appear to be placed at the lateral border of the oval shadow of pedicle. The shaft of the

Jamshidi needle is then adjusted to maintain parallel position with the superior endplate on AP image. The Jamshidi needle is then advanced into the pedicle bone for 2 cm in a proper angle such that the tip will not breach the medial wall of the pedicle (Fig. 21.4) [6]. The ideal trajectory of the Jamshidi needle on AP image is toward the medial border of the oval shadow of pedicle. The position of the beveled tip will have an influence on the direction of needle advancement. If the bevel is in the lateral position, the needle will tend to advance in a more slightly medial pathway due to the force vector. In the contrary, the needle will tend to move forward in a more lateral pathway when the bevel is positioned medially. The surgeon can manipulate the bevel position to gain a more desirable location of the needle tip during its advancement. After 2 cm of advancement, an AP image is obtained to show that position for the needle tip is just lateral to the medial border of the pedicle shadow and the needle shaft parallel to the superior endplate (Fig. 21.5).

The C-arm is then rotated to take lateral fluoroscopic images. An aforementioned superimposed line of superior and posterior border of vertebrae is critical to certify the bony structure is well-aligned. Once an optimal image is obtained, the tip of Jamshidi needle should be very close to the base of the pedicle. The K-wire is then introduced through the Jamshidi needle into the cancellous bone of the vertebral body. We recommend to advance the K-wire tip to the anterior half of the vertebral body on the lateral view. It is important to avoid penetration of the anterior cortex with the K-wire (Fig. 21.6).

The Jamshidi needle is then removed without displacing the K-wire. It is important to palpate the bottom of the K-wire and make sure it is inside the bone of the vertebral body. The pedicle bone and part of the posterior half of vertebral body is tapped over the K-wire (Fig. 21.7). Then, the cannulated screw is inserted through the guidewire in a usual manner. The tapping and the screw insertion should follow the trajectory of the guidewire (Fig. 21.8). Excessive bending of the guidewire during the tapping or screw insertion may result in the unfavorable complication of breakage and retention of the K-wire inside the bone.

After all the screws are placed, the percutaneous rod is passed. The proper rod length is selected, and the rod is bent as required to correct any angular deformities. It is important to pass

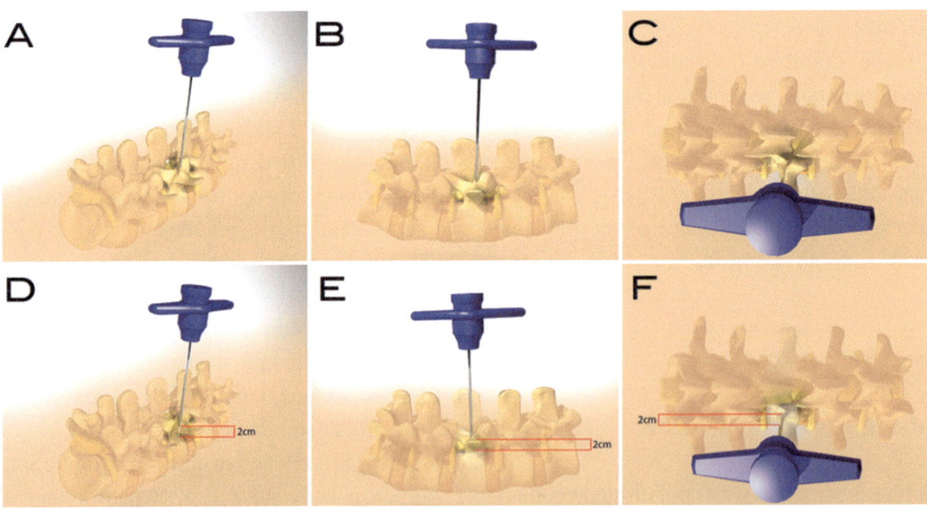

Fig. 21.4 Illustration for the true AP technique. A Jamshidi needle is docked on the bony surface at the junction of the lateral border of the facet joint and transverse process (**a**, oblique view; **b**, lateral view; and **c**, AP view). The needle is then advanced into the pedicle bone for 2 cm. The needle tip should not pass the medial border of the pedicle shadow under AP image (**d**, oblique view; **e**, lateral view; and **f**, AP view) (Adapted from Ref. [6])

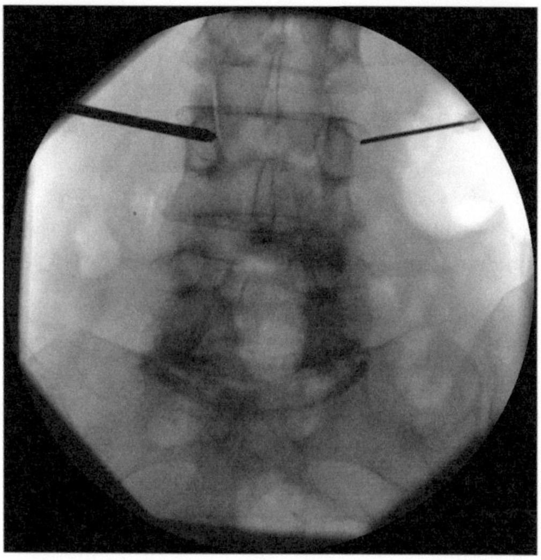

Fig. 21.5 The position of Jamshidi needle during cannulation. On the right side of the image, a small diameter needle is pointing at the 3 o'clock position of the pedicle, the ideal entry point. On the left side of the image, the tip of the Jamshidi needle already reaches the medial border of the pedicle shadow after 2 cm of advancement. This is the ideal end point for the needle tip

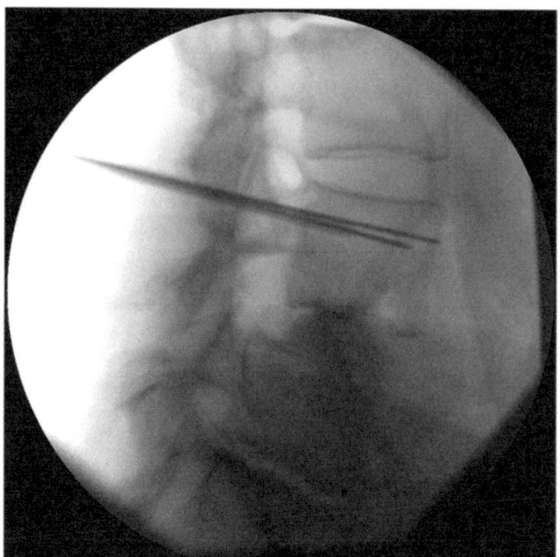

Fig. 21.6 The lateral view of K-wire cannulation

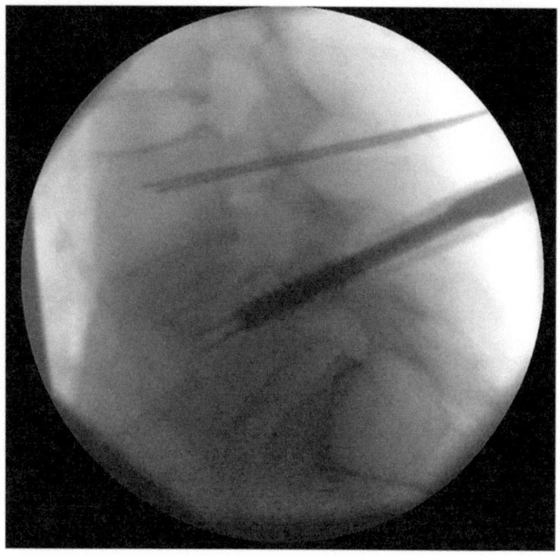

Fig. 21.7 The tapping of the pedicle bone and vertebral body along the axis of K-wire

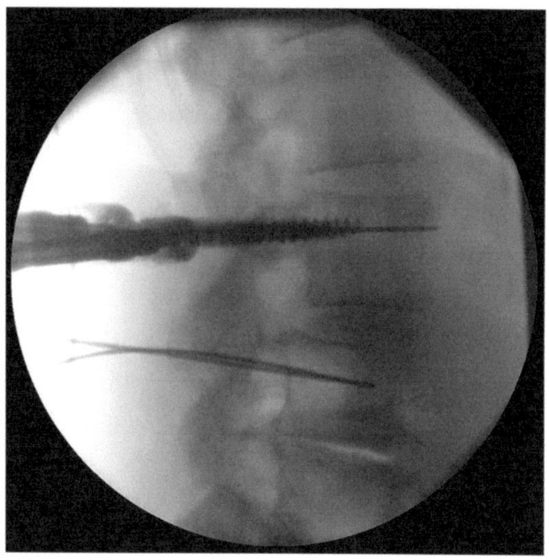

Fig. 21.8 Percutaneous screw insertion following the trajectory of the K-wire

the rod as deeply as possible so as to minimize the amount of muscle compressed underneath it (Fig. 21.9). There are several different methods to pass the rod depending on the system used. One of the common systems adopts a swinging arm rod inserter which swings the rod in through a geometrically constrained arc. In another system, the rod insertion is done through one of the percutaneous skin incisions under the muscular fascia with direct vision. In other circumstances, the rod passage for multilevel and deformity cases can be challenging but is out of the scope for this chapter. The set screws are then inserted and torqued as recommended by the manufacturer. If required, extension tabs are broken off.

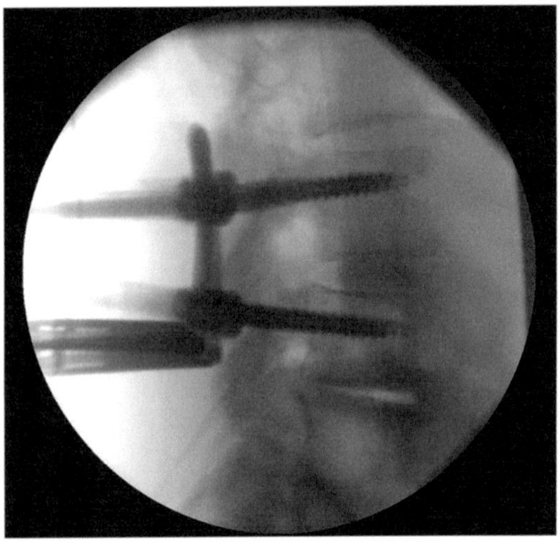

Fig. 21.9 Placement of the rods in the screw heads

Final AP and lateral X-rays are taken to ensure the construct is in proper place. In traditional open-pedicle screw insertion, stimulus-evoked electromyography (EMG) has been applied for the detection of screw breach and is considered a useful method to reduce the rate of screw misplacement. However, the utilization of EMG on percutaneous pedicle screw with insulated sleeve does not seem to be as reliable as it is in open cases. Using a typical stimulation threshold (<12 mA), the ability of detecting low-grade breached screw is low in percutaneous setting [7]. In our opinion, intraoperative imaging remains a more reliable assessment than EMG for percutaneous pedicle screw.

Alternative Targeting Methods

If the true AP technique is not feasible or the image quality is poor, an owl's eye image may be an alternative method. The owl's eye image, a.k.a. En face view, involves aligning the view directly with the long axis of the pedicle [8]. The owl's eye image is obtained by starting with an AP image, adjusting the sagittal angle, and centering on target vertebrae and then rotating the C-arm on the axial plane to align with the pedicle (Fig. 21.10). When the ideal view of the owl's eye image is achieved, the superior endplate shadows should be superimposed and the superior articular facet aligned properly with the medial border of the pedicle. The skin incision should be made directly over the projected image of the pedicle. Since the cannulation of the K-wire is parallel to the pedicle and X-ray beam, the wire usually appears as one spot on the owl's eye image. The depth of the cannulation is determined before surgery by measuring on the preoperative CAT scan or MRI. The process of tapping and screw insertion is similar to aforementioned AP image procedure. The owl's eye approach requires that the right and left pedicles at any given level be targeted independently.

The mini-open technique involves exposure of the pedicle screw entry site by splitting the paraspinal muscles and using an expandable tubular retractor to aid visualization. This method is most appropriate for short segment (one or two intervertebral discs) PPS placement [10, 11]. After serial muscle dilators and the retractor are set up properly, electrocautery is used to dissect the soft tissue around the facet joint and transverse process. This exposes the bone surface at the junction between transverse process and the lateral border of the facet joint. The junction is the ideal entry point for a gearshift probe or cannulation of guidewire. After the pedicle is probed or cannulated with a guidewire, the following procedure to tap the pedicle and insert the screw is very similar to that of open operation. The mini-open method serves as a well-combination and modification of minimally invasive technique and open screw placement with much less tissue destruction than the traditional open surgery (Fig. 21.11).

Percutaneous Facet Screws

Transfacet screw can be an alternative choice to pedicle screw. Percutaneous facet screws are performed less commonly and have a much shorter track record than pedicle screws. NSR – these screws are popular among some MIS surgeons. As with any percutaneous technique, facet screw placement relies heavily on intraoperative fluoroscopy for guidance. After a small skin incision, for an L4–L5 facet screw, a Jamshidi needle is placed

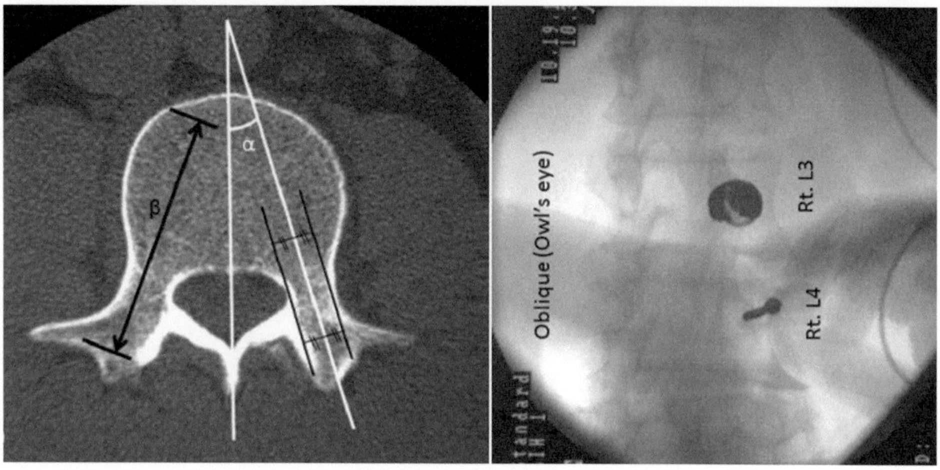

Fig. 21.10 The owl's eye image (*right*) is obtained by starting with an AP image, adjusting the sagittal angle, and centering on target vertebrae and then rotating the C-arm on the axial plane to align with the pedicle (α (angle, *left*) (Adapted from Ref. [9])

on the L4 lamina just medial to the inferior L4 facet. On the AP image, the starting point is at the junction of L4 lower endplate and the medial border of the L5 pedicle. The trajectory should aim toward the lateral tip of the L5 lower endplate on an AP image. On the lateral image, the trajectory should aim for the anterior tip of the L5 lower endplate (Fig. 21.12). Once the trajectory has been set, the Jamshidi needle can be replaced with guidewire or drill guide to establish the tract inside the bone. Then the procedure is followed by a standard percutaneous technique, including a cannulated tap and screws over the guidewire.

Percutaneous Iliac Screws

Besides percutaneous lumbar pedicle and facet screw, the technique of percutaneous iliac screw is also described in this chapter. Fluoroscopy is also used to perform percutaneous iliac screw insertion. The key step is to obtain the "teardrop" configuration on C-arm image. The body of the ischium is visualized by angling the fluoroscope in a "Ferguson" view in the sagittal plane and coronal plane. This allowed for the "teardrop" configuration of the ischial body to be used for K-wire cannulation (Fig. 21.13). This teardrop shape is visualized when the projection of the inner and outer tables of the ilium overlap both medially and laterally. Therefore, targeting the "teardrop" configuration provides a proper trajectory for percutaneous iliac screw placement. The entry point should be located just ventral to the posterior superior iliac spine to avoid hardware prominence. A drill is used to make a pilot hole on the cortical bone. A Jamshidi needle is then advanced with the tip of the needle kept within "teardrop" configuration under fluoroscopic guidance. The tract created with Jamshidi needle is exchanged with K-wire and followed by placement of a cannulated awl, tap, and iliac screw. Screw length and diameter are measured and planned according to the preoperative CT imaging.

Illustrative Case

History

A 70-year-old woman presented to our clinic with a complicated 20-year spinal history with chief complaint of progressively worsening lower back and anterior thigh pain for 5 months. The pain is bilateral; however, it is more severe on the

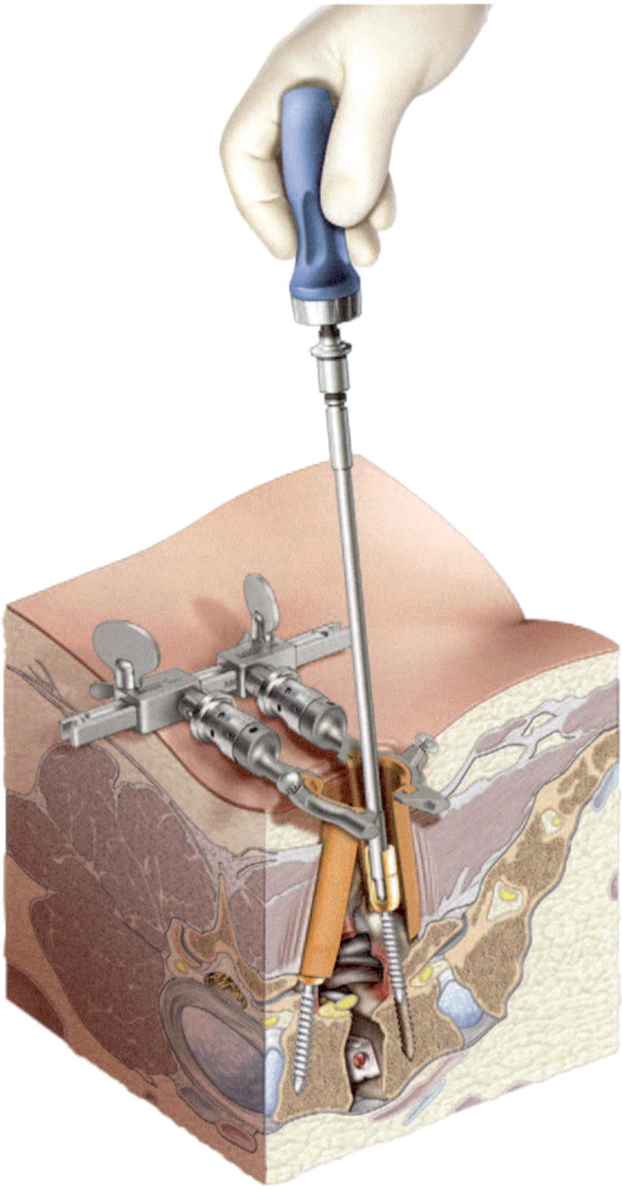

Fig. 21.11 Illustration of mini-open technique (Adapted from Ref. [10])

right side. Her leg pain is intermittent and can cause her legs to go weak and "give out at times." This hinders her ability to stand and ambulate normally. She has tried nonsteroidal anti-inflammatory drugs (NSAIDs) and physical therapy with no relief of symptoms. She denies any bladder or bowel dysfunction.

Her past surgical history is significant for three previous lumbar surgeries: an L5–S1 laminectomy 22 years ago, a L4–L5 laminectomy 20 years ago, and L3–L4 decompression and bilateral laminotomies 6 years ago. Preoperative imaging demonstrated an L3–L4 grade 2 spondylolisthesis (Fig. 21.14a). The decision was made to perform a L3–L4 right-sided minimally invasive transforaminal interbody fusion with intervertebral cage fixation and posterior L3–L4 percutaneous instrumentation.

Postoperatively she was noted to have significant improvement in her leg pain and ambulation (Fig. 21.14b, c).

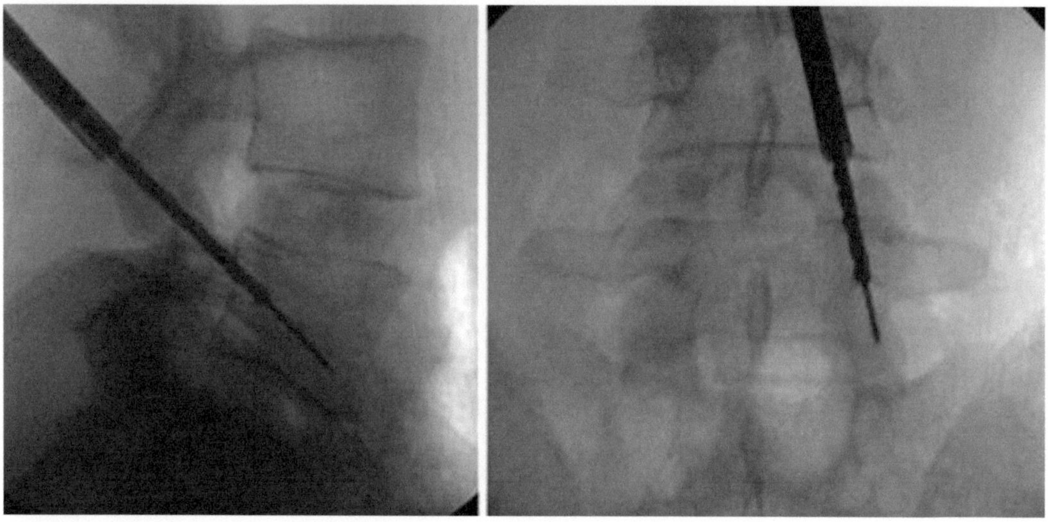

Fig. 21.12 The illustration of the trajectory for percutaneous facet screw on AP and lateral view (Adapted from Ref. [12])

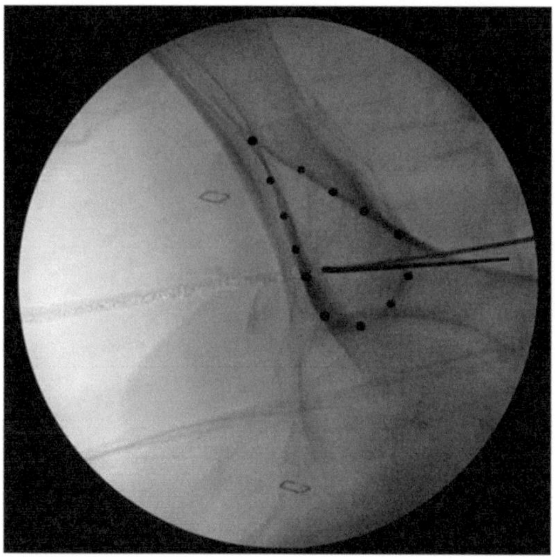

Fig. 21.13 The "teardrop" configuration (Adapted from Ref. [13])

Technical Pearls

- The entire percutaneous screw placement process relies heavily on a series of intraoperative fluoroscopic images. Satisfactory intraoperative fluoroscopic imaging is imperative for successful percutaneous screw placement in MIS surgery.
- To obtain properly aligned bony structures and avoid a distorted image, the fluoroscope should be manipulated to a certain position and angle in which the X-ray beam from the source lies perpendicular to the vertebrae of interest.
- A true anteroposterior (AP) fluoroscopic image is the first step and might be the most useful image when performing K-wire cannulation for percutaneous spinal fixation.
- The tip of the needle can be placed laterally to the lateral border of the pedicle shadow before skin incision, in order to estimate an appropriate entry point for Jamshidi needles on the skin under fluoroscopy.
- Jamshidi needles should dock on the junction between the transverse process and the lateral border of the facet joint in percutaneous pedicle screw placement.
- The length of the longest axis of lumbar pedicle is approximately 2 cm.
- The tapping and the screw insertion should follow the trajectory of the guidewire, in order to avoid excessive bending of the guidewire and possible breakage.
- The key factor of percutaneous iliac screw is to obtain the "teardrop" configuration on C-arm image and keep the cannulation and instrumentation procedure within the teardrop configuration.

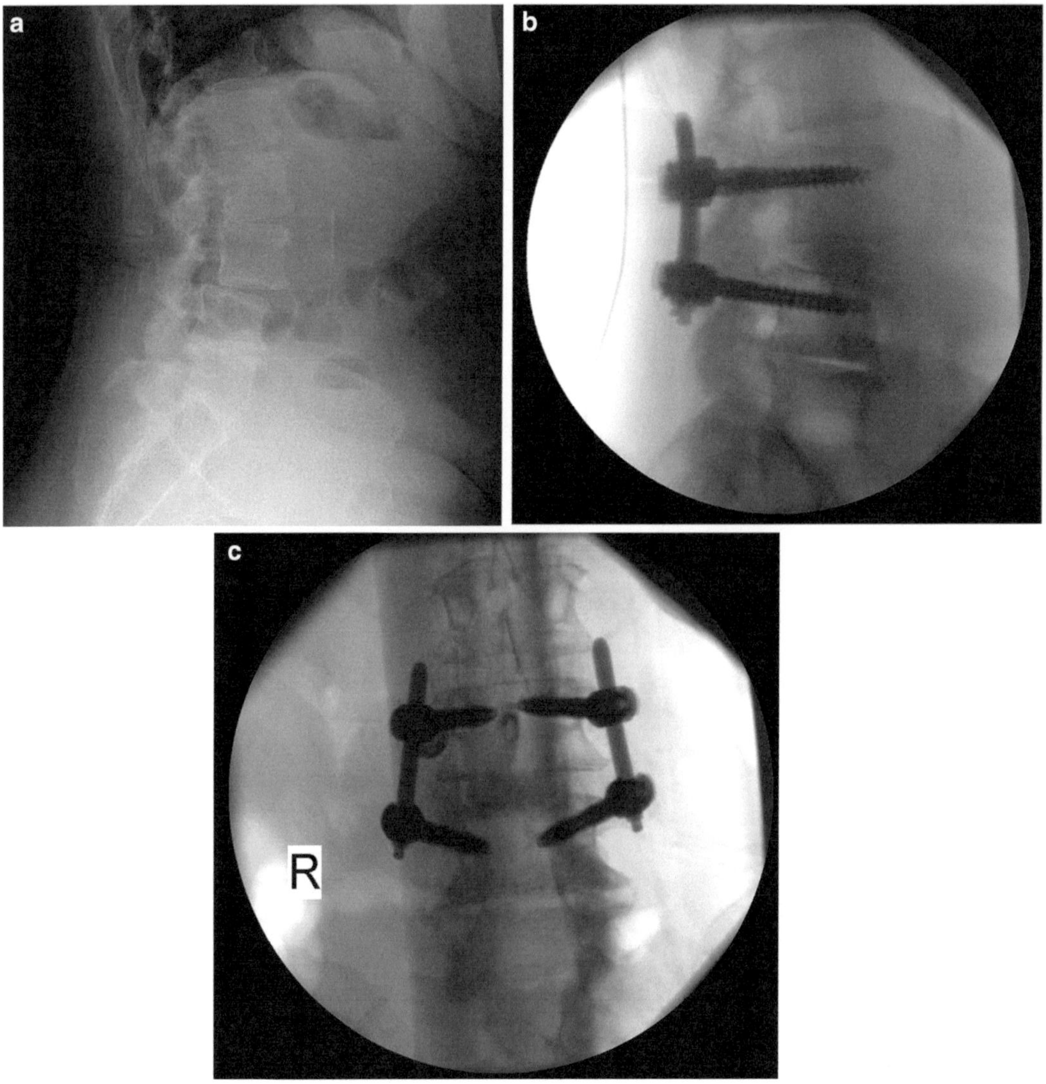

Fig. 21.14 (**a**) Preoperative lateral standing X-ray of a patient with L3–L4 grade I spondylolisthesis. (**b**) Postoperative lateral image status post L3–L4 MIS TLIF. The listhesis is almost completely reduced. (**c**) Postoperative AP image

Complications and Strategies for Avoidance

With the shift from open-pedicle screw fixation toward PPS, fixation advantages include preservation of posterior musculature, decreased intraoperative blood loss, shorter operative time, lower infection risk, decreased postoperative pain, shorter rehabilitation time, and hospital stay [14]. However, PPS fixation is associated with its own complication profile. The most common PPS fixation complications include screw misplacement, nerve root injury, and instrumentation malfunction.

The core limiting factor behind PPS fixation is the minimal surgical visibility compromising the identification of anatomic landmark grossly. The fundamental and most common complication for PPS fixation is inaccurate screw implants. Inaccurate placement can result in reoperation, subsequent instability, hardware malfunction, or neurologic sequelae like dura tear or nerve root injury. In some rare, yet severe, cases, misplacements can cause major vascular and visceral injury that can result in devastating consequence as limb amputation or even death [15]. A German study investigating PPS fixation accuracy demonstrated that 27 of 408 (6.6%) percutaneously placed screws were misplaced, with 19 medial pedicle violations, 6 lateral cortical defects, and only 1 cranial and 1 caudal displacement. Two misplacements resulted in nerve root injuries at levels L4 and L5 and required open revision. The S1 level showed the highest misplacement rate (12%) [16]. The L5 and sacral level are known to be associated with the higher rates of misplacement. This may be due to their proximity to the posterior iliac crest often causing screws to deviate medially. The other cause could be that the axis of L5 and S1 pedicle is much more medialized and steep than the other levels and the vertebral body tends to be more like a triangle on the axial plane. Occasionally an ideal AP image for the pedicle shadow at L5 or S1 is not feasible. In such cases, we recommend to start with a more lateral entry point and aim at a more medialized angle. This maneuver can prevent the screw from perforating the anterior wall of vertebral body as well as violating the spinal canal at the same time. L5 or sacral screw misplacement may also be avoided with lateral sacral screw placement, although this concurrently increases risk of injury to the lumbosacral trunk and internal iliac vein, thus making it an uncommon alternative [16].

The thoracic spine is a unique challenge for PPS fixation. The T1–T7, pedicles are often narrow, have varying angles, and decreased space from the medial border of the pedicle to the spinal cord [17]. For thoracic PPS fixation, physicians often use the "in-out-in" technique which adopts a more lateral entry point for screw placement in order to avoid a medial breach [17]. Additional studies report differing rates of accuracy, 6.7% of 104 were misplaced screws with no neurologic deficits [18] and 0.29% of 700 misplaced screws with one neurologic complication [4]. Accuracy rates rely heavily on spine location (thoracic, lumbar, or sacral), operator dependency, and the subsequent learning curve. Previous studies have found that the majority of misplaced screws were implanted in the trial's initial patients, attesting for the procedure's steep learning curve [4, 19]. Traversing this learning curve can be more feasible through the use of cadaveric training and intraoperative training under a physician competent in PPS [20].

Maintaining full control of the guidewire is crucial throughout the whole procedure. Once the guidewire is lost, it is difficult to re-cannulate. Surgeons must control the guidewire while manipulating the instrument along the wire. It is also critical to follow the trajectory of the guidewire during instrumentation and assure the trajectory is parallel to the K-wire. Otherwise, the K-wire may potentially break and then be retained within the bone.

One of the drawbacks of PPS fixation is radiation exposure due to intraoperative fluoroscopy and CT guidance. One study showed that PPS was associated with an average of 54% more radiation per pedicle screw compared to open-pedicle screw fixation [21]. Recent advances in CT computer navigation software aim to decrease the physician radiation burden, only taking images while the team is outside the operation room. However, these new 3D fluoroscopy and CT protocols depend on having specially equipped ORs with trained staff. Though these requirements initially increase the cost burden of PPS fixation, centers that perform at least 254 CT-navigated PPS cases a year offset these costs by avoiding reoperations [22].

Facet joint and pedicle bone that are sclerotic can be very difficult for the advancement and cannulation of Jamshidi needles. Occasionally the Jamshidi needles have to be replaced with direct cannulation of the pedicle with a high-speed drill. The tip of the drill is docked on the same entry point as a Jamshidi needle would place. With careful advancement of the drilling tip under X-ray monitoring, we will be able to create an accessible pathway into sclerotic bone (Fig. 21.15). The drill can then be removed and replaced with Jamshidi needles or cannulated pedicle probe. The remainder of the step is identical to usual PPS procedures.

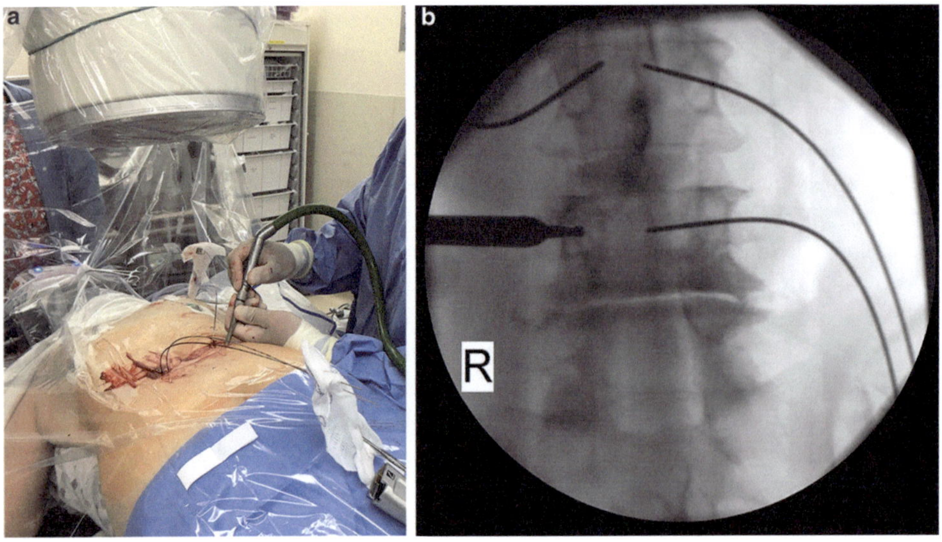

Fig. 21.15 (**a**) The drill is carefully controlled under X-ray monitoring and used to advance into sclerotic bone. (**b**) The trajectory of the drill is identical to that of a usual Jamshidi needle under fluoroscopic image

Other Considerations

Chapman et al. published a largest series of 1609 screws comparing the accuracy of PPS to open-pedicle screws. It appeared that the breach rate was lower with PPS. But the magnitude of breach was worse once the PPS had a breach. They reported the facet violation was similar between both methods [23]. Kwan et al. published a study of pedicle screw placement for cadaveric thoracic spine and concluded that the accuracy of PPS and open screws were similar [24]. This study concluded that the percutaneous technique with fluoroscopy guidance was safe and feasible for thoracic spine fixation. Most of the existing studies support these results and reinforce that PPS technique is safe and accurate compared to the open alternative.

Superior facet violation has also been reported with PPS. Superior facet violations may accelerate future adjacent segment degeneration [25, 26]. Some investigations suggest that poor visualization of anatomical landmarks during PPSF increases rates of facet violation reporting 12% in PPS fixation versus 5% in open [27] and 8.5% (PPS) versus 2% (open) for grade 3 violations, respectively [28]. However, other studies show no difference in the incidence (18.18% vs. 18.72%, $p = 0.62$) [29, 30]. Some studies have proposed that a high body mass index (BMI) is a risk factor for facet violation.

With the increasing popularity of minimally invasive procedures, the PPS technique has been used for spinal deformity, often regarded as the most difficult and high risk field in spine surgery, even in the open setting. Wang et al. evaluated 400 percutaneous screws using fluoroscopy guidance in a 5-year period with CAT scan, with a total breach rate of 7.1%. Two percent of the screws had high grade pedicle violation (>4 mm, either medial or lateral). Only two screws, in two respective patients, required revision. The overall rate of facet joint violation in this series was low (11.2%) compared to other percutaneous series. The results from this study demonstrated that the outcome and safety profile of PPS is favorable for deformity patients. However, more studies are required to reinforce this evidence of percutaneous screws for deformity [6].

3D image guide is another common option for percutaneous screws. The new technology of O-arm-guided screw placement provides surgeons with three-dimensional images, offering a clear perspective. During the procedure, the position of all the instruments is well presented in axial, coronal, and sagittal views on the O-arm monitor. Surgeons may feel more secure with comprehensive monitoring during the procedure. The downside is that new technology requires more OR space, expense, and trained personnel and creates more radiation. It should also be noted that the O-arm cannot provide real-time image as C-arm fluoroscopy does. During the step of tapping and screw insertion along the K-wire, the surgeon is not able to track the trajectory of the instrumentation and make sure it is parallel to that of the K-wire without fluoroscopic shots. There is some evidence showing that O-arm navigation can improve the accuracy and decrease superior facet violations for percutaneous screws [30, 31]. One study investigated accuracy of CT vs. fluoroscopy, with 96.4% vs. 93.9% accuracy for in the lumbar spine and 95.5% vs. 79.0% in thoracic spine [32]. Meta-analysis studies also support these findings [33, 34].

Another emerging technology has been robot-assisted spine surgery. The surgical robot is able to assist surgeons in both open and percutaneous settings. Preoperative thin-cut CT image is uploaded into the robot software and used for presurgical planning for screw placement. During the surgery, the robot "arm" can rotate and indicate a desirable trajectory according to the preoperative planning. Guidewire is used for cannulation with the trajectory provided, followed by tapping and screw insertion as the usual percutaneous technique. Early investigations suggest that robot-assisted methods are able to achieve excellent accuracy of percutaneous screw placement and reduce the radiation exposure [35, 36].

Conclusion

With the ubiquity of the minimally invasive spinal surgery, percutaneous spinal fixation has become a fundamental skill set. It is important for spinal surgeons to familiarize themselves with these percutaneous spinal instrumentation techniques. Among all of the methods, percutaneous lumbar pedicle screws remain the most popular and reliable procedure under fluoroscopic guidance. As with all new technologies, percutaneous spinal fixation will continue to evolve and become more precise and efficient over time.

References

1. Kabins MB, Weinstein JN. The history of vertebral screw and pedicle screw fixation. Iowa Orthop J. 1991;11:127–36.
2. Foley KT, Gupta SK. Percutaneous pedicle screw fixation of the lumbar spine: preliminary clinical results. J Neurosurg. 2002;97(1 Suppl):7–12.
3. McAnany SJ, Overley SC, Kim JS, Baird EO, Qureshi SA, Anderson PA. Open versus minimally invasive fixation techniques for thoracolumbar trauma: a meta-analysis. Global Spine J. 2016;6(2):186–94.
4. Mobbs RJ, Sivabalan P, Li J. Technique, challenges and indications for percutaneous pedicle screw fixation. J Clin Neurosci. 2011;18(6):741–9.
5. Rosen DS, Ferguson SD, Ogden AT, Huo D, Fessler RG. Obesity and self-reported outcome after minimally invasive lumbar spinal fusion surgery. Neurosurgery. 2008;63(5):956–60. discussion 960
6. Ahmad FU, Wang MY. Use of anteroposterior view fluoroscopy for targeting percutaneous pedicle screws in cases of spinal deformity with axial rotation. J Neurosurg Spine. 2014;21(5):826–32.
7. Wang MY, Pineiro G, Mummaneni PV. Stimulus-evoked electromyography testing of percutaneous pedicle screws for the detection of pedicle breaches: a clinical study of 409 screws in 93 patients. J Neurosurg Spine. 2010;13(5):600–5.
8. Wiesner L, Kothe R, Ruther W. Anatomic evaluation of two different techniques for the percutaneous insertion of pedicle screws in the lumbar spine. Spine (Phila Pa 1976). 1999;24(15):1599–603.
9. Yoshida G, Sato K, Kanemura T, Iwase T, Togawa D, Matsuyama Y. Accuracy of percutaneous lumbosacral pedicle screw placement using the oblique fluoroscopic view based on computed tomography evaluations. Asian Spine J. 2016;10(4):630–8.
10. Pakzaban P. Modified mini-open transforaminal lumbar interbody fusion: description of surgical technique and assessment of free-hand pedicle screw insertion. Spine (Phila Pa 1976). 2016;41(18):E1124–30.
11. Dhall SS, Wang MY, Mummaneni PV. Clinical and radiographic comparison of mini-open transforaminal lumbar interbody fusion with open transforaminal lumbar interbody fusion in 42 patients with long-term follow-up. J Neurosurg Spine. 2008;9(6):560–5.
12. Chin KR, Seale J, Cumming V. Mini-open or percutaneous bilateral lumbar transfacet pedicle screw fixation: a technical note. J Spinal Disord Tech. 2015;28(2):61–5.
13. Wang MY, Williams S, Mummaneni PV, Sherman JD. Minimally Invasive Percutaneous Iliac Screws: Initial 24 Case Experiences With CT Confirmation. Clin Spine Surg. 2016;29(5):E222–5.
14. Court C, Vincent C. Percutaneous fixation of thoracolumbar fractures: current concepts. Orthop Traumatol Surg Res: OTSR. 2012;98(8):900–9.
15. Lopera JE, Restrepo CS, Gonzales A, Trimmer CK, Arko F. Aortoiliac vascular injuries after misplacement of fixation screws. J Trauma. 2010;69(4):870–5.

16. Wiesner L, Kothe R, Schulitz KP, Ruther W. Clinical evaluation and computed tomography scan analysis of screw tracts after percutaneous insertion of pedicle screws in the lumbar spine. Spine. 2000;25(5):615–21.
17. Puvanesarajah V, Liauw JA, Lo S-F, Lina IA, Witham TF. Techniques and accuracy of thoracolumbar pedicle screw placement. World J Orthop. 2014;5(2):112–23.
18. Ni WF, Huang YX, Chi YL, et al. Percutaneous pedicle screw fixation for neurologic intact thoracolumbar burst fractures. J Spinal Disord Tech. 2010;23(8):530–7.
19. Sclafani JA, Kim CW. Complications associated with the initial learning curve of minimally invasive spine surgery: a systematic review. Clin Orthop Relat Res. 2014;472(6):1711–7.
20. Voyadzis J-M. The learning curve in minimally invasive spine surgery. Semin Spine Surg. 2011;23(1):9–13.
21. Wild MH, Glees M, Plieschnegger C, Wenda K. Five-year follow-up examination after purely minimally invasive posterior stabilization of thoracolumbar fractures: a comparison of minimally invasive percutaneously and conventionally open treated patients. Arch Orthop Trauma Surg. 2007;127(5):335–43.
22. Dea N, Fisher CG, Batke J, et al. Economic evaluation comparing intraoperative cone beam CT-based navigation and conventional fluoroscopy for the placement of spinal pedicle screws: a patient-level data cost-effectiveness analysis. Spine J. 2016;16(1):23–31.
23. Chapman TM, Blizzard DJ, Brown CR. CT accuracy of percutaneous versus open pedicle screw techniques: a series of 1609 screws. Eur Spine J. 2016;25(6):1781–6.
24. Kwan MK, Chiu CK, Lee CK, Chan CY. Comparison between percutaneous fluoroscopic-guided and conventional open pedicle screw placement techniques for the thoracic spine: a safety evaluation in human cadavers. Bone Joint J. 2015;97-B(11):1555–61.
25. Babu R, Park JG, Mehta AI, et al. Comparison of superior-level facet joint violations during open and percutaneous pedicle screw placement. Neurosurgery. 2012;71(5):962–70.
26. Lau D, Terman SW, Patel R, La Marca F, Park P. Incidence of and risk factors for superior facet violation in minimally invasive versus open pedicle screw placement during transforaminal lumbar interbody fusion: a comparative analysis. J Neurosurg Spine. 2013;18(4):356–61.
27. Jones-Quaidoo SM, Djurasovic M, Owens RK, Carreon LY. Superior articulating facet violation: percutaneous versus open techniques. J Neurosurg Spine. 2013;18(6):593–7.
28. Babu R, Park JG, Mehta AI, et al. Comparison of superior level facet joint violations during open and percutaneous pedicle screw placement. Neurosurgery. 2012;71(5):962–70.
29. Wang L, Wang Y, Yu B, Li Z, Li Y. Comparison of cranial facet joint violation rate between percutaneous and open pedicle screw placement: a systematic review and meta-analysis. Medicine. 2015;94(5):e504.
30. Yson SC, Sembrano JN, Sanders PC, Santos ER, Ledonio CG, Polly DW Jr. Comparison of cranial facet joint violation rates between open and percutaneous pedicle screw placement using intraoperative 3-D CT (O-arm) computer navigation. Spine (Phila Pa 1976). 2013;38(4):E251–8.
31. Ohba T, Ebata S, Fujita K, Sato H, Haro H. Percutaneous pedicle screw placements: accuracy and rates of cranial facet joint violation using conventional fluoroscopy compared with intraoperative three-dimensional computed tomography computer navigation. Eur Spine J. 2016;25(6):1775–80.
32. Waschke A, Walter J, Duenisch P, Reichart R, Kalff R, Ewald C. CT-navigation versus fluoroscopy-guided placement of pedicle screws at the thoracolumbar spine: single center experience of 4,500 screws. Eur Spine J. 2013;22(3):654–60.
33. Tian NF, Huang QS, Zhou P, et al. Pedicle screw insertion accuracy with different assisted methods: a systematic review and meta-analysis of comparative studies. Eur Spine J. 2011;20(6):846–59.
34. Kosmopoulos V, Schizas C. Pedicle screw placement accuracy: a meta-analysis. Spine (Phila Pa 1976). 2007;32(3):E111–20.
35. Kantelhardt SR, Martinez R, Baerwinkel S, Burger R, Giese A, Rohde V. Perioperative course and accuracy of screw positioning in conventional, open robotic-guided and percutaneous robotic-guided, pedicle screw placement. Eur Spine J. 2011;20(6):860–8.
36. Schatlo B, Molliqaj G, Cuvinciuc V, Kotowski M, Schaller K, Tessitore E. Safety and accuracy of robot-assisted versus fluoroscopy-guided pedicle screw insertion for degenerative diseases of the lumbar spine: a matched cohort comparison. J Neurosurg Spine. 2014;20(6):636–43.

22 Lumbar Osteotomy Techniques

Ryan Nazar, Jeffrey Gum, John Dimar, and Mladen Djurasovic

Introduction

Adult spinal deformity is becoming increasingly common in our aging US population [1]. In addition to degenerative etiologies, iatrogenic sagittal malalignment complications are more common with the increase in lumbar fusion procedures being performed. The critical goal in the surgical treatment of the adult deformity patient is two-fold: (1) restoration of anatomic alignment and (2) preservation of function.

Sagittal balance and overall global spinal alignment have been shown to be one of the most important factors associated with improvement in patient outcomes following adult deformity surgery [2]. In the past decade, studies have found that restoration of normal or near-normal spinopelvic parameters correlates closely with health-related quality of life (HRQOL) and pain measures in both deformity and degenerative patients [3]. Although coronal alignment has not been as important as sagittal alignment, fusing the spine such that the torso is balanced over the pelvis within the cone of economy in both planes does allow better global balance of the spine and is seen as an optimal goal [4]. Fusion of the spine with significant residual coronal or sagittal malalignment can place excessive stresses through both the instrumented segments and non-instrumented segments of the spine contributing to additional degeneration, instrumentation failure, and progression of the malalignment [5, 6].

In this chapter, we will review modern surgical corrective techniques for spinal deformity focusing on lumbar osteotomies that can be utilized to improve sagittal and coronal alignment and restore global spinal alignment in the adult patient. The origins of these techniques will be briefly reviewed to help frame and appreciate the advancement of correction methodology that has occurred. Utilizing the best available evidence, we then will review the indications and patient selection as a first step and also discuss the decision-making process and preoperative planning. Lastly, we detail the surgical technique of the most common osteotomy types with emphasis on complication avoidance. Although variations exist, three general categories of osteotomy have been described: (1) posterior column osteotomy (PCO), (2) pedicle subtraction osteotomy (PSO), and (3) vertebral column resection (VCR).

R. Nazar, MD
Department of Neurological Surgery, University of Louisville, Louisville, KY, USA
e-mail: Ryan.gregory.nazar@gmail.com

J. Gum, MD • J. Dimar, MD
M. Djurasovic, MD (✉)
Norton Leatherman Spine Center, Department of Orthopaedic Surgery, University of Louisville, Louisville, KY, USA
e-mail: djuraso@hotmail.com

L.T. Holly, P.A. Anderson (eds.), *Essentials of Spinal Stabilization*,
DOI 10.1007/978-3-319-59713-3_22

More recently, the Schwab classification describes six anatomically defined osteotomies that are commonly accepted and used [7].

History

The surgical techniques for restoration of spinal alignment continue to evolve (Fig. 22.1). The posterior column osteotomy (PCO) includes both the Smith-Petersen osteotomy (SPO) and the Ponte osteotomy. In 1945, Smith-Petersen et al. described a posterior extension or chevron-type osteotomy combined with anterior osteoclasis for single-level correction of kyphosis in the setting of ankylosing spondylitis [8]. The Smith-Petersen osteotomy involves bilateral removal of the facet joints or fusion mass allowing the spine to pivot along the middle column increasing segmental lordosis and causing an extension in length of the anterior column [9]. In modern practice, the SPO is usually performed across multiple segments for correction of a multi-segmental deformity [10]. The osteotomies can be performed asymmetrically to allow for some degree of coronal plane correction [11]. Because SPO requires lengthening of the anterior column, the patient must have a mobile anterior disc in theory; thus, it cannot be optimally effective across a fully ankylosed segment.

The Ponte-type osteotomy was first described by Ponte et al. in 1984 for Scheuermann kyphosis and is described as segmental osteotomies followed by posterior decompression along unfused regions of kyphotic deformity [12]. Although today the terms Smith-Petersen osteotomy and Ponte osteotomy are used interchangeably, the modern technique more closely resembles the procedure described by Alberto Ponte. In fact, these osteotomies have also become a mainstay in correction of coronal plane deformities, such as in adolescent idiopathic scoliosis.

Pedicle subtraction osteotomy (PSO) was first introduced by Thomasen in 1985 [13]. The PSO has further been referred to as a transpedicular wedge procedure, wedge osteotomy, and eggshell osteotomy. PSO has found widespread use for fixed, angular sagittal plane deformity resulting from multiple etiologies [14]. Like vertebral column resection (VCR), PSO has been associated with significant perioperative complications; however, modern advancements

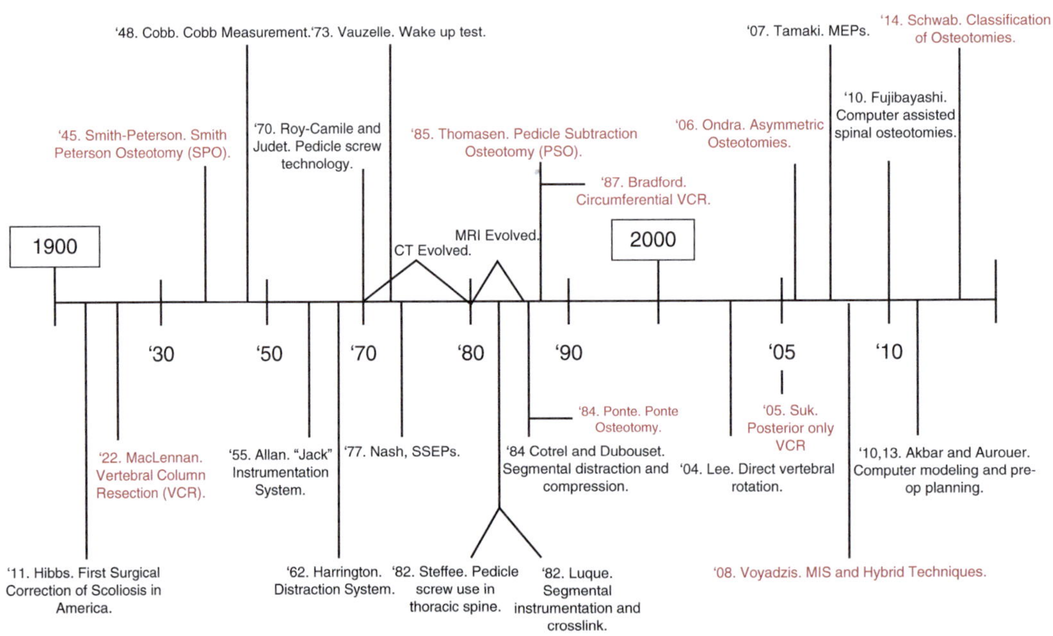

Fig. 22.1 Evolution of lumbar spinal osteotomies

in anesthetic management, surgical technique, and postoperative critical care have all led to improved patient outcomes [15]. Neurological injury is the most devastating complication when performing osteotomies; evolution from the "wake-up test" popularized by Vauzelle in 1973 to the use of somatosensory evoked potentials (SSEPs) by Nash and motor evoked potentials (MEPs) by Tamaki together has allowed direct feedback regarding spinal cord function with a high degree of accuracy to more widely perform these procedures safely [16–18]. Additionally, in part because of the aforementioned advancements, the utilization of these procedures has dramatically increased, as much as fourfold, over the last decade [19]. Although the complication rate with regard to neurological deficit is still significant, neurologic complications can be minimized with the use of modern neuromonitoring techniques [20–22].

Vertebral column resection (VCR) was first described by MacLennan in 1922 for the treatment of severe scoliosis via posterior vertebrectomy and postoperative casting [23]. The approach to VCR has undergone its own evolution in the past decades. Bradford described a circumferential approach when performing a VCR, performing a circumferential VCR with concave rib osteotomies, convex thoracoplasty, and segmental spinal instrumentation [24]. Often staging of anterior and posterior approaches was done due to long operative times [25]. Suk et al. reported on a posterior-only approach (PVCR) allowing for simultaneous control of the spinal column and access to the neural elements [26]. VCR consists of complete resection of at least one vertebral segment through either a posterior alone or combined anterior-posterior approach for multiplanar correction of severe rigid spinal deformity [24]. Often concomitant with the PVCR, posterior releases of the ligaments and facets via adjacent level PCO's are done [9].

At present, there are many variations of established techniques including hybrid and minimally invasive techniques [27]. Despite these variations, an anatomically based classification can provide a common language among spine surgeons to describe osteotomy types. A comprehensive and widely accepted classification has been described by Schwab and Lafage et al. [7]. This classification system is based on six anatomical grades of resection (1, 6, through) corresponding to the extent of bone resection and increasing degree of destabilizing potential. Grades 1 and 2 include PCOs and involve partial (Grade 1) or full (Grade 2) resection of the facet joints. Grades 3 and 4 represent PSO or extended PSO, thus involving resection of the pedicle, partial vertebral body (Grade 3), and possibly the cranial disc (Grade 4). Grades 5 and 6 represent VCR so that the complete vertebral body and disc are removed (Grade 5) or multiple vertebral bodies (Grade 6) and discs. In addition, a surgical approach modifier can be added (posterior approach or combined anterior and posterior approaches).

Indications and Patient Selection

In general, the type of osteotomy chosen should take many factors into consideration including but not limited to the severity of deformity and underlying pathology, flexibility of the spine, bone density/quality, operative goals, surgeon's experience and comfort level, and critical care support. Age, regional and global alignment, comorbidities, psychosocial status, and amount of postoperative activity also influence the decision-making process including whether surgical or conservative therapy is indicated. Furthermore, symptoms such as radiculopathy or axial back pain will also influence the extent of decompression and arthrodesis. Patients with radicular leg pain were more likely to proceed with surgery than those with back pain [28]. Furthermore, it has been demonstrated that sagittal spinopelvic alignment varies with age, and thus operative realignment goals should also account for age with younger patients requiring more rigorous alignment objectives [29].

The surgeon should develop an algorithmic approach to this complex decision-making process. The mnemonic TEAMS can aid in developing a comprehensive decision: (1) **T**ype of curve, (2) **E**nd points of deformity, (3) **A**pex of deformity,

Table 22.1 Criteria for selection of lumbar osteotomy

	Posterior column osteotomy (PCO)	Pedicle subtraction osteotomy (PSO)	Vertebral column resection (VCR)
Type	Gradual or sweeping kyphosis Typically degenerative causes; Scheuermann kyphosis 1° of correction per millimeter of bone resection	30 to 40° of correction in the sagittal plane at the level that it is performed Examples include post-traumatic or junctional kyphosis, ankylosing spondylitis, flat-back deformity	Fixed trunk translation, often congenital or neuromuscular origin, spondyloptosis, spinal tumor, rigid spinal deformity
End points	Multi-segment nature Roughly 10° of angular correction per level	Short, angular kyphosis	Correction over short segment Most effective for angular kyphosis
Apex	Harmonious correction over multiple segments Lengthening of anterior column Pivots at middle column	No lengthening of anterior column Shortening of posterior column Correction via three columns at a single level Ideal levels: L2–L4	Asymmetry between the length of the convex column and length of concave column of the deformity Closure pivots on anterior placed cage
Mobility	Mobile disc space	Mobile disc not required Fixed disc space Anterior ankylosis and lack of flexibility	Correction over levels with anterior ankylosis of lack of flexibility
Stable zone	Mild to moderate sagittal imbalance Less than 10 cm of sagittal imbalance	More than 10 cm of sagittal imbalance	More than 80° in the coronal plane Combined severe coronal and sagittal imbalance

(4) **M**obile disc segments, and (5) **S**table cone of economy. Table 22.1 provides a quick reference for selection of osteotomy procedure.

Posterior Column Osteotomy (PCO)

Indications for considering PCO's would include a deformity with a mobile anterior column, where adequate disc height and mobility of the disc space anteriorly can add to the corrective potential. The deformity may be either in the sagittal plane such as kyphosis or in the coronal plane. For sagittal plane deformity, typically symmetric shorting of the posterior column yields 1° of correction per millimeter of bone resected, thus requiring correction to be carried out over multiple levels [9]. This type of osteotomy lends itself very well to any mild to moderate malalignment that is degenerative in origin.

The PCO provides roughly 5–10° of angular correction per level. Three PCOs are able to achieve a degree of correction comparable to a single PSO with no difference in fusion rates or patient-reported outcome [9]. A PCO may be combined with an anterior release or performed as a stand-alone posterior approach. In a patient with combined sagittal and coronal deformity and shoulder angulation tilted to the concavity, an anterior release followed by multilevel PCOs can be a useful technique.

Fixed angular deformity and ossification of the anterior longitudinal ligament are relative contraindications to a posterior column osteotomy. Compression of instrumentation after multilevel PCO results in gradual, harmonious correction of a smooth kyphotic curve rather than angular correction. The classic indication for a PCO is a long smooth kyphosis such as in Scheuermann kyphosis. In adult deformities, PCO is often a good option if the patient has a flexible kyphotic deformity, as evidenced by correction on hyperextension films or supine positioning such as MRI or CT scanning (Fig. 22.2). Although an anterior gap may be created after SPO, there is typically no need for an anterior bone graft. The Zielke technique involves multiple PCOs at all levels from T10 to the sacrum [10].

Pedicle Subtraction Osteotomy (PSO)

PSOs can achieve approximately 30 to 40° of correction in the sagittal plane at the level that it is performed [30]. Closure of the osteotomy occurs in a wedge fashion, bringing kyphosis into correction via posterior shortening (Fig. 22.3). Briefly, the technique consists of resection of the entire posterior elements of the vertebral body, including pedicles, followed by a wedge-shaped removal of the posterior cortex and cancellous bone from the vertebral body. A variation includes the extended PSO which, in addition, incorporates resection of the cranial disc. The closure of the osteotomy hinges on the anterior column. In the lumbar spine, there is a broad anterior cortical surface that can function as a rigid pivot for PSO closure helping to prevent translation.

PSOs are not commonly used in the distal lumbar spine because of limited fixation points distally. However, more recent studies suggest the lower the PSO is performed, the more physiologic is the restoration of lumbar lordosis as the majority of lumbar lordosis is found between L4 and S1. This appears to also correlate with patient satisfaction [31]. The best candidates for a PSO are patients with the following conditions: [1] sagittal malalignment of more than 10 cm, [2] sharp angular kyphosis, and [3] fixed sagittal malalignment caused by anterior ankylosis or circumferential fusion between multiple segments [32]. Other indications would include flat-back deformity or fixed kyphotic deformity. It is the preferred osteotomy for patients with ankylosing spondylitis who have sagittal malalignment.

The most common levels for a PSO are L2, L3, and L4. Recent studies have shown that the level of the PSO (L3 versus L4) does not affect the degree of correction; but lower lumbar PSOs correlate with an increased correction in pelvic tilt [33]. Ideally, the PSO should be performed at the apical region of the kyphosis or at the epicenter of the junctional deformity. Recent advances in pelvic fixation techniques, such as S2 alar iliac screws, have allowed these osteotomies to be performed more distally. Although the overall complication rate is high, there is high success rate with fusion due to bone contact across three columns and low reported rates of pseudarthrosis [34]. An extended PSO has been described as the wedge of vertebral body resection to include the disc space above the decancellated segment. Typically an extended PSO is used for correction of thoracolumbar junctional kyphosis and focal junctional kyphosis including arthrodesis of the interspace after the cephalad disc is resected.

Vertebral Column Resection

The VCR is reserved for malalignment that is severe enough that other osteotomies cannot correct the deformity, especially in patients who have combined coronal and sagittal malalignment. It is also more commonly used for rigid deformities in the thoracic and thoracolumbar spine, whereas PSO is more likely used in the lumbar spine. The VCR can result in 40 to 60° of correction at a single level.

Indications for VCR include fixed trunk translation, severe scoliosis (often of a congenital or neuromuscular origin), spondyloptosis, spinal tumor, rigid spinal deformity of more than 80° in the coronal plane, and severe asymmetry between the length of the convex column and length of concave column of the deformity [24].

The VCR essentially is an extension of the three-column resection of the PSO, involving opening of the anterior column and closing of the posterior column after complete removal of the posterior elements and vertebral body, with placement of an anterior cage or strut graft to serve as the pivot (Fig. 22.4). Nerve roots can be ligated and sacrificed in the thoracic spine to improve exposure to the vertebral body. The vertebral body

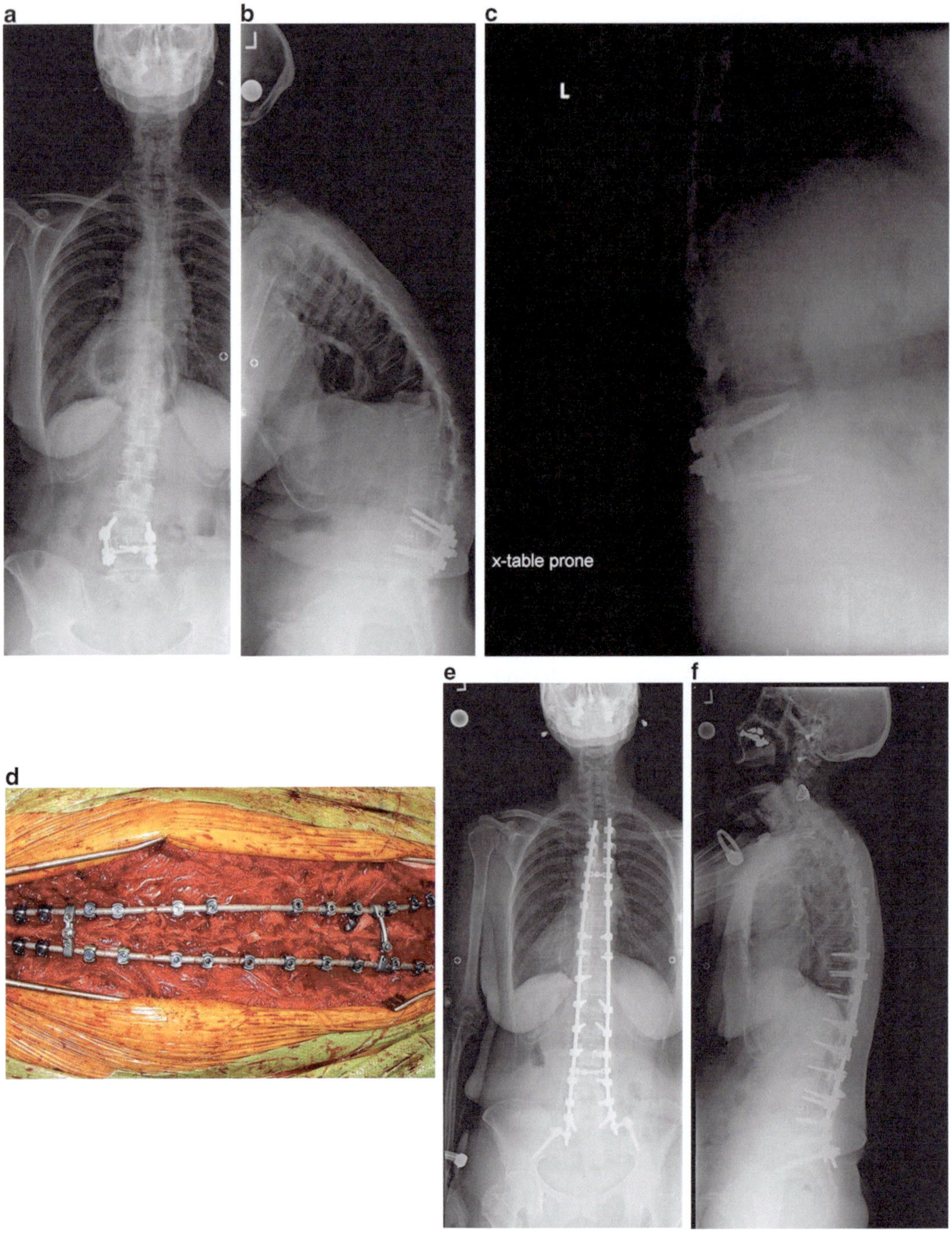

Fig. 22.2 Case example of Ponte osteotomies. (**a**) Standing AP 36-inch scoliosis x-ray of patient with prior L4–L5 TLIF. (**b**) Standing lateral 36-inch scoliosis x-ray demonstrates severe sagittal imbalance and rounded kyphosis. Disc spaces above L4–L5 fusion are still open. (**c**) Prone hyperextension lateral x-ray demonstrates significant correction and relatively mobile discs. (**d**) Instrumentation placed with multiple Ponte osteotomies through thoracolumbar junction and upper lumbar spine. (**e**) Standing postoperative AP 36-inch scoliosis x-ray demonstrates T4–ilium instrumented fusion. (**f**) Standing postoperative lateral 36-inch scoliosis x-ray demonstrates restoration of normal spinal alignment

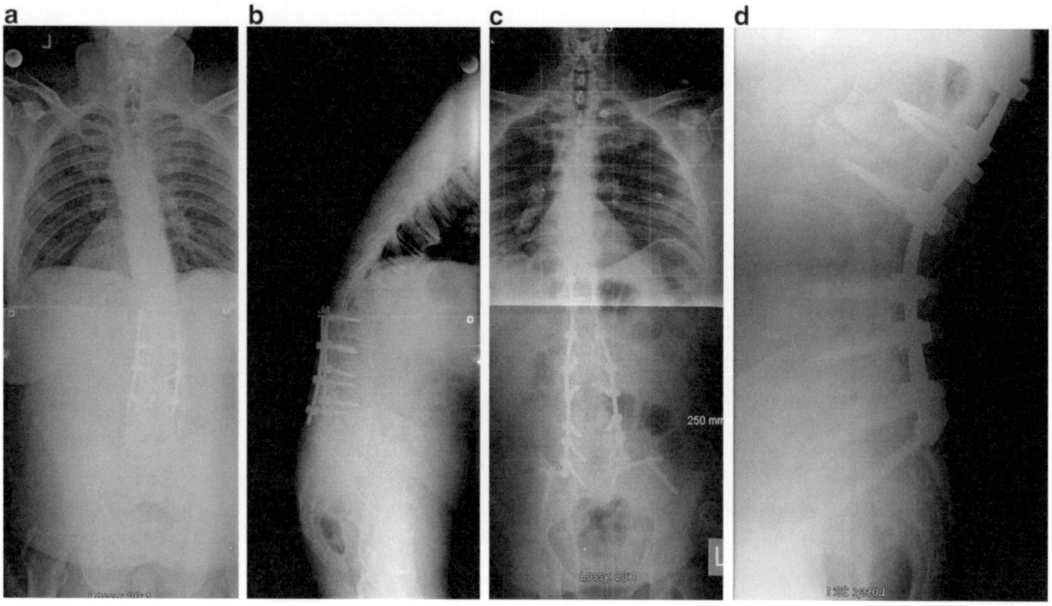

Fig. 22.3 Case example of pedicle subtraction osteotomy. (**a**) Standing AP 36-inch scoliosis x-ray of patient with prior L2–L5 posterior fusion. (**b**) Standing lateral 36-inch scoliosis x-ray demonstrates sagittal imbalance with angular kyphosis above prior fusion. (**c**) Standing postoperative AP 36-inch scoliosis x-ray demonstrates T10–ilium fusion with pedicle subtraction osteotomy through L3. (**d**) Standing postoperative lateral lumbar x-ray demonstrates significant correction through PSO

is then completely resected, including the anterior cortex. Because the entire vertebra is removed, this is a highly unstable osteotomy; the anterior cortex is not left as a pivot point, as in the PSO. Thus, some type of structural graft, typically a structural cage, must be placed in the vertebrectomy defect in order to create a pivot point. A closing of the posterior portion of the osteotomy is then done to correct kyphosis. The surgery can be performed by a posterior approach only or combined anterior-posterior approach. Additionally, more recent data suggest that a staged approach is acceptable because of the length and complexity of these procedures [35].

Preoperative Considerations

Scoliosis and other spinal deformities may be associated with various systemic diseases involving many different systems including cardiac, pulmonary, musculoskeletal, neurological, renal, and more. Furthermore, a patient may need optimization of other preexisting medical conditions including but not limited to asthma, diabetes, heart disease, tobacco abuse, any coagulopathies, nutrition, and bone health. Recognition of associated conditions and medical comorbidities, whether part of a syndrome or not, may benefit from consultation with a medical subspecialist.

It is important for the surgeon and patient to have an understanding about management and optimization of medical comorbidities before the decision is made to operate. Thus, some specific recommendations the surgeon (as well as the medical physicians) should make include the following: (1) pulmonary optimization, (2) cardiac optimization, (3) glycemic control, (4) bone health, and (5) nutritional support. *Respiratory system:* Thoracic curves can affect pulmonary function, and tobacco abuse is known to negatively affect spinal fusion and increase susceptibility to postoperative infection [36]. Also, smoking may place the patient at risk for perioperative respiratory infections. It is important to

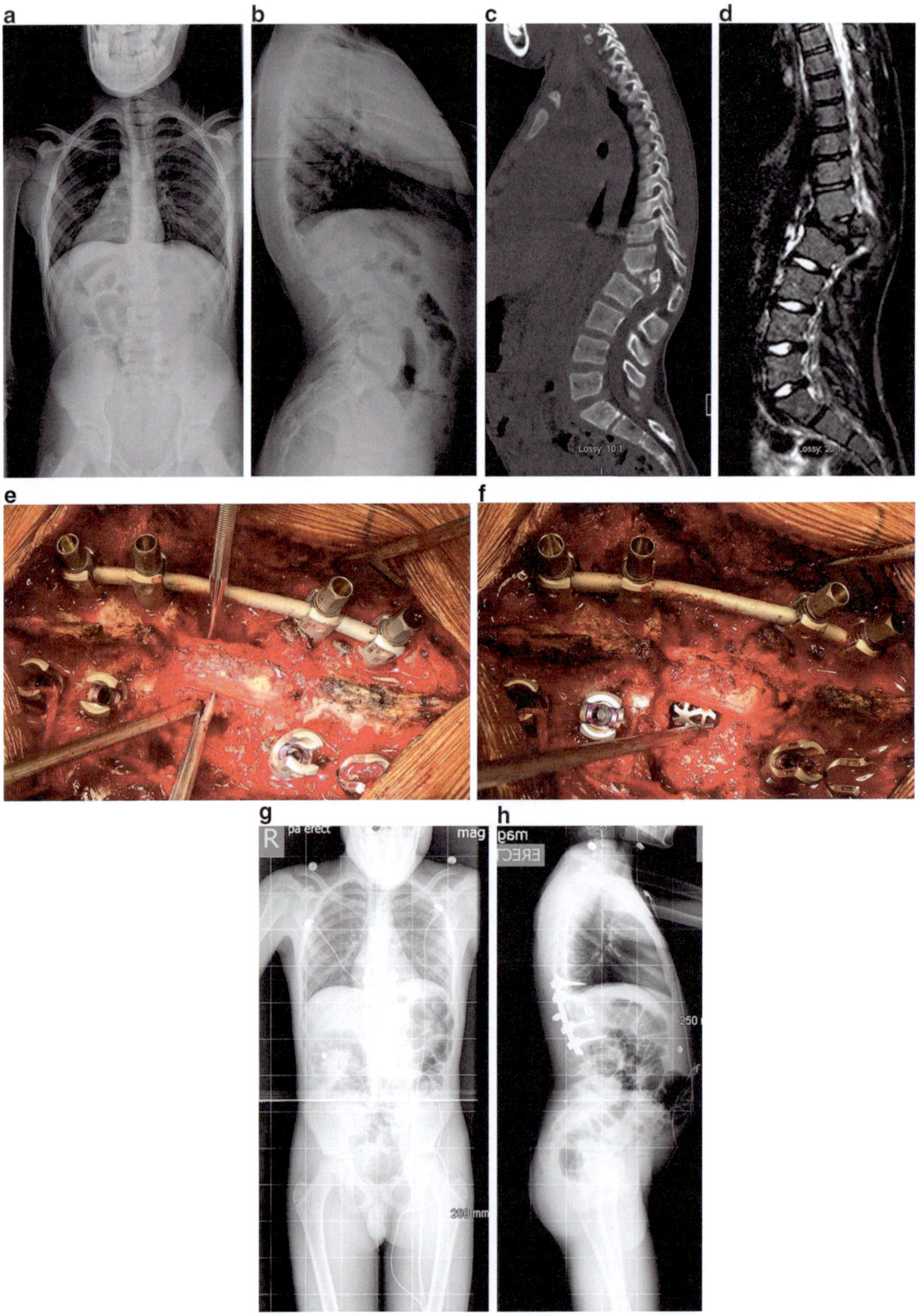

Fig. 22.4 Case example of vertebral column resection. (**a**) Standing AP 36-inch scoliosis x-ray of patient with congenital kyphosis. (**b**) Standing lateral 36-inch scoliosis x-ray demonstrates L1 dorsal hemivertebra with mild kyphosis. (**c**) CT scan sagittal reconstruction demonstrates L1 dorsal hemivertebra with significant encroachment

emphasize smoking cessation 4–6 weeks prior to surgery to allow recovery of the respiratory system [37]. Nicotine blood and urine testing is becoming more and more common in presurgical evaluation of patients undergoing spinal fusion. *Cardiac system*: High degree curves and pulmonary hypertension place a patient at risk for cor pulmonale. In patients with known or suspected cardiac compromise, consultation with a cardiologist during the perioperative period, as well as possible invasive cardiac monitoring during surgery, may be warranted [38]. *Glycemic control*: Uncontrolled diabetes mellitus has been found to be a risk factor for wound infection, nonunion, postoperative hemorrhage, acute renal failure, deep vein thrombosis, and mortality [39]. Despite the fact that even well-controlled diabetics have higher than normal complication rates, every effort should be made to maintain tight glycemic control in the perioperative setting. *Bone health*: Bone mineral density and physical preparation should be considered prior to surgery as well. The surgeon should always screen for osteoporosis clinically with a detailed history and obtain dual-energy x-ray absorptiometry (DEXA) testing if indicated. A useful tool, if already available, is the lumbar CT scan of the patient from which Hounsfield unit (HU) measurements can be obtained to provide both local and global bone density without additional cost and minimal effort [40]. When appropriate, it is important to initiate treatment for poor bone health or refer the patient for further management. The benefits of pre-habilitation are also becoming more evidence-based in terms of optimizing bone health, weight, function, and outcomes [41]. *Nutritional support*: Dietary optimization and adequate protein intake need to be considered as a serum albumin >3.5 g/L and total blood lymphocyte count >1500 cells/mm^3 are associated with a decreased risk of postoperative infection and wound breakdown [42].

It is also of great importance to review all of the patient's medications in detail prior to surgery. Try to wean patients off narcotic pain medications and muscle relaxants if possible to decrease tolerance to pain medication. Many prescription medications may be taken safely prior to and on the day of surgery such as blood pressure medications; however, several medications should be stopped prior to surgery such as blood thinners, aspirin, anti-inflammatories, herbal drugs, steroids, and some diabetic medications.

The overall clinical appearance and condition of a patient with spinal malalignment can help customize the surgical approach to individual patients. The surgeon and patient need to have specific goals for each stage of the surgery including decompression, fusion, and deformity correction. These goals should be individualized so as to obtain maximum benefit while minimizing complications. Table 22.2 summarizes general preoperative considerations prior to the day of surgery. The larger or more severe the curve and thus corresponding deformity, the more important significant correction is to the patient-reported outcome of the surgery. Recent studies have emphasized the importance of patient-perceived self-image with regard to outcomes [31, 43].

Preoperative surgical planning can be carried out using numerous modeling software systems [44]. Many mathematical models for determining the degree of correction needed through osteotomies to achieve sagittal alignment have been proposed [11, 45, 46]; however, one should note that formulas alone often underestimate the amount of correction needed.

The role of the pelvis in standing alignment is now well established, and spinopelvic parameters will need to be identified, including pelvic

Fig. 22.4 (continued) into the spinal canal. (**d**) Parasagittal MRI demonstrates severe stenosis at level of congenital deformity. (**e**) Intraoperative photograph of VCR with posterior resection of hemivertebra. (**f**) Placement of cage following complete L1 vertebrectomy. (**g**) Standing postoperative AP 36-inch scoliosis x-ray demonstrates L1 cage with posterior T11–L3 fusion. (**h**) Standing postoperative lateral 36-inch scoliosis x-ray shows cage reconstruction and neutral thoracolumbar alignment

Table 22.2 Preoperative considerations for lumbar osteotomies

Patient	Symptoms	Imbalance	Compensation	Imaging	Correction
Age	Back pain	Regional malalignment	Hip extension	Standing scoliosis radiograph	Sagittal vertical axis (SVA) < 5 cm
Medical Comorbidities	Radiculopathy	Global malalignment	Knee flexion	Side bending/ hyperextension radiograph	Lordosis/pelvic incidence Mismatch ±9°
Body Habitus	Claudication	Shoulder or waist asymmetry	Pelvic tilt (PT)	CT-myelogram	Pelvic tilt goal <25°
Tobacco use	Bowel/ bladder	Spinopelvic morphology	Sacral slope (SS)	MRI	Lumbar lordosis > thoracic kyphosis
Quality of life	Psychological distress	Curve stiffness			
Bone quality	Natural course				
Prior surgery					

incidence (PI) and lumbar lordosis (LL). Pelvic incidence is a fixed parameter for any given patient. Generally speaking, the goal of surgery is to restore lumbar lordosis to within +/−9° of the patient's pelvic incidence. Sacral slope (SS) and pelvic tilt (PT) are dynamic pelvic parameters that measure pelvic version that can change as a compensatory mechanism. Patients with spinal malalignment often compensate for lost lordosis with pelvic retroversion, hip extension, and knee flexion leading to the classic "crouched gait" [47]. Spinopelvic mismatch is an important driver in sagittal malalignment—pelvic retroversion becomes exhausted with increasing mismatch, at which point the compensation is transferred to the lower limbs with differential recruitment being affected by age [48].

In addition to gauging how much correction should be achieved, complication avoidance begins with preoperative planning. Multidisciplinary discussion involving the anesthesia team and neuromonitoring team should emphasize the importance of maintaining normal blood pressure throughout surgery to maintain adequate spinal cord perfusion and prevent blindness [49]. Patients benefit from arterial and central venous monitoring. The coagulation profile and normothermia should be monitored [50]. Neurophysiological monitoring with measurement of SSEPs and MEPs is often used for PCOs and routinely used for PSOs and VCRs. MEP monitoring consists of transcranial, spinal, neurogenic, and muscle MEPs to evaluate descending motor pathways; as such complexity exist in the pathway, there are variations in how various institutions monitor MEPs [51]. Obtaining good baseline neuromonitoring and being prepared to deal with any changes detected are of great importance [52]. Patients with preoperative myelopathy are difficult candidates for optimal neuromonitoring, but often require extensive osteotomies. Proper preoperative counseling of patients regarding the risks of this complex surgery is essential [53]. Despite patients undergoing spinal deformity surgery being well informed about potential risks, studies have shown that patients cannot recall most surgical risks discussed and recall declines over time [54].

Surgical Technique

General Principles

At the time of surgery, patients need to be appropriately padded and positioned on a radiolucent table that permits the abdomen to float freely to decrease epidural bleeding and allows gravity to assist pulling the lumbar spine back into lordosis. Placing additional chest pads can help to achieve further lordosis if the spine is flexible. It is recommended that the patient's head be placed level or higher than the heart [55]. Preoperatively, the amount of correction that will occur from general anesthesia and prone positioning with the abdomen dependent can be estimated on supine preoperative imaging such as MRI or CT. Furthermore, proper positioning and operating room setup can aid in closure of the osteotomy. For instance, the patient may be positioned on a four-poster frame with supports under the thighs and hips extended to assist in maintaining or increasing lumbar lordosis. Additionally, some operating tables allow a break in the table for initial positioning and the break in the table can be reduced to help close the osteotomy when it is complete. The four-poster frame can be positioned with its lower end at the break in the operating table, and the table is flexed to facilitate patient positioning. The flex is reduced and table straightened after the osteotomy is completed to assist in closure of the posterior wedge. Thus, the surgeon needs to be aware that the osteotomy gap can be closed while the operating table is brought from a flexed to a straight position. The level of the osteotomy should be aligned with the break in the operating table.

General Osteotomy Techniques

As previously stated, there are many different types of spinal osteotomies, but three general categories exist and more detailed techniques can be found below for each one. However, there are some generic steps that all osteotomies share, and we will review the general sequence of procedure here. It will be a surgeon's discretion as to whether or not to perform preoperative halo-gravity traction. Firstly, meticulous exposure is required including areas for grafting, decompression, and instrumentation. Secondly, insertion of pedicle screw at predetermined levels is completed. Decompression (laminectomies) can then be performed at indicated levels including the level of the osteotomy and adjacent levels. Any available bone graft is removed and saved for later use as fusion material. Care should be taken not to tear the dura. A temporary rod may be inserted on one side capturing three levels above and below the planned resection site to maintain alignment. Next, the planned osteotomy is carried out with further details provided below. It is important to avoid injury to the segmental artery and vein that lie just lateral to the vertebral body. Lastly, after closure of the osteotomy and hardware placement, bone grafting is completed to remaining facet joints and transverse processes.

Posterior Column Osteotomy

PCO includes both SPO and Ponte techniques. Furthermore, PCOs include Grade 1 or 2 osteotomies according to the comprehensive anatomical spinal osteotomy classification [7]. The inferior aspect of the spinous process is removed followed by removal of the interspinous ligament using a standard rongeur or osteotome. Next the ligamentum flavum (LF) is removed with a Kerrison rongeur; it is important to highlight that the LF arises from the lower half of the anterior surface of the cephalad lamina and attaches to the posterior surface and upper margin of the caudal lamina.

The surgeon must be vigilant not to penetrate deeply against the dura or tear the dura. The bilateral facet joints are removed either with a Kerrison rongeur, high-speed burr, or combination. One may choose to remove the LF intact during resection of bony elements to aid a barrier and protect the dura.

Partial facetectomy, complete facetectomy, or asymmetric facetectomy may be performed. For partial facetectomy, resection of the inferior facet and joint capsule at a given spinal level is done versus for a complete facet joint resection where both superior and inferior facets at a given spinal level are resected. This results in a V-shaped gutter with the width of the gutter typically between 10 and 15 mm.

Correction is performed gradually over multiple segments at the same time by compression of the pedicle screws closing the gap in the posterior elements. It is important to ensure that wider cranial and caudal laminectomies are performed so as not to trap or compress the thecal sac during osteotomy compression. This is done so as to redistribute corrective forces over a large area of the spinal column. Rods are set followed by decortication before wound closure. A cross table radiograph should be taken prior to closure.

Pedicle Subtraction Osteotomy

PSOs can be customized to patient-specific pathology depending on the amount of correction needed. The surgeon may resect bilateral pedicles and partial vertebral body; bilateral pedicles, partial vertebral body, and cephalad disc; or bilateral pedicles and asymmetric wedge of vertebral body. These osteotomies would include Grades 3 and 4 according to Schwab classification [7].

PCOs can be performed at the upper and lower level of the planned PSO vertebra. A wide laminectomy is performed from mid-pars region of the vertebra cephalad to the PSO vertebra distal to the lower-pars level of the PSO vertebra. The laminectomy should be in excess of the posterior element closure to minimize dural impingement. Furthermore, if there is extensive dural scarring from prior surgery, this will also need to be resected so that the plane between dura and scar is identified and mobilized cranially and caudally until normal dura is identified; otherwise, this can lead to compression upon closure.

The goal is to isolate and surround both pedicles so that they may be resected down to the base of the vertebral body. Of note, the surgeon must be careful to protect the exiting nerve roots that lie just against the medial and inferior aspect of the pedicle. The vertebral body is then decancellated of the cancellous bone to thin out the vertebral body and provide collapse and wedging of that segment. The surgeon needs to maintain the anterior vertebral body wall to act as the pivot point during closure of the osteotomy as well as maintain a protective barrier between the surgical field and viscera/major blood vessels. This will provide significant bone graft in addition to any graft harvested from prior PCOs. It is important to save all bone to be used later as fusion material. Additionally, if performing a traditional PSO, the vascularity of the remaining bone segment should be considered and preserved. Thus, if not removing the cranial disc, we recommend resection of the pedicle with the cranial cut just inside the pedicle itself.

Both lateral portions of the PSO vertebral body are exposed subperiosteally with Penfield 1 and Kittner dissectors, and a wedge of the lateral vertebral body is removed from superficial to deep. The subperiosteal dissection is of high importance to help protect and prevent injury to the segmental artery and vein that lie just lateral to the vertebral body. The lateral vertebral body cuts are made with straight osteotomes in a precise wedge based upon the desired closure so that the pivot point is the apex is the anterior vertebral wall. Of note, special retractor blades are available that allow access to the lateral wall and protect the segmental vessels. The cancellous bone is removed with a combination of curettes and rongeurs. Using angled curettes, the cancellous bone in the vertebra is pushed anteriorly to further create a cavity. Osteotomy contouring can be tailored using high-speed drill.

The final step involves dissecting the posterior vertebral body wall away from the ventral dural surface. An impaction technique is used with curettes or specialized impactors to push the posterior wall into the vertebral body, thus freeing up the entire ventral dural surface. If extensive anterior resection or thinning of the anterior cortex is performed, temporary rod stabilization is required to prevent translation. It is important not to place excessive stretch or tension on the dura during this portion of the procedure. PSO closure is performed by gentle compression across temporary rods. If excessive compression is required, the resection is likely inadequate. Temporary rods are then replaced with permanent rods that cover all instrumented segments: segmental pedicle screws at all predetermined levels at least three levels above and below the osteotomy site.

Vertebral Column Resection

VCR would include anatomic classification Grades 5 and 6 [7]. The extent of resection may include a complete vertebra with adjacent discs or multiple vertebrae and discs. Posterior alone or a combined anterior-posterior approach may be utilized. Please see the general steps for osteotomy above; we will begin this discussion as if exposure has been completed and pedicle screws have been placed.

PCOs are performed above and below the planned VCR level, and the posterior exposure is similar to the technique described for a PSO except that the laminectomy is done for the entire lamina of the VCR vertebrae and cephalad to the level of pars of the cranial lamina. Typically, the entire lamina of the level to be resected and the lamina cephalad to the pedicles above and caudad to the pedicles below are removed. Normally, for a one-level resection procedure, a posterior column laminectomy will result in a 5–6 cm exposure of the dura and neural elements. It is important not to minimize the posterior column exposure to gain thorough access to the spinal cord and/or cauda equina circumferentially, to aid in the resection procedure and also for visualizing any dural impingement during the correction.

In the thoracic spine, 5–6 cm of the medial rib associated with the level to be resected may be removed. Subperiosteal dissection of the medial aspect of the rib is performed. It is cut approximately 5–6 cm lateral to the vertebral attachment, and then as much of the rib as possible is removed down to the head anteriorly and is kept intact for later placement on top of the laminectomy defect. This is performed prior to the laminectomy to avoid canal intrusion if needed.

Pedicle screws have been placed at the predetermined levels. Prior to removing the anterior body, a temporary, stabilizing rod should be placed and attached to at least two or three pedicle screws both above and below the resection area. Classically, a unilateral rod is used; however, in severe angular kyphotic or kyphoscoliotic deformities, bilateral rods are recommended to prevent spinal subluxation. In the thoracic spine, the surgeon may elect to sacrifice one or both of the exiting nerve roots to provide increased exposure; however, this is generally not done in the lumbar spine, as nerve root function is critical to motor function of the lower extremities. Resection of the thoracic roots should be done medial to the dorsal root ganglia to reduce the chance of chronic pain. Sacrificing L1 or L2 in isolation will produce weakness, but over time many patients are able to compensate for the loss quite well. Nevertheless, sacrifice of these roots is not recommended. Loss of nerve root function below L2 will generally lead to a significant deficit.

The lateral vertebral body walls are subperiosteally dissected using protective instruments against the anterior and lateral margins to safely protect adjacent viscera and vasculature from harm. The lateral vertebral body walls are removed to allow entrance into the remainder of the vertebral body and to facilitate removal of all cancellous bone from endplate to endplate of the adjacent discs above and below. In primary procedures, super-periosteal dissection around the lateral aspect of the pedicles and vertebral body is performed using Penfield elevators. The soft tissues and the anterior vasculature are protected with either malleable retractors or special lateral wall vertebral body elevators. In revision cases, a subperiosteal dissection will be required due to previous scarring with a similar approach to gain access circumferentially around the vertebrae to be resected. In both circumstances, the segmental vessels are kept lateral in a soft tissue cuff and should not be violated if possible; otherwise, they may require ligation.

During resection of the pedicles, the surgeon must not only be careful of the exiting nerve roots but also of the spinal cord/dura when removing the concave pedicle as any coronal malalignment can allow this to rest against the pedicle. Careful dural protection with minimal retraction is the goal, and often using a high-speed burr to remove bone in high-risk areas is advised. For a scoliosis or kyphoscoliosis deformity, resecting the apical concave pedicle can be quite challenging since it is very cortical, and in a pure scoliosis deformity, the entire spinal cord/dural sac is resting on the medial concave pedicle which does not have any ventral vertebral body associated with it since the body is swung lateral and dorsal in its rotated position on the convexity. In this regard, using a small, high-speed burr is helpful to carefully burr away the cortical bone along this concave region.

The vertebral body is then decancellated of the cancellous bone in order to thin out the vertebra. Thus, in scoliosis and kyphoscoliosis deformities, the majority of the vertebral body will be removed from the convexity of the deformity since that is where the vertebral body is located. We prefer to perform the concave resection of the pedicle prior to the convex removal so there is no bleeding into this dependent concave region. This also allows the concave spinal cord to drift somewhat more medial and remove tension prior to going to the convexity for completion of the corpectomy. Again, it is important to save as much bone as possible to use in fusion later. Also, preservation of the cortices allows for temporary packing and tamponade of excess bleeding.

Both the anterior and posterior vertebral walls have been left intact thus far. The discs cephalad and caudad to the VCR are then removed using curettes. It is important not to violate the endplates of the superior and infero-adjacent regions as placement of a structural intracorporeal cage may be required. The last part of the vertebral resection is the posterior vertebral body wall. It is carefully dissected from the ventral dural surface and impacted into the vertebral body. Here it will be essential to control epidural bleeding with the judicious use of bipolar cauterization, topical hemostatic agents, and cottonoids. The dural sac must be circumferentially freed and exposed and then separated from the epidural venous complex as well as the posterior longitudinal ligament (PLL). The entire body is removed except for the anterior shell, as we like to keep a thin rim of bone intact on the anterior longitudinal ligament (ALL) for fusion purposes. However, if this bone is cortical, then it must be thinned to allow easy closure of the resection area. It is important not to place excessive stretch or tension on the dura during this step of the procedure. It is imperative that the ventral spinal cord is completely free of any bony prominences to avoid impingement during closure. This is especially true at the disc levels, especially above but also below, as there tends to be osteophytic lipping in that region which can cause ventral compression if not removed.

The deformity is then ready for correction by the temporary instrumentation always beginning with spinal shortening by convex rod compression to avoid excessive stretch on the spinal cord. This is performed either with individual pedicle screws in primary cases where a good bony grip of the vertebrae is found or in a construct-to-construct closure mechanism utilizing dominoes at the apex of the resected area. In this method, closing from a construct rod above to a construct rod below to distribute the forces of correction over several levels is performed. It is imperative to compress slowly as subluxation and/or dural impingement can occur along the way. In any deformity that has a degree of kyphosis, we place an anteriorly based structural cage to prevent over-shortening of the deformity, and it also acts as a hinge to provide further kyphosis correction. Typically, the spinal column will be shortened by 1 to 1.5 cm, an appropriate height and length cage will be inserted, and then further closure onto the cage to make it snug and fixed will be performed as a final correction maneuver. It is important to have the anesthesia team elevate the mean arterial pressure for cord perfusion and frequently communicate with the neuromonitoring team during this step.

Once closure has been fully performed, a permanent contralateral rod is placed with appropriate correction maneuvers performed. Then the temporary closing rod is removed and a permanent, final rod is placed on the contralateral side as well. Appropriate compression and distraction forces, in situ contouring, and other correction techniques may be performed always being mindful of any resultant effect on the resected area with respect to subluxation or dural impingement. Next, adequate alignment is confirmed by intraoperative radiographs. Decortication and bone grafting follow with copious amounts of local graft obtained from the resection procedure. The laminectomy defect is covered with the previously harvested ribs for the costotransversectomy approach. These ribs are split in half longitudinally with the cancellous surface placed along the entire laminectomy defect from the lamina above to the lamina below. This creates a rib "bridge" of bone to protect the dura, as well as to provide a posterior onlay fusion. The rib is held in place with sutures or a cross-link if there is room and no prominence. To confirm the absence of impingement, final implant security is documented as well as a final circumferential check of the exposed dura.

Illustrative Case (Fig. 22.4a–h)

History A 12-year-old young male presented with a visible dorsal prominence at the thoracolumbar junction with mild pain. His parents state that this "bump" had increased in size in the previous 2 years.

Physical Examination On inspection, a visible dorsal prominence was seen at the thoracolumbar junction. No tenderness. Patient had full motor strength in all lower extremity muscle groups, with normal sensation. Hyperreflexia was evident with patellar tendon reflex testing with 3–4 beats of clonus evident. Babinski reflex testing was equivocal.

Radiographic Imaging Standing AP (4a) and lateral (4b) 36-inch scoliosis x-rays demonstrate L1 dorsal hemivertebra with mild kyphosis. CT scan with sagittal reconstruction (4c) and MRI (4d) demonstrate significant encroachment into the spinal canal with stenosis and spinal cord compression.

Treatment He underwent a vertebral column resection (VCR) with posterior resection of the hemivertebra (4e). A structural cage was placed following completion of the L1 vertebrectomy (4f), prior to corrective maneuvers through the instrumentation.

Outcome Standing postoperative AP (4g) and lateral (4h) 36-inch scoliosis x-rays demonstrate L1 cage in place and posterior instrumented T11–L3 fusion. His thoracolumbar alignment has returned to neutral. At 2-year follow-up, he has maintained correction of deformity and has normal neurologic function.

Technical Pearls

General Principles

- A bear hugger placed underneath the operating table covering the free abdomen aids in maintaining normothermia. Preoperatively elevating room temperatures to excess levels while the patient is exposed aids with this as well.
- Placing the head 10° above the heart helps minimize the risk of visual complications [56].
- Special attention should always be applied to the intraoperative SSEP and MEPS at the time of osteotomy closure.
- At the time of closure, the surgeon should make sure that blood pressure and hematocrit are optimized.
- Patients with a mobile anterior column are often able to achieve correction of deformity by proper positioning alone.

Posterior Column Osteotomy

- Compression during closure of SPOs can lead to narrowing of the neural foramina which necessities a preceding wide facetectomy to prevent nerve root impingement. It is advised to palpate the foramina and nerve roots of levels involved prior to closure.
- Patients with anterior column fusion are unlikely to gain significant correction with multiple SPOs, and therefore a PSO may be a better option.

Pedicle Subtraction Osteotomy/ Vertebral Column Resection

- Most ideal in lumbar spine (L3 or L4) or in an ankylosed spine.
- Avoid leaving big open disc spaces (consider extended PSO, TLIF/PLIF below PSO, anterior fusion).
- Wide decompression of foramen and early identification of nerve roots.

- Leave anterior cortical wall intact to prevent translocation.
- Place temporary rods prior to removal of lateral and posterior cortical walls.
- Wide central canal decompression to accommodate dural buckling with resection of any scarred dura.
- A pedicle pilot hole created at the level of the PSO is useful to maintain orientation during bony removal.
- By performing the wider portion of the osteotomy on the convex side of the curve, coronal correction can be obtained at the same time as sagittal correction.

Complications and Strategies for Avoidance

PSO and VCR are technically more demanding and associated with longer operative times, greater blood loss, and higher risk of neurological complications than PCOs [57]. Complications related to the surgery include pseudarthrosis, proximal junctional kyphosis, instrumentation failure, adjacent spinal stenosis/adjacent segment disease, and infection. Postoperative medical complications include deep vein thrombosis, pulmonary embolus, small bowel ileus or obstruction, blindness, myocardial infraction, or stroke [58]. Table 22.3 reviews potential complications along with avoidance and management strategies.

Durotomies are sometimes unavoidable, especially in revision surgery. Emphasis should be placed on repair of the cerebrospinal fluid leak with direct repair or sealants, as it is important to prevent pseudarthrosis.

Neurological complications can be minimized with good intraoperative neuromonitoring and adequate bony resection; however, radiculopathy may be noted postoperatively due to compression of nerve roots as they exit the foramina; thus, care must be taken to perform a wide facetectomy and palpate the nerve roots after osteotomy closure.

Achievement of "ideal global sagittal realignment" has been shown to be protective against the development of reoperation and proximal junctional kyphosis [59]. Patients of concern may be evaluated with postoperative thin-cut CT scans to assess osteotomy closure and accuracy of implant placement. For all patients, standing AP and lateral 14 × 36 inch scoliosis radiographs are obtained before hospital discharge and at follow-up appointments, typically every 3 to 6 months. The patient should stand in a natural position without knee flexion or hip hyperextension. Correction of the osteotomy should be measured using preoperative and postoperative Cobb angles on lateral radiographs across the superior and inferior endplates of the vertebrae at which the osteotomies were performed. Global sagittal balance should be evaluated using a C7 plumb line and noting its relationship to the posterior superior corner of the sacrum.

Conclusion

The surgical treatment of spinal deformity is challenging. Traditionally, a circumferential approach with anterior releases via discectomies, followed by posterior instrumentation and fusion, has been the standard of care. However, the evolution of posterior approaches and osteotomies has allowed the modern era of spinal deformity surgery to promote posterior-only procedures. Currently, six anatomically defined osteotomies are accepted which fall into three general categories: (1) posterior column resection, (2) pedicle subtraction osteotomy, and (3) vertebral column resection. When considering an osteotomy for deformity correction, it is of great importance to match the correct osteotomy required by the malalignment. Thus, patient selection, preoperative planning, and decision-making are key to success. Restoration of satisfactory sagittal global alignment with thresholds of pelvic tilt <25°, sagittal vertical axis < 50 mm, and harmony between pelvic incidence and lumbar lordosis correlates with health-related quality-of-life scores. Furthermore, the surgeon needs to be aware of medical comorbidities and general health optimization prior to any surgery.

Table 22.3 Potential complications and avoidance strategies for lumbar osteotomies

General	Cardiopulmonary	Thromboembolic	CSF leak	Hemorrhage	Screw malposition	Neurologic	Infection	Revision
Medical optimization	Early mobilization	IVC filter (high-risk patient)	Careful dissection	Position (abdomen free)	Maximize exposure	Neuromonitoring	Preoperative decolonization	Smoking cessation
Careful padding	Pulmonary hygiene	Mechanical prophylaxis	High index	Meticulous hemostasis	Intraoperative Fluoroscopy	Normotension	Preoperative Antibiotics	Osteoporosis management
Normotension		Early mobilization	Primary repair	Blood salvage techniques	Spinal navigation	Wide decompression	Antibiotic powder	Consider biologics
Normothermia		Pharmacologic prophylaxis	CSF diversion	Intraoperative fibrinolytics		Resection of dural scar tissue	Excise tissue	Avoid NSAIDs
Identify high risk				Preoperative donation			Layered closure	
Patient education				Normothermia				

References

1. Cheng JS. The epidemiology of adult spinal deformity and the aging population. In: Wang YM, Lu Y, Anderson GD, Mummaneni VP, editors. Minimally invasive spinal deformity surgery: an evolution of modern techniques. Vienna: Springer Vienna; 2010.
2. Glassman SD, Berven S, Bridwell K, et al. Correlation of radiographic parameters and clinical symptoms in adult scoliosis. Spine (Phila Pa 1976). 2005;30(6):682–8.
3. O'Shaughnessy BA, Ondra SL. Measuring, preserving, and restoring sagittal spinal balance. Neurosurg Clin N Am. 2007;18(2):347–56.
4. Schwab F, Lafage V, Boyce R, Skalli W, Farcy JP. Gravity line analysis in adult volunteers: age-related correlation with spinal parameters, pelvic parameters, and foot position. Spine. 2006;31(25):E959–67.
5. Umehara S, Zindrick MR, Patwardhan AG, et al. The biomechanical effect of postoperative Hypolordosis in instrumented lumbar fusion on instrumented and adjacent spinal segments. Spine. 2000;25(13):1617–24.
6. Aebi M. The adult scoliosis. Eur Spine J. 2005; 14(10):925–48.
7. Schwab F, Blondel B, Chay E, et al. The comprehensive anatomical spinal osteotomy classification. Neurosurgery. 2013;74(1):112–20.
8. Smith-Petersen MN, Larson CB, Aufranc OE. Osteotomy of the spine for correction of flexion deformity in rheumatoid arthritis. Clin Orthop Relat Res. 1969;66:6–9.
9. Cho KJ, Lenke LG, Berra A, et al. Comparison of Smith-Petersen versus pedicle subtraction osteotomy for the correction of fixed sagittal imbalance. Spine. 2005;30(18):2030–7.
10. Hehne HJ, Zielke K, Bohm H. Polysegmental lumbar osteotomies and transpedicled fixation for correction of long-curved kyphotic deformities in ankylosing spondylitis. Clin Orthop Relat Res. 1990a;258:49–55.
11. Ondra SL, Marzouk S, Koski T, et al. Mathematical calculation of pedicle subtraction osteotomy size to allow precision correction of fixed sagittal deformity. Spine. 2006;31(25):E973–9.
12. Geck MJ, Macagno A, Ponte A, Shufflebarger HL. The Ponte procedure: posterior only treatment of Scheuermann's kyphosis using segmental posterior shortening and pedicle screw instrumentation. J Spinal Disord Tech. 2007;20(8):586–93.
13. Thomasen E. Vertebral osteotomy for correction of kyphosis in ankylosing spondylitis. Clin Orthop Relat Res. 1985;194:142–52.
14. Wang MY, Berven SH. Lumbar pedicle subtraction osteotomy. Neurosurgery. 2007;60(2 Suppl 1): ONS140–6.
15. Bridwell KH, Lewis SJ, Edwards C, et al. Complications and outcomes of pedicle subtraction osteotomies for fixed sagittal imbalance. Spine. 2003;28(18):2093–101.
16. Vauzelle C, Stagnara P, Jouvinroux P. Functional monitoring of spinal cord activity during spinal surgery. Clin Orthop Relat Res. 1973;93:173–8.
17. Nash CL, Loring RA, Schatzinger LA, et al. Spinal cord monitoring during operative treatment of the spine. Clin Orthop Relat Res. 1977;126:100–5.
18. Tamaki T, Kubota S. History of the development of intraoperative spinal cord monitoring. Eur Spine J. 2007;16(2):S140–6.
19. Gum JL, Buchowski JM, Lenke L, et al. Utilization trends of pedicle subtraction osteotomies compared to posterior spinal fusion for deformity: a national database analysis between 2008–2011. Scoliosis. 2016: In Press.
20. Sponseller PD, Jain A, Lenke LG, et al. Vertebral column resection in children with neuromuscular spine deformity. Spine (Phila Pa 1976). 2012;37(11): E655–61.
21. Kelly MP, Lenke LG, Shaffrey CI, et al. Evaluation of complications and neurological deficits with three column spine reconstructions for complex spinal deformity: a retrospective Scoli-risk 1 study. Neurosurg Focus. 2014;36(5):E17.
22. Lenke LG, Fehlings MG, Shaffrey CI, et al. Neurologic outcomes of complex adult spinal deformity surgery: results of the prospective, Multicenter Scoli-RISK-1 study. Spine. 2016;41(3):204–12.
23. MacLennan A. Scoliosis. Br Med J. 1922;2:865–6.
24. Bradford DS. Vertebral column resection for the treatment of rigid coronal decompensation. Spine. 1997;22(1):1590–9.
25. Dick J, Boachie-Adjei O, Wilson M. One-stage versus two-stage anterior and posterior spinal reconstruction in adults. Comparison of outcomes including nutritional status, complication rates, hospital costs, and other factors. Spine. 1992;17(Suppl):S310–6.
26. Suk SI, Chung ER, Kim JH, Kim SS, Lee JS, Choi WK. Posterior vertebral column resection for severe rigid scoliosis. Spine. 2005;30:1682–7.
27. Voyadzis JM, Gala VC, O'Toole JE, Eichholz KM, Fessler RG. Minimally invasive posterior osteotomies. Neurosurgery. 2008;63(3 Suppl):204–10.
28. Glassman SD, Schwab FJ, Bridwell KH, et al. The selection of operative versus nonoperative treatment in patients with adult scoliosis. Spine. 2007;32:93–7.
29. Lafage R, Schwab F, Challier V, et al. International spine study group. Defining Spino-pelvic alignment thresholds: should operative goals in adult spinal deformity surgery account for age? Spine (Phila Pa 1976). 2016;41(1):62–8.
30. Gill JB, Levin A, Burd T, et al. Corrective osteotomies in spine surgery. J Bone Joint Surg Am. 2008;90:2509–20.
31. Gum JL, Bridwell KH, Lenke LG, Bumpass DB, Sugrue PA, Karikari IO, Carreon LY. SRS22R appearance domain correlates most with patient satisfaction after adult deformity surgery to the sacrum at 5-year follow-up. Spine (Phila Pa 1976). 2015;40(16):1297–302.

32. Bridwell K. Decision-making regarding Smith-Petersen vs. pedicle subtraction osteotomy vs. vertebral column resection for spinal deformity. Spine. 2006;31(19 Suppl):S171–8.
33. Lafage V, Schwab F, Vira S, et al. Does vertebral level of pedicle subtraction osteotomy correlate with degree of spinopelvic parameter correction? J Neurosurg Spine. 2011;14(2):184–91.
34. Kim YH, Bridwell KH, Lenke LG, et al. Results of lumbar pedicle subtraction osteotomies for fixed sagittal imbalance: a minimum 5-year follow-up study. Spine. 2007;32(20):2189–97.
35. Gum, JL, Lenke LG, Bumpass D, et al. Does planned staging for posterior-only vertebral column resections in spinal deformity surgery increase perioperative complications? Spine Deform. 2016; 4(2):131–137.
36. Brown CW, Orme TJ, Richardson HD. The rate of pseudoarthrosis (surgical nonunion) in patients who are smokers and patients who are nonsmokers: a comparison study. Spine. 1986;11:942–3.
37. West J. Respiratory physiology: the essentials. 6th ed. Philadelphia: Lippincott Williams & Williams; 2000. p. 122.
38. Bertorini TE. Perisurgical management of patients with neuromuscular disorders. Neurol Clin. 2004;22: 293–313.
39. Shin JI, Phan K, Kathari P, et al. Impact of glycemic control on morbidity and mortality in adult idiopathic scoliosis patients undergoing spinal fusion. Clin Spine Surg. 2016: Oct 19. [Epub ahead of print].
40. Pickhardt PJ, Pooler BD, Lauder T, et al. Opportunistic screening for osteoporosis using abdominal computed tomography scans obtained for other indications. Ann Intern Med. 2013;158(8):588–95.
41. Snow R, Granata J, Ruhil AV, et al. Associations between preoperative physical therapy and post-acute care utilization patterns and cost in total joint replacement. J Bone Joint Surg Am. 2014;96(12):e165.
42. Jevsevar DS, Karlin LI. The relationship between preoperative nutritional status and complication after an operation for scoliosis in patients who have cerebral palsy. J Bone Joint Surg Am. 1993;75:880–994.
43. Tones MJ, Moss ND. The impact of patient self assessment of deformity on HRQL in adults with scoliosis. Scoliosis. 2007;2(1):1–9.
44. Aurouer N, Obeid I, Gille O, et al. Computerized preoperative planning for correction of sagittal deformity of the spine. Surg Radiol Anat. 2009;31(10):781–92.
45. Rose PS, Bridwell KH, Lenke LG, et al. Role of pelvic incidence, thoracic kyphosis, and patient factors on sagittal plane correction following pedicle subtraction osteotomy. Spine (Phila Pa 1976). 2009;34(8):785–91.
46. Akbar M, et al. Use of Surgimap spine in sagittal plane analysis, osteotomy planning, and correction calculation. Neurosurg Clin N Am. 2013;24(2):163–72.
47. Lafage V, Schwab F, Patel A, et al. Pelvic tilt and truncal inclination: two key radiographic parameters in the setting of adults with spinal deformity. Spine (Phila Pa 1976). 2009;34(17):E599–606.
48. Diebo BG, Ferrero E, Lafage R, et al. Recruitment of compensatory mechanisms in sagittal spinal malalignment is age and regional deformity dependent: a full-standing axis analysis of key radiographical parameters. Spine (Phila Pa 1976). 2015;40(9):642–9.
49. Turner JD, Eastlack RK, Mirzadeh Z, et al. Fluctuations in spinal cord perfusion during adult spinal deformity correction identify neurologic changes: proof of concept. World Neurosurg. 2016;85:365. e361–6.
50. Hart SR, Bordes B, Hart J, et al. Unintended perioperative hypothermia. Ochsner J. 2011;11(3):259–70.
51. Park J-H, Hyun S-J. Intraoperative neurophysiological monitoring in spinal surgery. World J Clin Cases. 2015;3(9):765–73.
52. Vitale MG, Skaggs DL, et al. Best practices in intraoperative Neuromonitoring in spine deformity surgery: development of an intraoperative checklist to optimize response. Spine Deform. 2014;2(5):333–9.
53. Biscevic M, Biscevic S, Ljuca F, Smrke BU, et al. Motor evoked potentials in 43 high risk spine deformities. Med Arch. 2014;68(5):345–9.
54. Saigal R, Clark AJ, Scheer JK, et al. Adult spinal deformity patients recall fewer than 50% of the risks discussed in the informed consent process Preoperatively and the recall rate worsens significantly in the postoperative period. Spine (Phila Pa 1976). 2015;40(14):1079–85.
55. Apfelbaum JL, Roth S, Connis RT, Domino KB, et al. Practice advisory for perioperative visual loss associated with spine surgery. Anesthesiology. 2012;116(2):274–85.
56. Emery SE, Daffner SD, France JC, et al. Effect of head position on intraocular pressure during lumbar spine fusion: a randomized, prospective study. J Bone Joint Surg Am. 2015;97(22):1817–23.
57. Daubs MD, Lenke LG, Cheh G, et al. Adult spinal deformity surgery: complications and outcomes in patients over age 60. Spine. 2007;32(20):2238–44.
58. Good CR, Auerbach JD, O'Leary PT, et al. Adult spinal deformity. Curr Rev Musculoskelet Med. 2011;4:159–67.
59. Maruo K, Ha Y, Inoue S, et al. Predictive factors for proximal junctional kyphosis in long fusions to the sacrum in adult spinal deformity. Spine. 2013;38(23):E1469–76.

Repair of Pars Defects and Spondylosis

23

Adam S. Kanter and Michael M. McDowell

Introduction

Defects of the pars interarticularis, or spondylolysis, represent a relatively common phenomenon in the lumbosacral spine creating the clinical dilemma of discerning whether its presence is of coincidental association or causative in a variety of clinical settings. Pars defects may be unilateral (20%) or bilateral (80%) and occur at the L5 vertebra in approximately 95% of cases [1–3]. Spondylolysis occurs in ~5–10% of the adult population but varies widely based on age and patient characteristics [1, 2, 4–7]. While there is a slight male predominance of spondylolysis, progression to spondylolisthesis occurs at a 2:1 ratio in women compared to men [1, 4].

Pathogenesis

The pars functions as a bony strut connecting the inferior and superior articulating processes of the vertebra to the pedicle and lamina. This results in a fulcrum-like phenomenon when loading, and translational forces are distributed through the axial spine. Biomechanical evidence suggests that the anterior aspect of the caudal pars is placed under the greatest stress during repetitive extension and rotation movements, particularly in bipedal positions [8, 9.] This is supported by CT findings that incomplete pars fractures typically involve the caudal pars with preservation of the rostral section [10]. The L5 vertebra serves as the point of maximal stress as force is transferred to the pelvis from the axial skeleton, thus the overwhelming prevalence of L5 pars defects in comparison to rostral levels (Fig. 23.1) [11].

Risk factors associated with developing spondylolysis and subsequent spondylolisthesis include a family history of pars defects, congenital spinal defects, and high-level athletics, particularly in childhood [2, 12]. It is considered to be predominantly an acquired defect with early childhood rates of pars defects being essentially nonexistent until after ambulation begins and with gradual increases in prevalence with increasing age [4, 5]. Inherent fragility due to an underlying dysplastic pars has been postulated to be present in many cases, as evidenced by a high rate of familial associations with pars defects [13]. In contrast, the higher prevalence in certain athletes suggests that repetitive stress may result in microfractures gradually resulting in spondylolysis. A combination of both predisposed weakness and repetitive trauma is likely in most cases [2, 14, 15].

A.S. Kanter, MD, FAANS (✉) • M.M. McDowell, MD
Department of Neurological Surgery, University of Pittsburgh Medical Center, Pittsburgh, PA, USA
e-mail: kanteras@upmc.edu; mcdowellmm2@upmc.edu

L.T. Holly, P.A. Anderson (eds.), *Essentials of Spinal Stabilization*,
DOI 10.1007/978-3-319-59713-3_23

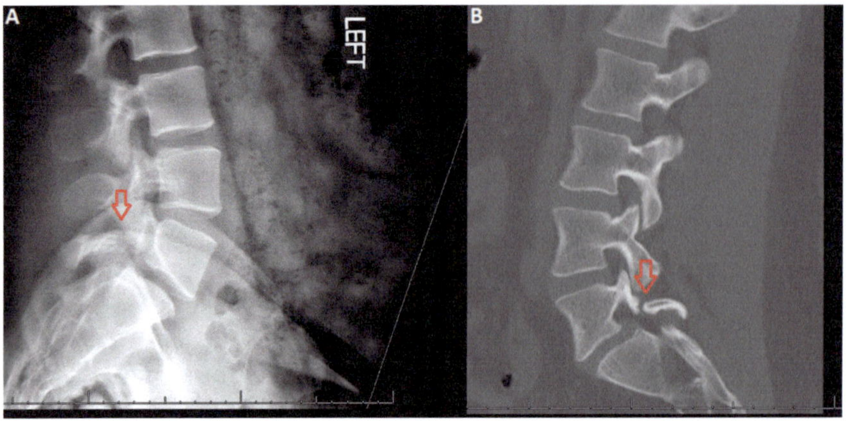

Fig. 23.1 Lateral lumbar radiograph (**a**) and sagittal CT of the lumbar spine (**b**) demonstrating an L5 pars defect (*arrows*)

Isthmic spondylolisthesis, or vertebral body slippage associated with pars defects, is the most common type of spondylolisthesis. Approximately 70% of adult patients with spondylolysis develop some level of slippage; however, in most cases, it remains stable and asymptomatic [1, 4, 5]. Typically, if the slippage of one vertebra relative to the adjacent vertebra is <30%, it rarely progresses, and the likelihood lessens even further with increasing age [4, 5, 16]. Patients with higher degrees of spondylolisthesis, particularly those with slippage >50%, have a much higher rate of progression and subsequent potential for neurological compromise [16]. Of note, isthmic spondylolisthesis comprises the largest proportion of patients who will develop high-grade slippage, potentially secondary to the inherent reduction in bony structural integrity [17]. Several subclassification models have postulated for high-grade spondylolisthesis based on etiology and pelvic parameters but to date have not been found to consistently conform with clinical decision-making to any greater extent than radiographic characteristics alone [17–21].

Symptomology

A defect in the pars frequently has no direct consequences, presumably due to the redundancy provided by adjacent ligamentous and bony structures. However, in a subset of this cohort, the lack of a rigid connection between articulating joints allows for slippage to occur and chronic wear and tear on overburdened adjacent structures resulting in spondylosis/degenerative changes, both of which may result in pain or neurological dysfunction. Spondylolysis, spondylosis, and spondylolisthesis may all be asymptomatic but, when not, are most often associated with low back pain exacerbated by hyperextension and relieved by rest [22]. These symptoms frequently start in adolescence. Spondylolysis represents approximately 50% of identifiable causes of insidious low back pain in pediatric patients but in less than 5% of adult patients [23, 24]. Radiculopathy and progressive spinal deformity may also be present, most typically associated with a high-grade progressive slip [25, 26].

While numbness and weakness in a radicular distribution is highly concerning, it is infrequent relative to the prevalence of pars defects. When radiculopathy is present in patients with an L5 pars defect, it typically involves the L5 nerve root [6, 27]. In rare instances of higher-level involvement, cauda equina or cord compression is possible. Patients may stand with a hyperlordotic posture and flexed knees and hips, known as the Phalen-Dickson sign, in order to mitigate low back pain [28]. Patients with severe spondylolisthesis may have discontinuity of the alignment of spinous processes upon palpation. Chronic spondylolisthesis, particularly high grade, may gradually lead to scoliotic deformity, hamstring contracture, abnormal gait, or a combination thereof [29–35].

Surgical Indications and Patient Selection

Spondylolysis and isthmic spondylolisthesis are primarily chronic conditions, so it is critical that careful consideration be given as patients are evaluated and intervention considered. The following are frequent indications for operative intervention:

Failure of Conservative Management

Barring acute, progressive, or severe neurological deficits, a trial of conservative management is often sufficient to allow symptomatic improvement and return to their prior level of activity in many patients with pars defects and spondylolisthesis [36, 37]. Recommended interventions include bracing if tolerated, rehabilitation, avoidance of activities that induce hyperextension or heavy loading of the lumbar spine, and restriction from competitive sports when applicable. Symptomatic control, not radiographic improvement, is the primary goal of management. Conservative management is most successful at relieving symptoms in patients with less than 50% slippage; however, osseous fusion of the spondylolysis may not occur despite symptomatic resolution [24, 38–42]. In the absence of persistent symptoms after a course of conservative management, long-term improvement is often durable, and patients do not require permanent activity restrictions or surgical intervention [38, 39, 41, 43]. Osseous regeneration is most likely to occur in adolescent patients, particularly in cases of unilateral or partial pars defects [36, 42]. Athletic adolescent patients with pars defects and low-grade spondylolisthesis are frequently successful in returning to their prior activity level without surgical intervention [36, 44, 45].

High-Grade Isthmic Spondylolisthesis

The degree of spondylolisthesis has been found to predict response to conservative management. The majority of patients with symptomatic pars defects and either no or low-grade (I or II) spondylolisthesis are often responsive to conservative treatment. However, both adolescent and adult patients with symptomatic high-grade (III or higher) spondylolisthesis tend to ultimately necessitate surgical intervention. In a study of 11 patients with symptomatic high-grade slippage, only one was found to have satisfactory pain relief with conservative management [46–48]. This asymptomatic high-grade slippage may be monitored, with surgical consideration if attributable symptoms develop [49].

Progressive Spondylolisthesis

Progression of spondylolisthesis is more common in juvenile patients who have not yet reached skeletal maturity. Adults, even with higher-grade slippage, will more frequently remain stable due to gradual autofusion and soft tissue hypertrophy. If progressive slippage is noted on interval imaging, controversy exists as to whether or not operative management is indicated in the asymptomatic patient [17, 46, 47]. Patients with progressive spondylolisthesis and intractable back pain and/or neurological deficits frequently benefit from surgical intervention.

Spinopelvic Alignment

Pelvic parameters and global spinal alignment have become increasingly recognized as important clinical considerations in patients being evaluated with pars defects [50–52]. Sagittal imbalance associated with spondylolisthesis may require a multilevel corrective procedure should a progressive deformity develop [35]. Careful assessment of relevant radiographic parameters is required and discussed further below.

Neurological Symptoms

High-grade slippage may result in traction injury to the L5 nerve root in the absence of foraminal stenosis. Radicular weakness in the L5 distribution, although uncommon, warrants decompression of the nerve root. Fusion and, when indicated, reduction may improve nerve root function and prevent future stretch injury. Numbness does not resolve as consistently as other radicular symptoms following decompressive surgery.

Preoperative Considerations

Imaging

Plain lumbar radiographs are recommended as the initial step in the evaluation of patients with nonurgent symptomology including low back and radicular pain. Flexion-extension views are routinely included to assess for dynamic instability, particularly in the presence of a preexisting spondylolisthesis. Historically, radiographs are performed in the anterior-posterior, lateral, right-oblique, and left-oblique orientations, but the increased availability of computed tomography (CT) imaging and its sensitivity for spondylolysis detection have limited plain imaging diagnoses [53]. When performed, pars defects are identified in > 95% of cases, with the classic "scotty dog" sign marred by a "broken neck" classical finding (Fig. 23.2) [54, 55]. Other findings on plain radiographs suggestive of spondylolysis, particularly unilateral defects, may include sclerosis of the contralateral pedicle or a rotated spinous process with the superior aspect of the process pointing toward the defect [56].

Simple lateral radiographs are sufficient for assessment of the degree of accompanying spondylolisthesis. The most widespread grading system is the Meyerding classification system [57]. This system divides the degree of slippage by 25% increments relative to the adjacent vertebral body (grade I slippage < 25%, grade II 25% to 50%, grade III 50% to 75%, and grade IV 75% to 100%); slippage >100% is termed spondyloptosis [57]. This classification schema has been strongly associated with prognosis and surgical necessity [11]. Meyerding grade 3 and higher slips are more often found to be unstable on dynamic imaging [11, 52].

Spinopelvic parameters have been found to play an important role in spondylolisthesis occurrence and progression. The effect of spondylolisthesis on global spinal alignment should be

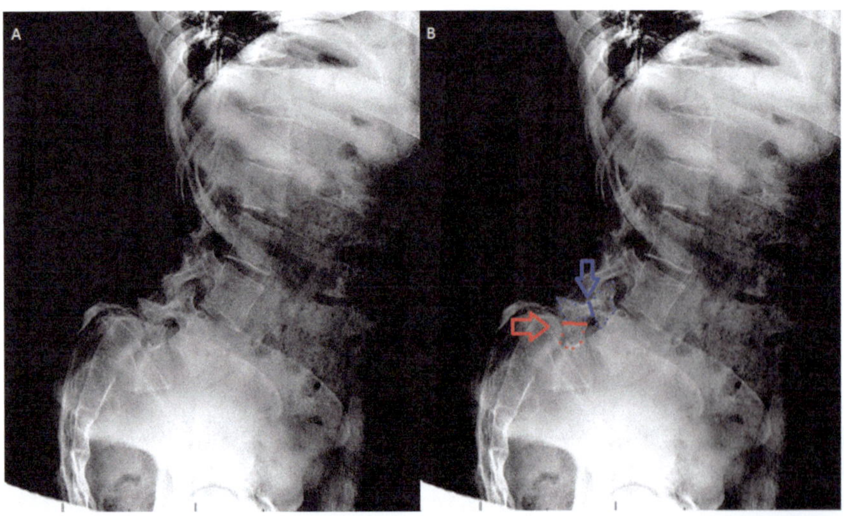

Fig. 23.2 Lateral lumbar radiograph depicting Meyerding grade 5 spondylolisthesis: spondyloptosis. The *blue* outline indicates an intact pars interarticularis in the shape of the "scotty dog sign" with intact neck at L4. The *red* outline indicates the broken off "head" of the scotty dog at L5

considered and corrected when applicable. Sacral inclination, the angle between the posterior border of the sacrum and a vertical line, has been associated with progressive spondylolisthesis when the angle is greater than 60 degrees [52]. Pelvic incidence, the angle of a line from the femoral head to the middle of the sacral endplate and a line perpendicular from the same point, has been found to increase in an approximately linear relationship to the severity of spondylolisthesis [50]. A high pelvic incidence is associated with higher shear stress at the L5–S1 junction and may increase the likelihood of slippage over time [17]. While most patients with pars defects and spondylolisthesis have lordotic spinal alignment, as slip grade progresses, there tends to be a tendency toward lumbosacral kyphosis at the L5–S1 junction. Some data suggest that severe lumbosacral kyphosis plays a causative role in slip progression, and restoration of normal lordosis may be useful to correct sagittal balance of the global spine [35, 58, 59].

Measurement of the lumbosacral angle, the angle of a line parallel to the superior endplate of L5 and a line to the posterior aspect of the S1 body (Fig. 23.3), has a strong correlation with kyphosis and avoids the need to measure the degenerated L5–S1 junction [30]. In a study comparing 20 patients without spondylolisthesis to 20 patients with high-grade spondylolisthesis by Glavas et al., the mean angle was found to be 119 and 71 degrees, respectively [59].

Long-cassette x-rays, or "scoliosis films," are increasingly valuable when considering patients with significant spondylolisthesis to assess for global sagittal alignment as well as the aforementioned pelvic parameters. CT imaging can be useful in detecting partial pars defects or in circumstances where severe degenerative changes make interpretation of radiographs difficult [53]. Non-dynamic spinal parameters can be detected by CT imaging as well, but supine imaging may not accurately reflect erect spinal alignment. Single-photon emission computed tomography (SPECT) scans have been used to assess pars defects in younger patients who have greater potential for bony repair and remodeling. Increased uptake on SPECT scans with the presence of a partial or small pars defect on CT is suggestive of local repair processes that may occur with conservative management [52, 53]. Magnetic resonance imaging (MRI) should be obtained in patients with neurological deficits or radicular symptoms to rule out other explanations.

Age

Spondylolysis is an interesting phenomenon in that the pathology can become symptomatic in patients ranging from adolescence to senescence. The underlying mechanism is presumed to be more due to acute injury and joint instability (or,

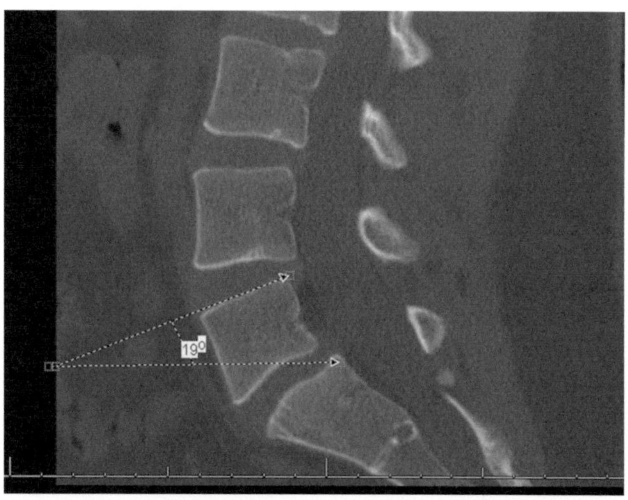

Fig. 23.3 CT of the lumbar spine in the sagittal plane depicting the measurement of the lumbosacral angle via drawing a line from the superior endplate of L5 to the posterior aspect of the S1 vertebral body

at least, hypermobility) in younger patients, whereas arthritic degeneration is frequently cited as the root cause in older patients. In contrast to the younger cohort, degenerative changes found in older symptomatic patients often necessitate bony decompression and stabilization to address the pars defect and spondylolisthesis. Adult patients with comorbidities, particularly those with a tobacco history, have a higher rate of pseudarthrosis and often require interbody fusion graft procedures. In patients with high-grade spondylolisthesis, reduction of the slippage can be performed to induce spinal realignment and nerve decompression. Spinal reduction is easier in the athletic adolescent cohort with minimal arthritic change; in adults, chronicity of the deformity and degenerative changes reduce the mobility of the spine and may not be feasible based on intraoperative findings. As previously noted, adults tend to have a lower frequency and degree of slip progression when spondylolisthesis is present. As such, a lower threshold for observation in asymptomatic patients, even when mild progression is noted, is generally recommended when compared to a young patient with progressive changes.

Reduction

Reduction of high-grade spondylolisthesis remains an area of contention, with early authors citing neurological injury as a common reason to avoid reduction maneuvers, particularly given the high rate of excellent outcomes with fusion alone [17, 60]. With the growing value of global spinal alignment and advances in instrumentation and technique, renewed interest in reduction techniques to maximize positive, durable outcomes has evolved [61–64]. Reduction of slippage has since proven biomechanically advantageous in correcting lumbosacral kyphosis and promoting an appropriate upright posture. Failure to reduce in the setting of severe lumbosacral kyphosis subjects the construct to additional shear forces that may increase the risk of pseudarthrosis, non-fusion, and ultimately slip progression [65–67]. In high-grade spondylolisthesis and spondyloptosis, the angulation of the vertebral body plays an even greater role in spinal imbalance than the slippage itself, necessitating dramatic reduction in order to maximize correction and spinal realignment [50, 51, 58].

New-onset neurological deficits following reduction remain the preeminent concern among surgical practitioners; however, recent data suggests that carefully selected patients have a lower risk of new-onset deficit than in early reports. A review of the Scoliosis Research Society morbidity and mortality database conducted by Kaswliwal et al. determined that permanent neurological deficit after high-grade spondylolisthesis reduction ranged from 5% to 10% of patients in most participating centers, and this rate was not statistically higher than permanent neurological deficits occurring after in situ decompression and fusion alone [68]. Partial reduction to decrease the slip angulation may be sufficient to reduce the risk of reoperation and restore spinal alignment and may reduce the likelihood of a neurological deficit in high-risk patients [69].

Surgical Technique

General indications for surgery include failure of conservative management as described above, persistent or worsening back pain in conjunction with pars non-union or spondylolisthesis, progressive slippage on repeat imaging, and new or progressive neurological deficits [70].

There is tremendous heterogeneity in the surgical management of pars defects and spondylolisthesis, in part due to multiple procedures all yielding excellent clinical outcomes. The wide range of age at presentation and the degree of degenerative and deformational changes remain important considerations in the surgical decision-making process.

Direct Repair

Symptomatic patients who fail conservative management can be considered for direct pars repair alone where preservation of ligamentous and muscular attachments is desired, such as in younger patients, and where complicating factors such as diffuse arthritic changes, spondylolisthesis, and abnormal spinal alignment are absent. In this subset of patients, excellent results can be obtained in greater than 75% of patients [71].

Direct repair of a pars defect via Buck's procedure or a variant has been frequently reported as an attractive alternative to fusion procedures [72, 73]. Briefly, this procedure is performed by a standard lumbar exposure of the lamina and defective pars. Fibrotic material in the vicinity of the pars is debrided and bony edges decorticated. It is critical to prevent disruption of the facet capsules during exposure to prevent future joint dysfunction. A screw is inserted from the inferior lamina into the pars at a trajectory aimed superior and slightly lateral from the starting point under direct visualization approximately 1 centimeter deep to the pars into the pedicle. Unilateral or bilateral defects can be packed with autograft, allograft, or other fusion-stimulating material. This procedure is best performed in patients with minimal degenerative disease at the level in question. Drazin et al. recommend that the intervertebral disc at the level of slippage (L5–S1 typically) be at least two-thirds the height of adjacent discs and recommend limiting the procedure to patients with spondylolisthesis of less than 1 centimeter [74]. A variant of this technique can be performed in a minimally invasive setting under fluoroscopy [75].

Alternatives to this technique are abundant and include the placement of pedicle screws with a sublaminar hook attached (Fig. 23.4) and segmental wire fixation [76–78]. Segmental wire fixation is performed by dissection of the L5 spinous process, lamina, and transverse process with careful avoidance of exposing the facet joints. A wire may be wrapped around the circumference of each transverse process and secured. Bone graft may be pressed into the wire to promote subsequent fusion [79]. For sublaminar hook technique, pedicle screws are placed in typical fashion after dissection and debridement as described in Buck's procedure. Laminar hooks attached to short rods are inserted at the level of the inferior aspect of the L5 lamina and then secured to the pedicle screws. This has also been described using minimally invasive dilators to access the L5–S1 interlaminar space [80]. Newer techniques in development include the use of intralaminar screws at the junction of the spinous process and the lamina, with one screw placed slightly more superior in order to allow for bilateral placement. These screws are then connected via a titanium rod to adjacent pedicle screws without the need to transverse the fractured pars [81].

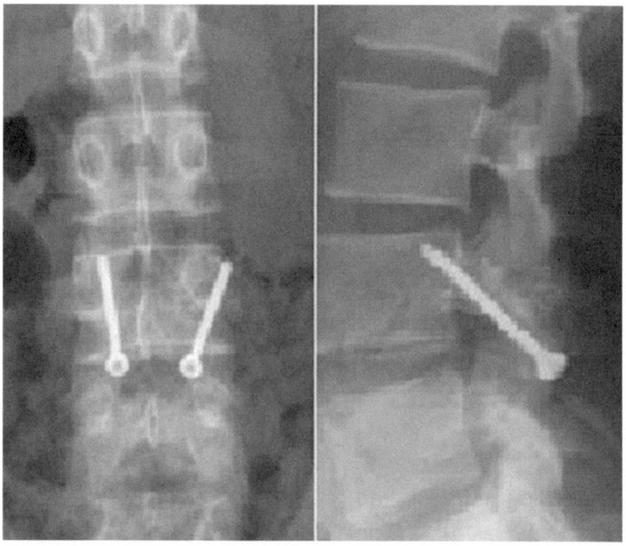

Fig. 23.4 Postoperative lateral x-ray demonstrating pars repair via direct repair

Posterolateral Fusion

The most common intervention for the repair of pars defects with spondylolisthesis is the posterolateral fusion and fixation [70, 82]. This versatile procedure, though more invasive, is useful in older patients in the setting of degeneration and severe vertebral body slippage. It also can be performed in the setting of a bony decompression via laminectomy, whereas direct repair typically relies upon intact adjacent structures. Bony decompression is frequently necessary in the setting of radicular symptoms such as pain or weakness, in which case posterolateral fusion is preferable over direct repair even in young athletic patients. The surgical details of standard posterolateral fusion are discussed elsewhere in this book. Non-instrumented fusion in patients with spondylolysis alone or with low-grade spondylolisthesis may be considered in younger patients with immobile slips, but in high-grade spondylolisthesis, instrumentation is recommended with or without reduction as above.

A common issue that can arise with posterolateral fusion with high-grade slippage is the difficulty in achieving appropriate transpedicle L5 screw placement. One alternative is to place transsacral S1 pedicle screws of sufficient length to extend across the sacral promontory into the L5 vertebral body to provide stability via tricortical purchase utilizing fluoroscopy or image guidance. Fibular dowels or, if the L5 vertebral body has slipped anterior to the sacrum, a fibular strut via a reamed canal can be inserted through the sacrum into L5 for added stability [83]. This is particularly useful when there is limited trajectory to reach the L5–S1 disc space without osteotomy or when there is no adjacent contact between the L5 and S1 bodies to enable interbody graft placement. In extreme cases, such as severe spondyloptosis, an L5 vertebral resection, also known as a vertebrectomy or spondylectomy, can be performed [84]. The lack of bony contact and the tendency of the L5 vertebra to descend below the superior sacral endplate make this challenging from a posterior approach. An anterior, retroperitoneal approach can be used to resect the L5 vertebral body, with subsequent instrumentation of the L4 vertebral body to S1 and placement of an interbody device when appropriate [85, 86]. Partial resection of the sacral dome may be sufficient to access L5 for instrumentation and partial reduction, foregoing the need for spondylectomy [87].

Interbody Fusion

For simple spondylosis or pars defects with mild spondylolisthesis, posterolateral fusion is typically sufficient to ensure lasting symptom resolution and adjacent level stability. However, in patients with high-grade slippage, interbody support may improve deformity correction and provide greater lumbosacral stability by diverting shear forces from that of the instrumented construct [17, 67, 83]. In addition, patients with symptomatic pars defects with associated degeneration such as disc herniations with dynamic instability or radicular symptoms may also benefit from interbody fusion in order to address both problems simultaneously [88]. Anterior column support via an interbody graft can be obtained via a posterior or anterior approach, based upon the anatomy of the slippage itself. The technique for interbody insertion is discussed elsewhere in this book.

Illustrative Case

History and Physical Exam

A 36-year-old gentleman with bilateral pars defects presented with 1 year of progressively severe mechanical back pain refractory to anti-inflammatory medications, oral steroids, injections, and intensive physical therapy. He endorsed increasing radicular pain in the left lateral leg to his toes, including numbness in the same distribution. Bending and lifting objects at work significantly exacerbated his symptoms. His physical examination remained neurologically intact, with full motor and sensory function and symmetric reflexes; however, extensive postures elicited severe midline pain that caused him to buckle at the knees.

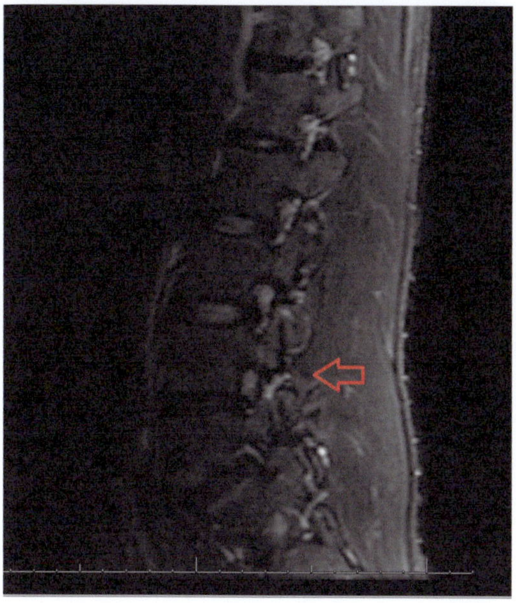

Fig. 23.5 Sagittal cut of the T1 sequence of an MRI of the lumbar spine demonstrating the presence of an L5 pars defect (*arrow*)

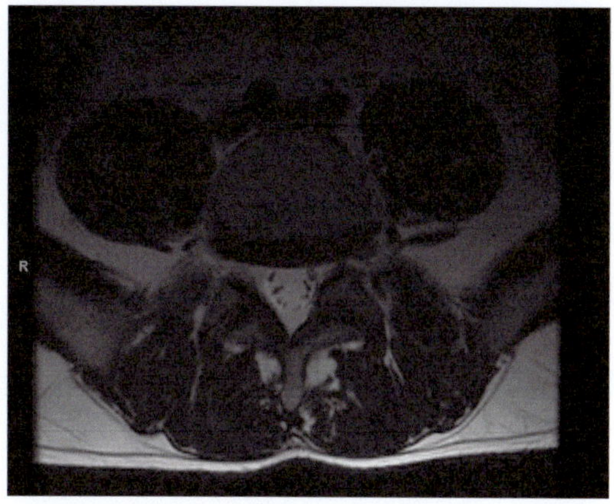

Fig. 23.6 Axial cut of the T2 sequence of an MRI of the lumbar spine demonstrating the presence of a large, broad-based disc bulge at L5–S1 resulting in moderate left-sided foraminal stenosis

Imaging

MR imaging revealed bilateral L5 pars defects (Fig. 23.5) with grade 1 spondylolisthesis and a broad-based disc bulge with mild left foraminal narrowing when supine (Fig. 23.6). Dynamic x-ray imaging revealed the listhesis was grossly immobile, and CT confirmed the findings of isthmic spondylolisthesis.

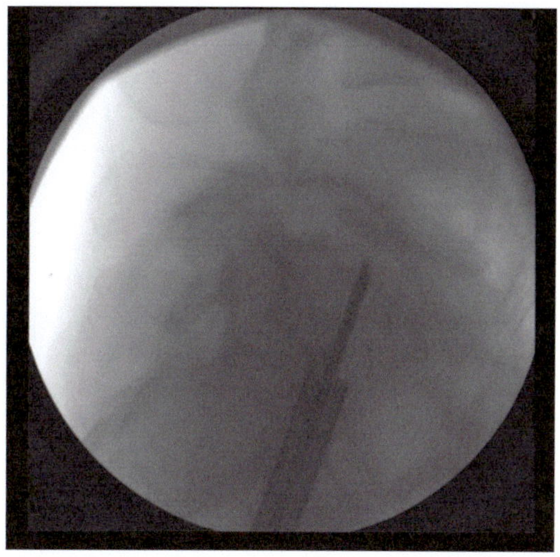

Fig. 23.7 Intraoperative lateral x-ray demonstrating the entry of the presacral guide pin into the L5–S1 disc space and the advancement of a dilator halfway to target

Treatment

The patient was counseled on various operative options and ultimately underwent interbody fusion to address his radicular and mechanical symptomatology. A minimally invasive presacral approach was chosen given his young age and normal spinal alignment in order to minimize long-term consequences from ligamentous and muscular disruption. The patient was brought to the operating room and placed in the prone position after appropriate induction of general anesthesia. After being prepped and draped, an incision was made to the left of his coccyx, and the presacral space was approached and then bluntly dissected. Using a guide pin, the sacrum was pierced and the disc space entered using sequential dilators (Fig. 23.7). A discectomy was performed, and the L5 and S1 endplates were curetted. A guide pin was then inserted through the disc space into L5, and a 15 mm cage was inserted (Fig. 23.8). Percutaneous pedicle screws were placed at L5 and S1 under fluoroscopy (Fig. 23.9).

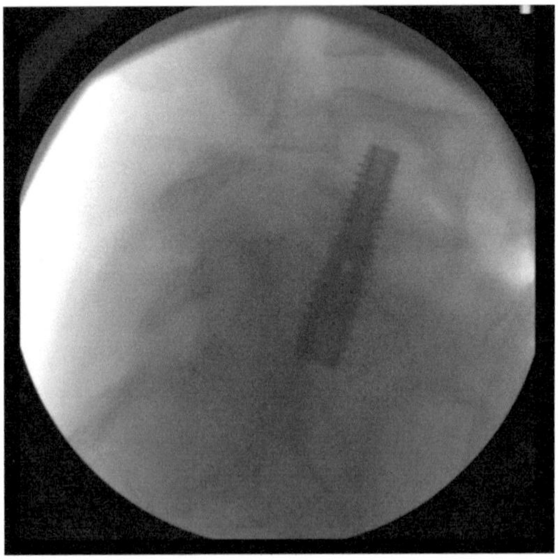

Fig. 23.8 Intraoperative lateral x-ray demonstrating the successful placement of a L5–S1 interbody graft via the minimally invasive presacral approach

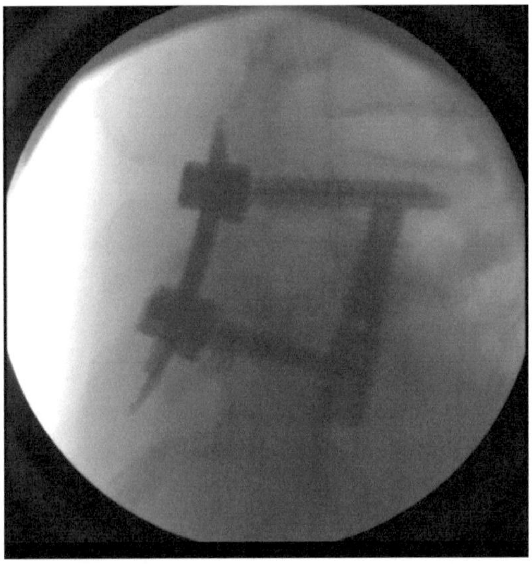

Fig. 23.9 Intraoperative lateral x-ray demonstrating the completed minimally invasive construct of a L5–S1 interbody fusion via the presacral approach

Outcome

The patient was followed for 2 years postoperatively. He reported complete resolution of his radicular pain and approximately 80% reduction in his mechanical back pain at last follow-up. Final imaging revealed a solid fusion mass.

Technical Pearls

- Minimal disruption of ligamentous connections and preservation of facet capsules should be attempted in young patients undergoing direct repair of spondylolysis with minimal or no spondylolisthesis to reduce risk of reoperation.
- High-grade spondylolisthesis implies greater instability. Instrumentation at L4–S1 is often recommended for patients undergoing posterolateral fusion.
- Partial reduction of high-grade slippage in the presence of a significant degree of slip angle reduces the shear stress on instrumentation and will relieve L5 nerve root tension with a low risk of iatrogenic injury.
- If pedicle screw placement across L5 is insufficient or technically infeasible, tricortical purchase via an S1 pedicle screw extending into the listhesed L5 vertebral body provides stability when incorporated into a construct extending rostral to L4.
- Extension of decompression and fusion may be required in order to achieve appropriate correction of sagittal imbalance and other parameters of spinal alignment.

Complications and Strategies for Avoidance

The degree and complication profile is associated with the type of surgical procedure chosen to address the pars defect and slip [68, 89]. For minimally disruptive procedures such as Buck's procedure for direct repair of spondylolysis, the primary concern is the disruption of soft tissue attachments and facet capsules which increase the risk of adjacent level disease and reoperation. Instrumented fusion has the inherent risk of pseudarthrosis and other instrumentation failure such as rod fracture or pedicle screw malposition. Judicious use of intraoperative imaging to ensure appropriate instrumentation is recommended. When combined with bony decompression, durotomy and neurological injury can be minimized with careful dissection and exposure. As with all spine surgery, there is a risk of wound infection, deep vein thrombosis, pulmonary embolism, and pneumonia. Early mobilization, fastidious wound care, and appropriate pulmonary toilet should be aggressively encouraged in the postoperative period. Reduction should be performed with caution, due to the association with permanent neurological deficit in up to 10% of patients. Prior to reduction, a thorough decompression with unroofing of bilateral nerve root foramen should be achieved. Partial reduction can be considered when complete reduction is anatomically limited. Neuro-monitoring is intraoperatively performed in almost all cases.

Conclusion

Pars defects can be a source of significant mechanical back pain and can predispose patients to secondary spinal disorders, such as spondylolisthesis and instability. Both direct and indirect methods of repair are available. Direct repair is ideal for younger symptomatic patients with isolated pars defects, whereas indirect methods including posterolateral fusion and interbody techniques allow for management of the pars defect in combination with secondary disease processes. Critical evaluation needs to be given when determining if symptomatology is the result of the spondylolysis, particularly in chronic situations without neurological compromise or progressive radiologic disease or instability.

References

1. Belfi LM, Ortiz AO, Katz DS. Computed tomography evaluation of spondylolysis and spondylolisthesis in asymptomatic patients. Spine. 2006;31(24):E907–10.
2. Harvey CJ, Richenberg JL, Saifuddin A, Wolman RL. The radiological investigation of lumbar spondylolysis. Clin Radiol. 1998;53(10):723–8.
3. Gurd DP. Back pain in the young athlete. Sports Med Arthrosc. 2011;19(1):7–16.
4. Fredrickson BE, Baker D, McHolick WJ, Yuan HA, Lubicky JP. The natural history of spondylolysis and spondylolisthesis. J Bone Joint Surg Am. 1984;66(5):699–707.
5. Beutler WJ, Fredrickson BE, Murtland A, Sweeney CA, Grant WD, Baker D. The natural history of spondylolysis and spondylolisthesis: 45-year follow-up evaluation. Spine. 2003;28(10):1027–35. discussion 35
6. Cassidy RC, Shaffer WO, Johnson DL. Spondylolysis and spondylolisthesis in the athlete. Orthopedics. 2005;28(11):1331–3.
7. Toueg CW, Mac-Thiong JM, Grimard G, Parent S, Poitras B, Labelle H. Prevalence of spondylolisthesis in a population of gymnasts. Stud Health Technol Inform. 2010;158:132–7.
8. Terai T, Sairyo K, Goel VK, Ebraheim N, Biyani A, Faizan A, et al. Spondylolysis originates in the ventral aspect of the pars interarticularis: a clinical and biomechanical study. J Bone Joint Surg Br. 2010;92(8):1123–7.
9. Wiltse LL. The etiology of spondylolisthesis. J Bone Joint Surg Am. 1962;44-A:539–60.
10. Dunn AJ, Campbell RS, Mayor PE, Rees D. Radiological findings and healing patterns of incomplete stress fractures of the pars interarticularis. Skelet Radiol. 2008;37(5):443–50.
11. Foreman P, Griessenauer CJ, Watanabe K, Conklin M, Shoja MM, Rozzelle CJ, et al. L5 spondylolysis/spondylolisthesis: a comprehensive review with an anatomic focus. Childs Nerv Syst. 2013;29(2):209–16.
12. Lonstein JE. Spondylolisthesis in children. Cause, natural history, and management. Spine. 1999;24(24):2640–8.
13. Niethard FU, Pfeil J, Weber M. Etiology and pathogenesis of spondylolytic spondylolisthesis. Orthopade. 1997;26(9):750–4.
14. Albanese M, Pizzutillo PD. Family study of spondylolysis and spondylolisthesis. J Pediatr Orthop. 1982;2(5):496–9.
15. Wynne-Davies R, Scott JH. Inheritance and spondylolisthesis: a radiographic family survey. J Bone Joint Surg Br. 1979;61-B(3):301–5.
16. Seitsalo S, Osterman K, Hyvarinen H, Tallroth K, Schlenzka D, Poussa M. Progression of spondylolisthesis in children and adolescents. A long-term follow-up of 272 patients. Spine. 1991;16(4):417–21.
17. Kasliwal MK, Smith JS, Kanter A, Chen CJ, Mummaneni PV, Hart RA, et al. Management of high-grade spondylolisthesis. Neurosurg Clin N Am. 2013;24(2):275–91.
18. Hammerberg KW. New concepts on the pathogenesis and classification of spondylolisthesis. Spine. 2005;30(6 Suppl):S4–11.
19. Hresko MT, Labelle H, Roussouly P, Berthonnaud E. Classification of high-grade spondylolistheses based on pelvic version and spine balance: possible rationale for reduction. Spine. 2007;32(20):2208–13.
20. Mac-Thiong JM, Duong L, Parent S, Hresko MT, Dimar JR, Weidenbaum M, et al. Reliability of the spinal deformity study group classification of lumbosacral spondylolisthesis. Spine. 2012;37(2):E95–102.

21. Mac-Thiong JM, Labelle H, Parent S, Hresko MT, Deviren V, Weidenbaum M, et al. Reliability and development of a new classification of lumbosacral spondylolisthesis. Scoliosis. 2008;3:19.
22. Kim HJ, Green DW. Adolescent back pain. Curr Opin Pediatr. 2008;20(1):37–45.
23. Micheli LJ, Wood R. Back pain in young athletes. Significant differences from adults in causes and patterns. Arch Pediatr Adolesc Med. 1995;149(1):15–8.
24. Standaert CJ, Herring SA. Expert opinion and controversies in sports and musculoskeletal medicine: the diagnosis and treatment of spondylolysis in adolescent athletes. Arch Phys Med Rehabil. 2007;88(4):537–40.
25. Tsirikos AI, Garrido EG. Spondylolysis and spondylolisthesis in children and adolescents. J Bone Joint Surg Br. 2010;92(6):751–9.
26. Smith JA, Hu SS. Management of spondylolysis and spondylolisthesis in the pediatric and adolescent population. Orthop Clin North Am. 1999;30(3):487–99. ix
27. Herman MJ, Pizzutillo PD, Cavalier R. Spondylolysis and spondylolisthesis in the child and adolescent athlete. Orthop Clin North Am. 2003;34(3):461–7. vii
28. Rapala K, Jagielak MJ. A case of Phalen-Dickson syndrome. Wiad Lek. 1992;45(23–24):931–3.
29. Barash HL, Galante JO, Lambert CN, Ray RD. Spondylolisthesis and tight hamstrings. J Bone Joint Surg Am. 1970;52(7):1319–28.
30. Arlet V, Rigault P, Padovani JP, Touzet P, Finidori G, Guyonvarch G. Scoliosis, spondylolysis and lumbosacral spondylolisthesis. A study of their association apropos of 82 cases in children and adolescents. Rev Chir Orthop Reparatrice Appar Mot. 1990;76(2):118–27.
31. Bozdech Z. Scoliosis and spondylolisthesis. Acta Chir Orthop Traumatol Cechoslov. 1962;29:224–8.
32. Chang KW, McAfee PC. Degenerative spondylolisthesis and degenerative scoliosis treated with a combination segmental rod-plate and transpedicular screw instrumentation system: a preliminary report. J Spinal Disord. 1988;1(4):247–56.
33. Fisk JR, Moe JH, Winter RB. Scoliosis, spondylolysis, and spondylolisthesis. Their relationship as reviewed in 539 patients. Spine. 1978;3(3):234–45.
34. Mau H. Scoliosis and spondylolysis-spondylolisthesis. Arch Orthop Trauma Surg. 1981;99(1):29–34.
35. Lenke LG, Bridwell KH. Evaluation and surgical treatment of high-grade isthmic dysplastic spondylolisthesis. Instr Course Lect. 2003;52:525–32.
36. Miller SF, Congeni J, Swanson K. Long-term functional and anatomical follow-up of early detected spondylolysis in young athletes. Am J Sports Med. 2004;32(4):928–33.
37. Alvarez-Diaz P, Alentorn-Geli E, Steinbacher G, Rius M, Pellise F, Cugat R. Conservative treatment of lumbar spondylolysis in young soccer players. Knee Surg Sports Traumatol Arthrosc. 2011;19(12):2111–4.
38. Iwamoto J, Sato Y, Takeda T, Matsumoto H. Return to sports activity by athletes after treatment of spondylolysis. World J Orthod. 2010;1(1):26–30.
39. Iwamoto J, Takeda T, Wakano K. Returning athletes with severe low back pain and spondylolysis to original sporting activities with conservative treatment. Scand J Med Sci Sports. 2004;14(6):346–51.
40. Debnath UK, Freeman BJ, Grevitt MP, Sithole J, Scammell BE, Webb JK. Clinical outcome of symptomatic unilateral stress injuries of the lumbar pars interarticularis. Spine. 2007;32(9):995–1000.
41. El Rassi G, Takemitsu M, Woratanarat P, Shah SA. Lumbar spondylolysis in pediatric and adolescent soccer players. Am J Sports Med. 2005;33(11):1688–93.
42. Sys J, Michielsen J, Bracke P, Martens M, Verstreken J. Nonoperative treatment of active spondylolysis in elite athletes with normal X-ray findings: literature review and results of conservative treatment. Eur Spine J. 2001;10(6):498–504.
43. El Rassi G, Takemitsu M, Glutting J, Shah SA. Effect of sports modification on clinical outcome in children and adolescent athletes with symptomatic lumbar spondylolysis. Am J Phys Med Rehabil. 2013;92(12):1070–4.
44. Sutton JH, Guin PD, Theiss SM. Acute lumbar spondylolysis in intercollegiate athletes. J Spinal Disord Tech. 2012;25(8):422–5.
45. Menga EN, Kebaish KM, Jain A, Carrino JA, Sponseller PD. Clinical results and functional outcomes after direct intralaminar screw repair of spondylolysis. Spine. 2014;39(1):104–10.
46. Pizzutillo PD, Hummer CD 3rd. Nonoperative treatment for painful adolescent spondylolysis or spondylolisthesis. J Pediatr Orthop. 1989;9(5):538–40.
47. Pizzutillo PD, Mirenda W, MacEwen GD. Posterolateral fusion for spondylolisthesis in adolescence. J Pediatr Orthop. 1986;6(3):311–6.
48. Cavalier R, Herman MJ, Cheung EV, Pizzutillo PD. Spondylolysis and spondylolisthesis in children and adolescents: I. Diagnosis, natural history, and nonsurgical management. J Am Acad Orthop Surg. 2006;14(7):417–24.
49. Harris IE, Weinstein SL. Long-term follow-up of patients with grade-III and IV spondylolisthesis. Treatment with and without posterior fusion. J Bone Joint Surg Am. 1987;69(7):960–9.
50. Labelle H, Roussouly P, Berthonnaud E, Transfeldt E, O'Brien M, Chopin D, et al. Spondylolisthesis, pelvic incidence, and spinopelvic balance: a correlation study. Spine. 2004;29(18):2049–54.
51. Labelle H, Roussouly P, Berthonnaud E, Dimnet J, O'Brien M. The importance of spino-pelvic balance in L5-s1 developmental spondylolisthesis: a review of pertinent radiologic measurements. Spine. 2005;30(6 Suppl):S27–34.

52. Hu SS, Tribus CB, Diab M, Ghanayem AJ. Spondylolisthesis and spondylolysis. Instr Course Lect. 2008;57:431–45.
53. Leone A, Cianfoni A, Cerase A, Magarelli N, Bonomo L. Lumbar spondylolysis: a review. Skelet Radiol. 2011;40(6):683–700.
54. Amato M, Totty WG, Gilula LA. Imaging rounds #96. Spondylolysis—laminal fragmentation on the AP view. Orthop Rev. 1988;17(9):925–31.
55. Amato M, Totty WG, Gilula LA. Spondylolysis of the lumbar spine: demonstration of defects and laminal fragmentation. Radiology. 1984;153(3):627–9.
56. Maldague BE, Malghem JJ. Unilateral arch hypertrophy with spinous process tilt: a sign of arch deficiency. Radiology. 1976;121(3 Pt. 1):567–74.
57. Meyerding HW. Spondylolisthesis; surgical fusion of lumbosacral portion of spinal column and interarticular facets; use of autogenous bone grafts for relief of disabling backache. J Int Coll Surg. 1956;26(5 Part 1):566–91.
58. Tanguay F, Labelle H, Wang Z, Joncas J, de Guise JA, Mac-Thiong JM. Clinical significance of lumbosacral kyphosis in adolescent spondylolisthesis. Spine. 2012;37(4):304–8.
59. Glavas P, Mac-Thiong JM, Parent S, de Guise JA, Labelle H. Assessment of lumbosacral kyphosis in spondylolisthesis: a computer-assisted reliability study of six measurement techniques. Eur Spine J. 2009;18(2):212–7.
60. Nachemson A, Wiltse LL. Editorial: spondylolisthesis. Clin Orthop Relat Res. 1976;117:2–3.
61. Goyal N, Wimberley DW, Hyatt A, Zeiller S, Vaccaro AR, Hilibrand AS, et al. Radiographic and clinical outcomes after instrumented reduction and transforaminal lumbar interbody fusion of mid and high-grade isthmic spondylolisthesis. J Spinal Disord Tech. 2009;22(5):321–7.
62. Poussa M, Remes V, Lamberg T, Tervahartiala P, Schlenzka D, Yrjonen T, et al. Treatment of severe spondylolisthesis in adolescence with reduction or fusion in situ: long-term clinical, radiologic, and functional outcome. Spine. 2006;31(5):583–90. discussion 91-2
63. Poussa M, Schlenzka D, Seitsalo S, Ylikoski M, Hurri H, Osterman K. Surgical treatment of severe isthmic spondylolisthesis in adolescents. Reduction or fusion in situ. Spine. 1993;18(7):894–901.
64. Ruf M, Koch H, Melcher RP, Harms J. Anatomic reduction and monosegmental fusion in high-grade developmental spondylolisthesis. Spine. 2006;31(3):269–74.
65. Martiniani M, Lamartina C, Specchia N. "In situ" fusion or reduction in high-grade high dysplastic developmental spondylolisthesis (HDSS). Eur Spine J. 2012;21(Suppl 1):S134–40.
66. Pawar A, Labelle H, Mac-Thiong JM. The evaluation of lumbosacral dysplasia in young patients with lumbosacral spondylolisthesis: comparison with controls and relationship with the severity of slip. Eur Spine J. 2012;21(11):2122–7.
67. Boxall D, Bradford DS, Winter RB, Moe JH. Management of severe spondylolisthesis in children and adolescents. J Bone Joint Surg Am. 1979;61(4):479–95.
68. Kasliwal MK, Smith JS, Shaffrey CI, Saulle D, Lenke LG, Polly DW Jr, et al. Short-term complications associated with surgery for high-grade spondylolisthesis in adults and pediatric patients: a report from the scoliosis research society morbidity and mortality database. Neurosurgery. 2012;71(1):109–16.
69. Petraco DM, Spivak JM, Cappadona JG, Kummer FJ, Neuwirth MG. An anatomic evaluation of L5 nerve stretch in spondylolisthesis reduction. Spine. 1996;21(10):1133–8. discussion 9
70. Radcliff KE, Kalantar SB, Reitman CA. Surgical management of spondylolysis and spondylolisthesis in athletes: indications and return to play. Curr Sports Med Rep. 2009;8(1):35–40.
71. Logroscino G, Mazza O, Aulisa G, Pitta L, Pola E, Aulisa L. Spondylolysis and spondylolisthesis in the pediatric and adolescent population. Childs Nerv Syst. 2001;17(11):644–55.
72. Buck JE. Direct repair of the defect in spondylolisthesis. Preliminary report. J Bone Joint Surg Br. 1970;52(3):432–7.
73. Tonino A, van der Werf G. Direct repair of lumbar spondylolysis. 10-year follow-up of 12 previously reported cases. Acta Orthop Scand. 1994;65(1):91–3.
74. Drazin D, Shirzadi A, Jeswani S, Ching H, Rosner J, Rasouli A, et al. Direct surgical repair of spondylolysis in athletes: indications, techniques, and outcomes. Neurosurg Focus. 2011;31(5):E9.
75. Widi GA, Williams SK, Levi AD. Minimally invasive direct repair of bilateral lumbar spine pars defects in athletes. Case Rep Med. 2013;2013:659078.
76. Songer M. Repair of the pars interarticularis defect with a cable-screw construct. Spine. 1998;23(2):284.
77. Morscher E, Gerber B, Fasel J. Surgical treatment of spondylolisthesis by bone grafting and direct stabilization of spondylolysis by means of a hook screw. Arch Orthop Trauma Surg. 1984;103(3):175–8.
78. Tokuhashi Y, Matsuzaki H. Repair of defects in spondylolysis by segmental pedicular screw hook fixation. A preliminary report. Spine. 1996;21(17):2041–5.
79. Hioki A, Miyamoto K, Sadamasu A, Nozawa S, Ogawa H, Fushimi K, et al. Repair of pars defects by segmental transverse wiring for athletes with symptomatic spondylolysis: relationship between bony union and postoperative symptoms. Spine. 2012;37(9):802–7.
80. Noggle JC, Sciubba DM, Samdani AF, Anderson DG, Betz RR, Asghar J. Minimally invasive direct repair of lumbar spondylolysis with a pedicle screw and hook construct. Neurosurg Focus. 2008;25(2):E15.
81. Patel RD, Rosas HG, Steinmetz MP, Anderson PA. Repair of pars interarticularis defect utilizing a pedicle and laminar screw construct: a new technique based on anatomical and biomechanical analysis. J Neurosurg Spine. 2012;17(1):61–8.

82. Li Y, Hresko MT. Lumbar spine surgery in athletes: outcomes and return-to-play criteria. Clin Sports Med. 2012;31(3):487–98.
83. Bohlman HH, Cook SS. One-stage decompression and posterolateral and interbody fusion for lumbosacral spondyloptosis through a posterior approach. Report of two cases. J Bone Joint Surg Am. 1982;64(3):415–8.
84. Gaines RW. L5 vertebrectomy for the surgical treatment of spondyloptosis: thirty cases in 25 years. Spine. 2005;30(6 Suppl):S66–70.
85. Gaines RW, Nichols WK. Treatment of spondyloptosis by two stage L5 vertebrectomy and reduction of L4 onto S1. Spine. 1985;10(7):680–6.
86. Papanastassiou ID, Jain S, Baaj AA, Eleraky M, Papagelopoulos PJ, Vrionis FD. Vertebrectomy and expandable cage placement via a one-stage, one-position anterolateral retroperitoneal approach in L5 tumors. J Surg Oncol. 2011;104(5):552–8.
87. Gandhoke GS, Kasliwal MK, Smith JS, Nieto JARN, Ibrahimi D, Park P, Lamarca F, Shaffrey C, Okonkwo DO, Kanter AS. A multicenter evaluation of clinical and radiographic outcomes following highgrade spondylolisthesis reduction and fusion. Clin Spine Surg. 2017;30(4):E363–9.
88. Tobler WD, Gerszten PC, Bradley WD, Raley TJ, Nasca RJ, Block JE. Minimally invasive axial presacral L5-S1 interbody fusion: two-year clinical and radiographic outcomes. Spine. 2011;36(20):E1296–301.
89. Ogilvie JW. Complications in spondylolisthesis surgery. Spine. 2005;30(6 Suppl):S97–101.

Surgical Management of Lumbar Spondylolisthesis

24

Jad G. Khalil, Jeffrey S. Fischgrund, and Richard V. Roberts

Introduction

Spondylolisthesis, from the Greek roots of *spondylos*, meaning vertebrae, and *olisthesis*, meaning to slip, refers to the anterior or posterior translational displacement of the vertebral body compared to the level inferior to the defect [1, 2]. In terms of the adult lumbar spine, this displacement results from a causative defect in bony architecture, trauma, or degenerative changes over time [3–6]. Spondylolisthesis was first described by Herbiniaux, a Belgian obstetrician, in 1782 as a bony prominence anterior to the sacrum [7]. Later in 1853 a German physician Robert reported on specific defects in the pars interarticularis, which were first labeled in 1854 by Killian as spondylolysis [2, 8]. Then in 1881 Neugebauer suggested that lysis, the elongation and angulation of the pars interarticularis, could lead to spondylolisthesis [9]. Following in 1888, the phenomenon spondyloptosis, Greek root of *ptosis* meaning falling off or down, was termed by Neugebauer to describe a vertebra that is completely displaced [1, 9]. It was then in 1893 that Lane posited that spondylolisthesis was due to the modification of the interarticular part of the fifth lumbar vertebra by pressure from both the inferior facet of the fourth lumbar vertebra above and the superior sacral process below [1].

J.G. Khalil, MD (✉) • J.S. Fischgrund, MD
R.V. Roberts, MD
Department of Orthopaedic Surgery,
William Beaumont Hospital, 3535 West
13 Mile Rd., Suite 744, Royal Oak, MI 48073, USA
e-mail: jadkhalil@gmail.com;
jsfischgrund37@gmail.com;
richardrobertsmd@gmail.com

Classification

The most widely used classification system today was described by Wiltse (Fig. 24.1), in which he divided spondylolisthesis into five main categories [10–13]. Type I (congenital spondylolisthesis) is derived from an inherited defect of either the superior sacral facet, the inferior facet, or both, with a gradual anterior translation of the vertebra, most commonly seen in L5-S1. Type II (isthmic spondylolisthesis) implies the defect to be in the isthmus, also known as the pars interarticularis. This type is further subdivided into three subtypes: type IIA denotes a stress fracture of the pars region, referred to as a spondylolysis; type IIB refers to an elongated pars that is the product of bony remodeling from repetitive stresses; and type IIC, the rarest of the isthmic spondylolistheses, is due to an acute traumatic fracture of the pars leading to anterolisthesis. Type III (degenerative spondylolisthesis) is a disease of the aging spine that progresses due to facet arthritis and remodeling that can result in anterolisthesis, retrolisthesis, or rotational deformities and instability. Type IV (post-traumatic

L.T. Holly, P.A. Anderson (eds.), *Essentials of Spinal Stabilization*,
DOI 10.1007/978-3-319-59713-3_24

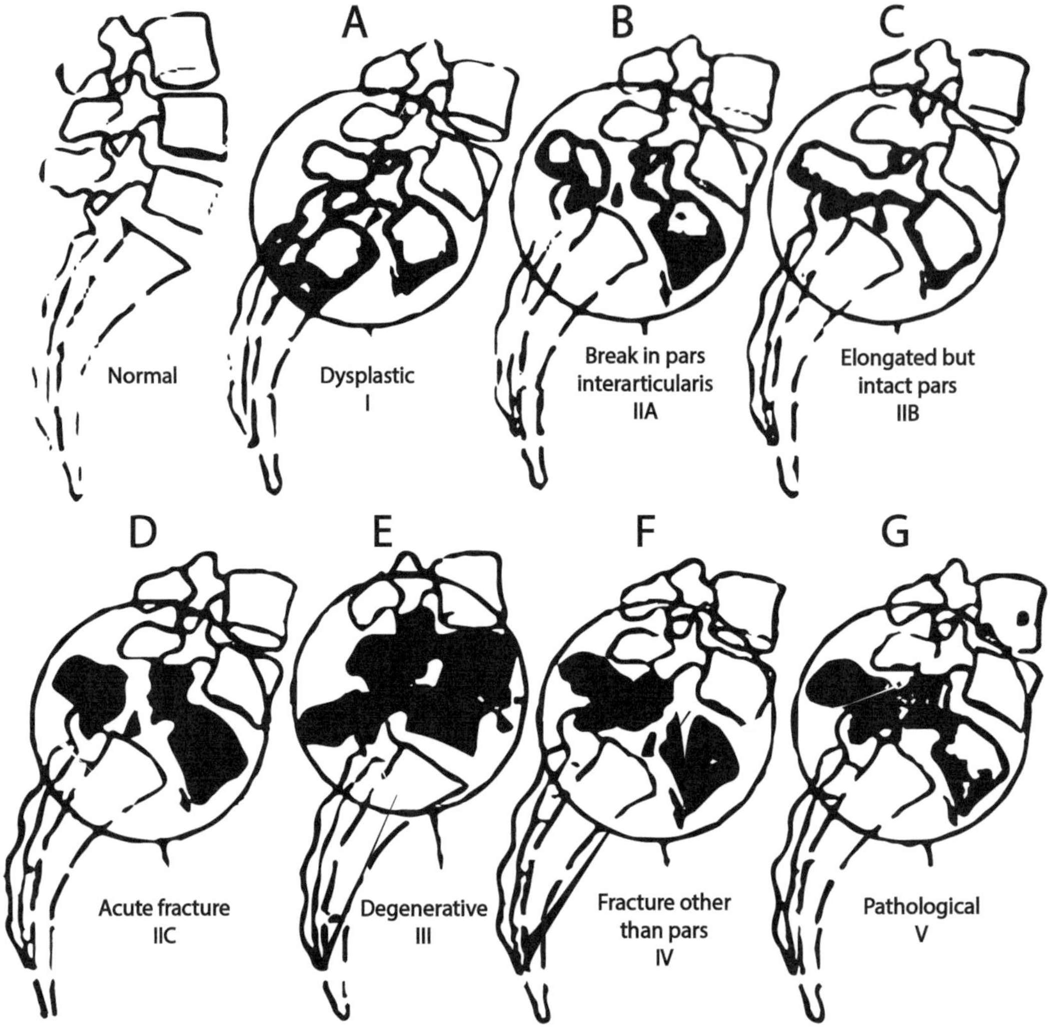

Fig. 24.1 Wiltse classification (From Wiltse et al. [10])

spondylolisthesis) results from acute trauma and failure to the posterior elements; in contrast to isthmic, traumatic spondylolisthesis is not related to a direct pars injury. Type V (pathologic spondylolisthesis) is a result of the destructive nature of posterior elements from a pathologic process, i.e., chronic disorders, infections, malignancy, or iatrogenic processes, over a period of time.

In 1982 Marchetti and Bartolozzi then categorized spondylolisthesis into developmental and acquired subtypes [14]. The acquired etiologies contained iatrogenic (now considered postsurgical), pathologic, traumatic, and degenerative conditions, whereas the developmental etiologies comprised of the elongation of the pars or lytic lesions. In 1994 a revised classification system further organized the developmental group based on the grade of dysplasia, either high or low dysplasia [1]. Degenerative spondylolisthesis, reported initially by MacNab and later by Newman and Stone, is a subtype of the acquired form later described by Marchetti and Bartolozzi [14, 15]. In that classification, degenerative spondylolisthesis may be either primary or secondary. Primary is typically seen in middle-aged women presenting with clinical signs of spinal stenosis, while secondary is related to a predisposing factor, such as adjacent segment degeneration, causing a slip above a preexisting fusion [1, 14, 15].

In combination with developmental susceptibilities, certain activities place patients at risk for spondylolysis because of the nature of the biomechanical stresses imparted on the pars interarticularis [1]. Biomechanical analyses have shown that hyperextension and persistent lordosis increases shear stresses at the neural arch [16–19]. This stress during hyperextension of the lumbar spine can be seen in activities such as gymnastics, weightlifting, diving, football, soccer, cricket, and volleyball [19–29], as well as Scheuermann kyphosis, owing to the exaggerated lumbar lordosis [30]. The progression of slippage during adolescence and the observation that females are several times more likely to have an increase in deformity suggests a hormonal role in the development of spondylolisthesis [31]. The slippage can occur as the lumbar spine rotates around the sacral dome due to the body's center of gravity being anterior to the lumbosacral joint [1]. The age of the patient when these defects occur and the individual's sagittal alignment of the spine influence the degree of deformity progression. Pelvic incidence seems to play an important role in the progression of the spondylolisthesis, with a statistically significant increase in the chance of slippage as the pelvic incident angle increases [32, 33].

Adult spondylolisthesis presents in predominately two patterns: the isthmic type, resulting from abnormalities of the pars intra-articularis; and the degenerative type, an outcome of lumbar spondylosis with its disc degeneration and instability causing a physiologic uncoupling of the facets in the sagittal plane [34–36].

Incidence

The incidence of defects in the pars interarticularis is seen in 4% to 6% in the general population, which can progress to isthmic spondylolisthesis. Isthmic spondylolisthesis, with a reported incidence between 2.6% and 4.4% of general population, is more common in males [37]. It is most frequently seen at the L5-S1 level [38–40]. Around 50% of patients presenting with a pars defect do not show evidence of anterior listhesis [1]. Female patients exhibit a lower incidence of isthmic defects; however they show a higher propensity for slip progression [1]. The incidence of isthmic spondylolisthesis also varies according to race with 6.4% in white American males, 2.8% in black males, 2.3% in white females, and 1.1% in black females [1]. Eskimos have been shown to have a rate as high as 50% [1, 3]. Additionally, spina bifida occulta has been associated with spondylolysis of the lumbar spine in 11.8–35% of patients [41–43]. Although there are reports of greater frequency of posterior spine defects connected to isthmic spondylolisthesis, no etiologic link has been accepted [10, 44, 45]. The risk of spondylolisthesis progressing is greater in patients that have a midline lumbosacral defect due to the decreased stabilizing effects associated with the lack of attachment of the multifidus muscles to the deficient spinous processes [45, 46]. Hence, the deficient or dysplastic posterior elements in spina bifida defects actually increase the amount of pars loading, leading to the development of isthmic spondylolisthesis and thus serve as a risk factor to high-grade (>50%) olisthesis progression [41, 47–49].

Degenerative spondylolisthesis is approximately four to five times more common in females than in males (8.4% in females and 2.7% in males) and more common in black females than in white females [3, 34]. This female prevalence is thought to be due to greater ligamentous laxity and hormonal effects [50–52]. Degenerative spondylolisthesis rarely affects those younger than 40 years of age and most frequently involves the L4-L5 level. Unlike isthmic spondylolisthesis, degenerative spondylolisthesis occurs much less frequently at the L5-S1 level [1]. Factors that have been reported to predispose to anterolisthesis at the lumbosacral junction include: a fifth lumbar vertebral body that is less deeply seated within the pelvis, slim transverse processes of the fifth lumbar vertebral body, and an increased sacral inclination, all of which are more common in women than men [53]. The factors associated with an increased risk in women were elevated body mass index (BMI), increased age, and increased angle of lordosis, whereas in men only an increased age was associated with a higher risk of degenerative spondylolisthesis [54]. The effect of facet joint orientation is also seen as a potential factor in the development of degenerative spondylolisthesis with a more sagittal orientation at the L4-L5 facet joints being associated as a cause [55–57]. Even in the absence of symptoms from the pars defects themselves, spondylolisthesis may lead to clinically significant radiculopathy and progressive neurologic deficits secondary to nerve root impingement [1].

Imaging

Initial imaging of the patient can be established with plain radiographs, including anteroposterior, lateral, and oblique views. For the anteroposterior views, a Ferguson view of 15° of inclination optimizes the evaluation of lumbar transverse process size and disc height at the L5-S1 level [58]. When the lateral view is obtained with the patient standing, it allows for ideal appreciation of the degree of olisthesis in spondylolisthesis; additionally, the flexion-extension in lateral views helps evaluate the presence of instability [1]. The benefits of an oblique lateral view are the increased ability to detect the pars defect, with an oblique lateral view detecting the pars defect in 84% of cases [59], whereas the standard lateral view is able to identify it 19% of the time [60, 61]. Oblique radiographs are associated with significant radiation exposure, and they should be sparingly used, as directed by a specialist; this holds especially true in the adolescent population. Furthermore, unless the preoperative lateral radiographs are obtained with the patient standing, it cannot be determined if the presence of postoperative spondylolisthesis in a patient with poor pain relief after surgery was the result of destabilization from the surgery or if it was a preexisting condition [1]. Relying only on supine MRI imaging for the identification of degenerative spondylolisthesis has been demonstrated to miss the diagnosis in almost one third of cases [62]. Table 24.1 [1, 63–67] reviews the different choices of imaging techniques and their associated benefits in outlining various findings in cases of patients with suspected spondylolisthesis.

There have been several biomechanical studies that have successfully recognized that lumbosacral facet joint disease and degenerative disc disease may cause degenerative spondylolisthesis [68–72]. While standing lateral flexion-extension lumbar radiographs are used to identify lumbar spine instability, supine lumbosacral MRI is routine in evaluating various lumbar disorders. Though degenerative spondylolisthesis is not always present in the supine position, the axial T2-weighted MRI can detect increased fluid in the lumbar facet joints [73–76]. Extensive facet effusion (>1.5 mm) is highly predictive of degenerative spondylolisthesis at the L4-L5 level in the absence of measureable anterolisthesis on the supine MRI [74].

In 1932 Meyerding proposed a radiographic grading system for spondylolisthesis [77] (Fig. 24.2), which is now the most common system in use, with the degree of slippage being measured as the percentage of distance the anteriorly translated vertebral body has moved forward [38]. This classification by Meyerding grades the olisthesis as it increases from grades I to IV. Spondyloptosis, in which the fifth lumbar vertebra has slipped forward over 100% of the gliding plane past the sacral promontory, is given a grade V; instances of spondylolysis without olisthesis is noted as a grade 0 [1]. Other important measurements to quantify the sagittal rotation of a vertebral body that may also exist in spondylolisthesis are the slip angle and pelvic tilt which, like the Meyerding classification, are best analyzed using standing lateral radiographs. Calculation of the slip angle is achieved by measuring the angle formed by the intersection of two lines: the first being a line perpendicular to the posterior cortex of the sacrum and the second being a line paralleling the inferior end plate of L5 [1]. In the normal spine, slip angle values should be close to zero, whereas a slip angle greater than 55° is associated with a high probability and increased rate of progression [78]. Pelvic tilt, also known as sacral inclination, denotes the vertical position of the sacrum. It is

Table 24.1 Imaging modalities

Imaging modality	Benefits	Notes
Radionuclide (Technetium 99 mm) Bone Imaging [1]	Identify pars interarticularis stress fractures without a visible bony defect	Recent trauma/symptomatic with strenuous activity: increased uptake in spondylolytic area Chronic LBP: normal scan if defect is chronic, sclerotic, and avascular
SPECT (Single Photon Emission Computed Tomography) [63–65]	More sensitive than plain radiographs or technetium bone scan	"Hot scan" suggests increased activity (orthotic immobilization may be beneficial) "Cold scan" suggests chronic lesion/not metabolically active (unlikely to respond only to orthotic immobilization)
CT (Computed Tomography) [66, 67]	Gauge degree of spondylolisthesis Assess healing potential of identified pars defect	Superior to plain radiographs in revealing dysplastic facets, pars defects, changes in apophyseal joints
MRI (Magnetic Resonance Imaging) [1]	Soft tissue Neural structures	No exposure to radiation

Imaging techniques and their relative roles in assessing patients with spondylolisthesis [1, 63–67]

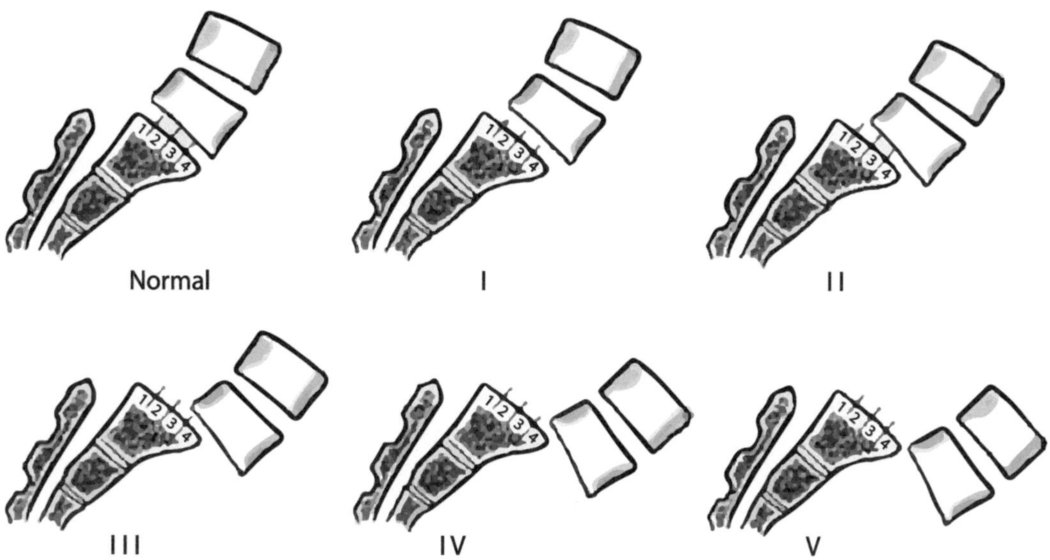

Fig. 24.2 The five grades of the Meyerding grading system [77]. Grade 1, 0–25% of the vertebral body; grade II, 26–50%; grade III, 51–75%; grade IV, 76–100%; grade V, spondyloptosis

the angle formed by the intersection of two lines: (a) a line perpendicular to the floor and (b) a line parallel to the posterior cortex of the sacrum [1]. Normal values usually are greater than 30°; yet with an increasing slip, the lumbosacral kyphosis is increased; therefore the sacrum is forced into a more vertical orientation and decreases the pelvic tilt [1]. Proper documentation of the Meyerding class, slip angle, and pelvic tilt are advocated as part of evaluation of the progression of the deformity [79] (Figs. 24.3 and 24.4).

Indications and Patient Selection

Initial treatment should consist of pain relief, strengthening of core muscle groups, and return of range of motion in the lumbar spine. This is

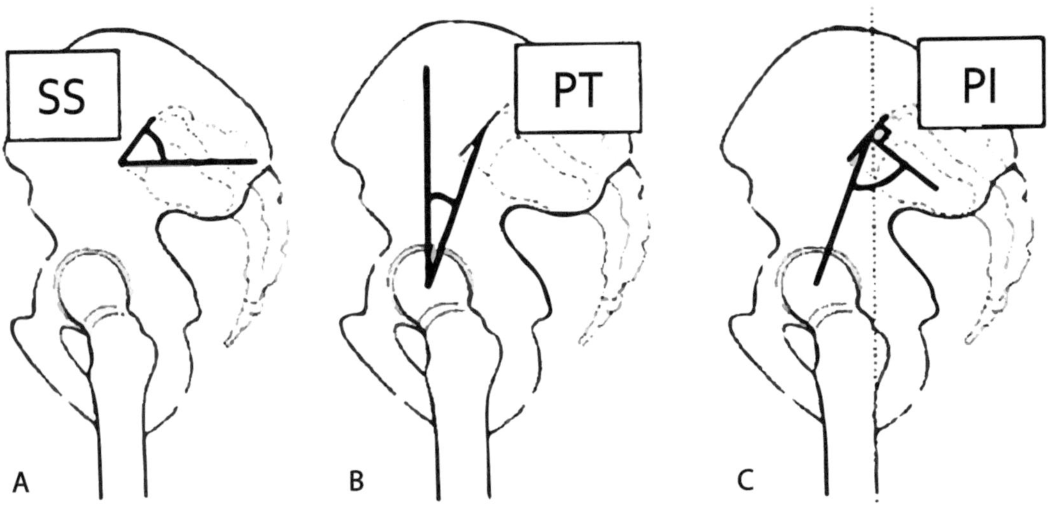

Fig. 24.3 Pelvic parameters. *SS* sacral slope; *PT* pelvic tilt; *PI* pelvic incidence (From Oh et al. [79], with permission)

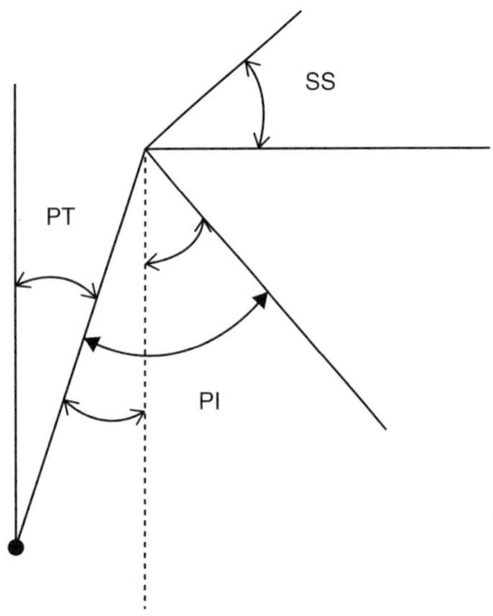

Fig. 24.4 Mathematical relation between pelvic parameters [79]. PI = PT + SS (From Oh et al. [79], with permission)

typically initiated with nonsteroidal anti-inflammatory drugs (NSAIDs), pain management, and physiotherapy. Steroid injections into the facet joint and epidural space are helpful in the acute phase but not recommended for prolonged usage, as there are potential complications of this medication with long-term use [1]. This is similarly true with the use of narcotic medications, as their prolonged use can adversely affect recovery, lead to continued disability, and increase the risk of addiction [1]. The conservative management of spondylolysis includes cessation of strenuous activity, rehabilitation with strengthening of the abdominal and paraspinal musculature, minimization of pelvic tilt, and perhaps anti-lordotic bracing [80]. There are many factors that influence potential treatment protocols. Conservative management protocols also depend on several factors, such as disease involvement (spondylolysis vs. spondylolisthesis), the level and laterality of the defect (unilateral vs. bilateral pars defects), duration since injury (acute vs. chronic), and the age of the patient [81]. Exercises should be focused on strengthening the abdominal and paraspinal musculature, as the local muscular system that controls the lumbar spine consists of lumbar multifidus, internal oblique, and transversus abdominis [82]. Along with exercises that target specific core muscle groups with the spine in neutral position, a stretching program to improve flexibility and strengthening of hip flexors and hamstring stretching is frequently recommended [83–85]. Weight loss and aerobic conditioning programs are added as necessary. Individual patient goals may vary, but in general the ability to return to normal activity without restrictions is the main objective. The severity of symptoms tends to dictate the management of spondylolysis and spondylolisthesis, as most lesions do not heal with bony union, but rather become a stable fibrous union that remains relatively asymptomatic [1]. Patients with low-grade dysplastic spondylolisthesis are less likely than patients with isthmic spondylolisthesis to benefit from conservative methods; however conservative therapy is still recommended as the initial modality [37].

Surgical Treatment

The main goals of surgical treatment in spondylolisthesis consist of stabilization of the affected levels and decompression of the involved neural elements. Surgery should be considered in patients who have failed a full course of conservative treatment and have persistent severe back and predominant leg pain, evidence of instability on imaging, documented progressive spondylolisthesis, a progression of the neurologic deficit, or cauda equina symptoms [1]. Surgical treatment options may be broadly divided into two categories: direct repair of the pars defects versus arthrodesis of the involved segments to prevent slip progression with or without decompression of affected neural structures.

Direct Pars Repair

Procedures for direct fixation of pars defects (Fig. 24.5) include the Buck's technique [86], Scott wiring [87], repair with an ipsilateral pedicle screw and hook [88, 89], and U-rod technique [90, 91]. The Buck's method is an open technique in which the fibrous tissue at the pars defect is identified, thoroughly debrided, and stabilized with a 4.5 mm stainless steel cortical screw in compression [86]. In the Scott wiring technique, a stainless steel wire is looped from the transverse processes to the spinous process of the level involved and tightened, in conjunction with local iliac crest bone graft [87]. In the U-rod technique, bilateral pedicle screws are connected through a U-shaped rod around the spinous process, thus applying compressive forces to enhance healing of the bone graft across the defect [90, 91].

Posterior Fusion with Pedicle Instrumentation

Transpedicular fixation has been shown to increase the rate of fusion, and a positive correlation has been reported between successful fusion and clinical outcomes [93–99]. A trend for improved clinical outcome with increased rigidity of fixation has been noted [94]. Pedicle screw fixation systems have been shown to be mechanically superior to other fixation devices, while allowing for the selective segmental force without extension to adjacent levels [100].

High-Grade Spondylolisthesis

Multiple factors must be considered in the treatment of high-grade spondylolisthesis [1]. Symptomatic patients with high-grade spondylolisthesis do not seem to achieve a satisfactory outcome with non-operative treatment as compared to those with low-grade spondylolisthesis [101]. In high-grade spondylolisthesis, reduction of the slip angle rather than the degree of anterior listhesis should be the main concern [1]. While studies show that patients with greater than 50% of slippage may have a poor non-operative outcome, fusion is in general the treatment of choice among spinal surgeons [102]. In determining the most appropriate procedure, one must take into account all presenting symptoms, neurologic function, radiographic findings, clinical deformity, age of the patient, and the surgeon experience. Treatment approach is influenced by the level of spinal maturity, degree of slippage, symptoms, the patient's activity level, and expected progression [1]. Surgical stabilization through arthrodesis of the affected segment can result in improvement and even resolution of the neural deficit by alleviating impingement of neural elements and increasing the stability [103]. While the treatment of an asymptomatic adult is very rarely surgical, an asymptomatic adolescent

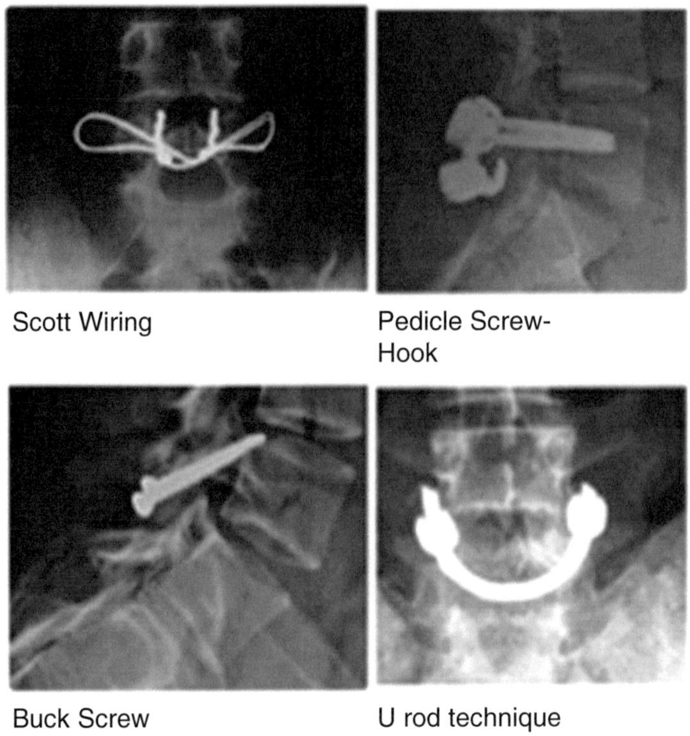

Fig. 24.5 Procedures for direct fixation of pars defects (From Warner and Leahy [92])

may be a candidate for surgical intervention because of expected progression of deformity in a high-grade slip, which may lead to mechanical and neurologic dysfunction [1]. The long-term effects of fusion in a young patient must be considered due to the potential for future adjacent segment degeneration [104, 105]. In a skeletally immature patient with slippage greater than 50% or a mature adolescent with a slip greater than 75%, operative intervention is recommended even if the patient is asymptomatic [106–108]. Surgical decompression is also indicated when a patient has neural compromise, with a severe radiculopathy or bowel/bladder dysfunction [109–111].

Reduction of spondylolisthesis has been a controversial topic. It has been shown that partial slip reduction occurs with the positioning and administration of general anesthetic/muscle relaxation [112]. Active reduction can also be performed after placement of the instrumentation. There has not been a compelling indication to perform an active reduction in cases of degenerative spondylolisthesis. In isthmic spondylolisthesis partial reduction that aims to correct the slip angle has been associated with improved postoperative outcomes [113]. Reducing a spondylolisthesis also has limitations and drawbacks. The most common postoperative complication is neurapraxia of the L5 nerve root. It has been suggested that a wide decompression and thorough excision of the Gill fragment may decrease the incidence [113–115].

Fusion of the involved level has been widely advocated as the definitive treatment of symptomatic spondylolysis [106, 116]. In the Spine Patient Outcomes Research Trial (SPORT), a prospective evaluation of the 2-year [117] and 4-year [118, 119] outcomes of 607 patients with degenerative spondylolisthesis, patients were divided into two enrollment groups, with 50% in a randomized cohort and 50% in an observational cohort. Pre-enrollment non-operative care was not specified, and the type of surgery or non-operative treatment during the study period was left to the discretion of the treating physicians. The study was laden with a significant crossover and nonadherence to treatment between the two groups, leading to both an as-treated and an intent-to-treat analysis of the data. When both the randomized and observational cohorts were combined, the as-treated analysis revealed that the surgically treated patients had significantly better outcome for both pain and function at 2-year and 4-year follow-ups. This study did not allow comparison of types of treatments; therefore it did not answer the question of which surgical treatments provided better outcomes.

Treatment options in isthmic spondylolisthesis consist of a direct repair of the pars intra-articularis [120–123], decompression of the neural elements alone [109, 110, 124, 125], decompression of the neural elements in conjunction with an in situ posterior lateral fusion [96, 122, 126, 127], decompression of posterior lateral fusion with associated pedicular instrumentation [96, 128, 129], and decompression and reduction of the spondylolisthesis with instrumentation and interbody fusion [130–132].

Although all patients should be initially treated with non-operative management, large multi-institutional studies have demonstrated that surgical treatment tends to result in more favorable outcomes [117]. While a fusion is firmer and solid with instrumentation, prior to these large multi-institutional studies, the incremental benefits of instrumentation on clinical outcome were not as clear. Although it had seemed rational with radiographic imaging showing evidence of instability, the direct stability offered by instrumentation was found to increase surgical time, expense, and potential morbidity [1]. On the other hand, indications for using instrumentation in a patient with a collapsed disc space, no motion at the spondylolisthetic level, or the presence of osteoporotic bone are not as clear [1]. The SPORT study successfully recognized an advantage of surgical treatment over nonsurgical treatment in stenotic patients who had degenerative lumbar spondylolisthesis. A comparison of surgically treated patients and the control cohort demonstrated improved outcomes of the surgically treated patients at intervals of 3 months and 12 months, with marginally reduced improvement at 24 months [117]. Additional breakdown of this data from the SPORT trial gave insight to significant findings. It was demonstrated that operatively treated patients with degenerative lumbar spondylolisthesis had better outcomes than symptomatic stenosis without spondylolisthesis [133]. Furthermore, surgical outcome was superior in patients with predominately leg pain compared to those that presented with primarily back pain [134].

In a prospective, randomized study by Herkowitz, the comparison of decompression alone versus decompression and non-instrumented posterolateral spinal fusion in the treatment of lumbar spine levels L3-L4 and L4-L5 degenerative spondylolisthesis with spinal stenosis reported superior clinical results when concomitant fusion was performed with the decompression [135]. They found that a satisfactory outcome was more than twice as common in the fused group (96%) as compared to the decompression without fusion group (44%). The authors concluded that the results of surgical decompression with in situ arthrodesis were superior to those of decompression alone.

Lumbar fusion for spondylolisthesis can be accompanied by unintended consequences. In elderly patients, either vertebral compression fractures of adjacent levels or stress fracture due to the bone stock in the osteoporotic bone can occur [1]. Instrumentation may also directly harm the superior facet by either capsular disruption or articular facet damage; thus the use of less rigid instrumentation or no instrumentation may be of interest because of the theoretical reduction of stress on adjacent levels by the presence of a less rigid fusion or even a stable pseudarthrosis [1]. A multi-level decompression without any fusion is certainly a sensible option for some patients, depending on age and comorbidities, even though the literature generally supports concomitant fusion. A multilevel non-instrumented fusion increases the incidence of pseudarthrosis at one or more levels, as well as the possibility of flat-back deformity; therefore, in some cases, it may be appropriate to decompress all of the stenotic levels that are symptomatic and perform an instrumented fusion at the spondylolisthetic level only [1].

The role of anterior column support in the surgical management of spondylolisthesis has been debated. Anterior column support can be provided by a posterior lumbar interbody fusion (PLIF), a transforaminal lumbar interbody fusion (TLIF), or an anterior lumbar interbody fusion (ALIF). Newer techniques using lateral transpsoas or anterior oblique approaches are also being utilized. Possible choices for interbody fusion device materials are metallic cages, carbon fiber cages, polyetheretherketone (PEEK) cages, or bone [1]. Anterior column support can be used for treatment of isthmic spondylolisthesis as well as degenerative spondylolisthesis [136–140]. Proposed advantages of using interbody fusion with PLIF or TLIF as compared to posterior instrumented fusion without an interbody fusion includes an increased likelihood of fusion, better indirect foraminal decompression, better reduction of the spondylolisthesis, and better restoration of lordosis [137, 138, 140]. Oda et al. reported that when anterior column support was deficient, the addition of posterior stabilization with pedicle screws alone provided inadequate stability and resulted in a high level of implant strain. In these situations, the addition of an interbody cage significantly increased the construct stiffness and decreased hardware strain, although it resulted in increased motion at the adjacent segment [141].

The Spine Patient Outcomes Research Trial (SPORT) performed a cost-effectiveness analysis of conservative to surgical treatment of spondylolisthesis at 2-year follow-up [142]. The study found that surgery significantly improved the quality of life in surgical patients compared with non-operative treatment. Two-year follow-up surgery was not deemed cost effective; however at longer follow-up, the procedure is likely to meet current cost-effectiveness standards [142].

Surgical Technique

Patient Positioning

The patient is placed in the prone position on the Jackson table with hips fully extended to improve lumbar lordosis. This position also minimizes epidural venous distention from abdominal compression; additionally it can aid in the reduction of spondylolisthesis. A partial correction of both the slip angle and the spondylolisthesis can be occasionally seen with patient positioning alone. The patient should have padding over all areas. Once positioning is satisfactory, neuromonitoring signals should be checked for baseline comparisons. The intraoperative neurophysiologic monitoring (IONM) techniques that are commonly used during surgery include both upper and lower SSEPs (somatosensory evoked potentials) as well as continuous and triggered EMG activity [143].

Pedicle Screw Placement

We prefer to place the pedicle screws prior to performing the decompression. Dissection should provide full exposure of the transverse process with meticulous removal of the soft tissues in the region of the segment to be fused. Once the external landmarks of the pedicles have been identified, fluoroscopic confirmation can be obtained for pedicle identification, hole preparation, and proper screw placement. There are two well-known methods for pedicle screw placement, the Roy-Camille method and the Magerl method. Roy-Camille's screw entrance point is situated at the crossing of two lines on a typical bony crest with the horizontal line passing through the middle of the transverse process and the vertical line given by the articular process 1 mm under the facet joint [144]. Magerl's direction of the pedicle screw is 10–20° convergent toward the sagittal plane [145]. The point of entry is in the central axis of the pedicle, indicated by the intersection of the two lines with the vertical line touching the lateral border of the superior articular process and the horizontal line bisecting the base of the transverse process [145]. Confirmatory identification of the facet complex can be accomplished by using a towel clamp to move the spinous process and identify the facet joint and then removal of the soft tissues from the surface of the superior facet. For the external landmarks of the first sacral pedicle, the inferolateral portion of the superior S1 facet can be utilized. There are two common sacral screw placements: anterolaterally into the ala and anteromedially into the promontory. Each pedicle screw is placed beginning with the burr, providing a localization screw for the curved pedicle probe, starting with the curve directed laterally and then positioned medially once the probe is in the vertebral body. The continuous tactile confirmation, using a pedicle feeler, prevents breaching of the lateral and medial wall cortex. The depth of the channel can be established with a depth gauge. Tapping the pedicles for subsequent insertion of the screw also requires tactile confirmation of wall stock in the pedicles. Pedicle screw size can be determined on preoperative CT scans, but intraoperative modifications are common. Placement of the screw along the same trajectory as the pedicle probe and the tap are vital to prevent breaching of the lateral and, more importantly, the medial wall of the pedicle. The optimal length of the screw is one in which about 75% of the depth of the vertebral body is obtained, with a critical understanding of not penetrating the anterior portion of the vertebral body to avoid injury to both vascular and visceral structures in the retroperitoneum. After all of the appropriate pedicle screws are placed, verification of their exact position can be done intraoperatively with fluoroscopy.

Decompression

Decompressive laminectomy alone is mostly recommended in patients without spondylolisthesis, yet it is also a choice in patients with a low-grade, static spondylolisthesis [146]. In order to attain a successful decompression, there are three stages suggested that are most often seen as a continuous procedure intraoperatively. Central laminectomy is performed and extended pedicle to pedicle. The lateral recess is then decompressed, confirming thorough bony removal of the medial part of the facet joint complex, and the hypertrophied ligamentum is then detached. Foraminotomies are performed to safeguard full decompression of the exiting and traversing nerve roots, while preserving most of the facet joint and at least 8 mm of pars interarticularis [147]. An aggressive decompression can result in iatrogenic disruption of the facet joint or pars, which could lead to accelerated degeneration or instability, respectively [148]. In patients with advanced age or comorbid conditions that preclude an extended surgical procedure, we recommend decompression of only the levels with critical stenosis. In patients presenting with unilateral symptomatology, particularly radicular instead of claudication, a hemilaminectomy can be a viable option [149].

Spondylolisthesis Reduction

Surgical techniques for reduction of spondylolisthesis are dependent upon the understanding of biomechanics, implant materials, and the goal of the surgery. Being mindful not to over- or undertreat the patient requires an understanding of the approach and proper techniques to accomplish a reduction that is satisfactory with the appropriate construct and planning. Figure 24.9 shows the preoperative, intraoperative, and postoperative images from a patient with an L5-S1 isthmic spondylolisthesis that had a grade III slip. An L4-S1 posterolateral arthrodesis was performed with L4-S1 posterior instrumentation with pedicle screws and an L5-S1 Gill laminectomy. In this case, a rod persuader was used with a cantilever method to carefully reduce the spondylolisthesis so not to lose the lordosis and cause a subsequent flat-back deformity.

Correction of high-grade isthmic spondylolisthesis poses several challenges. In order to minimize complications, proper understanding of the correct and altered anatomy must be mastered [150]. We recommend full decompression (Gill type laminectomy) prior to any active reduction attempt. Special attention should be turned to removing all "Gill fragment" pieces from the foramen and ensuring full decompression of the exiting nerve root; i.e., in a case of L5-S1 isthmic spondylolisthesis, we focus our attention to obtaining full decompression of the L5 nerve root. This nerve root is visualized from takeoff, all the way to the extraforaminal region. In cases of high-grade L5-S1 isthmic spondylolisthesis, we recommend placing bicortical screws in the sacrum. Alternatively, iliac screws can be placed. In cases where the L5 pedicles are dysplastic and rigid fixation is not assured, we recommend placing pedicle screws in L4.

Posterolateral Fusion

A posterolateral fusion is considered standard in cases of posterior arthrodesis. Once the proper placement of the pedicle screws and rods has been achieved, with reduction being noted on intraoperative fluoroscopic imaging, and an interbody cage/implant has been placed, posterolateral fusion can be started with decortication. Decortication promotes the fusion process, offers a source of vascular supply from the underlying cancellous bone, and allows access to pluripotent stem cells within the marrow [151]. In posterolateral intertransverse process fusions, the transverse processes and lateral facets are essential areas to be decorticated, whereas the pars interarticularis is less beneficial [151]. After the fusion sites have been properly decorticated, the graft should be placed directly on the sites so as to create a fusion mass between the selected levels. Recommended grafts to use are maximization of the local bone that is properly prepared with removal of soft tissues and crushed cancellous or demineralized bone matrix (DBM). DBM in the form of fiber "boats" filled with local bone and/or crushed cancellous grafts can be used to contain the graft and allow for exact placement.

TLIF

Transforaminal lumbar interbody fusion (TLIF) techniques have a learning curve that can be overcome with experience. Depending on the surgeons' comfort level, training, and expertise in performing TILF, there are two main choices of either open TLIF or MIS TLIF. Open TLIF indications vary, depending on the surgeon's experience, comfort level, and training. Open TLIF has the benefit of broader exposure with multilevel disease that requires multiple levels of fixation or decompression where a minimally invasive technique would not be advantageous with time, visualization, or high grade of spondylolisthesis. As stated previously in an earlier paragraph, the possible choices for interbody fusion device materials are metallic cages, carbon fiber cages, polyetheretherketone (PEEK) cages, or bone [1].

Open TLIF Technique

It is the author's preference to perform TLIF after screws are placed and the decompression is completed. The inferior articular process of the cephalad vertebra is removed with an osteotome or burr. The superior portion of the superior articular process of the caudal vertebrae is then resected. The exiting and traversing nerve roots are identified and protected. We prefer to use a Penfield dissector to protect the exiting root superiorly and a Love nerve root retractor to protect the traversing nerve root medially. After complete removal of disc material, cartilaginous end plates are scraped using curets, ensuring removal of as much cartilage as possible. It is important to make sure the cortical bone surface is not breach to minimize the occurrence of end plate fracture and cage subsidence. We recommend packing of graft material prior to cage insertion; it should be noted here that graft volume is of utmost importance in obtaining adequate fusion, and the authors recommend packing of at least 15 cc of graft material. Following that, the interbody cage is inserted and its position checked with fluoroscopy.

Minimally Invasive Techniques

Minimally invasive techniques have recently gained popularity in the treatment of spondylolisthesis with the growing technology that allows the percutaneous placement of instrumentation. The appeal for minimally invasive surgery stems from evidence showing lower rates of complications, diminished blood loss, and faster return to function [152]. Minimally invasive transforami-

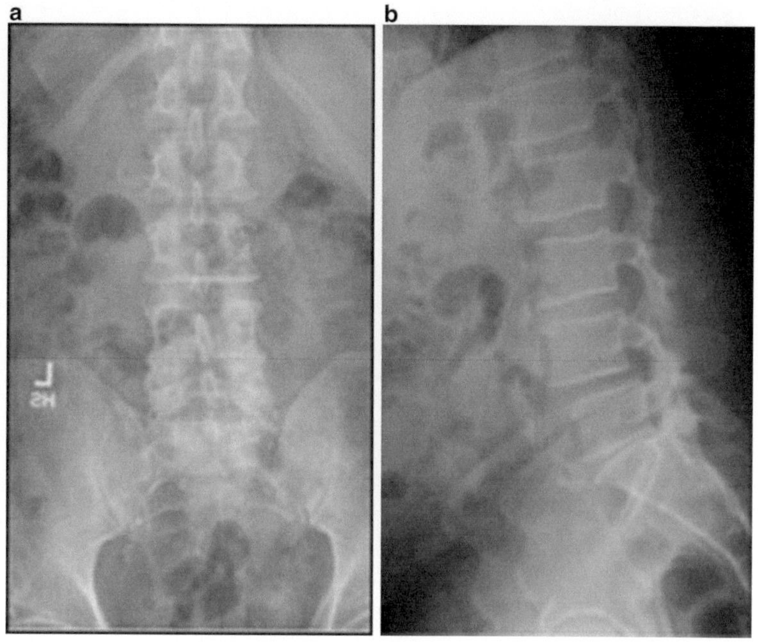

Fig. 24.6 Standing AP and lateral radiograph. Degenerative lumbar spondylolisthesis

nal lumbar interbody fusion (MIS TLIF) has been popularized as an alternative to open posterior fusion techniques. This approach seems particularly useful in cases of degenerative as well as isthmic spondylolisthesis.

MIS Technique [153–156]

MIS TLIF surgery makes use of rigid or expandable tubular retractors. The patient is positioned on a Jackson frame with hips extended and knees flexed to 20–30°. Fluoroscopic guidance allows localization of the disc space and corresponding facet joint. It is our preference to place guidewires prior to decompression and TLIF. After adequate placement of guidewires is verified, a 22 mm tubular retractor is docked on the ipsilateral facet joint. Although loupe magnification and headlight can be used, we prefer to utilize the operating microscope for the remainder of the procedure. Facetectomy is performed using a high-speed burr. The interval between thecal sac, exiting and traversing nerve roots, is then identified. Disc preparation is then performed followed by bone grafting and insertion of an interbody device. If a bilateral laminectomy needs to be performed, we prefer to do so after the spacer is inserted. The table is tilted and a series of burr and Kerrison rongeurs can be used to achieve full bilateral decompression. Screws and rods can then be placed.

The majority of the fusion (contralateral facet can be decorticated and grafted) occurs within the intervertebral disc space. For this reason, meticulous discectomy and preparation of the cartilaginous surfaces on both end plates is critical. Bone grafting is the cornerstone of a successful MIS TLIF procedure. Care must be taken to place a maximum amount of bone graft within the disc space. We prefer to pack 20–30 cc of bone graft material prior to cage insertion.

Although the learning curve is steep, proficiency offers the advantage of faster surgical time, diminished blood loss, and lower infection rate. Multiple case series have demonstrated shorter hospital stay and faster return to function [153, 154, 157–160]. In the setting of spondylolisthesis, minimally invasive technique can be used for the treatment of degenerative (Figs. 24.6, 24.7, and 24.8) as well as isthmic (Fig. 24.9) variants [161, 162]. Active reduction is usually not recommended, and it is the authors' prefer-

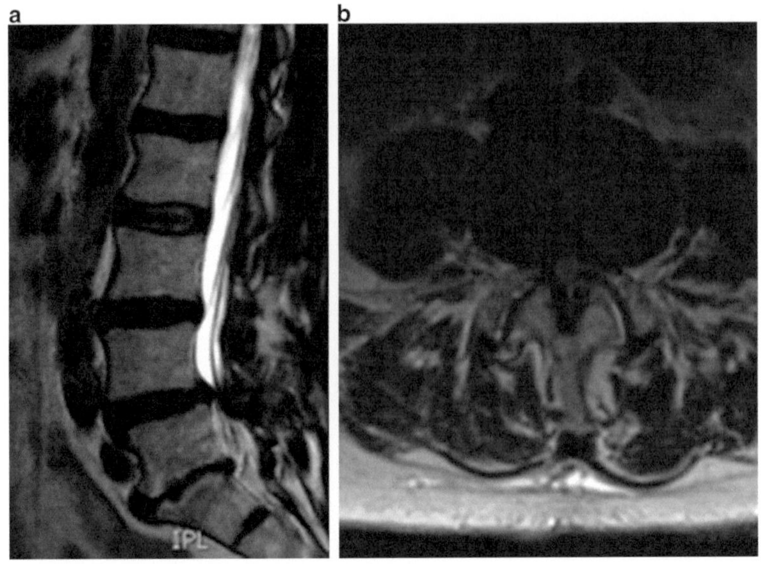

Fig. 24.7 Sagittal and axial MRI. Degenerative lumbar spondylolisthesis

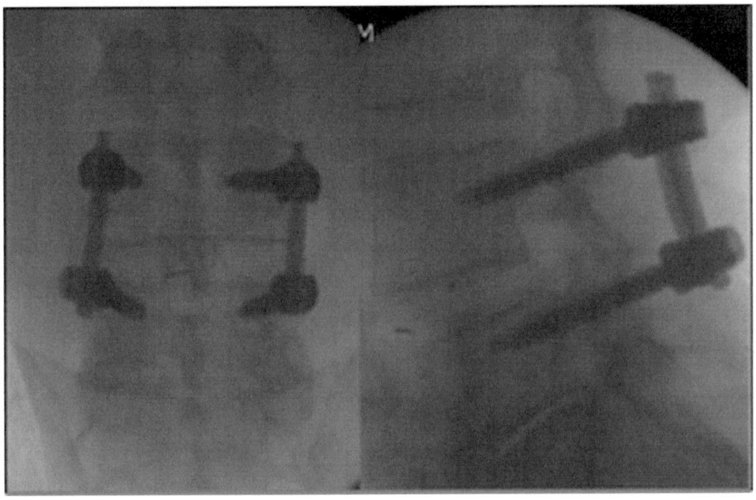

Fig. 24.8 Intraoperative fluoroscopy. MIS TLIF for degenerative lumbar spondylolisthesis

ence not to perform active reduction, whether in an open or minimally invasive setting.

Illustrative Case

History and Physical Examination

The patient is a 45-year-old male who presents to our clinic with a history of chronic bilateral L5 radiculopathy. Symptoms are worsened by standing and walking and are relieved by lying down. He had undergone physical therapy for 6 months and numerous epidural steroid injections (both interlaminal and foraminal). On a physical exam, the patient was noted to be obese, with calculated BMI of 39. The patient had a normal sensory examination, and a normal motor examination in all major muscle groups with intact reflexes; overall neurovascularly intact.

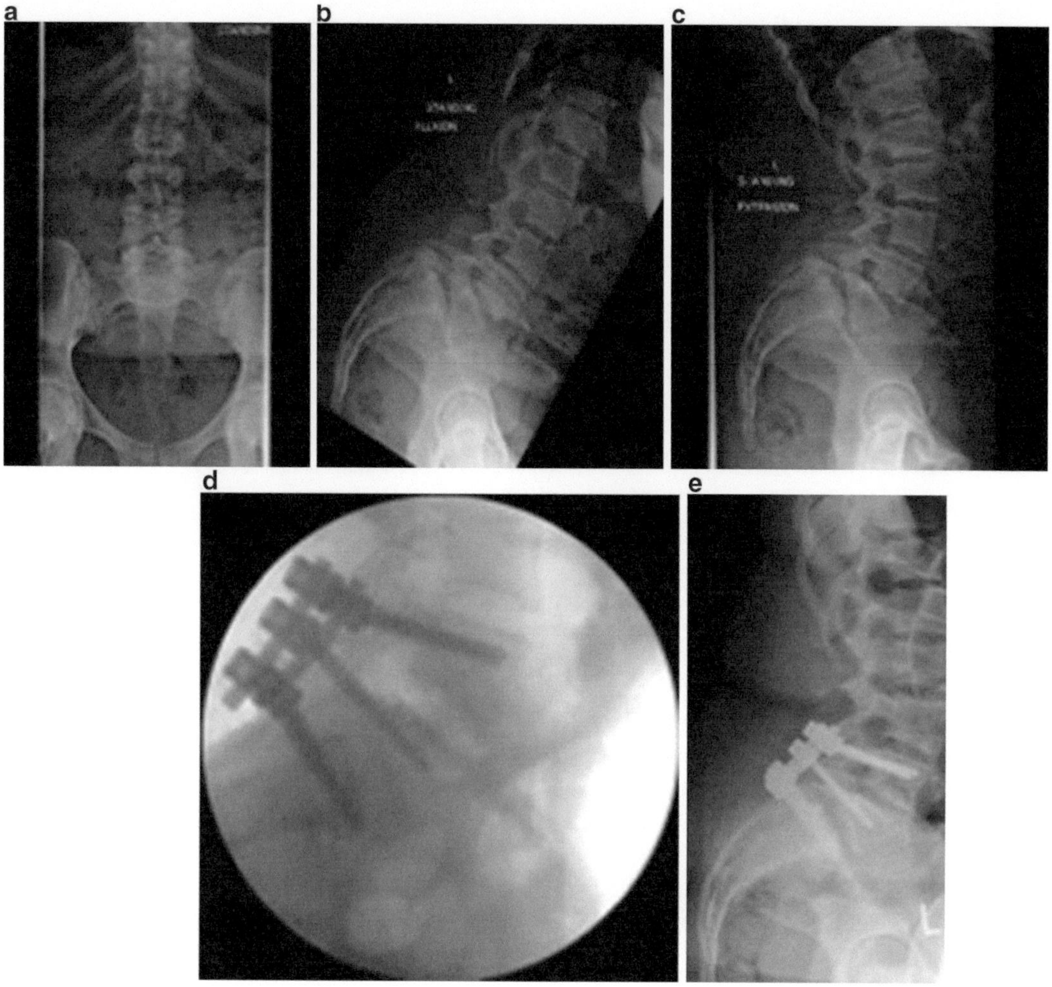

Fig. 24.9 Radiographic images from L5-S1 isthmic spondylolisthesis, grade III slip. Preoperative standing AP, flexion, and extension. Intraoperative lateral. Postoperative lateral

Pre-operative Radiographic Imaging (Fig. 24.10)

Standing AP and lateral radiographs as well as flexion-extension radiographs show a sacralized L5 vertebra with a dynamic grade II/III isthmic spondylolisthesis at L5-S1.

Treatment

The patient underwent MIS TLIF with expandable cage at L5-S1.

Outcome: Follow-up with Post-operative Radiographic Imaging (Fig. 24.10)

Patient's follow-up at 6 months states he is doing well, no complaints of pain with activity or mechanical instability. Radiographic imaging at follow-up shows proper placement of cage without subsidence or shifting, no hardware loosening or lucency around hardware. The patient was pleased with his outcome and was able to resume his activities with no persistent symptoms.

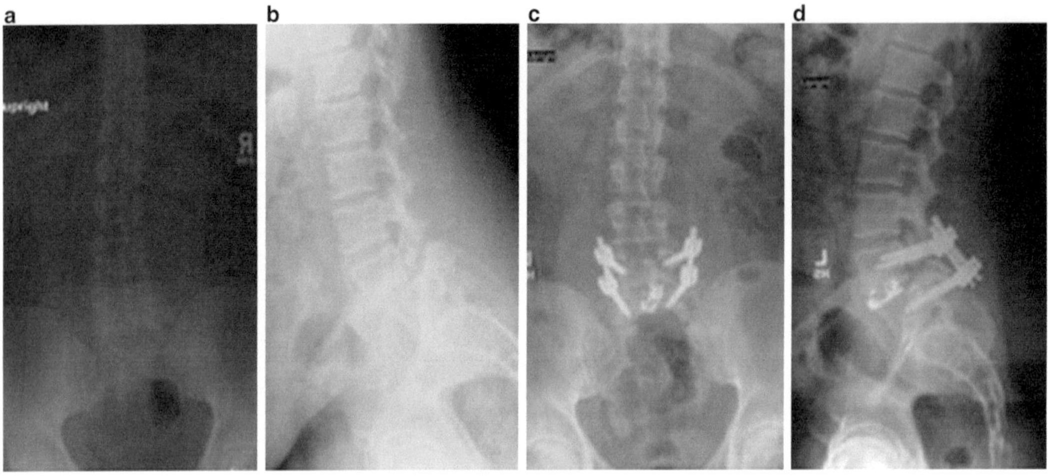

Fig. 24.10 Standing AP and lateral radiographs, preoperative, and postoperative imaging of sacralized L5 vertebra with an isthmic spondylolisthesis at L5-S1 treated with MIS TLIF and an expandable cage

Technical Pearls

- The use of the prone Jackson frame allows lordosis restoration and partial reduction of spondylolisthesis. Maximal lordosis should be achieved on the table through the use of thigh and hip pads and leg boards.
- Good clinical outcomes can be obtained with partial reduction and fusion in the adult isthmic spondylolisthesis patients.
- If active reduction is desired, we recommend extensive decompression of the exiting and traversing nerve roots through a Gill laminectomy.
- Active reduction can be achieved by locking the distal screws and reducing the rod into the proximal screws.
- MIS TLIF can achieve similar outcomes to open procedures; however the technique requires a learning curve estimated to be between 30–40 cases [163–165].
- We recommend the use of a 22 mm rigid tube and use of the microscope for the MIS TLIF.
- Arthrodesis in minimally invasive fusions is largely depended on interbody fusion; therefore, we recommend thorough disc preparation and bone grafting of at least 15 cc. We typically use demineralized bone matrix to pack the disc space and local bone graft (harvested from facet joint and morcellized) to pack the interbody spacer.

Complications and Strategies for Avoidance

The most common complication seen in any lumbar fusion surgery is pseudarthrosis, with rates that vary from 0% to 39% [166–170]. The frequency of pseudarthrosis increases in fusions performed for the type IIA (lytic) spondylolisthesis [171]. Radiographic evidence of pseudarthrosis includes a lack of bridging bone, lucency around the pedicle screws, instrumentation failure, the progression of slip angle, or an increased vertebral displacement [1]. There have been accounts of postoperative worsening of spondylolisthesis even with a non-instrumented solid arthrodesis [10, 39, 106, 169, 172, 173]. The majority of these reports utilized radiographs and not CT to assess the fusion mass; therefore, pseudarthroses might have been attributed to many of these cases. An increase in the olisthesis has been reported in non-instrumented fusions, providing a sound argument for instrumented fusion.

Radiculopathy and neurapraxia are common complications. The Scoliosis Research Society reported the percentage of neurologic complications that occurred with lytic spondylolisthesis surgery is 3.1% [174]. The most common surgical complication following reduction is a radiculopathy. The manipulation during surgery can cause direct dural trauma and damage to multiple sacral and lumbar nerve roots, resulting in postoperative neurological deficit [1]. The most commonly involved nerve roots are the L5 nerve roots, with reports showing variable rates of recovery. The highest risk of nerve root injury appears to be associated with aggressive reductions of high-grade listhesis [175–177]. We recommend wide decompression and Gill laminectomy in cases of isthmic spondylolisthesis. As previously mentioned, it is important in these cases to ensure full decompression of not only the traversing but also of the exiting nerve root.

Dural tears are also a common surgical complication [157, 178]. Although small durotomies can usually be addressed with placement of fibrin sealant, larger durotomies need to be addressed by primary closure. In our experience, the occurrence of persistent dural leaks is relatively infrequent.

Conclusion

The optimal surgical management of lumbar spondylolisthesis is highly dependent upon the symptomatology, radiographic anatomy, and surgeon's comfort level. The goals of surgical treatment are to alleviate neurologic symptoms from nerve impingement and to stabilize spinal segments that exhibit abnormal motion.

Decompression typically relies on laminectomy, the removal of all bony and ligamentous structures causing stenosis; decompression can also be achieved by indirect means through vertebral segment height restoration with interbody device insertion.

Stabilization is achieved through arthrodesis of unstable motion segments. Arthrodesis can be achieved through anterior or posterior means. The use of instrumentation has been standard since multiple reports emerged in the past two decades showing superior outcomes. The addition of interbody grafting and support has gained popularity with reports showing increased fusion rates when interbody grafting was added. Although it was shown to achieve higher fusion success and foraminal height decompression, clinical studies have not consistently shown superior clinical results.

We recommend that surgeons be familiar with more than one treatment modality. Careful examination of the specifics of each case should point toward the most appropriate technique.

References

1. Herkowitz HN, Garfin SR, Eismont FJ, Bell GR, Balderston RA. Rothman-Simeone The Spine. 6th ed. Philadelphia PA: Saunders; 2011.
2. Killian HF. Schilderungen neuer beckenformen and ihres verhaltens im leben. Mannheim: Verlag von Bassermann & Mathy; 1854.
3. Wiltse LL. Spondylolisthesis: classification and etiology. Symposium on the Spine, American Academy of Orthopaedic Surgeons. St. Louis: CV Mosby; 1969. p. 143–68.
4. Fredrickson BE, Baker D, McHolick WJ, et al. The natural history of spondylolysis and spondylolisthesis. J Bone Joint Surg. 1984;66A:699–707.
5. Gaines R, Nichols W. Treatment of spondyloptosis by two-stage L5 vertebrectomy and reduction of L4 onto S1. Spine. 1985;10:680–6.
6. Schlenzka D, Remes V, Helenius I, et al. Direct repair for treatment of symptomatic spondylolisthesis in young patients: no benefit in comparison to segmental fusion after a mean follow-up of 14.8 years. Eur Spine J. 2006;15:1437–47.
7. Herbiniaux G. Traite sur divers accouchemens labprieux, et sur polypes de la matrice. DeBoubers: Bruxelles; 1782.
8. Robert C. Eine cigenthumliche Angeborene lodose, Wahrscheinlich Bedingt durch eine Verschiebung des Korpers des letzen Lendenwirbels auf die Vordere fiache des ersten Kreuzbeinwirbels (spondylolisthesis killian) nebst Bemerkungen uber die Mechanic diser Bekenformation. Monatsschr Beburtskund Frauenkrankheiten, 2nd ed. 1853, pp 429–432.
9. Neugebauer FL. Aetiologie der sogenannten Spondylolisthesis. Arch Gynakol. 1882;20:133.
10. Wiltse L, Newman PH, Macnab I. Classification of spondylolysis and spondylolisthesis. Clin Orthop Relat Res. 1976;117:23–9.

11. Wiltse L, Rothman S. Spondylolithesis: classification, diagnosis, and natural history. Semin Spine Surg. 1989;1:78–94.
12. Wiltse L, Rothman S. Spondylolisthesis: classification, diagnosis, and natural history. Semin Spine Surg. 1993;5:264–80.
13. Wiltse L, Winter RB. Terminology and measurement of spondylolisthesis. J Bone Joint Surg Am. 1983;65:768–72.
14. Marchetti PG, Bartolozzi P. Classification of spondylolisthesis as a guidance for treatment. In: DeWald RL, Bridwell KH, editors. The textbook of spinal surgery, vol. 2. Philadelphia: Lippincott Wilkins & Williams; 1997. p. 1211–54.
15. Hammerberg KW. New concepts on the pathogenesis and classification of spondylolisthesis. Spine. 2005;30(Suppl):S4–11.
16. Dietrich M, Kurowski P. The importance of mechanical factors in the etiology of spondylolysis: a model analysis of loads and stresses in human lumbar spine. Spine (Phila Pa 1976). 1985;10:532–42.
17. Krenz J, Troup JD. The structure of the pars interarticularis of the lower lumbar vertebrae and its relation to the etiology of spondylolysis, with a report of a healing fracture in the neural arch of a fourth lumbar vertebra. J Bone Joint Surg Br. 1973;55:735–41.
18. Letts M, Smallman T, Afanasiev R, et al. Fracture of the pars interarticularis in adolescent athletes: a clinical-biomechanical analysis. J Pediatr Orthop. 1986;6:40–6.
19. Schulitz KP, Niethard FU. Strain on the interarticular stress distribution: measurements regarding the development of spondylolysis. Arch Orthop Trauma Surg. 1980;96:197–202.
20. Jackson DW, Wiltse LL, Cirincoine RJ. Spondylolysis in the female gymnast. Clin Orthop Relat Res. 1976;117:68–73.
21. Ciullo JV, Jackson DW. Pars interarticularis stress reaction, spondylolysis, and spondylolisthesis in gymnasts. Clin Sports Med. 1985;4:95–110.
22. Semon RL, Spengler D. Significance of lumbar spondylolysis in college football players. Spine (Phila Pa 1976). 1981;6:172–4.
23. Soler T, Calderon C. The prevalence of spondylolysis in the Spanish elite athlete. Am J Sports Med. 2000;28:57–62.
24. Wimberly RL, Lauerman WC. Spondylolisthesis in the athlete. Clin Sports Med. 2002;21:133–45.
25. Stinson JT. Spondylolysis and spondylolisthesis in the athlete. Clin Sports Med. 1993;12:517–28.
26. Standaert CJ. Spondylolysis in the adolescent athlete. Clin J Sport Med. 2002;12:119–22.
27. Lundin DA, Wiseman DB, Shaffrey CI. Spondylolysis and spondylolisthesis in the athlete. Clin Neurosurg. 2002;49:528–47.
28. Herman MJ, Pizzutillo PD, Cavalier R. Spondylolysis and spondylolisthesis in the child and adolescent athlete. Orthop Clin North Am. 2003;34:461–7.
29. MacDonald J, D'Hemecourt P. Back pain in the adolescent athlete. Pediatr Ann. 2007;36:703–12.
30. Ogilvie JW, Sherman J. Spondylolysis in Scheuermann's disease. Spine (Phila Pa 1976). 1987;12:251–3.
31. Newman PH. Degenerative spondylolisthesis. Orthop Clin North Am. 1975;6:197–9.
32. Labelle H, Roussouly P, Berthonnaud E, et al. Spondylolisthesis, pelvic incidence, and spinopelvic balance: a correlation study. Spine. 2004;15(29):2049–54.
33. Hanson DS, Bridwell KH, Rhee JM, et al. Correlation of pelvic incidence with low-and high-grade isthmic spondylolisthesis. Spine. 2002;27:2026–9.
34. Rosenberg NJ. Degenerative spondylolisthesis: surgical treatment. Clin Orthop. 1976;117:112–20.
35. Rowe GG, Roche MB. The etiology of separate neural arch. J Bone Joint Surg. 1953;35A:102–9.
36. Iguchi T, Wakami T, Kurihara A, et al. Lumbar multilevel degenerative spondylolisthesis: radiological evaluation and factors related to anterolisthesis and retrolisthesis. J Spinal Disord Tech. 2002;15:93–9.
37. Ganju A. Isthmic spondylolisthesis. Neurosurg Focus. 2002;13:E1.
38. Meyerding H. Spondylolisthesis: surgical treatments and results. Surg Gynecol Obstet. 1932;54:371–7.
39. Boxall D, Bradford DS, Winter RB, et al. Management of severe spondylolisthesis in children and adolescents. J Bone Joint Surg. 1979;61A:479–95.
40. Taillard W. Etiology of spondylolisthesis. Clin Orthop. 1976;115:30–9.
41. Burkus JK. Unilateral spondylolysis associated with spina bifida occulta and nerve root compression. Spine. 1990;15:555–9.
42. Lonstein JE. Spondylolisthesis in children. Spine. 1999;24:2640–8.
43. Seitsalo S. Progression of spondylolisthesis in children and adolescents. Spine. 1991;16:417–21.
44. Wynne-Davies R, Scott JHS. Inheritance and spondylolisthesis. J Bone Joint Surg Br. 1979;61:301–5.
45. Hennrikus WL. Incidence of spondylolisthesis in ambulatory cerebral palsy patients. J Pediatr Orthop. 1993;13:317–40.
46. Blackburne JS, Velikas EP. Spondylolisthesis in children and adolescents. J Bone Joint Surg Br. 1977;59:490–4.
47. Maurer SG. Iatrogenic spondylolysis leading to contralateral pedicular stress fracture and unstable spondylolisthesis. Spine. 2000;25:895–8.
48. Wiltse LL. Fatigue fracture: the basic lesion in isthmic spondylolisthesis. J Bone Joint Surg Am. 1975;57:17–22.
49. Kumar R. Spina bifida occulta in isthmic spondylolisthesis: a surgical trap. Eur Spine J. 2002;11:159–61.
50. Bird HA, Eastmond CJ, Hudson A, Wright V. Is generalized joint laxity a factor in spondylolisthesis? Scand J Rheumatol. 1980;9:203–5.
51. Kee-Yong H, Cheong-Ho C, Ki-Won K, et al. Expression of estrogen receptor of the facet joints in degenerative spondylolisthesis. Spine. 2005;30:562–6.

52. Sanderson PL, Fraser RD. The influence of pregnancy on the development of degenerative spondylolisthesis. J Bone Joint Surg Br. 1996;78:951–4.
53. Hosoe H, Ohmori K. Degenerative lumbosacral spondylolisthesis: possible factors which predispose the fifth lumbar vertebra to slip. J Bone Joint Surg Br. 2008;90:356–9.
54. Jacobsen S, Sonne-Holm S, Rovsing H, et al. Degenerative lumbar spondylolisthesis: an epidemiological perspective: the Copenhagen osteoarthritis study. Spine. 2007;32:120–5.
55. Boden SD, Riew KD, Yamaguchi K, et al. Orientation of the lumbar facet joints: association with degenerative disc disease. J Bone Joint Surg Am. 1996;78:403–11.
56. Grobler LJ, Robertson PA, Novotny JE, Pope MH. Etiology of spondylolisthesis: assessment of the role played by lumbar facet joint morphology. Spine. 1993;18:80–91.
57. Love TW, Fagan AB, Fraser RD. Degenerative spondylolisthesis: developmental or acquired? J Bone Joint Surg Br. 1999;81:670–4.
58. Lowe RW, Hayes TD, Kaye J, et al. Standing roentgenograms in spondylolisthesis. Clin Orthop Relat Res. 1976;117:80–4.
59. Standaert CJ, Herring SA. Spondylolysis: a critical review. Br J Sports Med. 2000;34:415–22.
60. Amato M, Totty WG, Gilula LA. Spondylolysis of the lumbar spine: demonstration of defects and laminal fragmentation. Radiology. 1984;153:627–9.
61. Libson E, Bloom RA, Dinari G. Symptomatic and asymptomatic spondylolysis and spondylolisthesis in young adults. Int Orthop. 1982;6:259–61.
62. Segebarth PB, Kurd MF, Haug PH, Davis R. Routine upright imaging for evaluating degenerative lumbar stenosis: incidence of degenerative spondylolisthesis missed on supine MRI. J Spinal Disord Tech. 2015; 28(10): 394–97.
63. Bodner RJ, Heyman S, Drummond DS, et al. The use of single photon emission computed tomography (SPECT) in the diagnosis of low-back pain in young patients. Spine (Phila Pa 1976). 1988;13:1155–60.
64. Bellah RD, Summerville DA, Treves ST, et al. Low-back pain in adolescent athletes: detection of stress injury to the pars interarticularis with SPECT. Radiology. 1991;180:509–12.
65. Luhmann S, O'Brien MF, Lenke L. Spondylolysis and spondylolisthesis. In: Morrissy RT, Weinstein SL, editors. Lovell and Winter's pediatric orthopaedics, vol. Vol 2. 6th ed. Philadelphia: Lippincott Williams & Wilkins; 2006. p. 839–70.
66. Congeni J, McCulloch J, Swanson K. Lumbar spondylolysis: a study of natural progression in athletes. Am J Sports Med. 1997;25:248–53.
67. Teplick JG, Laffey PA, Berman A, et al. Diagnosis and evaluation of spondylolisthesis and/or spondylolysis on axial CT. AJNR Am J Neuroradiol. 1986;7:479–91.
68. Fujiwara A, Lim T, An HS, et al. The effect of disc degeneration and facet joint osteoarthritis on segmental flexibility of the lumbar spine. Spine. 2000;23:3036–44.
69. Schellinger D, Wener L, Ragsdale BD, et al. Facet joint disorders and their role in the production of back pain and sciatica. Radiographics. 1987;7:923–44.
70. Adams MA, Hutton WC. The mechanical function of the lumbar apophyseal joints. Spine. 1983;8:327–30.
71. Tencer AF, Mayer TG. Soft tissue strain and facet face interaction in the lumbar intervertebral joint. Part II: calculated results and comparison with experimental data. J Biomech Eng. 1983;105:210–5.
72. Yang KH, King AI. Mechanism of facet load transmission as a hypothesis for low back pain. Spine. 1984;9:557–65.
73. Rihn JA, Lee JY, Khan M, et al. Does lumbar facet fluid detected on magnetic resonance imaging correlate with radiographic instability in patients with degenerative lumbar disease? Spine. 2007;14:1555–60.
74. Chaput C, Padon D, Rush J, et al. The significance of increased fluid signal on magnetic resonance imaging in lumbar facets in relationship to degenerative spondylolisthesis. Spine. 2007;17:1883–7.
75. Schinnerer KA, Katz LD, Grauer JN. MR findings of exaggerated fluid in facet joints predicts instability. J Spinal Disord Tech. 2008;21:468–72.
76. Cho BY, Murovic JA, Park J. Imaging correlation of the degree of degenerative L4–5 spondylolisthesis with the corresponding amount of facet fluid. J Neurosurg Spine. 2009;11:614–9.
77. Lasanianos N, Triantafyllopoulos GK, Pneumaticos SG. Spondylolisthesis grades. Trauma and Orthopaedic Classifications, Part IV. London: Springer; 2015. p. 239–42.
78. Boxall D, Bradford DS, Winter RB, et al. Management of severe spondylolisthesis in children. J Bone Joint Surg Am. 1979;61:479–95.
79. Oh SK, Chung SS, Lee CS. Correlation of pelvic parameters with isthmic spondylolisthesis. Asian Spine J. 2009;3(1):21–6.
80. O'Sullivan PB, Phyty GD, Twomey LT, et al. Evaluation of specific stabilizing exercise in the treatment of chronic low back pain with radiologic diagnosis of spondylolysis or spondylolisthesis. Spine (Phila Pa 1976). 1997;22:2959–67.
81. Fujii K, Katoh S, Sairyo K, et al. Union of defects in the pars interarticularis of the lumbar spine in children and adolescents: the radiological outcome after conservative treatment. J Bone Joint Surg Br. 2004;86:225–31.
82. Panjabi MM. The stabilizing system of the spine. Part I. Function, dysfunction, adaptation, and enhancement. J Spinal Disord. 1992;5:383–9.
83. Steiner ME, Micheli LJ. Treatment of symptomatic spondylolysis and spondylolisthesis with the modified Boston brace. Spine (Phila Pa 1976). 1985;10:937–43.
84. Blanda J, Bethem D, Moats W, et al. Defects of pars interarticularis in athletes: a protocol for nonoperative treatment. J Spinal Disord. 1993;6:406–11.

85. Kurd MF, Patel D, Norton R, et al. Nonoperative treatment of symptomatic spondylolysis. J Spinal Disord Tech. 2007;20:560–4.
86. Buck JE. Direct repair of the defect in spondylolisthesis: preliminary report. J Bone Joint Surg Br. 1970;52:432–7.
87. Nicol RO, Scott JH. Lytic spondylolysis: repair by wiring. Spine (Phila Pa 1976). 1986;11:1027–30.
88. Ivanic GM, Pink TP, Achatz W, et al. Direct stabilization of lumbar spondylolysis with a hook screw: mean 11-year follow-up period for 113 patients. Spine (Phila Pa 1976). 2003;28:255–9.
89. Lundin DA, Wiseman D, Ellenbogen RG, et al. Direct repair of the pars interarticularis for spondylolysis and spondylolisthesis. Pediatr Neurosurg. 2003;39:195–200.
90. Gillet P, Petit M. Direct repair of spondylolisthesis using a rod-screw construct and new bone grafting of the pars defect. Spine. 1999;24:1252–6.
91. Ulibarri JA, Anderson PA, Escarcega T, Mann D, Noonan KJ. Biomechanical and clinical evaluation for surgical repair of spondylolysis in adolescents. Spine. 2006;31:2067–72.
92. Warner WC, Leahy, M. Treating spondylolysis in the adolescent athlete. Academic News AAOS http://www.aaos.org.
93. Yuan HA, Garfin SR, Dickman CA, et al. A historical cohort study of pedicle screw fixation in thoracic, lumbar, and sacral spinal fusions. Spine (Phila Pa 1976). 1994;19(20 Suppl):2279S–96S.
94. Zdeblick TA. A prospective, randomized study of lumbar fusion: preliminary results. Spine (Phila Pa 1976). 1993;18:983–91.
95. Bjarke Christensen F, Stender Hansen E, Laursen M, et al. Long-term functional outcome of pedicle screw instrumentation as a support for posterolateral spinal fusion: randomized clinical study with a 5-year follow-up. Spine (Phila Pa 1976). 2002;27:1269–77.
96. Deguchi M, Rapoff AJ, Zdeblick TA. Posterolateral fusion for isthmic spondylolisthesis in adults: analysis of fusion rate and clinical results. J Spinal Disord. 1998;11:459–64.
97. Bono CM, Lee CK. Critical analysis of trends in fusion for degenerative disc disease over the past 20 years: influence of technique on fusion rate and clinical outcome. Spine (Phila Pa 1976). 2004;29:455–463.; discussion Z5.
98. Chang P, Seow KH, Tan SK. Comparison of the results of spinal fusion for spondylolisthesis in patients who are instrumented with patients who are not. Singap Med J. 1993;34:511–4.
99. Ricciardi JE, Pflueger PC, Isaza JE, et al. Transpedicular fixation for the treatment of isthmic spondylolisthesis in adults. Spine (Phila Pa 1976). 1995;20:1917–22.
100. Shirado O, Zdeblick TA, McAfee PC, et al. Biomechanical evaluation of methods of posterior stabilization of the spine and posterior lumbar interbody arthrodesis for lumbosacral isthmic spondylolisthesis: a calf-spine model. J Bone Joint Surg Am. 1991;73:518–26.
101. Frennered AK, et al. Midterm follow-up of young patients fused in situ for spondylolisthesis. Spine (Phila Pa 1976). 1991;16:409–16.
102. Beutler WJ, Fredrickson BE, Murtland A, et al. The natural history of spondylolysis and spondylolisthesis: 45-year follow-up evaluation. Spine (Phila Pa 1976). 2003;28:1027–1035.; discussion 1035.
103. Wiltse LL. Spondylolisthesis and its treatment. In: Finneson BE, editor. Low back pain. 2nd ed. Philadelphia: JB Lippincott; 1980. p. 451–93.
104. Lehmann TR, Spratt KF, Tozzi JE, et al. Long-term follow-up of lower lumbar fusion patients. Spine (Phila Pa 1976). 1987;12:97–104.
105. Lee CK. Accelerated degeneration of the segment adjacent to a lumbar fusion. Spine (Phila Pa 1976). 1988;13:375–7.
106. Hensinger RN. Spondylolysis and spondylolisthesis in children and adolescents. J Bone Joint Surg Am. 1989;71:1098–107.
107. Harris IE, Weinstein SL. Long-term follow-up of patients with grade-III and IV spondylolisthesis: treatment with and without posterior fusion. J Bone Joint Surg Am. 1987;69:960–9.
108. Bell DL, Ehrlich MG, Zaleske DJ. Brace treatment for symptomatic spondylolisthesis. Clin Orthop Relat Res. 1988;236:192–8.
109. Gill GG, Manning JG, White HL. Surgical treatment of spondylolisthesis without spine fusion: excision of the loose lamina with decompression of the nerve roots. J Bone Joint Surg Am. 1955;37:493–520.
110. Gill GG. Long-term follow-up evaluation of a few patients with spondylolisthesis treated by excision of the loose lamina with decompression of the nerve roots without spinal fusion. Clin Orthop Relat Res. 1984;182:215–9.
111. Schoenecker P, Cole HO, Herring J, et al. Cauda equina syndrome after in situ arthrodesis for severe spondylolisthesis at the lumbosacral junction. J Bone Joint Surg Am. 1990;72:369–77.
112. Mikheal M, Shapiro G, Wang J. High-grade adult isthmic L5-S1 spondylolisthesis: a report of intraoperative slip progression treated with surgical reduction and posterior instrumented fusion. Global Spine J. 2012;2(2):119–24.
113. Passias P, Poorman C, Yang S, Boniello A, Jalai C, Worley N, Lafage V. Surgical treatment strategies for high-grade Spondylolisthesis: a systematic review. Int J Spine Surg. 2015;9:50.
114. Shufflebarger HL, Geck MJ. High-grade isthmic dysplastic spondylolisthesis: monosegmental surgical treatment. Spine. 2005;30:S42–S8.
115. Sasso RC, Shively KD, Reilly TM. Transvertebral transsacral strut grafting for high-grade isthmic spondylolisthesis L5-S1 with fibular allograft. J Spinal Disord Tech. 2008;21:328–33.
116. Nachemson A. Repair of the spondylolisthetic defect and intertransverse fusion for young patients. Clin Orthop Relat Res. 1976;117:101–5.
117. Weinstein JN, Lurie JD, Tosteson TD, et al. Surgical versus nonsurgical treatment for lum-

bar degenerative spondylolisthesis. N Engl J Med. 2007;356:2257–70.
118. Watters WC, Bono CM, Gilbert TJ, et al. An evidence-based clinical guideline for the diagnosis and treatment of degenerative lumbar spondylolisthesis. Spine J. 2009;9:609–14.
119. Weinstein JN, Lurie JD, Tosteson TD, et al. Surgical compared with nonoperative treatment for lumbar degenerative spondylolisthesis. J Bone Joint Surg. 2009;91-A:1295–304.
120. Schlenzka D, Seitsalo S, Poussa M, et al. Operative treatment of symptomatic spondylolysis and mild spondylolisthesis in young patients: direct repair of the defect or segmental spinal fusion. Eur Spine J. 1993;2:104–12.
121. Hambly M, Lee CK, Gutteling E, et al. Tension band wiring-bone grafting for spondylolysis and spondylolisthesis: a clinical and biomechanical study. Spine. 1989;14:455–60.
122. Buck J. Direct repair of the defect in spondylolisthesis: preliminary report. J Bone Joint Surg. 1970;52B:432–7.
123. Buck J. Further thoughts on direct repair of the defect in spondylolysis. J Bone Joint Surg. 1979;61B:123.
124. Osterman K, Lindholm TS, Laurent LE. Late results of removal of the loose posterior element (Gill's operation) in the treatment of lytic lumbar spondylolisthesis. Clin Orthop. 1976;117:121–8.
125. Van Rens JG, Van Horn JR. Long-term results in lumbosacral interbody fusion for spondylolisthesis. Acta Orthop Scand. 1982;53:383–92.
126. Ekman P, Moller H, Hedlund R. The long-term effect of posterolateral fusion in adult isthmic spondylolisthesis: a randomized controlled study. Spine J. 2005;5:36–44.
127. Watkins MB. Posterolateral bone-grafting for fusion of the lumbar and lumbosacral spine. J Bone Joint Surg. 1989;41A:388–96.
128. Carragee E. Single-level posterolateral arthrodesis, with or without posterior decompression, for the treatment of isthmic spondylolisthesis in adults. A prospective, randomized study. J Bone Joint Surg Am. 1997;79:1175–80.
129. McGuire RA, Amundson GM. The use of primary internal fixation in spondylolisthesis. Spine (Phila Pa 1976). 1993;15:1662–72.
130. Kim NH, Lee JW. Anterior interbody fusion versus posterolateral fusion with transpedicular fixation for isthmic spondylolisthesis in adults. A comparison of clinical results. Spine. 1999;24:812–7.
131. McPhee IB, O'Brien JP. Reduction of severe spondylolisthesis. Spine. 1979;4:430–4.
132. Csecsei GI, Klekner AP, Dobai J, et al. Posterior interbody fusion using laminectomy bone and transpedicular screw fixation in the treatment of lumbar spondylolisthesis. Surg Neurol. 2000;53:2–6.; discussion 6–7.
133. Pearson A, Blood E, Lurie J, et al. Degenerative spondylolisthesis versus spinal stenosis: does a slip matter? Comparison of baseline characteristics and outcomes (SPORT). Spine. 2010;35:298–305.
134. Pearson A, Blood E, Lurie J, et al. Predominant leg pain is associated with better surgical outcomes in degenerative spondylolisthesis and spinal stenosis: results from the Spine Patient Outcomes Research Trial (SPORT). Spine. 2011;36:219–29.
135. Herkowitz H, Kurz L. Degenerative lumbar spondylolisthesis with spinal stenosis: a prospective study comparing decompression with decompression and intertransverse process arthrodesis. J Bone Joint Surg Am. 1991;73:802–8.
136. Malmivaara A, Slätis P, Heliövaara M, et al. Surgical or nonoperative treatment for lumbar spinal stenosis? A randomized controlled trial. Spine. 2007;32:1–8.
137. Jagannathan J, Sansur C, Oskouian R Jr, et al. Radiographic restoration of lumbar alignment after transforaminal lumbar interbody fusion. Neurosurgery. 2009;64:955–963.; discussion 963–4.
138. Park P, Foley KT. Minimally invasive transforaminal lumbar interbody fusion with reduction of spondylolisthesis: technique and outcomes after a minimum of 2 years' follow-up. Neurosurg Focus. 2008;25:E16.
139. Xu H, Tang H, Li Z. Surgical treatment of adult degenerative spondylolisthesis by instrumented transforaminal lumbar interbody fusion in the Han nationality. J Neurosurg Spine. 2009;10:496–9.
140. McAfee PC, DeVine JG, Chaput CD, et al. The indications for interbody fusion cages in the treatment of spondylolisthesis: analysis of 120 cases. Spine. 2005;30(Suppl):S60–5.
141. Oda I, Abumi K, Yu BS, et al. Types of spinal instability that require interbody support in posterior lumbar reconstruction: an in vitro biomechanical investigation. Spine. 2003;28:1573–80.
142. Tosteson AN, Lurie JD, Tosteson TD, et al. Surgical treatment of spinal stenosis with and without degenerative spondylolisthesis: cost-effectiveness after 2 years. Ann Intern Med. 2008;149:845–53.
143. Stecker M. A review of intraoperative monitoring for spinal surgery. Surg Neurol Int. 2012;3(Suppl 3):S174–87.
144. Roy-Camille R, Saillant G, Mazel C. Internal fixation of the lumbar spine with pedicle screw plating. Clin Orthop. 1986;203:7–17.
145. Magerl FP. Stabilization of the lower thoracic and lumbar spine with external skeletal fixation. Clin Orthop. 1989;1984:125–41.
146. Epstein N, Epstein J. Decompression in the surgical management of degenerative spondylolisthesis: advantages of a conservative approach in 290 patients. J Spinal Disord. 1998;11:116–22.
147. Sengupta DK, Herkowitz HN. Lumbar spinal stenosis. Treatment strategies and indications for surgery. Orthop Clin North Am. 2003;34(2):281–95.
148. Smorgick Y, Park DK, Baker KC, Lurie JD, Tosteson TD, Zhao W, Herkowitz HN, Fischgrund JS, Weinstein JN. Single- versus multilevel fusion for single-level degenerative spondylolisthesis and multilevel lumbar stenosis. Four-year results of the Spine Patient Outcomes Research Trial. Spine. 2013;38(10):797–805.

149. Park JH, et al. A comparison of unilateral laminectomy with bilateral decompression and fusion surgery in the treatment of grade I lumbar degenerative spondylolisthesis. Acta Neurochir. 2012;154(7):1205–12.
150. Rengachary S, Balabhandra R. Reduction of spondylolisthesis. Neurosurg Focus. 2002;13(1):1–3.
151. Slappey G, Toribatake Y, Ganey TM, Ogden JA, Hutton WC. Guidelines to decortication in posterolateral spine fusion. J Spinal Disord. 1998 Apr;11(2):102–9.
152. Park Y, Lee SB, Seok SO, et al. Perioperative surgical complications and learning curve associated with minimally invasive transforaminal lumbar interbody fusion: a single-institute experience. Clin Orthop Surg. 2015;7:91–6.
153. Ahn J, Tabaraee E, Singh K. Minimally invasive transforaminal lumbar Interbody fusion. J Spinal Disord Tech. 2015;28:222–5.
154. Rhee JM, Boden SD, Flynn JM, editors. Operative techniques in spine surgery. Philadelphia: Lippincott Williams & Wilkins; 2013.
155. Singh K, Vaccaro AR, editors. Minimally invasive spine surgery: advanced surgical technique. Philadelphia: Jaypee Brothers Medical Publishers ® Ltd.; 2016.
156. Elboghdady IM, Naqvi A, Jorgenson AY, et al. Minimally invasive transforaminal lumbar interbody fusion for lumbar spondylolisthesis. Ann Transl Med. 2014;2:99.
157. Wang J, Zhou Y, Zhang ZF, et al. Comparison of one-level minimally invasive and open transforaminal lumbar interbody fusion in degenerative and isthmic spondylolisthesis grades 1 and 2. Eur Spine J. 2010;19:1780–4.
158. Khan NR, Clark AJ, Lee SL, et al. Surgical outcomes for minimally invasive vs open transforaminal lumbar interbody fusion: an updated systematic review and meta-analysis. Neurosurgery 2015 Dec; 77(6):847–74.
159. Phan K, Rao PJ, Kam AC, et al. Minimally invasive versus open transforaminal lumbar interbody fusion for treatment of degenerative lumbar disease: systematic review and meta-analysis. Eur Spine J. 2015;24:1017–30.
160. Adogwa O, Parker SL, Bydon A, et al. Comparative effectiveness of minimally invasive versus open transforaminal lumbar interbody fusion: 2-year assessment of narcotic use, return to work, disability, and quality of life. J Spinal Disord Tech. 2011;24:479–84.
161. Scheer JK, Auffinger B, Wong RH, et al. Minimally invasive Transforaminal lumbar Interbody fusion (TLIF) for Spondylolisthesis in 282 patients: in situ arthrodesis versus reduction. World Neurosurg. 2015;84:108–13.
162. Kim JY, Park JY, Kim KH, et al. Minimally invasive transforaminal lumbar interbody fusion for spondylolisthesis: comparison between isthmic and degenerative spondylolisthesis. World Neurosurg 2015 Nov; 84(5):1284–93.
163. Silva PS, Pereira P, Monteiro P, et al. Learning curve and complications of minimally invasive transforaminal lumbar interbody fusion. Neurosurg Focus. 2013;35:E7.
164. Lee JC, Jang HD, Shin BJ. Learning curve and clinical outcomes of minimally invasive transforaminal lumbar interbody fusion: our experience in 86 consecutive cases. Spine. 2012;37:1548–57.
165. Lee KH, Yeo W, Soeharno H, et al. Learning curve of a complex surgical technique: minimally invasive transforaminal lumbar interbody fusion (MIS TLIF). J Spinal Disord Tech. 2014;27:E234–40.
166. Seitsalo S, Osterman K, Poussa M. Scoliosis associated with lumbar spondylolisthesis: a clinical survey of 190 young patients. Spine (Phila Pa 1976). 1988;13:899–904.
167. Hensinger RN, Lang JR, MacEwen GD. Surgical management of spondylolisthesis in children and adolescents. Spine (Phila Pa 1976). 1976;1:207–16.
168. Burkus JK, Lonstein JE, Winter RB, et al. Long-term evaluation of adolescents treated operatively for spondylolisthesis: a comparison of in situ arthrodesis only with in situ arthrodesis and reduction followed by immobilization in a cast. J Bone Joint Surg Am. 1992;74:693–704.
169. Newton PO, Johnston CE 2nd. Analysis and treatment of poor outcomes following in situ arthrodesis in adolescent spondylolisthesis. J Pediatr Orthop. 1997;17:754–61.
170. Lamberg T, Remes V, Helenius I, et al. Uninstrumented in situ fusion for high-grade childhood and adolescent isthmic spondylolisthesis: long-term outcome. J Bone Joint Surg Am. 2007;89:512–8.
171. Lee C, Dorcil J, Radomisli TE. Nonunion of the spine: a review. Clin Orthop Relat Res. 2004;419:71–5.
172. Grzegorzewski A, Kumar SJ. In situ posterolateral spine arthrodesis for grades III, IV, and V spondylolisthesis in children and adolescents. J Pediatr Orthop. 2000;20:506–11.
173. Pizzutillo PD, Mirenda W, MacEwen GD. Posterolateral fusion for spondylolisthesis in adolescence. J Pediatr Orthop. 1986;6:311–6.
174. Montgomery D, SRS morbidity and mortality committee: report of changing surgical treatment trends for spondylolisthesis. Presented at Scoliosis Research Society Pre-Meeting Course, Quebec City, Quebec, 2003.
175. Albrecht S, Kleihues H, Gill C, et al. Repositioning injuries of nerve root L5 after surgical treatment of high degree spondylolistheses and spondyloptosis—in vitro studies. Z Orthop Ihre Grenzgeb. 1998;136:182–91.
176. Ogilvie JW. Complications in spondylolisthesis surgery. Spine (Phila Pa 1976). 2005;30(6 Suppl):S97–S101.
177. Petraco DM, Spivak JM, Cappadona JG, et al. An anatomic evaluation of L5 nerve stretch in spondylolisthesis reduction. Spine (Phila Pa 1976). 1996;21:1133–1138.; discussion 1139.
178. Seng C, Siddiqui MA, Wong KP, et al. Five-year outcomes of minimally invasive versus open transforaminal lumbar interbody fusion: a matched-pair comparison study. Spine. 2013;38:2049–55.

Lumbar Interspinous Devices: Fusion and Motion Sparing

25

Dean G. Karahalios and Michael J. Musacchio Jr.

Introduction

Lumbar spinous process fixation for stabilization is a technique that has been used for several decades. Many early techniques involved wire and plate fixation [1–5]. These were intended to facilitate arthrodesis; however, they did not gain widespread adoption as a result of early failures and the perception that they did not provide adequate stiffness and durability. More contemporary strategies for fixation were subsequently developed, such as pedicle screw fixation (PSF), that proved to be more effective. However, mastery of PSF was found to require substantial subspecialty training as it involved anatomic structures less familiar than seen in the traditional posterior midline approaches. In addition, PSF increased the potential risk of injury to critical neurovascular and visceral structures [6–9]. Despite these drawbacks, PSF techniques rapidly became the gold standard for thoracolumbar fixation [10–13].

D.G. Karahalios, MD (✉)
Advocate Medical Group, Advocate Health Care, Downers Grove, IL, USA
e-mail: dean.karahalios@advocatehealth.com

M.J. Musacchio Jr., MD
North Shore University Health System, Neurosurgery and Spine Center, Evanston, IL, USA
e-mail: mmusacchio@northshore.org

With the advent of percutaneous minimally invasive surgical (MIS) techniques for decompression and arthrodesis, PSF was adapted for internal fixation in these procedures. The lateral to medial axis of the pedicles required early generation of MIS procedures to use a *lateral* transmuscular approach [14–17]. With the refinement of newer fixation technologies, including facet screws [18, 19], translaminar facet screws [20, 21], cortical screws [22–24], and spinous process fixation (SPF) [25–28], both open and MIS *midline* techniques for decompression and arthrodesis have regained popularity. In addition to rigid fixation, a number of motion-preserving technologies have also been developed for this space and will be discussed in the second half of this chapter.

Midline stabilization technologies (MSTs), whether for rigid fixation to promote arthrodesis or motion preserving, may have advantages over more lateral approaches. These include greater surgeon familiarity with the midline anatomy, improved direct visualization of critical structures, multiple fixation options, flatter learning curve, less need for imaging, and the ability to easily extend constructs to adjacent levels (may be off label in some cases).

However, there are several theoretical disadvantages of interspinous devices [29]. The spinous processes must be preserved which may limit the extent of the decompression. Further, the midline approach requires muscle stripping

L.T. Holly, P.A. Anderson (eds.), *Essentials of Spinal Stabilization*,
DOI 10.1007/978-3-319-59713-3_25

that may be more painful, leading to a longer recovery and protracted use of pain medications [30, 31]. Rigid interspinous fixation devices may have less capability to restrict motion and may not be as durable as PSF and consequently not as effective in promoting arthrodesis [29]. In addition, these devices may increase interspinous flexion and result in sagittal plane imbalance. For the motion-preserving technologies, the failure of early dynamic devices to prevent progression of degenerative disease and/or protect adjacent levels from accelerated changes has indicted the entire class [32, 29, 33–37]. Newer iterations of MSTs have proven to be much more effective than their predecessors and in many cases approach and even surpass PSF and lateral approaches [27, 28, 38].

Rigid Interspinous Fixation for Fusion

Early techniques for interspinous stabilization were performed to limit motion in order to promote arthrodesis. These techniques commonly involved the wiring of adjacent spinous processes. Unfortunately, these techniques were prone to failure due to breakage or tearing out of the wires, fracture of the spinous processes, and pseudoarthrosis secondary to the inability to effectively restrict motion. Fixation devices such as the Daab [1] and Wilson [2] plates were an improvement but were bulky and also prone to failure. With the subsequent development of PSF techniques, attention shifted away from the midline.

More recently, a number of spinous process appliances for *rigid* fixation to promote arthrodesis have been developed (Table 25.1). The Spire plate (Medtronic, Memphis TN) was the first to come to market with a device consisting of a pair of plates with spikes that could easily be applied to the spinous processes to provide immediate rigid stability [25]. The adoption of this device was limited, most likely related to its perceived similarity to the X-stop motion preserving device (Medtronic, Memphis, TN) that was associated with a fairly high rate of failure [32, 29, 33–37].

The Aspen device (Zimmer-Biomet, Broomfield, CO) brought design improvements over the Spire plate, including a graft-containing cylinder of varying diameters that would fill the interspinous space. A biomechanical test compared the Aspen device to PSF in transforaminal interbody fusion (TLIF) [28] and anterior lumbar interbody fusion (ALIF) [27] constructs. In the TLIF construct, the interspinous device was as effective as PSF in limiting flexion-extension but was less effective in axial rotation and lateral bending. Similar results were seen in the ALIF construct but with an overall reduction in range of motion (ROM) that was statistically equivalent to bilateral PSF. The excellent performance of this device, especially in flexion-extension, is likely related to the large cylinder that fills the interspinous space and acts as an extension block. It has also been shown that while there is typically some associated flexion at the index level, there is also a compensatory extension at the adjacent levels and as such there is no significant change in overall sagittal balance [27, 39]. There is also an advantage of increased foraminal height that can be effective in addressing associated radicular issues.

One criticism of the Aspen device is its inability to provide compression on an interbody device and may promote stress shielding and eventual pseudoarthrosis. However, fusion rates have been shown to be comparable to PSF [40]. To further address this potential shortcoming, a newer Aspen-like device called Alpine was developed (Zimmer-Biomet, Broomfield, CO). This translating device allows for distraction and compression and also provides a mechanism that can expand and fit snugly within the interspinous space. A similar device named BridgePoint has been also been developed by Alphatec Spine (Carlsbad, CA).

Despite the encouraging biomechanical results seen with SPF devices [27, 28, 26], their performance in clinical practice has been the subject of debate [29]. Radiographic evidence of successful arthrodesis has been demonstrated [40, 38]. In our own experience, we typically not only see robust fusion mass in the disc space and posterolaterally but also between the spinous

Table 25.1 Select rigid interspinous fixation devices (listings are not comprehensive, nor an endorsement of any individual device)

Device	Company	Prominent feature(s)
Affix	NuVasive, San Diego, CA	Small footprint, zero-step locking
Aileron, Aileron Expandable, Aileron-TRX	LifeSpine, Huntley, IL	Custom fit, multiple sizes, large graft containment, bullet tip, facilitates anterior placement
Aspen	Zimmer Biomet, Broomfield, CO	Integrated interspinous graft chamber, contoured for optimal ventral positioning, wide range of sizes
Alpine	Zimmer Biomet, Broomfield, CO	Provides distraction and compression across interspace
BacFuse	Pioneer Surgical, Marquette, MI	Wide range of sizes
Bridgepoint	Alphatec, Carlsbad, CA	Provides distraction and compression across interspace, large bone graft window, large bone contact area
Interbridge	LDR Spine (now Zimmer Biomet), Broomfield, CO	Facilitates preservation of supraspinous ligament, simplified insertion instruments and technique
SP-Fix	Globus Medical, Audubon, PA	PEEK interspinous barrels, zero-step locking
Spire, Spire Z	Medtronic, Memphis, TN	First to market in modern era. Spire Z with revised shape to better accommodate anatomy
UniVise	Stryker, Kalamazoo, MI	One-piece implant, streamlined instrumentation and locking

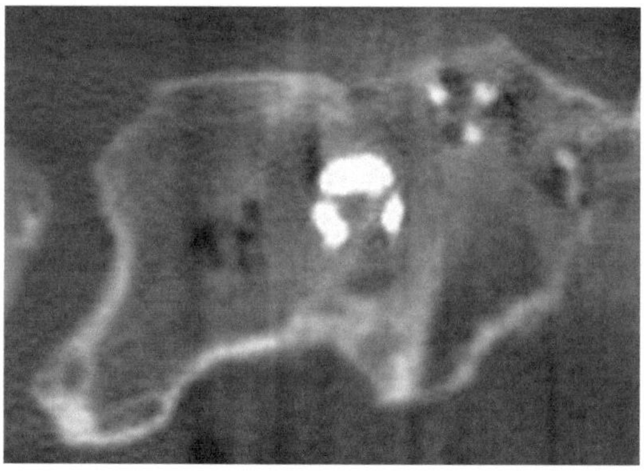

Fig. 25.1 Sagittal reconstructed computed tomographic (CT) view of an SPF construct demonstrating robust bone growth bridging between adjacent spinous processes (Alpine, Zimmer-Biomet, Broomfield, CO)

processes (Fig. 25.1). Radiographic success does not necessarily relate to good clinical outcomes. However, in the case of SPF, there is evidence to suggest that clinical outcomes are favorable and comparable to PSF [1, 2, 41, 25, 40].

There are some potential advantages of SPF over PSF technologies. As previously discussed, the anatomy is familiar to all surgeons. As such, very little in the way of training is required and the learning curve is relatively flat. There is also some evidence to suggest that operative times are shorter, there is less blood loss, less pain, and quicker recovery [40]. The technique is also safer in that there is less risk of injury to neurovascular and visceral structures. Typically, less imaging is required and thus the dose of radiation to the patient is less. The positioning of SPF devices places them medial and inferior to the cephalad facet complexes (Fig. 25.2a–b), which may have implications for mitigating the acceleration of adjacent level degenerative changes [40].

Surgical Indications

Spinous process fixation devices are versatile and can be utilized to provide stabilization to promote fusion in a number of clinical scenarios. These

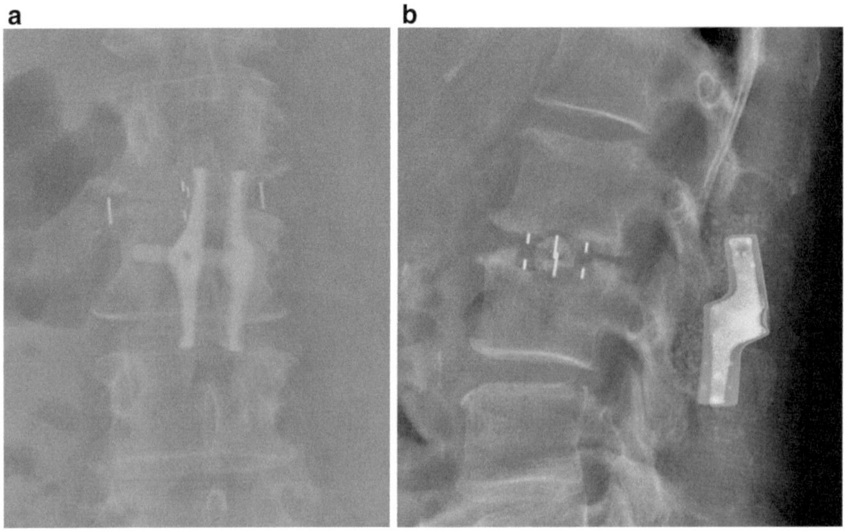

Fig. 25.2 (**a**). Anteroposterior (AP) and (**b**). lateral plain radiographic images demonstrating an SPF device (Medtronic Spire Z, Memphis, TN) used to stabilize a direct lateral interbody arthrodesis (DLIF) procedure (Medtronic Clydesdale system, Memphis, TN). Note that the SPF device is centered just below the index disc space

include posterior interlaminar fusion, posterolateral fusion, ALIF, TLIF alone, TLIF with unilateral pedicle screws, direct lateral fusion, topping off long PSF constructs, and in revisions addressing adjacent level degeneration.

Preoperative Considerations

The technique for SPF is relatively straightforward as the anatomy is familiar and the application of the device is not typically challenging. However, there are some important considerations in planning, technical nuances, and some minor variations depending on the particular device. Contraindications include pars defects and osteoporosis. However, in the aging spine, there may be a significant differential between the density of the posterior elements and the vertebral bodies, favoring posterior fixation (Table 25.2).

Table 25.2 Main contraindications to the placement of rigid spinous process fixation devices for the purpose of arthrodesis

Posterior spinal elements weakened or missing due to prior surgery, trauma, or congenital defect
Pars defect
Morbid obesity
Osteopenia or osteoporosis
Neuromuscular disorder
Smoking
Infection
Contact with other implants of varying metallurgy
Allergy to titanium

Surgical Technique

A midline incision 4–5 cm in length is planned over the rostral and caudal spinous processes to be fixated. It is important to remember that the rostral spinous process will be in the axial plane of the interspace that represents the level to be fused (Fig. 25.2a–b). The paraspinal musculature is then reflected off of the spinous processes and lamina. The facets and transverse processes may also be exposed for decompression and arthrodesis purposes.

Partial laminectomies can be performed along the inferior aspect of the rostral segment and the superior aspect of the caudal segment. Redundant ligamentum flavum can be resected with Kerrison punches. Partial medial facetectomies and foraminotomies can also be performed. In the setting of a TLIF procedure, a total facetectomy can be performed unilaterally. Care must be taken to not weaken or fracture the spinous processes during decompression or application of the SPF device.

The supraspinous ligament may be removed or left intact based on the surgeon's preference. Preservation of this structure is important for the application of some motion-sparing devices like X-Stop that require it to remain contained within the interspinous space. However, for SPF devices that provide rigid stabilization by attaching to the spinous processes themselves, it may be resected. Further, for translating SPF devices that provide distraction and compression, it is removed with a Leksell rongeur. Next, the interspinous space is measured with calipers or trials in order to select the appropriately sized device that will maximally fill the space. For the translating SPF devices, this is not necessary, since the device may be expanded to fit this space prior to engaging the spinous processes (Fig. 25.3a). In either case, the instruments used to prepare the interspinous space or the translating SPF devices can be used to apply distractive forces. Careful visual inspection, tactile feedback, and the surgeon's judgment are all critical in preventing fracture or weakening of the spinous processes through these maneuvers. The plates on either side of the midline are then compressed so that the spikes integral to the medial aspect of the plates engage the cortical bone of the spinous processes (Fig. 25.3b). Care must be taken to avoid overcompression, as this may fracture or weaken these structures as well. At this point, some devices are self-locking and others require subsequent steps to lock the device to the spinous processes.

The translating fixation devices can be distracted and subsequently collapsed and/or compressed rostrocaudally (Fig. 25.3a) and locked to secure an interbody graft or device (Fig. 25.3c). Many devices have integral graft containment capability in the portion of the device that passes through the interspinous space. These can be pre- or post-packed with graft material. Additional graft can be placed over remaining decorticated lamina, facets, and/or transverse processes (Fig. 25.3d). Final anterior posterior (AP) and lateral fluoroscopic imaging is typically performed to confirm adequate placement of the instrumentation over the appropriate levels.

Illustrative Case (Rigid Fixation for Arthrodesis)

History A 58-year-old male underwent an L3-4 microdiscectomy. Initially he responded well, but approximately 1 year after surgery, he developed new symptoms that were slightly different than the previous unilateral L4 radicular pattern. He failed conservative management that included physical therapy, epidural injections, and facet blocks.

Physical Examination His examination was consistent with a bilateral L3 radiculopathy.

Radiographical Imaging MR imaging revealed accelerated changes at the L3-4 level with disc space collapse, Modic changes, and foraminal stenosis (Fig. 25.4a).

Treatment He was taken to surgery for an instrumented TLIF procedure with spinous process fixation (Figs. 25.4b–c).

Outcome Postoperatively, his radicular pain resolved as did his mechanical back pain. At 2-year follow-up, he remains asymptomatic.

Technical Pearls

- Preoperative CT scans are helpful to confirm that the relevant bony anatomy is sound, that there are no pars defects, and for S1 that there is a spinous process that is large enough for the device to engage.
- Preoperative bone density studies may be misleading and should be interpreted with caution, as the posterior elements may be relatively sclerotic compared to the vertebral bodies.
- Care should be taken to advance the device as far ventrally as possible, so that it rests on the lamina rostrally and caudally. It may be

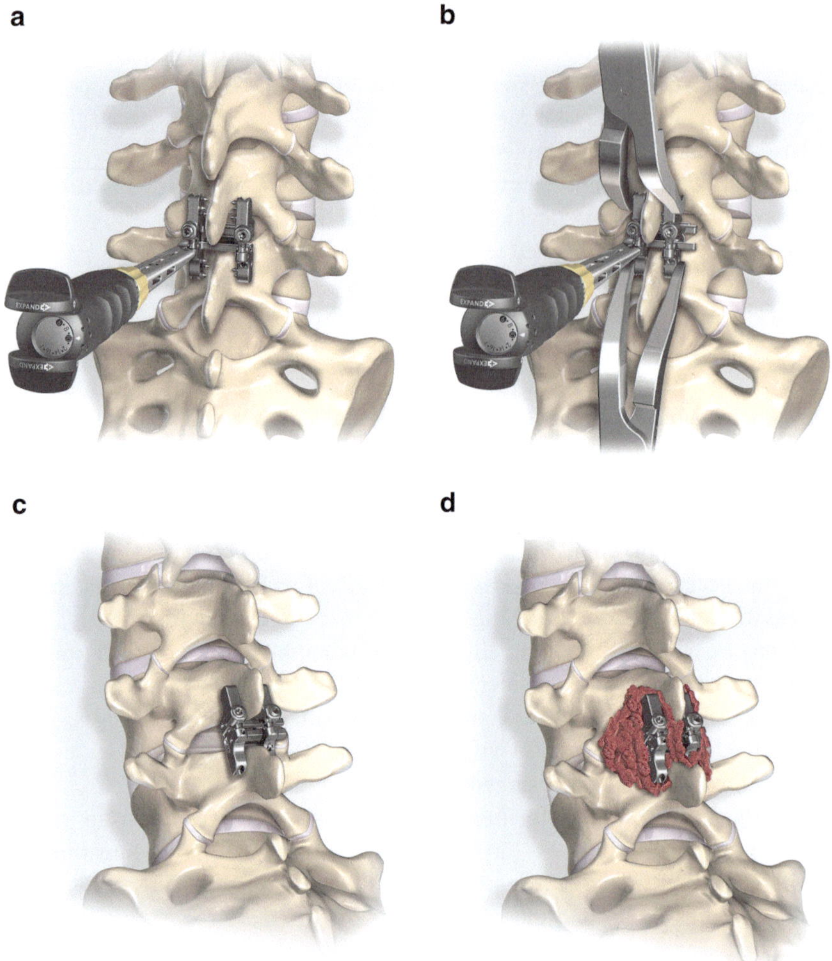

Fig. 25.3 Schematic drawing of Alpine XC device placement. (**a**). The device is inserted into the interspinous space and expanded provisionally by rotating the knob on the inserter until the graft containment portion of the device passing across the midline fills the space. (**b**). Compression is applied securing the spikes along the inner aspect of the plates to the spinous processes. (**c**). Final implant configuration. (**d**). Graft material is packed over the exposed decorticated bony elements, around the device, and through the interspinous space

necessary to drill down the medial aspects of the facet complexes to achieve proper positioning.

- Avoid excessive compression when engaging the spiked plates to the spinous processes as this may cause a fracture or weakening. The spikes, but not the plates, should sink into the cortical bone.
- For the devices that allow for distraction and compression across the interspace, forces should be applied with caution to avoid fracture or weakening of the spinous processes.

Complications and Strategies for Avoidance

The most common serious complication that can occur is the fracture of the spinous processes. This can lead to pain, migration of interbody implants, and pseudoarthrosis leading to the need for revision. Fractures can occur intraoperatively during placement of the device due to excessive compression of the spiked plates into the spinous processes or by excessive distraction and compression across the interspace.

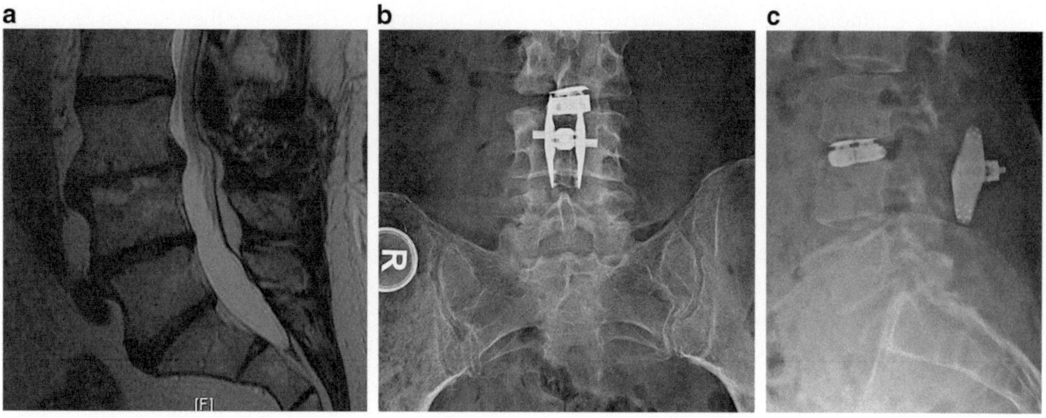

Fig. 25.4 (**a**). Sagittal T2-weighted magnetic resonance image of the lumbar spine demonstrating advanced degenerative and post-operative changes involving the L3-4 disc space. There is marked loss of disc space height and Modic changes. (**b**). AP and (**c**). lateral plain radiographic views of a Stryker UniVise spinous process fixation device (Stryker, Kalamazoo, MI) used to stabilize a Stryker AccuLIF expandable interbody device (Stryker, Kalamazoo, MI) in a TLIF construct

This can be avoided by careful visual inspection of the spinous processes as these forces are applied and attention to tactile feedback that provides a subjective but meaningful assessment of bony element strength. The risk of fracture can also be mitigated by positioning the device as ventral as possible, where the spinous processes are usually wider and stronger as they transition to the lamina. The surgeon must also counsel the patient preoperatively that if the anatomy is not conducive or a fracture occurs an alternative fixation technique may be required.

Postoperative fractures can occur due to excessive activity or trauma/falls. Patients should be carefully selected for compliance to activity restrictions. In addition, bracing may be used as well to limit excessive motion.

Wound dehiscence may occur at a slightly higher rate than in other fixation techniques, and is likely related to the relatively close proximity of the device to the midline and skin surface. This risk can be mitigated by performing a meticulous multi-layered closure, with coverage of the device by muscle and a tight closure of the fascia.

Interlaminar/Interspinous Motion Preservation

The concept of *motion sparing interspinous technology was developed* as a means to relieve symptoms of degenerative spinal disease with MIS and without fusion. While multiple devices have been introduced, only a limited number are available in the US market. The two most influential dynamic MSTs, the Wallis Interspinous Device (Abbott Spine, Abbott Park, IL) introduced for treatment of patients with recurrent disc herniations and the X-stop Interspinous Spacer (Medtronic, Memphis, TN) for mild to moderate stenosis, are no longer available for clinical use. Another device, Diam (Medtronic, Memphis, TN), intended for use as an indirect decompression device for spinal stenosis, failed to receive FDA clearance for use in the USA. Despite these early failures, there are significant benefits to be gained by exploiting the posterior midline for motion preserving stabilization devices.

Interlaminar and interspinous motion-preserving devices represent an evolution of stabilization technology for the posterior lumbar midline approach. Traditional means of spinal segmental stabilization include instrumented and non-instrumented fusion, including the interspinous fusion devices discussed earlier in this chapter. While stabilization via fusion accomplishes clinical goals of improved back pain, slowing of the degenerative cascade, reduction in intradiscal pressures, and preservation of foraminal height, it does so at the potential expense of adjacent level degeneration and the possibility of need for further treatments and intervention [42–44]. In analogous fashion to artificial disc replacement technology, the theory behind interspinous and interlaminar motion-preserving stabilization is to accomplish the goals of fusion stabilization without the downside of adjacent level degeneration and dependence on solid bony fusion for clinical efficacy.

Currently in the US market, there are only two FDA-approved and commercially available devices for interlaminar and interspinous motion-preserving stabilization. They are Coflex Interlaminar Stabilization (ILS) (Paradigm Spine, New York, NY) and Superion Interspinous Spacer System (ISS) (VertiFlex, San Clemente, CA). These devices have different mechanisms of action and insertion techniques but share the common goal of addressing clinically relevant elements of the disease state of lumbar spinal stenosis, while still allowing the index level to maintain some degree of motion, thereby minimizing impact on adjacent spinal levels. In the case of Coflex, the device is designed to preserve normal motion of the spinal segment while reducing back pain by offloading the facets and slowing the degenerative cascade. In contrast, Superion is designed as an extension blockade to relieve symptoms of neurogenic claudication but allow normal flexion.

Lumbar stenosis is not a discrete disease but is instead a part of a larger spinal degenerative cascade. Beyond symptoms of neural compression, patients with stenosis often progress to develop segmental degeneration that is associated with facet degeneration, disc collapse, foraminal narrowing, and mechanical back pain with or without instability. Therefore, there is not a single surgical solution that may address the totality of the disease spectrum.

While many patients with lumbar stenosis will benefit from laminectomy alone, there are many who will still have mechanical back pain or develop recurrent disease [45–47]. In these patients, stabilization may offer additional benefits. In the case of Coflex, decompression may be performed. Clinical evidence supports significant advantages in clinical outcomes, maintenance of spinal motion, reduced back and leg pain, and preservation of foraminal height in the Coflex procedure over decompression alone and decompression with fusion [48–53]. In the case of Superion, the primary goal is to relieve symptomatic lumbar stenosis in patients with moderate stenosis. By virtue of lack of surgical fixation, this device allows some degree of maintenance of motion but, unlike interlaminar stabilization, the maintenance of motion is not the intended mechanism of action.

Indications and Patient Selection

The primary diagnosis in candidates for posterior midline motion preserving stabilization is lumbar stenosis. These techniques may be considered for patients with moderate to severe stenosis without gross instability, generally defined as up to grade 1 spondylolisthesis with sagittal translation less than 4 mm on flexion vs. extension, and who have failed conservative treatment options. A major distinction between the two techniques is that patients who have significant back pain in addition to stenosis have been shown to benefit from Coflex after direct decompression, whereas Superion is intended to address only the symptoms associated with intermittent neurogenic claudication.

Coflex is intended to be an adjunct to direct surgical decompression via laminectomy, as opposed to the indirect decompression of Superion, which does not involve performing a laminectomy. Both techniques are aimed at addressing stenosis, but in the case of Coflex, more severe stenosis can be addressed via the laminectomy than could potentially be relieved by indirect distraction alone. By definition, the degree of stenosis in Superion must not be so severe that the patients are beyond relief by leaning forward or sitting. Additionally, a primary goal of Coflex is to relieve the mechanical back pain of the diseased segment, particularly as it relates to facetogenic disease, as it offloads the facets after the direct decompression, while the primary goal of ISS is to relieve the neurogenic claudication associated with stenosis.

Patients who have symptoms of back and/or buttock and leg pain with radiographic confirmation of at least moderate lumbar stenosis at one or two contiguous levels from L1 to L5 may be candidates for either of these procedures. Table 25.3 lists notable contraindications for motion-sparing procedures. Generally speaking, motion sparing is contraindicated in patients who have greater than grade 1 spondylolisthesis, gross instability on flexion/extension X-rays, moderate to high grade deformity or scoliosis, and more than two segments of disease requiring surgical decompression. Relative contraindications may also include previous back surgeries at index levels, osteopenia/osteoporosis, or other severe medical or systemic diseases.

Table 25.3 Contraindications for interspinous motion sparing device placement

Prior fusion or decompressive laminectomy at any index lumbar level
Radiographically compromised vertebral bodies at any lumbar level(s) caused by current or past trauma or tumor (e.g., compression fracture)
Severe facet hypertrophy that requires extensive bone removal which would cause instability
Grade II or greater spondylolisthesis
Isthmic spondylolisthesis or spondylolysis (pars fracture)
Degenerative lumbar scoliosis (Cobb angle of greater than 25°)
Osteoporosis
Back or leg pain of unknown etiology
Axial back pain only, with no leg, buttock, or groin pain
Active or chronic infection – systemic or local
Known allergy to titanium alloys or MR contrasting agents

Preoperative Considerations

When considering the appropriateness of ILS vs. ISS motion-preserving devices, one must consider whether a direct decompression will be required or if an indirect decompression will suffice. In the case of ISS, the entire success of the procedure hinges on whether the implantation of the device itself will provide enough indirect decompression to provide sustainable symptomatic relief. A broad distinction of whether direct decompression will be required or if indirect decompression will suffice is whether a patient gains relief of symptoms with sitting or bending forward. For patients who fail to gain symptom relief with flexion, indirect decompression will not be adequate, and the surgeon should consider direct decompression. The surgeon must also evaluate whether there is adequate spinous process anatomy to support the implant as poor bone quality or anatomic variance may compromise the integrity of the implantation.

With ILS, the decompression will be accomplished via direct laminectomy. Therefore, the preoperative considerations center around whether the patient would benefit from post-laminectomy stabilization to improve mechanical back pain and prevent recurrent stenosis and foraminal collapse. In the case of grossly unstable patients or patients with moderate to severe spinal deformity, fusion remains the gold standard for stabilization. Also, if the act of decompression will destabilize the spinal segment or if the degree of decompression requires excessive laminar removal, then ILS may not be feasible.

Surgical Technique: Interlaminar Stabilization

Coflex is the only ILS device FDA approved for use in the USA. The surgical technique for ILS begins with a modified segmental laminotomy and bilateral medial facetectomies with special attention paid toward creating a parallel space between the adjacent spinous processes and preserving portions of the lamina for engagement with the U-shaped Coflex device. The ligamentum flavum is resected as part of the decompression and to ensure the device can seat properly in the interlaminar space. It is recommended that the decompression be performed with the patient in a prone neutral position to ensure that the decompression is adequate for symptomatic relief but not so extensive as to preclude placement of the device.

When the decompression is completed, the proper-sized implant is selected using trials of increasing height inserted into the interlaminar space. Once selected, the one-piece titanium implant with superior and inferior wings is gently tapped into the interlaminar position with the ventral aspect within 1–2 mm of the dura. Once position is confirmed visually, and radiographically if so desired, the wings are then crimped against the superior and inferior spinous processes to prevent shearing or loosening. When sizing the interlaminar implant, the device should fit snugly within the interlaminar space but not over-distract the facets by more than 1–2 mm. It should not introduce kyphosis at the segment, as it is intended to stabilize motion after direct decompression, not create indirect decompression. Ultimately, the Coflex device will serve as a stabilizer of segmental motion while offloading the facet and posterior intradiscal pressures without causing significant alteration in spinal motion.

Surgical Technique: Interspinous Process Distraction

The Superion interspinous process spacer is the only interspinous motion-preserving device currently available for use in the USA. The surgical technique relies upon an indirect decompression of the spinal canal via the introduction of segmental distraction by leveraging off the spinous processes. The patient is placed in a prone position and a midline skin incision is made over the segment of interest. An incision is made through the fascia and supraspinous ligament, and dilators are used to introduce a cannula into the midline interspinous space. An intraspinous gauge is then passed through the cannula and used to select the appropriate size for implantation. The titanium implant is then inserted through the cannula and has two cam lobes which are deployed inferiorly and superiorly to encompass the corresponding spinous processes. Figure 25.5 provides an illustration of the surgical technique.

Illustrative Case (Interlaminar/Interspinous Motion Preservation)

History A 63-year-old male presents with complaints of progressive mechanical low back pain and neurogenic claudication. On a scale of 0 to 10, he rates both back and leg pain at a maximum of 8/10. His pain is significantly worse with

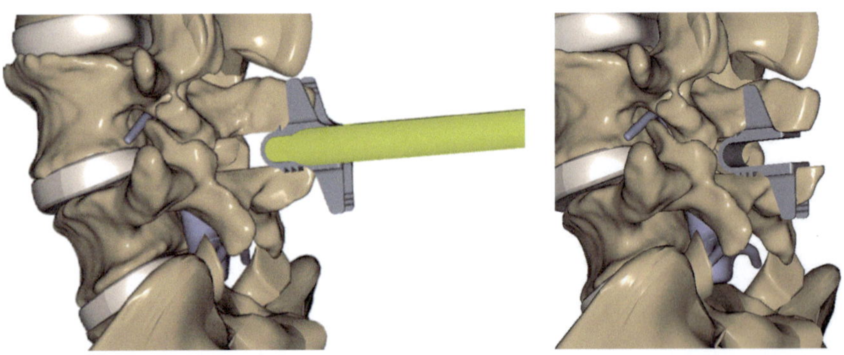

Fig. 25.5 Illustration showing insertion technique for interlaminar stabilization. A parallel channel is created in the interspinous process space seen on the left. The device is then inserted within this space and the ventral aspect is engaged within the interlaminar space, as seen in the image on the right.

standing and walking and is only partially abated with sitting.

Physical Examination Well-developed male with appropriate interactions and affect. Strength is 5/5 throughout. Gait is antalgic. Sensory is intact and reflexes are 2+/5 throughout.

Imaging Upright lumbar radiographs with flexion/extension views reveal a Grade 1 spondylolisthesis at L4-5 with less than 4 mm of translation on flexion vs. extension. MRI of his lumbar spine reveals severe L4-5 central spinal stenosis (Fig. 25.6a, b).

Treatment After failure of conservative treatment, he underwent a segmental laminotomy and bilateral medial facetectomy at L4-5 with insertion of an interlaminar stabilization device (Fig. 25.6c).

Outcome At 2-year postop, he rates his maximum back pain at 2/10 episodically and leg pain at 0/10.

Technical Pearls

Motion Sparing Interspinous Devices

- These procedures are motion-preserving, not motion-creating. Preoperating imaging, including dynamic flexion/extension X-rays, should be obtained to determine the absence of gross instability
- If the surgical decompression results in instability, then motion-sparing technologies are unlikely to be successful
- Careful attention to the extent of spinous process, laminar, and facet removal is important to ensure proper implantation and functioning of the implant.
- For motion-preserving devices depending on indirect decompression, ensure that the patient gets symptomatic relief when sitting or forward flexion
- If patient does not obtain symptomatic relief from sitting or forward flexion, consider direct decompression.

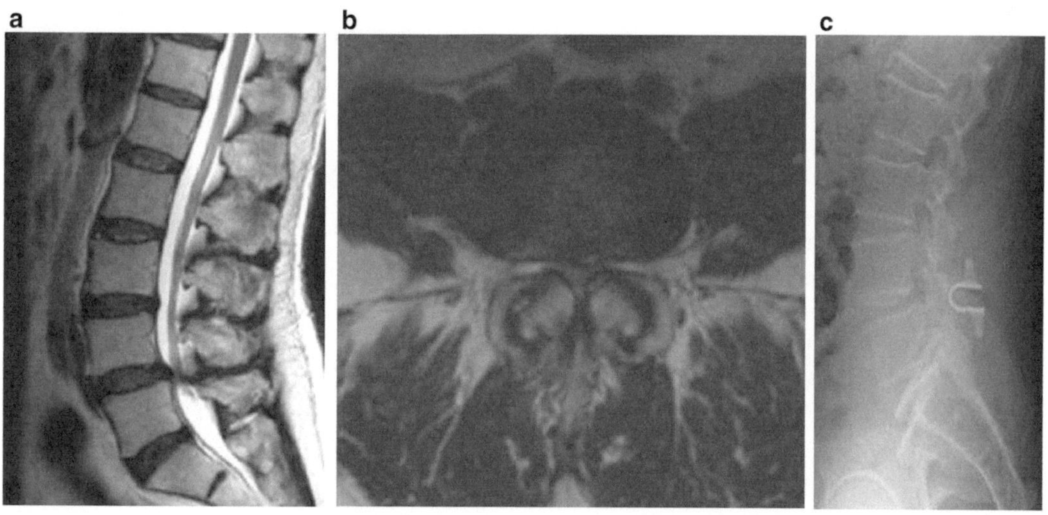

Fig. 25.6 (**a**). Sagittal and (**b**). axial T2-weighted magnetic resonance images revealing severe stenosis at L4-5 and Grade 1 spondylolisthesis. (**c**). The lateral plain radiographic image reveals proper placement of a dynamic lumbar interlaminar device at L4-5 inserted after direct segmental decompression (Coflex, Paradigm Spine, New York, NY)

Complications and Strategies for Avoidance

Motion Sparing Interspinous Devices

Coflex

The complications associated with this technique include wound related issues, inadequate laminectomy and decompression, and poor patient selection including those who ultimately require a fusion due to their instability. Less common adverse events include a 2.8% incidence of device-related failures requiring revision and a 4.2% incidence of late-term ineffective treatment requiring revision for a total of 7% of patients requiring revision at 5-year postop due to ineffective treatment [53]. In comparison, in the fusion control cohort of the FDA trial 5-year outcomes data, there was a 12.1% revision rate due to ineffective treatment. Complication avoidance in this technique includes standard precautions taken with standard laminectomy procedures, with the addition of carefully evaluating the patient preoperatively for preexistent instability or the possibility of the development of instability from the act of direct decompression.

Superion

Potential adverse events of this procedure primarily involve ineffective treatment and/or spinous process fracture. At 2-year follow-up, there was a 23.2% incidence of reoperations or revisions reported in the FDA trial data. Additionally, there was a 12.1% incidence of spinous process fracture and a 13.2% incidence of postoperative epidural steroid injection or nerve block at index level [54, 55]. Avoidance of therapeutic failure is most likely tied to proper patient selection and dependence on bone integrity to maintain spinal distraction.

Conclusion

The posterior midline anatomy of the lumbar spine is familiar to spine surgeons and presents opportunities for rigid and mobile stabilization techniques. There are distinct advantages that may be gained through use of MSTs over other stabilization techniques. MSTs are generally performed using less invasive surgical techniques when compared to other methods of spinal stabilization, and they typically do not introduce significant morbidity to the surgical procedure. Additionally, they may offer greater versatility in the case of revision surgeries and limited impact or interference with adjacent levels. Two types of devices are available including those that are intended to result in arthrodesis and those that preserve motion. The former are indicated as adjuncts to decompression and fusion while the later are for treatment of spinal stenosis and attempt to avoid fusion.

Disclosures DK serves as a consultant and derives royalties for products developed and commercialized by Medtronic and Zimmer-Biomet (including devices mentioned in this chapter). MM serves as a consultant for Medtronic and Paradigm Spine.

References

1. Böstman O, Myllynen P, Riska EB. Posterior spinal fusion using internal fixation with the Daab plate. Acta Orthop Scand. 1984 Jun;55(3):310–4.
2. Cobey MC. The value of the Wilson plate in spinal fusion. Clin Orthop Relat Res. 1971 May;76:138–40.
3. Drummond D, Guadagni J, Keene JS, Breed A, Narechania R. Interspinous process segmental spinal instrumentation. J Pediatr Orthop. 1984 Aug;4(4):397–404.
4. Heller KD, Prescher A, Schneider T, Block FR. Stability of different wiring techniques in segmental spinal instrumentation. Archives of orthopaedic [Internet]. 1998. Available from: http://link.springer.com/article/10.1007/BF00703452.
5. Tencer AF, Self J, Allen BL, Drummond D. Design and evaluation of a posterior laminar clamp spinal fixation system. Spine. 1991;16(8):910–8.
6. Esses SI, Sachs BL, Dreyzin V. Complications associated with the technique of pedicle screw fixation. A selected survey of ABS members. Spine. 1993;18(15):2231–8. discussion 2238–9
7. Jutte PC, Castelein RM. Complications of pedicle screws in lumbar and lumbosacral fusions in 105 consecutive primary operations. Eur Spine J. 2002;11(6):594–8.
8. Lonstein JE, Denis F, Perra JH, Pinto MR, Smith MD, Winter RB. Complications associated with pedicle screws. J Bone Joint Surg Am. 1999;81(11):1519–28.
9. Rivet DJ, Jeck D, Brennan J, Epstein A, Lauryssen C. Clinical outcomes and complications associated

with pedicle screw fixation-augmented lumbar interbody fusion. J Neurosurg Spine. 2004;1(3):261–6.
10. Dickman CA, Fessler RG, MacMillan M, Haid RW. Transpedicular screw-rod fixation of the lumbar spine: operative technique and outcome in 104 cases. J Neurosurg. 1992;77(6):860–70.
11. Karahalios DG, Apostolides PJ, Sonntag VK. Degenerative lumbar spinal instability: technical aspects of operative treatment. Clin Neurosurg. 1997;44:109–35.
12. Masferrer R, Gomez CH, Karahalios DG, Sonntag VK. Efficacy of pedicle screw fixation in the treatment of spinal instability and failed back surgery: a 5-year review. J Neurosurg. 1998;89(3):371–7.
13. Zdeblick TA. A Prospective, randomized study of lumbar fusion: preliminary results. Spine. 1993;18(8): 983.
14. Ozgur BM, Hughes SA, Baird LC, Taylor WR. Minimally disruptive decompression and transforaminal lumbar interbody fusion. Spine J. 2006 Jan;6(1):27–33.
15. Holly LT, Schwender JD, Rouben DP, Foley KT. Minimally invasive transforaminal lumbar interbody fusion: indications, technique, and complications. Neurosurg Focus. 2006;20(3):E6.
16. Slucky AV, Brodke DS, Bachus KN, Droge JA, Braun JT. Less invasive posterior fixation method following transforaminal lumbar interbody fusion: a biomechanical analysis. Spine J. 2006;6(1):78–85.
17. Tuttle J, Shakir A, Choudhri HF. Paramedian approach for transforaminal lumbar interbody fusion with unilateral pedicle screw fixation. Technical note and preliminary report on 47 cases. Neurosurg Focus. 2006;20(3):E5.
18. Kandziora F, Schleicher P, Scholz M, Pflugmacher R, Eindorf T, Haas NP, et al. Biomechanical testing of the lumbar facet interference screw. Spine. 2005;30(2):E34–9.
19. Mahar A, Kim C, Oka R, Odell T, Perry A, Mirkovic S, et al. Biomechanical comparison of a novel percutaneous transfacet device and a traditional posterior system for single level fusion. J Spinal Disord Tech. 2006;19(8):591–4.
20. Best NM, Sasso RC. Efficacy of translaminar facet screw fixation in circumferential interbody fusions as compared to pedicle screw fixation. J Spinal Disord Tech. 2006;19(2):98–103.
21. Boucher HH. A method of spinal fusion. J Bone Joint Surg Br. 1959;41-B(2):248–59.
22. Mitchell SM, Hsu WK. Lumbar pedicle cortical bone trajectory screw: indications and surgical technique. Contemporary Spine Surgery. 2016;17(1):1–5.
23. Neal MT, Rodriguez A, Branch CL Jr. Cortical bone trajectory pedicle screw fixation mast technique. In: Landriel F, Vecchi E, editors. Frontiers in Neurosurgery. Sharjah: Bentham Science Publishers; 2016. p. 327–34.
24. Dabbous B, Brown D, Tsitlakidis A, Arzoglou V. Clinical outcomes during the learning curve of MIDline lumbar fusion (MIDLF®) using the cortical bone trajectory. Acta Neurochir. 2016;158(7):1413–20.
25. Wang JC, Haid RW Jr, Miller JS, Robinson JC. Comparison of CD HORIZON SPIRE spinous process plate stabilization and pedicle screw fixation after anterior lumbar interbody fusion. J Neurosurg Spine. 2006;4(2):132–6.
26. Wang JC, Spenciner D, Robinson JC. SPIRE spinous process stabilization plate: biomechanical evaluation of a novel technology: invited submission from the joint section meeting on disorders of the spine …. J Neurosurg Spine [Internet]. 2006. Available from: http://thejns.org/doi/abs/10.3171/spi.2006.4.2.160.
27. Karahalios DG, Kaibara T, Porter RW, Kakarla UK, Reyes PM, Baaj AA, et al. Biomechanics of a lumbar interspinous anchor with anterior lumbar interbody fusion. J Neurosurg Spine. 2010;12(4):372–80.
28. Kaibara T, Karahalios DG, Porter RW, Kakarla UK, Reyes PM, Choi SK, et al. Biomechanics of a lumbar interspinous anchor with transforaminal lumbar interbody fixation. World Neurosurg. 2010;73(5):572–7.
29. Lopez AJ, Scheer JK, Dahdaleh NS, Patel AA, Smith ZA. Lumbar spinous process fixation and fusion: a systematic review and critical analysis of an emerging spinal technology. Clin Spine Surg [Internet]. 2016. doi:10.1097/BSD.0000000000000411.
30. Street J, DiPaola CP, Dvorak MF, Fisher CG, Dea N. Comparison of Wiltse muscle splitting approach to midline for fusion of the lumbar spine. Spine J. 2012;12(9):S156.
31. Anand N, Bray R Jr. P145. Comparison of traditional midline approach versus muscle splitting Paraspinal approach for posterior non-fusion stabilization of the lumbar spine – an analysis of functional outcome. Spine J. 2006;6(5):153S.
32. Kim DH, Tantorski M, Shaw J, Martha J, Li L, Shanti N, et al. Occult spinous process fractures associated with interspinous process spacers. Spine. 2011;36(16):E1080–5.
33. Tuschel A, Chavanne A, Eder C, Meissl M, Becker P, Ogon M. Implant survival analysis and failure modes of the X-stop interspinous distraction device. Spine. 2013;38(21):1826–31.
34. Barbagallo G, Olindo G, Corbino L. Analysis of complications in patients treated with the x-stop interspinous process decompression system: proposal for a novel …. Neurosurgery [Internet]. 2009. Available from: http://journals.lww.com/neurosurgery/Abstract/2009/07000/Analysis_of_Complications_in_Patients_Treated_With.23.aspx.
35. Verhoof OJ, Bron JL, Wapstra FH, van Royen BJ. High failure rate of the interspinous distraction device (X-stop) for the treatment of lumbar spinal stenosis caused by degenerative spondylolisthesis. Eur Spine J. 2008;17(2):188–92.
36. Bowers C, Amini A, Dailey AT, Schmidt MH. Dynamic interspinous process stabilization: review of complications associated with the X-stop device. Neurosurg Focus. 2010;28(6):E8.

37. Epstein NE. A review of interspinous fusion devices: high complication, reoperation rates, and costs with poor outcomes. Surg Neurol Int. 2012;3:7.
38. Vokshoor A, Khurana S, Wilson D, Filsinger P. Clinical and radiographic outcomes after spinous process fixation and posterior fusion in an elderly cohort. Surg Technol Int. 2014;25:271–6.
39. Schulte LM, O'Brien JR, Matteini LE, Yu WD. Change in sagittal balance with placement of an interspinous spacer. Spine. 2011;36(20):E1302–5.
40. Kim HJ, Bak KH, Chun HJ, Oh SJ. Posterior interspinous fusion device for one-level fusion in degenerative lumbar spine disease: comparison with pedicle screw fixation-preliminary report of at .... Journal of Korean [Internet]. 2012. Available from: http://synapse.koreamed.org/search.php?where=aview&id=10.3340/jkns.2012.52.4.359&code=0032JKNS&vmode=FULL.
41. Fidler MW. Spinal fusion: a combined anterior and supplementary interspinous technique. Eur Spine J. 1997;6(3):214–8.
42. Deyo RA, Ciol MA, Cherkin DC, Loeser JD, Bigos SJ. Lumbar spinal fusion. A cohort study of complications, reoperations, and resource use in the Medicare population. Spine. 1993;18(11):1463–70.
43. Deyo RA, Mirza SK, Martin BI, Kreuter W, Goodman DC, Jarvik JG. Trends, major medical complications, and charges associated with surgery for lumbar spinal stenosis in older adults. JAMA. 2010;303(13):1259–65.
44. Martin BI, Mirza SK, Comstock BA, Gray DT, Kreuter W, Deyo RA. Are lumbar spine reoperation rates falling with greater use of fusion surgery and new surgical technology? Spine. 2007;32(19):2119–26.
45. Modhia U, Takemoto S, Braid-Forbes MJ, Weber M, Berven SH. Readmission rates after decompression surgery in patients with lumbar spinal stenosis among Medicare beneficiaries. Spine. 2013;38(7):591–6.
46. Weinstein JN, Tosteson TD, Lurie JD, Tosteson A, Blood E, Herkowitz H, et al. Surgical versus nonoperative treatment for lumbar spinal stenosis four-year results of the spine patient outcomes research trial. Spine. 2010;35(14):1329–38.
47. Kleinstück FS, Grob D, Lattig F, Bartanusz V, Porchet F, Jeszenszky D, et al. The influence of preoperative back pain on the outcome of lumbar decompression surgery. Spine. 2009;34(11):1198–203.
48. Kumar N, Shah SM, Ng YH, Pannierselvam VK, Dasde S, Shen L. Role of coflex as an adjunct to decompression for symptomatic lumbar spinal stenosis. Asian Spine J. 2014;8(2):161–9.
49. Davis R, Auerbach JD, Bae H, Errico TJ. Can low-grade spondylolisthesis be effectively treated by either coflex interlaminar stabilization or laminectomy and posterior spinal fusion? Two-year clinical and .... J Neurosurg Spine [Internet]. 2013. Available from: http://thejns.org/doi/abs/10.3171/2013.4.spine12636.
50. Davis RJ, Errico TJ, Bae H, Auerbach JD. Decompression and Coflex interlaminar stabilization compared with decompression and instrumented spinal fusion for spinal stenosis and low-grade degenerative .... Spine [Internet]. 2013. Available from: http://journals.lww.com/spinejournal/Abstract/2013/08150/Decompression_and_Coflex_Interlaminar.2.aspx.
51. Bae HW, Davis RJ, Lauryssen C, Leary S, Maislin G, Musacchio MJ Jr. Three-year follow-up of the Prospective, randomized, controlled trial of Coflex Interlaminar stabilization vs instrumented fusion in patients with lumbar stenosis. Neurosurgery. 2016;79(2):169–81.
52. Bae HW, Lauryssen C, Maislin G, Leary S, Musacchio MJ Jr. Therapeutic sustainability and durability of coflex interlaminar stabilization after decompression for lumbar spinal stenosis: a four year assessment. Int J Spine Surg. 2015;9:15.
53. Musacchio MJ, Lauryssen C, Davis RJ, Bae HW, Peloza JH, Guyer RD, et al. Evaluation of decompression and Interlaminar stabilization compared with decompression and fusion for the treatment of lumbar spinal stenosis: 5-year follow-up of a Prospective, randomized. Controlled Trial Int J Spine Surg. 2016;10:6.
54. Patel VV, Whang PG, Haley TR, Bradley WD. Superion interspinous process spacer for intermittent neurogenic claudication secondary to moderate lumbar spinal stenosis: two-year results from a randomized .... Spine [Internet]. 2015. Available from: http://journals.lww.com/spinejournal/Abstract/2015/03010/Superion_Interspinous_Process_Spacer_for.2.aspx.
55. Patel VV, Whang PG, Haley TR, Bradley WD, Nunley PD, Miller LE, et al. Two-year clinical outcomes of a multicenter randomized controlled trial comparing two interspinous spacers for treatment of moderate lumbar spinal stenosis. BMC Musculoskelet Disord. 2014;15:221.

The Minimally Invasive Retroperitoneal Transpsoas Approach

26

Jacob Januszewski and Juan S. Uribe

Introduction

Minimally invasive retroperitoneal transpsoas approach or lateral interbody fusion (MIS LIF) was first introduced by Luiz Pimenta in 2001. It is a safe and effective alternative to anterior or posterior approaches for lumbar fusion such as anterior lumbar interbody fusion (ALIF), posterior lumbar interbody fusion (PLIF), or transforaminal lumbar interbody fusion (TLIF) procedures [1, 2]. Advantages include indirect neurological decompression with less tissue trauma, minimal blood loss, shorter operation times, fewer wound issues, placement of a larger cage, and early patient mobilization [3–6]. In addition, normal stabilizing ligaments are not sacrificed as compared to other interbody techniques.

MIS LIF was an adaptation of an endoscopic lateral transpsoas approach to lumbar fusion as described by Bergey et al. [7]. The authors have found that the endoscopic lateral transpsoas approach to the lumbar spine was a safe method to fuse the lumbar vertebrae, which allowed for exposure of the lumbar spine without mobilization of the great vessels or sympathetic plexus. The endoscopic approach led to the development of several systems from various manufacturers that allow for an MIS lateral retroperitoneal transpsoas approach under direct visualization.

Clinical applications of the retroperitoneal transpsoas MIS LIF include a wide range of spinal conditions including trauma, adult degenerative scoliosis, degenerative disc disease, spondylosis with instability, lumbar stenosis, spondylolisthesis, tumor, and adjacent segment failure. Research on MIS LIF is very active and clinical outcomes appear to be promising. However, success of this technique relies heavily on careful patient positioning, gentle retroperitoneal dissection, meticulous psoas splitting with directional EMG monitoring, and short retraction time.

Anatomic Considerations

The lateral approach is increasingly becoming popular among minimally invasive spine surgeons but as a relatively new procedure may still be unfamiliar to many trained traditionally in the open technique. Because of this, a review of key anatomic structures encountered with the lateral approach is paramount. In the order encountered, the muscles include the external oblique, the internal oblique, and the transversus abdominis muscle. Once the retroperitoneal space is entered,

J. Januszewski, DO (✉) • J.S. Uribe, MD
Department of Neurosurgery, Barrow Neurological Institute, Phoenix, AZ, USA
e-mail: Januszewski@health.usf.edu; juribe@health.usf.edu

L.T. Holly, P.A. Anderson (eds.), *Essentials of Spinal Stabilization*,
DOI 10.1007/978-3-319-59713-3_26

the quadratus lumborum and psoas muscle are then encountered. The details of blunt dissection, as opposed to electrocautery, are discussed later, but careful attention must be paid in order to avoid injuring a traversing lumbar plexus nerve, which could lead to postoperative deficits.

Psoas Muscle

The psoas major (or psoas) muscle is the key muscle traversed with blunt dissection during the MIS LIF approach. The psoas muscle is a long muscle that originates from the anterolateral aspect of the lumbar vertebral bodies, transverse processes, and their intervening disc spaces [8–11]. It is comprised of superficial and deep parts with the lumbar plexus lying between them. The psoas muscle descends anterolaterally, deep to the inguinal ligament, where it is joined by the iliacus muscle and together they insert into the lesser trochanter of the femur. Together they are referred to as iliopsoas muscle. As it progresses inferiorly from approximately the L1 level, the diameter of the psoas muscle steadily increases as it is contributed to by insertions at each subsequent level. The psoas major muscle receives innervations from the second to fourth lumbar spinal nerves as tiny intrinsic branches off the femoral nerve. The main action of the psoas muscle is hip flexion. In approximately 50% of the population, there is a smaller accompanying muscle lying on its ventromedial surface known as the psoas minor. It originates from the anterolateral surface of the twelfth thoracic and first lumbar vertebrae and the intervertebral disc between them. The psoas minor muscle ends in a long flat tendon that inserts into the superior ramus of the pubis. A branch of the first or second lumbar spinal nerve innervates it, and its action is to assist in upward rotation of the hip.

The Lumbar Plexus

The lumbar plexus is found within the substance of the psoas muscle. It is a part of the lumbosacral plexus, and it is made of the primary ventral rami of the first four lumbar nerves and a contribution of the subcostal nerve (T12), the last thoracic nerve. Multiple motor and sensory nerves are given off. The major motor branches consist of the femoral (L2–4) and obturator (L2–4) nerves. The major cutaneous, sensory branches consist of the iliohypogastric (L1), ilioinguinal (L1), genitofemoral (L1–2), lateral femoral cutaneous (L2–3), and anterior femoral cutaneous (L2–4) nerves. Most nerves are mixed motor and sensory. The intrinsic psoas nerves are the only purely motor nerves, and the lateral femoral cutaneous nerve is the only purely sensory nerve.

Motor Nerves

The femoral nerve is a mixed motor and sensory nerve that arises from the lateral border of the psoas muscle. It has two divisions, anterior and posterior. The anterior division gives off the anterior cutaneous nerve and muscular branches. It gives motor innervation to the pectineus and sartorius muscles. The posterior division gives off the saphenous nerve (sensory) and muscular branches. It gives motor innervation to the quadriceps femoris which is composed of the rectus femoris, vastus lateralis, vastus medialis, and vastus intermedius.

The obturator nerve is a mixed motor and sensory nerve that arises from the medial border of the psoas muscle. It innervates the adductor muscles of the lower extremity. These include the external obturator, adductor longus, adductor brevis, adductor magnus, gracilis, and the pectineus (inconstant) muscles. It does not innervate the obturator internus. It also supplies the sensory innervation of the skin of the medial aspect of the proximal thigh.

Sensory Nerves

The ilioinguinal nerve innervates the skin at the base of the penis and upper scrotum in males and the skin of the mons pubis and labia majora in females.

The iliohypogastric nerve consists of two branches that innervate the skin of the lower abdominal wall. The lateral cutaneous branch innervates the skin of the gluteal region. Of note, this nerve can also be injured when harvesting an anterior iliac crest bone graft. The anterior cutaneous branch innervates the hypogastric or lower abdominal region.

The genitofemoral nerve consists of two branches, the genital and femoral branches. The genital branch innervates the cremaster muscle and scrotal skin in males and the skin of the mons pubis and labia majora in females. The femoral branch innervates the skin over the femoral triangle. This nerve is distinct from the other sensory nerves in that it does not follow a lateral trajectory to the site of innervation but rather emerges on the anterior surface of the psoas and descends on the ventral surface.

The lateral femoral cutaneous nerve innervates the lateral aspect of the thigh. It consists of an anterior and a posterior branch. The anterior branch innervates the skin of the anterior and lateral surfaces of the thigh, as far as the knee. The posterior branch innervates the lateral and posterior surfaces of the thigh, from the level of the greater trochanter to the middle of the thigh.

The anterior femoral cutaneous nerve innervates the anterior and medial aspect of the thigh.

Subcostal Nerve

The most cranial nerve that contributes to the lumbar plexus is the subcostal nerve. It originates from the twelfth spinal nerve (T12) root and accompanies the subcostal vessels along the inferior border of the 12th rib. It passes behind the lateral arcuate ligament and kidney and travels anterior to the upper part of the quadratus lumborum. The subcostal nerve then perforates the aponeurosis of the origin of the transversus abdominis muscle and travels between the transversus abdominis and internal oblique muscles in a medial and inferior course. A lateral cutaneous branch pierces the internal and external obliques before reaching the costal angle. The subcostal nerve continues its course within the abdominal wall medially until it reaches the edge of the rectus abdominis where it perforates to give rise to the anterior cutaneous branches. It supplies the muscles of the anterior abdominal wall, especially the external oblique, and provides sensation to the anterior gluteal skin. Irritation or injury to this nerve, the potential for which may exist when treating the upper lumbar levels with lateral transpsoas interbody fusion, may result in abdominal wall paresis and pseudohernia [12]. It also occasionally communicates with the iliohypogastric nerve to give off a branch to the pyramidalis muscle.

Furcal Nerve

The furcal (meaning forked) nerve is an independent nerve with its own ventral and dorsal rootlets. It most commonly arises at the L4 level followed by L3 level as the second most common location, but it can be present at any lumbar level except for L1. It generally follows the L4 nerve in parallel through the neural foramina and is located superior and ventral to it extraforaminally. It forks and gives off branches to the obturator nerve, the femoral nerve, and the lumbosacral trunk serving as a link between lumbar and sacral plexus (Fig. 26.1). Compression of this nerve is responsible for atypical presentation of sciatica/radicular symptoms or for double nerve root contribution in unilateral radiculopathy [13]. Clinical presentation may differ from radiographic imaging on the CT myelogram or MRI. Sensory distribution may not exactly follow dermatomal patterns corresponding to the appropriate level of disc herniation. Because of its location, it can be easily injured during lateral transpsoas approaches.

Safe Zones

Early anatomic work related to the retroperitoneal transpsoas approach by Moro et al. helped to establish a safe zone to prevent nerve injuries when operating [14]. Specifically, they found that

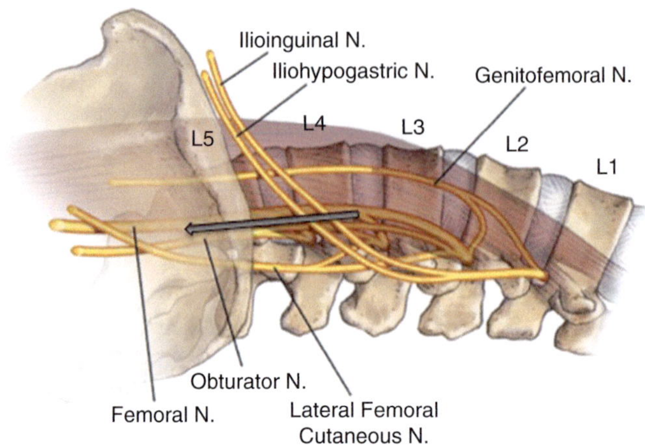

Fig. 26.1 Lumbar plexus and furcal nerve trajectory. The *black arrow* is located approximately where the furcal nerve serves as a link between the lumbar and the sacral plexus. Note the close location to the femoral nerve and the dorsal L4/L5 disc space

it was safe to traverse the psoas muscle at levels L4/L5 and above, with the exception of the genitofemoral nerve, which is at risk between L3 and L4.

Further studies described the course of the plexus and found that the plexus lies within the substance of the psoas muscle between the junction of the transverse process and vertebral body, while exiting along the medial edge of the psoas distally [15]. It is most dorsally positioned at the posterior endplate of L1/L2 with a general trend of progressive ventral migration down to the level of L4/L5. When a ratio of the distance from the posterior vertebral body wall to the total disc space length was calculated, it was found that there was a 0, 0.11, 0.18, and 0.28 ratio for L1/L2, L2/L3, L3/L4, and L4/L5, respectively. These findings suggest that an overly posterior placement of the dilator and/or retractor can lead to nerve injuries, especially at L4/L5 where the ventral migration is nearly one third of the disc space from the posterior vertebral body wall.

A cadaveric study by Uribe et al. established four different zones and described safe working zones for MIS LIF (Fig. 26.2) [10]. The four zones represent different quartiles of the vertebral body with zone I representing the most anterior and zone IV representing the most posterior quartile. The lumbar plexus, along with nerve roots, lies within the substance of the psoas muscle and dorsal to zone IV. The genitofemoral nerve was the only structure found to be ventral to zone III, starting at L2/L3 and progressing caudally to L3/L4 and L4/L5.

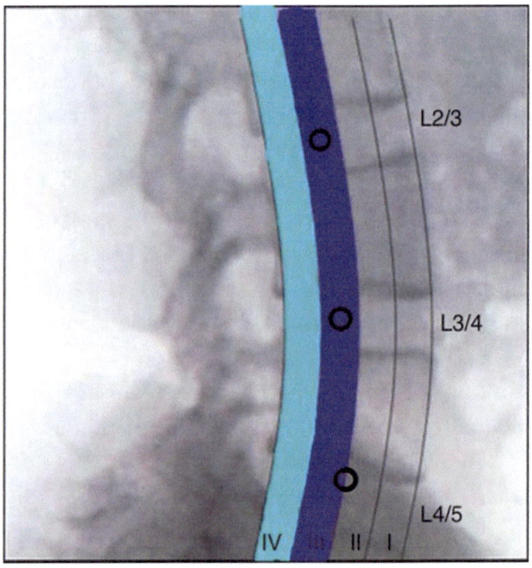

Fig. 26.2 Safe anatomical zones for MIS LIF. There are four quartiles, I–IV, from anterior to posterior. The *open circles* indicate a "safe zone" for placement of the retractor and for subsequent exposure. From L1/L2 to L3/L4, the posterior third is generally safe. At L4/L5, placement at the midpoint between zone II and III is generally safe since this will decrease the risk of injuring the femoral nerve

It was determined that the safe anatomical zones to avoid nerve injury from L1/L2 to L3/L4 are the midpoint of zone III (posterior third of the disc space) and the safe zone for L4/L5 is at the zone II/III junction (mid disc space). The genitofemoral nerve is at risk in zone II at L2/L3 and in zone I at L3/L4 and L4/L5. The ilioinguinal, iliohypogastric, and lateral femoral cutaneous nerves in the retroperitoneal space are also at risk since they travel obliquely, inferiorly, and anteriorly to reach the iliac crest and the abdominal wall outside of the psoas in the retroperitoneal space.

The femoral nerve is formed from the branches of the L2, L3, and L4 roots found deep in the substance of the psoas muscle and descending in a gradual posterior to anterior fashion. Thus, the most likely location of femoral nerve injury is at the L4/L5 disc space if the retractor is placed too close to zone 3 or zone 4. Injury to the femoral nerve in this location would result in a stereotypical hip flexion weakness, paralysis of knee extension, loss of patellar reflex, and sensory dermal zone III deficit [16]. It is important, however, to recognize a true neurological weakness from pain limited hip flexion weakness secondary to psoas "bruising" from muscle splitting during placement of the dilators and the retractor. Pain limited hip flexion weakness is isolated to only hip flexion and resolves within several hours to up to 72 h postoperatively.

There is a chance of lumbar plexus injury even in the early stages of the operation while obtaining access to the retroperitoneal space. Four nerves, the subcostal, iliohypogastric, ilioinguinal, and lateral femoral cutaneous nerves, are at risk of injury at this stage of the operation.

In addition to nerve injury, visceral and vascular structures should also be considered. The importance of meticulous preoperative planning was illustrated by Regev et al. in their morphometric study looking at the relationship of vascular structures as it relates to MIS LIF, where they found that the safe corridor for performing a discectomy and intervertebral cage placement progressively narrows from L1/L2 to L4/L5 [17]. In the presence of scoliosis, these corridors can potentially be further narrowed. One should also keep in mind that the kidneys are in the retroperitoneal space.

Indications for the Lateral Approach

Patient Selection

Once the decision to proceed with surgical intervention is made, selecting the most appropriate and patient-specific approach can be challenging. There are no "one-size-fits-all" constructs for spinal deformity. Stand-alone lateral constructs should be reserved for patients who are at an unacceptably high operative risk for alternative conventional or MIS combined approaches and free of any spinal instability. Patients with unrelievable pain, progressive degenerative scoliosis with advanced age, significant comorbidity, and significant anesthetic risk should be considered for less invasive interventions. Additionally, to consider a lateral stand-alone construct, the radiographic evaluation should exhibit reasonable coronal/sagittal balance. Finally, all patients being considered for stand-alone constructs should be evaluated for the degree of osteopenia or osteoporosis. The vertebral body endplate strength is greatly dependent on bone density [18]. Patients with osteoporosis or advanced osteopenia should not be considered for stand-alone lateral fusion but rather nonoperative treatment options or a limited decompression. However, this can lead to a deformity progression and worsening of symptoms.

Surgical considerations for MIS LIF include trauma, adult degenerative scoliosis, degenerative disc disease, spondylosis with instability, lumbar stenosis, spondylolisthesis, and adjacent segment failure. Early outcome studies have demonstrated that MIS LIF is associated with shorter operative times, minimal blood loss, few complications, minimal hospital length of stay, and quicker recovery [19, 20]. Long-term outcomes are generally favorable, with maintained improvements in patient-reported pain and function scores, as well as radiographic parameters, including high rates of fusion.

Degenerative Spine Disease and Deformity

Minimally invasive surgery was initially developed to address morbidity associated with traditional, open spinal surgery. As the field has continued to progress, MIS techniques are increasingly used to treat degenerative spine disease and deformity. The factors that make MIS LIF appealing as mentioned above are an obvious draw to surgeons trying to minimize the morbidity associated with traditional open deformity correction [21, 22]. Using this technique, coronal Cobb angles can be improved [19, 23–25]. Since a positive global sagittal imbalance is most closely linked to a decreased quality of life, health status outcomes, and function, the effect of MIS on sagittal Cobb angles, lumbar lordosis, and pelvic tilt has been increasingly investigated [26]. Sagittal imbalance can lead to higher energy requirements to stand and ambulate, leading to early fatigue, intolerance to standing, and walking with compensation through other joints.

The clinical outcomes data regarding deformity correction are encouraging thus far, with improved radiographic parameters as well as improved clinical results with a lower complication profile compared to traditional open approaches [27]. Up until recently, the main critique of MIS surgery in deformity correction was its inability to improve sagittal balance to the same extent as traditional open techniques. Sagittal imbalance was traditionally managed with posterior shortening osteotomies (such as Smith-Petersen osteotomies, pedicle subtraction osteotomies, extended pedicle subtraction osteotomies, or vertebral column resection), which have been reported to have at least 40% complication rate in adjacent segment degeneration (ASD) [28, 29]. Anterior longitudinal ligament release (ALR) via the MIS lateral transpsoas approach with placement of a hyperlordotic cage has been shown to have similar radiographic and clinical outcomes as the open techniques, while at the same time minimizing complications such as blood loss and CSF leak [30].

The learning curve for successful ALR release is fairly steep however, and cadaveric dissection as well as review of safe zones of the lateral approach prior to attempting this procedure in vivo is strongly recommended. Injury to the great vessels is a major complication of this procedure and could result in a fatal outcome if attention to detail is not observed. After performing the discectomy with careful attention to endplate preparation, a slight curved custom retractor is gently passed along the anterior edge of the anterior longitudinal ligament (ALL) and positioned between the large vessels/sympathetic plexus and the ventral aspect of the disc. Dissection is performed dorsal to the great vessels in order to avoid a catastrophic complication at this point. It is also important to avoid mistaking the sympathetic plexus for the lateral edge of the ALL at this step, which would lead to sectioning of the plexus. The ligament is sectioned in a sequential fashion using a ligament blade on a long handle, easing the curved retractor across to the contralateral side of the disc space. Upon complete release of the ALL, there is immediate mobilization and "fish-mouthing" of the adjacent vertebral body endplates. An appropriate hyperlordotic poly-ether-ether-ketone (PEEK) cage is selected at this point and packed with allograft. The cage is anchored to the adjacent vertebral body with one or two screws to prevent ventral migration into the peritoneal cavity. ALR is further backed with posteriorly placed pedicle screws for total stability.

Segmental lordosis after ALR is increased by 14° when posterior elements (spinous process, facets, posterior ligaments) are left intact. A facetectomy increases this lordosis to 21–27°. In order to match the cage lordosis, a spinous process can be resected along with bilateral facetectomy, achieving segmental lordosis of up to 30° with 30° cages. The intradiscal angle can be as great as 20–24° when posterior elements are resected and a 30° cage is used [31]. These results are equivalent to open pedicle subtraction osteotomies.

As the role of MIS LIF in spinal deformity correction is further clarified through further research, it is important to keep in mind that the ultimate end goal should still be to reestablish spinopelvic harmony or the proportional relationships of one regional parameter to another as it relates to global spinopelvic alignment, as spinopelvic harmony has been directly linked to a satisfactory postsurgical outcome as assessed by health-related quality-of-life instruments [26, 32]. Four basic radiographic targets to aim for in order to achieve spinopelvic harmony include: (1) sagittal vertical axis of <50 mm or T1-SI < 0°, (2) pelvic tilt of <20°, (3) coronal Cobb angle <10, and (4) lumbar lordosis-pelvic incidence mismatch ±9° [26, 30]. Attention to these four goals serves as the foundation for individual, patient-specific, spinopelvic realignment in the sagittal and coronal plane. Even partial improvements of these parameters may translate to better clinical outcomes. Addition of ALR to the MIS armamentarium allows for greater deformity correction and different MIS surgical approaches to be used depending on deformity severity (Fig. 26.9).

Adjacent segment failure is a common complication encountered in patients with prior lumbar fusions. Operations to address this issue can often involve further posterior muscle dissection and revision of the existing instrumentation, all while negotiating through previous scar tissue, leading to risks of infection and cerebrospinal fluid (CSF) leaks. The MIS LIF is an option for treatment of adjacent segment failure. A virgin corridor is traversed with placement of an intervertebral cage which avoids some of the pitfalls of reoperations as mentioned above. In addition, if further internal fixation is desired, then a lateral plate could be placed without much additional difficulty. Literature regarding the specific use of the lateral retroperitoneal transpsoas approach is lacking for adjacent segment failure revision surgeries, but studies related to revision surgery using this approach for revision and explantation of lumbar total disc replacements have shown its effectiveness and low rate of complications by avoiding a previous, scarred approach [33–35].

Trauma

Another area with increased interest for the use of the lateral approach is in traumatic thoracolumbar fractures. Traumatic burst fractures commonly occur in the thoracic and lumbar spine, with many occurring at the thoracolumbar junction. The decision of whether or not to treat with nonoperative management with external orthoses or bedrest versus surgical decompression, instrumentation, and fusion is beyond the scope of this discussion. However, when surgical treatment is planned for situations where there is instability with neurologic deficit, a minimally invasive retroperitoneal transpsoas approach is an option.

In a study by Smith et al. with a follow-up of 2 years, patients treated with lateral corpectomies with supplemental instrumentation were found to have very favorable operating room times, estimated blood loss, and hospital length of stay [36]. None of the patients required reoperations, and there was a significant improvement in the neurologic status based on the American Spinal Injury Association categorization, with none experiencing a neurologic decline.

Preoperative Considerations

The preoperative planning is critical to ensure that the patient is a good surgical candidate. Preoperative magnetic resonance imaging (MRI) is evaluated to ensure that abdominal blood vessels will not hinder access to the desired disc space. The psoas muscle must also be carefully examined on the axial MRI as it will elucidate the best side for the approach. Psoas muscle that starts to migrate ventrally on the disc space at L4/L5 as it normally would at L5/S1 is called a transitional psoas. The muscle bulk (and therefore the lumbar plexus) of a transitional psoas is more ventral and therefore puts the femoral nerve at risk during retraction. It is not recommended to attempt MIS LIF when a transitional psoas is encountered on a preoperative MRI. A preoperative AP radiograph is also evaluated as it also may determine which side will provide the best access to the desired level, especially at L4/L5, in relation to the iliac crest (Fig. 26.3).

Surgical Technique

The technique of the retroperitoneal transpsoas MIS LIF by our team has evolved with time and experience. Significant changes were made to our technique in 2010, and these changes have been the standard method we currently use for every patient. Specifically, the technique below refers to use of the transpsoas procedure with a special

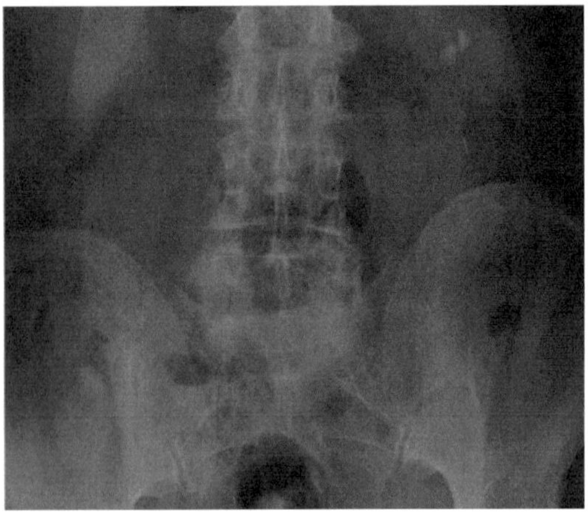

Fig. 26.3 AP radiograph of the lumbar spine. It is crucial to evaluate the clearance of the iliac crest (IC) preoperatively to determine positioning and operative feasibility

retractor system. In general, the main principles apply to any lateral access system; however, a significant difference that will not apply to other systems is the use of a directional, triggered EMG (t-EMG), which will be explained further in this discussion.

The patient is then placed in a true 90° lateral decubitus position with the optimal side facing up. If a scoliotic deformity is present, the patient is placed with the concave side facing up. The reasoning for this is that this usually provides better access to the L4/L5 disc space if that is an operative level. In addition, positioning the concave side up will allow for access to multiple levels through potentially fewer and smaller incisions.

At our institution, patients are placed on a Cmax® table (Steris, Mentor, OH), but any radiolucent operating table that allows for adjustment of flexion, extension, Trendelenburg/reverse Trendelenburg, as well as lateral tilting will suffice. The iliac crest is placed at the level of the table break where table flexion occurs. The legs are flexed maximally at the knee and hip to relax tension on the psoas muscle. A roll is placed beneath the axilla to prevent brachial plexus injury, and a roll is placed under the iliac crest to promote flexion at the iliac crest for improved access to the L4/L5 level.

Intraoperative fluoroscopy is then used to position the patient in such a manner that a symmetric AP image with the pedicles equidistant from the spinous processes is achieved. It is essential that these images be as accurate and symmetric as possible to prevent inadvertently dissecting too far anteriorly or posteriorly. Caution should be exercised if a prior laminectomy exists over the desired level and spinous processes cannot be visualized.

Once properly positioned, the patient is taped and secured into place at the iliac crest and chest. The ipsilateral hip and leg are then taped to pull the iliac crest inferiorly and then secured to the table to prevent the patient from moving during surgery. The patient is then taped and secured into position (Fig. 26.4).

A repeat AP fluoroscopic image is taken to ensure that good images are still obtainable, and the bed is tilted slightly if correction of the image is needed. To ensure exact position of the cage, it is imperative that the AP image show perfectly parallel endplates of the level being operated on and the spinous processes are exactly in the midline and equal distance from each pedicle (Fig. 26.5). The relationship of the ipsilateral iliac crest and the lowest level to be approached are then evaluated. The angle of the disc space in relation to the iliac crest should ideally allow direct access to the disc space. At this point, the table is flexed at the level of the iliac crest just enough to give access to the disc space. If there is good access to the disc space without needing to flex the table, then it is advisable to perform the operation without flexing the table. Too much flexion of the table can put tension on the lumbar plexus and potentially cause nerve injury, so the table is flexed as minimally as possible while still achieving good access to the disc space.

Lateral fluoroscopy is then used, and the patient's position is modified with Trendelenburg or reverse Trendelenburg to obtain images clearly displaying the endplates, posterior vertebral cortex, and pedicle, as well as to evaluate the relationship of the disc space of interest to the ipsilateral iliac crest. A guide wire or cross can be placed on the patient's skin to localize the plane of the disc space (Fig. 26.6). Palpation of this area confirms that the iliac crest will not obstruct the pathway to the disc space.

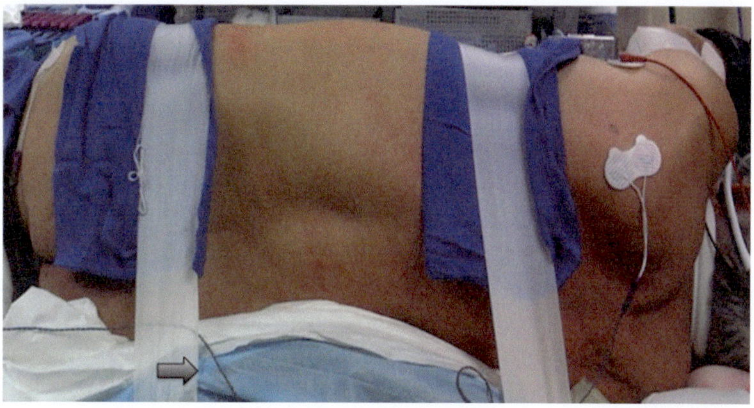

Fig. 26.4 Lateral decubitus positioning for MIS LIF. The patient is placed on an adjustable operative table and secured with silk tape. There is a bend in the table (*arrow*) to allow for better access during surgery

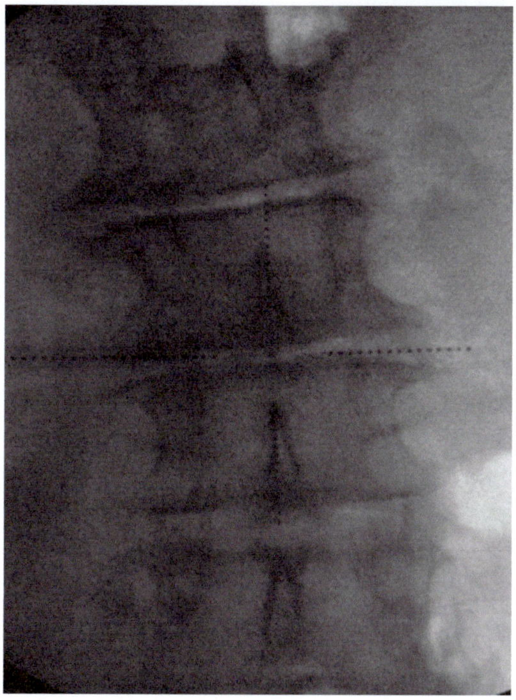

Fig. 26.5 Fluoroscopic AP image through the L3/L4 disc space. Note the center of the fluoro image must be at the operative level. The superior and inferior endplates are perfectly lined up and parallel to each other. Spinous processes are in the exact midline

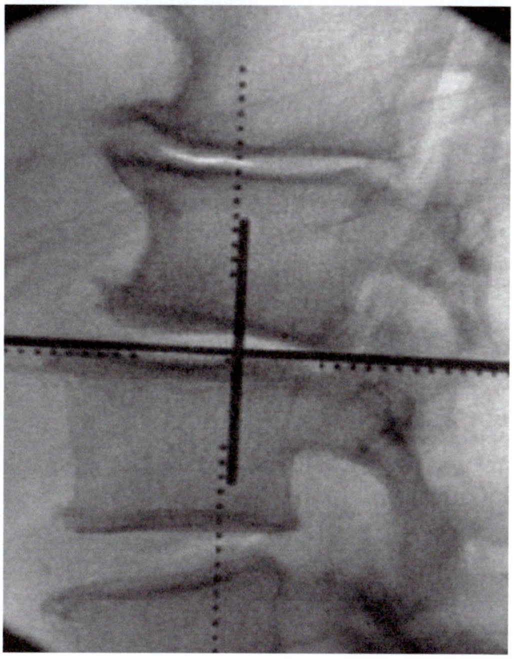

Fig. 26.6 Lateral fluoroscopic image showing a cross at the perfect docking location for the retractor. Note that both superior and inferior endplates are exactly parallel to each other. Iliac crest is completely out of the way

An AP image for final positioning is then obtained to ensure there has not been any significant patient movement and that the images are still acceptable. Lateral fluoroscopy is then obtained to mark the disc space transversely and the posterior third of the disc space vertically. An exception is at L4/L5, where the vertical mark is at the middle of the disc space based on the anatomic safe zones [10]. If one level is to be approached, a single transverse incision approximately 5 cm is used. If more than one level is to be approached, a single vertical incision or multiple transverse incisions are used depending on the length of the incisions and cosmetic concerns.

Operative Procedure

The area is then prepped and draped. An incision is made with a #10 scalpel blade to the subcutaneous fat. A second posterior incision is routinely not used as originally described as this route of access may cause injury to the ilioinguinal or iliohypogastric nerves [1]. A self-retaining retractor is used to help dissect subcutaneous fat transversely along the original incision line with monopolar cautery until fascia is encountered. A transverse incision is then made in the fascia with monopolar cautery in line with the disc space. If multiple disc spaces are being approached, separate fascial incisions are made for each disc space to help stabilize the retractor.

Once the fascial incision over the area of interest is completed and muscle is encountered, two tonsil hemostats are used to dissect through the muscle gently in the plane of the disc space through as small an access as possible. Great care is taken to ensure the dissection is performed in line with the original skin marking for the posterior third of the disc space (or at the mid-vertebral body at L4/L5) and that the dissection is not carried too anteriorly (to avoid bowel injury) or too posteriorly (to avoid nerve injury). The external oblique, internal oblique, and transversus abdominis muscles are identified and dissected until the transversalis fascia and retroperitoneal space are encountered.

Once in the retroperitoneal space, the quadratus lumborum can be palpated posterolaterally. The quadratus can then be followed medially until the transverse process of the vertebra of interest can be palpated. Then, proceeding further medially, the psoas muscle can be palpated.

The first dilator can be inserted at this point, guided with the surgeon's finger anterior to the dilator to avoid peritoneal injury. The dilator is docked gently on the psoas without traversing the psoas. Lateral fluoroscopy is obtained to check the position of the dilator to ensure it is in correct position (posterior third of the disc space, except for L4/L5, in which case the middle of the disc space is the target), and the dilator position is adjusted as needed. The dilator is stimulated for triggered EMG (t-EMG), and the dilator is then rotated 360° to check for activity. Typically, anything ≥11 mA indicates a safe distance from any surrounding neural structure (Table 26.1). The dilator is then advanced through the psoas muscle until it is docked onto the spine. The dilator is again stimulated for t-EMG and rotated 360° to check for activity. Lateral fluoroscopy is again obtained to confirm position of the dilator in relation to the disc space as mentioned previously. If the stimulation of the initial dilator did not reveal any concerning t-EMG responses, a guide wire is placed through the dilator into the disc space to maintain position. Sequential dilators are then used to dilate the psoas muscle and stimulated in a similar fashion as described above. Once the final dilator is placed, it is stimulated for t-EMG and the responses are analyzed.

Sharp decreases in the threshold are not uncommon at this portion of the procedure. In fact, finding these sharp decreases is advantageous. The position of the femoral nerve can be estimated by the location of the sharp decreases in the t-EMG threshold. Ideally, the sharp decreases will be present when stimulating with the dilator posteriorly and increased thresholds present anteriorly; thus the femoral nerve can be estimated to be posterior to the dilators. This orientation will allow placement and opening of the retractor with minimal risk of nerve injury. If decreased thresholds are obtained anteriorly, the guide wire and dilators are removed and advanced more anteriorly so that the dilators are positioned anterior to the femoral nerve. The sequence for dilator and guide wire placement described above is again carried out.

Once the t-EMG stimulation with the final dilator verifies decreased threshold responses posteriorly and increased threshold responses anteriorly, the retractor is then placed over the dilators with the retractor blades oriented superiorly, inferiorly, and posteriorly. Downward pressure is applied to the retractor during the procedure until final placement of the shim blade to prevent psoas muscle fibers from creeping into the surgical field. The retractor is locked into place with the articulating arm while maintaining downward pressure. The dilators are removed

Table 26.1 Triggered EMG interpretation

Numeric reading (mA)	Color displayed	Interpretation
≥11	Green	Acceptable
5–10	Yellow	Caution
<5	Red	Alert

while the guide wire is kept in place. A light source is attached to the inferior blade and used in conjunction with suction to visualize the disc space while maintaining downward pressure on the retractor. The surgeon should be able to visualize "red and white" indicating the disc space and small amounts of psoas muscle fibers that have crept into the surgical field. If only "red" is seen, then too much psoas muscle is in the field to visualize the disc space. If only "white" is seen, it is possible that the fascia of the psoas muscle has not been penetrated which may cause the retractor to shift if it slides off the fascia during the procedure. The field is also inspected for evidence of nerves that could be injured with the procedure. Anything suspicious for being a nerve is stimulated with manual t-EMG to check for EMG activity. Sensory nerves will not stimulate with t-EMG, so a high index of suspicion must be maintained for an object that does not trigger EMG response.

Once it is confirmed that disc space is visualized and no nerves are present in the surgical field, lateral fluoroscopy is obtained to check the position of the retractor in relation to the disc space. The shim blade is engaged into the posterior blade of the retractor but not deep into the disc space yet.

The retractor, while maintaining downward pressure, is adjusted into the correct position. The articulating arm is loosened, and moving the retractor in relation to the guide wire helps to maintain proper orientation. Once proper position is attained on lateral fluoroscopy, AP fluoroscopy is used to show the superior-inferior relation of the retractor blades to the disc space. The shim blade is advanced into the disc space and malleted into position firmly with image guidance using AP fluoroscopy. The articulating arm is then attached and tightened to lock the retractor into position. Lateral fluoroscopy is then used to "look down" the posterior blade to ensure the proper pathway for the remainder of the procedure. The manual t-EMG stimulator is used to stimulate the entire surgical field and behind the posterior blade. Decreased thresholds elicited posterior to the posterior blade are expected and desired to ensure the working area is anterior to the femoral nerve, which is now protected by the posterior blade. The guide wire is then removed.

Once the retractor is in final position, the rest of the procedure must be performed as efficiently and quickly as possible to reduce the duration of retraction of the lumbar plexus. It is recommended that the total retraction time be under 20 min for a typical interbody placement and under 30 min for anterior column reconstruction where anterior longitudinal ligament is cut. The retractor is now opened minimally to just allow discectomy and placement of the interbody graft.

The position of the anterior longitudinal ligament can be estimated by visualizing the slope of the anterior vertebral body. The procedure should remain as posterior as possible to this slope to prevent unwanted rupture of the anterior longitudinal ligament. A wide rectangular annulotomy is then made with an annulotomy knife. A pituitary rongeur is then used to remove disc material. A curved Cobb elevator is placed into the disc space with the handle vertically oriented and malleted under AP fluoroscopy guidance until the contralateral annulus is broken. This procedure is repeated with the curve of the Cobb elevator in the opposite orientation. The box cutter disc shaver is then placed in the disc space. Vertical orientation of the handle is confirmed, and the box cutter is malleted flush with the posterior blade under AP fluoroscopy guidance to ensure the endplates are not violated. Once the box cutter is removed, AP fluoroscopy is used to confirm position of the shim blade in the disc space which can be malleted into the disc space to guarantee the stability of the retractor. Again, a pituitary rongeur is used to remove disc material.

Depending on the preoperative radiograph, a straight or lordotic poly-ether-ether-ketone (PEEK) or titanium interbody cage can be filled with a variety of biologics. Our practice now is to pack approximately 5 cc of cadaveric cancellous bone mixed with mesenchymal stem cells (Osteocel Plus®, NuVasive, San Diego, CA) into the cage. A graft retainment device is used to retain the packed contents in the cage, and the cage is then placed in the disc space with a vertical orientation of the handle. It is malleted into position until the medial radiographic marker is in line with the spinous process. The graft is then released and the retainment device removed. The surgical field is inspected for any graft that may have become dislodged during placement and removed if identified. The area is inspected for any bleeding, and bipolar cautery can be used to obtain hemostasis. The articulating arm is loosened and the retractor is then closed. The retractor is removed slowly from the surgical field while inspecting for any bleeding.

Once the retractor is completely removed, final AP and lateral fluoroscopic images are obtained to ensure proper placement of the graft. The operating table is then leveled to assist with incision closure. Fascia is closed with interrupted 0 Vicryl sutures and the subcutaneous layer closed with 3-0 Vicryl sutures. The skin is approximated with 4-0 subcuticular Monocryl suture and dressed with Dermabond®.

Biomechanics

PEEK Interbody Cage

An essential component of MIS LIF is the placement of a large interbody cage. Traditionally, implant materials have been autograft or allograft bone, but issues with fracture, migration, and pseudoarthrosis led to the development of synthetic cages such as titanium, carbon fiber, and PEEK [37]. Among the synthetic cage materials, PEEK has been found to be favorable since it shares the same modulus of elasticity as bone [38–40]. In addition, it is also nonabsorbable, elicits a minimal cellular response, and allows for a clear, unobstructed view of new bone formation during follow-up exams [41, 42]. The placement of a large interbody cage, as accommodated by the lateral approach, is an advantage of MIS LIF. Large-diameter solid implants are less likely to subside compared to small-diameter cages, possibly related to a more efficient transfer of force to the endplate [43–45].

Lateral Plate

The MIS LIF can be supplemented with a lateral plate that spans across the disc space (Fig. 26.7). The titanium plate has a rostral and caudal screw hole, and it can come in varying lengths (there is also a four-screw hole type which we do not routinely use due to its larger profile). It is seated on two bicortical titanium screws that are placed across the width of the vertebral body parallel to the adjacent endplate.

Biomechanical comparisons between the lateral plate and stand-alone, unilateral pedicle screw, and bilateral pedicle screw constructs have demonstrated its increased rigidity compared to a stand-alone construct to promote arthrodesis [46, 47]. The greatest biomechanical advantage of a lateral plate is its very favorable range of motion restriction in lateral bending with only bilateral pedicle screws offering slightly more rigidity. In total, however, lateral plates still fall short of unilateral and bilateral pedicle screws, which are much more rigid overall.

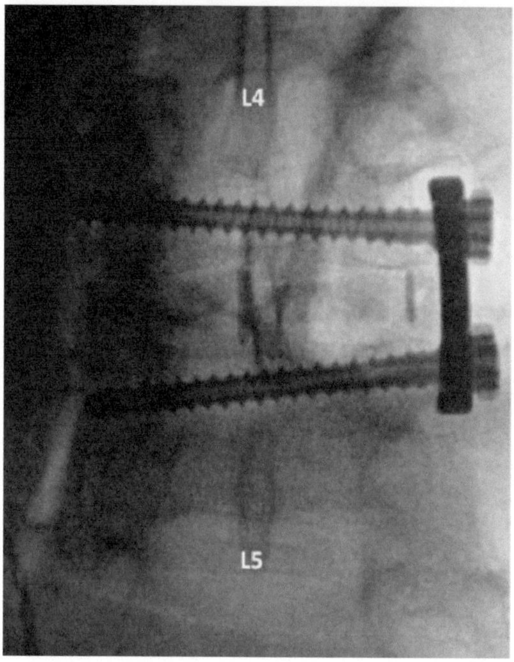

Fig. 26.7 Lateral plate fixation. This is an AP fluoroscopic view. Note the intervertebral cage placed spanning the entire vertebral body. The screws are placed near the subchondral bone

Good candidates for a lateral plate supplementation should be free of any significant gross instability, since bilateral pedicle screws would be best in that situation. For similar reasons, lateral plates may not be optimal for deformity correction. In addition, bilateral pedicle screws are preferred in this situation because lateral plates only stabilize one segment at a time compared to multilevel stabilization offered by a unified, multilevel, pedicle screw and rod construct.

Illustrative Case

History A 67-year-old retired man presented with chronic back pain for several years with intermittent radiating symptoms in his right leg. Walking and standing aggravated the symptoms. Pain appeared to be progressively worse throughout the day. Only sitting slightly relieved the pain. He had tried nonoperative therapies including physical therapy, epidural steroid injections, trigger point injections, and pain management for at least 1 year without success. He denied any weakness or urinary incontinence.

Physical Examination His focused neurological examination was benign. He had full Sunderland grade 5/5 strength in bilateral hip flexion/extension, hip abduction/adduction, knee extension, extensor hallucis longus, and dorsi and plantarflexion. His sensory dermal zones (SDZ), as previously described, were fully examined next [16]. He had full sensation in subcostal, iliohypogastric, ilioinguinal, and genitofemoral (SDZ zone 1) nerve distribution, full sensation in lateral femoral cutaneous (SDZ zone 2) nerve distribution, full sensation in femoral and saphenous (SDZ zone 3) nerve distribution, and full sensation in the obturator (SDZ zone 4) nerve distribution. His patellar and Achilles reflexes were 2+ bilaterally. His muscle tone was normal in both lower extremities.

Imaging Preoperatively, full scoliosis computed radiography (CR) 15 × 34 inch radiographs were ordered including lateral bending films. Lumbar and thoracic CT and MRI were also reviewed. Preoperative parameters were severe dextroscoliosis with a coronal Cobb angle of 54°, CSVL 2 cm, SVA 12 cm, PT 40°, PI 71°, and LL 35° (Fig. 26.8). His dual x-ray absorptiometry scan was within normal limits. MRI was reviewed to rule out a transitional psoas or abnormal segmental vessels that could potentiate unexpected bleeding. CT was used to evaluate degenerated disc spaces and pedicle size.

Treatment He underwent lateral interbody fusion from T12 to L5 and an ALIF at L5/S1. He had two levels of ALL release at L2/L3 and L3/L4. This was followed by a second stage posterior percutaneous pedicle screw fixation from T10 to the sacrum (Fig. 26.9).

Outcome Postoperative imaging demonstrated a coronal Cobb angle of 29°, CSVL 6 cm, SVA 5 cm, PT 26°, PI 71°, and LL 74°. His PI-LL mismatch was corrected from 36° preoperatively to 4° postoperatively. His postoperative course was uneventful, and at the 12-month follow-up evaluation, his

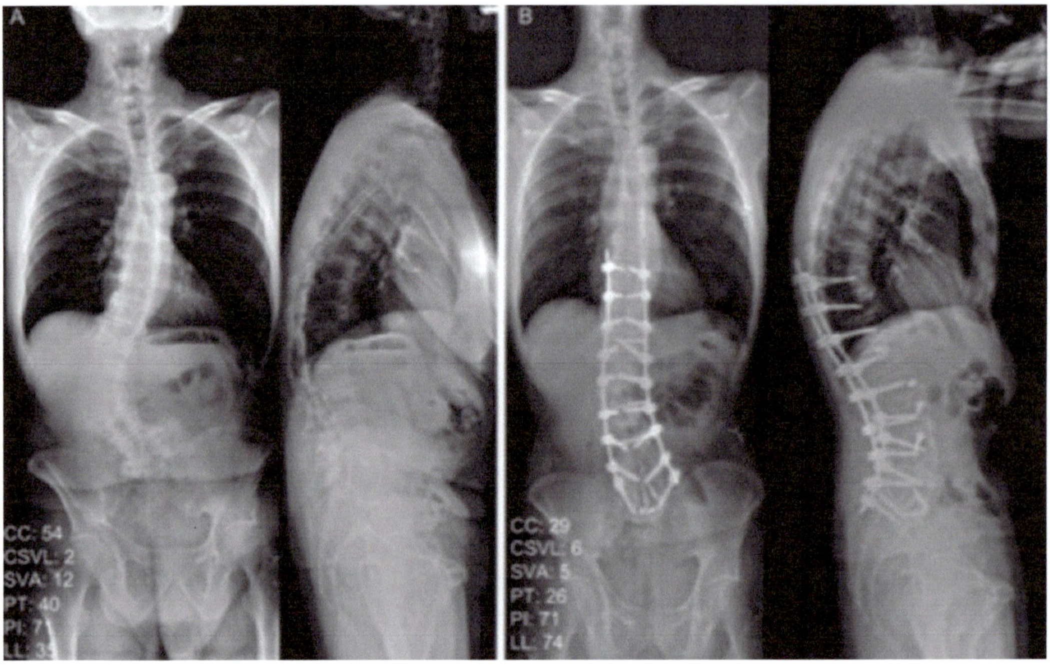

Fig. 26.8 Anteroposterior and lateral 36-inch radiographs of a patient with severe deformity (red group). (**a**) Preoperative images of a patient with severe deformity. (**b**) Postoperative images obtained after T10/S1 open posterior arthrodesis with osteotomies and with MIS lateral interbody fusion with multilevel ALL release showing restoration of disc height and improvement in spinopelvic parameters

	Mild	Moderate	Severe
CCA	<30°	>30	>30
PI-LL	<20°	20° - 30°	>30°
SVA	<5cm	5 - 9cm	>10cm
PT	<25°	25 - 30°	>30°
Anterior arthrodesis	Limited MIS-LIF consider standalone if PT<20°	MIS-LIF to neutral vertebrae + ALLR	MIS-LIF to neutral vertebrae ± ALLR
Posterior fixation	Percutaneous fixation	Percutaneous fixation ± facetectomy	Pedicle screw fixation + osteotomy

Fig. 26.9 Radiographic subgroups and related surgical intervention. *Green* represents radiographic parameters of patients with mild symptomatic deformity and spinopelvic compensation. *Yellow* represents radiographic parameters of patients with moderate symptomatic deformity and associated lack of sagittal balance with SVA between 5 and 9 cm. *Red* represents radiographic parameters of patients with severe symptomatic deformity and associated lack of sagittal balance with SVA greater than 10 cm despite maximal pelvic tilt (PT). *ALLR* ALL release, *CCA* coronal Cobb angle, *LIF* lateral interbody fusion

VAS score had improved from 76 to 53, and his ODI score had improved from 50 to 30. There was no sign of interbody graft subsidence or proximal junctional kyphosis (PJK).

Technical Pearls

- Minimally invasive lateral interbody fusion through a retroperitoneal transpsoas approach has gained popularity as an alternative to anterior, posterior, and transforaminal interbody fusion.
- The approach is straightforward but detail oriented with a need to systematically evaluate surgical corridor anatomy and follow stepwise surgical steps in order for it to be reproducible and predictable
- Beyond thorough understanding of surgical anatomy, proper patient selection and preoperative workup is paramount for success of the procedure. Detailed history and physical examinations cannot be underscored enough as the most important part of the patient care. Not all surgical pathologies can benefit from the MIS LIF approach. For example, pathology at L5/S1 usually cannot be reached with this technique due to the anatomical constraint of the iliac crest. Indirect decompression may not be adequate for patients with severe spinal canal or foraminal stenosis. Previous abdominal surgery might preclude a safe retroperitoneal approach.
- Preoperative imaging used for surgical planning and surgical approach includes plain radiographs including flexion and extension views along with standing scoliosis and lateral bending films, CT, MRI, and/or dual energy x-ray absorptiometry (DEXA) scan depending on patients' age and smoking status.
- The relative anatomic position of pathologic levels with respect to the ribs and iliac crest should be assessed on radiographs. A high iliac crest on one side may prompt the surgeon to change the surgical approach to the contralateral side. In patients with coronal deformity requiring multilevel surgery, the preferred approach is from the concave side, as this will allow easier access to multiple levels through fewer and smaller incisions. For L1/L2 and L2/L3 levels, mobilization of the rib may be necessary. If not possible, resection of a rib may be required for access, although it is usually not necessary.
- MRI provides detailed anatomy of great vessels, psoas morphology, and the lumbar plexus within. Position of other retroperitoneal structures like location of the colon can also be appreciated. Ventral migration of the psoas muscle (aka transitional psoas or "Mickey mouse ear" psoas) similarly contains a ventrally located lumbar plexus and may pose an increased risk of femoral injury. Lateral approach should be avoided in such cases.
- When the goal of surgery is indirect decompression, several MRI and CT findings can be helpful to evaluate for success of lateral transpsoas approach. Severely decreased disc height, vacuum disc phenomenon on CT, and T2 hyperintensity in facets on axial MRI signify relatively mobile disc/facet joints and are associated with restoration of postoperative spinal alignment.
- Stepwise and detailed surgical technique is described earlier in the chapter; however several important technical pearls should be underscored. For patient positioning, in general, the side without prior surgery and/or the side with more favorable psoas and lumbar plexus anatomy is chosen. If a scoliotic deformity is present, the patient is placed with the concave side facing up.
- The patient should be positioned in a true 90° lateral decubitus position with the top of the crest just inferior to the table break. Legs should be bent at a 45° angle.
- Care must be taken to ensure the patient is not rotated. Each level operated on has to be in perfect AP and lateral projection. Intraoperative fluoroscope is used to ensure the pedicles are equidistant from the spinous

processes in the AP projection with clearly displayed endplates in both AP and lateral projections.

- Once the skin is incised and fascia opened, two tonsil hemostats are used to dissect through muscle gently in the plane of the disc space through as small an access as possible. The transversalis fascia is also breached and opened with the tonsils.
- Finger dissection should be used to separate retroperitoneal fat and adhesions off the belly of the psoas muscle. The psoas muscle and the transverse process should be palpated.
- It is important that the first dilator is positioned in the bulkiest part of the psoas so as not to have too much psoas anteriorly or posteriorly. Once lateral fluoroscopy confirms dilator position in the center of the disc space, it is advanced until it is docked onto the lateral border of the disc.
- The triggered EMG stimulation is delivered posteriorly, superiorly, anteriorly, and inferiorly to locate the position of the femoral nerve. The distance to the nerve is determined by the energy required to elicit a discrete threshold response, with lower thresholds indicating closer proximity. Femoral nerve should always be located behind (posterior to) the dilator. If t-EMG stimulation has no directionality or is somehow questionable, the first dilator should be repositioned more anteriorly.
- Total retraction time from the time retractor is placed to the time retractor is removed should be under 20 min for a routine case or under 30 min when ACR is performed.

Complications and Strategies for Avoidance

The importance of meticulous attention to detail throughout the perioperative period is crucial as it may reduce the risk of complications [48]. Complications can arise from the result of inadequate preoperative planning. For instance, neurovascular structures may be in the way of the intended exposure, which may preclude a safe corridor for operating. Transitional psoas may bring the femoral nerve closer to the docking site of the retractor causing irreversible damage from nerve root retraction or direct damage. Close attention to preoperative MRIs can help avoid this from happening. In addition, positioning mistakes leading to placement of the nonoptimal side positioned up can make access to the L4/L5 disc space, for example, much more difficult, leading to an increased risk of postoperative motor or sensory deficits.

Numbness, Paresthesia, and Weakness

The lateral retroperitoneal transpsoas approach is a technique that can be challenging since it is a nontraditional approach for many spine surgeons who are more accustomed to a posterior approach. Because of this, it does have a learning curve, and the skill at which it is performed is very dependent on experience with the regional anatomy and with the approach itself. Small changes in technique with this approach can result in dramatic changes in patient outcome due to the proximity of the lumbar plexus. Real-time EMG monitoring is critical to minimize the chance of motor nerve injury [5]. However, sensory nerves cannot be monitored, thus leaving them susceptible to iatrogenic injury if there is not a thorough understanding of the regional anatomy.

The current literature is inconsistent with its reporting of postoperative “thigh” symptoms which could range from numbness, paresthesias, dysesthesias, or weakness. While injury can occur at any level of approach, the rate of femoral nerve injury is highest at the L4/L5 segment. Reports of motor weakness from femoral nerve injury have varied ranging from 3.4% to 23.7% [48–50]. The rate of paresthesias following MIS LIF can range from 0.7% to 30% [7, 48, 49, 51], and numbness has been reported in 8.3–42.4% [19, 49, 50]. The specific nerve distribution may vary as well, but commonly affected nerves are the genitofemoral, lateral femoral cutaneous, and anterior femoral cutaneous nerves. On the postoperative examination, it is important to distinguish between the different dermatomes of these sensory nerves and not to simply report that a patient has thigh pain or numbness.

It is important to realize that most motor and sensory deficits are transient and do recover with 50% recovery at 90 days and 90% recovery at 1 year [49]. This may be a result of the muscles and nerves recovering from manipulation, inflammation, and irritation during the operation. As a result, it is advisable to fully disclose to patients preoperatively that there is a chance of motor or sensory deficit following the operation, but that the vast majority of cases are transient in nature.

As previously stated in this chapter, it is also important to recognize a true neurological weakness from pain limited hip flexion weakness secondary to psoas "bruising" from muscle splitting during placement of the dilators and the retractor. Pain limited hip flexion weakness is isolated to only hip flexion and resolves within several hours to up to 72 h postoperatively.

Abdominal Wall Paresis and Bowel Perforation

Abdominal wall paresis, also referred to as a "pseudohernia," has been identified as a potential complication of the MIS lateral approach [12]. The mechanism is attributed to iatrogenic nerve injury during the initial dissection of the abdominal wall. Consequences include denervation, paresis, and bulging of the anterior abdominal wall. Associated signs and symptoms include swelling, pain, hyperesthesia, or other sensory abnormalities. If suspected, it is important to rule out a true abdominal hernia in these instances. In many cases, spontaneous recovery can occur.

Ogilvie's syndrome (OS), delayed ileus from colonic pseudo-obstruction potentially leading to bowel perforation, is another possible complication [52]. While etiology is not completely understood, it must be differentiated from acute bowel perforation that may be a result of retractor insertion. OS is clinically identified as diminished gastric motility that does not resolve on its own in a matter of several days. Radiographically it is characterized by dilatation of cecum greater than 9 cm and lack of mechanical obstruction on abdominal CT. If not diagnosed and treated early, it may lead to colon rupture with an associated mortality rate between 50% and 71% [53–55]. Initial management may consist of bowel rest, indirect decompression with a nasogastric tube, a rectal tube, and in some cases colonoscopy for direct decompression. Best evidence for medical therapy is available for neostigmine, an acetylcholinesterase inhibitor [54, 56]. However, side effects may include bradycardia and hypotension requiring patient monitoring in an intensive care setting or at least a telemetry floor.

Hardware-Related Complications

There have been few reports of complications attributed to the hardware implanted such as the interbody cage or lateral plate. Dua et al. reported a 15% rate of hardware-related complications based on a series of 13 patients [57]. These cases consisted of two atraumatic coronal plane fractures at L4/L5 in the first 6 weeks of the postoperative period.

Our own series has demonstrated a hardware-related complication rate of 5.9% in a series of 101 consecutive cases [58]. The complications included three hardware failures and three vertebral body fractures. All cases were atraumatic. All cases presented with recurrent back pain except one which was identified incidentally. All hardware failures involved a dislodged lateral plate and lock nut(s). The mechanism is unclear but may involve a cage subsidence with a fixed angle screw, resulting in the screws cutting through the vertebral bodies in a coronal plane, a stress riser in the area of stress concentration, a violation of the endplate during preparation or screw insertion, or a malplacement of the hardware lock nuts [57–59].

Subsidence

As with any technique used for lumbar fusion, subsidence of the cage can occur at one or both endplates. The subsequent progressive deformity and compression of neural elements can lead to a loss of indirect decompression with reduced chance of successful fusion and possible reoperation [43, 60].

In a study that included 140 patients and 238 levels fused in the lumbar spine with a mean follow-up of 9.6 months, we have recently found subsidence to be present in 14.3% of the cases and in 8.8% of the total levels fused [61]. Only 2.1% of the patients had symptomatic subsidence, however. Subsidence appears to correlate with construct length.

The most important finding, however, was that there was a 14.1% rate of subsidence with smaller 18 mm cages versus only 1.9% with larger 22 mm cages, leading to the conclusion that the largest interbody cage should be used whenever feasible.

Rhabdomyolysis

Rhabdomyolysis is a rare, but known, complication of spinal surgery. In severe cases, acute renal failure may result. The first cases of rhabdomyolysis and acute renal failure have recently been reported following MIS LIF [62]. This potential complication should be suspected in appropriate cases especially in morbidly obese patients and in procedures associated with prolonged operative times.

Contralateral Psoas Hematoma

The contralateral psoas hematoma is a rare complication suspected to occur from segmental vessel injury during contralateral annulus release [63]. Careful preoperative MRI review should be performed to assess the contralateral disc space for segmental vessels that may be torn during annulotomy. Contralateral leg weakness can occur as a result of this complication as a large hematoma can compress the femoral nerve causing symptomatic neuropraxia. Prompt evacuation is recommended to prevent permanent injury to the lumbar plexus.

Lateral Incisional Hernia

Lateral incisional hernia came to attention very recently and has been often missed or overlooked. It likely happens due to inadequate closure of the fascia and herniation of the peritoneum through a fascial defect. Occasionally loops of small bowel may also herniate through the defect along with the peritoneum; however, incarceration or strangulation of the bowel has never been reported. It is recommended that careful attention be paid to fascial closure at the end of the procedure. Unbreaking of the operative table may be of benefit in a good closure as it releases some of the tension and makes approximation of the fascia easier.

Conclusions and Key Points

The retroperitoneal transpsoas approach is a safe and effective alternative to traditional posterior, open lumbar techniques. It can be utilized for a variety of clinical applications including trauma, adult degenerative scoliosis, degenerative disc disease, spondylosis with instability, lumbar stenosis, spondylolisthesis, and adjacent segment failure. As with most minimally invasive techniques, there is a learning curve to be overcome in order to minimize the risk of iatrogenic nerve injuries. An integral aspect of this curve is to always be aware of the regional anatomy encountered. It is important to stay within the "safe zones" when performing an MIS LIF, staying in the posterior third of the disc space at L1/L2, L2/L3, and L3/L4 or at the midpoint of the vertebral body at L4/L5. The patient should be positioned in a true 90° lateral decubitus position with the top of the crest just inferior to the table break. Care must be taken to ensure the patient is not rotated. Directional t-EMG can help guide the surgeon and alert of any critical distances from surrounding motor nerves. Even with this, transient sensory deficits and, on occasion, weakness may occur. It is important to discuss this potential with surgical candidates preoperatively.

References

1. Ozgur BM, Aryan HE, Pimenta L, Taylor WR. Extreme Lateral Interbody Fusion (XLIF): a novel surgical technique for anterior lumbar interbody fusion. Spine J Off J North Am Spine Soc. 2006;6:435–43.
2. Pimenta L. Lateral endoscopic transpsoas retroperitoneal approach for lumbar spine surgery. In: VIII Brazilian Spine Society meeting. Belo Horizo te, Minas Gerais; 2001.
3. Benglis DM, Elhammady MS, Levi AD, Vanni S. Minimally invasive anterolateral approaches for the treatment of back pain and adult degenerative deformity. Neurosurgery. 2008;63:191–6.
4. Eck JC, Hodges S, Humphreys SC. Minimally invasive lumbar spinal fusion. J Am Acad Orthop Surg. 2007;15:321–9.
5. Uribe JS, Vale FL, Dakwar E. Electromyographic monitoring and its anatomical implications in minimally invasive spine surgery. Spine. 2010;35:S368–74.
6. Wang MY, Anderson DG, Poelstra KA, Ludwig SC. Minimally invasive posterior fixation. Neurosurgery. 2008;63:197–203.
7. Bergey DL, Villavicencio AT, Goldstein T, Regan JJ. Endoscopic lateral transpsoas approach to the lumbar spine. Spine. 2004;29:1681–8.
8. Dakwar E, Vale FL, Uribe JS. Trajectory of the main sensory and motor branches of the lumbar plexus outside the psoas muscle related to the lateral retroperitoneal transpsoas approach. J Neurosurg Spine. 2011;14:290–5.
9. Netter FH. Atlas of human anatomy. Philadelphia: Saunders Elsevier; 2006.
10. Uribe JS, Arredondo N, Dakwar E, Vale FL. Defining the safe working zones using the minimally invasive lateral retroperitoneal transpsoas approach: an anatomical study. J Neurosurg Spine. 2010;13:260–6.
11. Gray H, Williams PL, Bannister LH. Gray's anatomy: the anatomical basis of medicine and surgery. New York: Churchill Livingstone; 1995.
12. Dakwar E, Le TV, Baaj AA, Le AX, Smith WD, Akbarnia BA, Uribe JS. Abdominal wall paresis as a complication of minimally invasive lateral transpsoas interbody fusion. Neurosurg Focus. 2011;31:E18.
13. Harshavardhana NS, Dabke HV. The furcal nerve revisited. Orthop Rev. 2014;6:5428.
14. Moro T, Kikuchi S, Konno S, Yaginuma H. An anatomic study of the lumbar plexus with respect to retroperitoneal endoscopic surgery. Spine. 2003;28:423–8. discussion 427–428
15. Benglis DM, Vanni S, Levi AD. An anatomical study of the lumbosacral plexus as related to the minimally invasive transpsoas approach to the lumbar spine. J Neurosurg Spine. 2009;10:139–44.
16. Ahmadian A, Deukmedjian AR, Abel N, Dakwar E, Uribe JS. Analysis of lumbar plexopathies and nerve injury after lateral retroperitoneal transpsoas approach: diagnostic standardization. J Neurosurg Spine. 2013;18:289–97.
17. Regev GJ, Chen L, Dhawan M, Lee YP, Garfin SR, Kim CW. Morphometric analysis of the ventral nerve roots and retroperitoneal vessels with respect to the minimally invasive lateral approach in normal and deformed spines. Spine. 2009;34:1330–5.
18. Oxland TR, Lund T. Biomechanics of stand-alone cages and cages in combination with posterior fixation: a literature review. Eur. Spine J Off Publ Eur Spine Soc Eur Spinal Deform Soc Eur Sect Cerv Spine Res Soc. 2000;9(Suppl 1):S95–101.
19. Dakwar E, Cardona RF, Smith DA, Uribe JS. Early outcomes and safety of the minimally invasive, lateral retroperitoneal transpsoas approach for adult degenerative scoliosis. Neurosurg Focus. 2010;28:E8.
20. Youssef JA, McAfee PC, Patty CA, Raley E, DeBauche S, Shucosky E, Chotikul L. Minimally invasive surgery: lateral approach interbody fusion: results and review. Spine. 2010;35:S302–11.
21. Carreon LY, Puno RM, Dimar JR 2nd, Glassman SD, Johnson JR. Perioperative complications of posterior lumbar decompression and arthrodesis in older adults. J Bone Joint Surg Am. 2003;85-A:2089–92.
22. Okuda S, Miyauchi A, Oda T, Haku T, Yamamoto T, Iwasaki M. Surgical complications of posterior lumbar interbody fusion with total facetectomy in 251 patients. J Neurosurg Spine. 2006;4:304–9.
23. Anand N, Rosemann R, Khalsa B, Baron EM. Mid-term to long-term clinical and functional outcomes of minimally invasive correction and fusion for adults with scoliosis. Neurosurg Focus. 2010;28:E6.
24. Tormenti MJ, Maserati MB, Bonfield CM, Okonkwo DO, Kanter AS. Complications and radiographic correction in adult scoliosis following combined transpsoas extreme lateral interbody fusion and posterior pedicle screw instrumentation. Neurosurg Focus. 2010;28:E7.
25. Wang MY, Mummaneni PV. Minimally invasive surgery for thoracolumbar spinal deformity: initial clinical experience with clinical and radiographic outcomes. Neurosurg Focus. 2010;28:E9.
26. Schwab F, Patel A, Ungar B, Farcy JP, Lafage V. Adult spinal deformity-postoperative standing imbalance: how much can you tolerate? An overview of key parameters in assessing alignment and planning corrective surgery. Spine. 2010;35:2224–31.
27. Mundis GM, Akbarnia BA, Phillips FM. Adult deformity correction through minimally invasive lateral approach techniques. Spine. 2010;35:S312–21.
28. Glassman SD, Hamill CL, Bridwell KH, Schwab FJ, Dimar JR, Lowe TG. The impact of perioperative complications on clinical outcome in adult deformity surgery. Spine. 2007;32:2764–70.
29. Yadla S, Maltenfort MG, Ratliff JK, Harrop JS. Adult scoliosis surgery outcomes: a systematic review. Neurosurg Focus. 2010;28:E3.
30. Deukmedjian AR, Dakwar E, Ahmadian A, Smith DA, Uribe JS. Early outcomes of minimally invasive anterior longitudinal ligament release for

correction of sagittal imbalance in patients with adult spinal deformity. TheScientificWorldJournal. 2012;2012:789698.
31. Uribe JS, Harris JE, Beckman JM, Turner AW, Mundis GM, Akbarnia BA. Finite element analysis of lordosis restoration with anterior longitudinal ligament release and lateral hyperlordotic cage placement. Eur. Spine J Off Publ Eur Spine Soc Eur Spinal Deform Soc Eur Sect Cerv Spine Res Soc. 2015;24(Suppl 3):420–6.
32. Lafage V, Schwab F, Vira S, Patel A, Ungar B, Farcy JP. Spino-pelvic parameters after surgery can be predicted: a preliminary formula and validation of standing alignment. Spine. 2011;36:1037–45.
33. Leary SP, Regan JJ, Lanman TH, Wagner WH. Revision and explantation strategies involving the CHARITE lumbar artificial disc replacement. Spine. 2007;32:1001–11.
34. Patel AA, Brodke DS, Pimenta L, Bono CM, Hilibrand AS, Harrop JS, Riew KD, Youssef JA, Vaccaro AR. Revision strategies in lumbar total disc arthroplasty. Spine. 2008;33:1276–83.
35. Wagner WH, Regan JJ, Leary SP, Lanman TH, Johnson JP, Rao RK, Cossman DV. Access strategies for revision or explantation of the Charite lumbar artificial disc replacement. J Vasc Surg. 2006;44:1266–72.
36. Smith WD, Dakwar E, Le TV, Christian G, Serrano S, Uribe JS. Minimally invasive surgery for traumatic spinal pathologies: a mini-open, lateral approach in the thoracic and lumbar spine. Spine. 2010;35:S338–46.
37. Yang JJ, Yu CH, Chang BS, Yeom JS, Lee JH, Lee CK. Subsidence and nonunion after anterior cervical interbody fusion using a stand-alone polyetheretherketone (PEEK) cage. Clin Orthop Surg. 2011;3:16–23.
38. Brantigan JW, Steffee AD. A carbon fiber implant to aid interbody lumbar fusion. Two-year clinical results in the first 26 patients. Spine. 1993;18:2106–7.
39. Cho DY, Lee WY, Sheu PC. Treatment of multilevel cervical fusion with cages. Surg Neurol. 2004;62:378–85. discussion 385–376
40. Matge G. Cervical cage fusion with 5 different implants: 250 cases. Acta Neurochir. 2002;144:539–49. discussion 550
41. Boakye M, Mummaneni PV, Garrett M, Rodts G, Haid R. Anterior cervical discectomy and fusion involving a polyetheretherketone spacer and bone morphogenetic protein. J Neurosurg Spine. 2005;2:521–5.
42. Vaidya R, Sethi A, Bartol S, Jacobson M, Coe C, Craig JG. Complications in the use of rhBMP-2 in PEEK cages for interbody spinal fusions. J Spinal Disord Tech. 2008;21:557–62.
43. Closkey RF, Parsons JR, Lee CK, Blacksin MF, Zimmerman MC. Mechanics of interbody spinal fusion. Analysis of critical bone graft area. Spine. 1993;18:1011–5.
44. Lowe TG, Hashim S, Wilson LA, O'Brien MF, Smith DA, Diekmann MJ, Trommeter J. A biomechanical study of regional endplate strength and cage morphology as it relates to structural interbody support. Spine. 2004;29:2389–94.
45. Pearcy MJ, Evans JH, O'Brien JP. The load bearing capacity of vertebral cancellous bone in interbody fusion of the lumbar spine. Eng Med. 1983;12:183–4.
46. Bess RS, Cornwall G, Vance R, Bachus KN, Brodke DS. Biomechanics of lateral arthrodesis. St. Louis: Quality Medical Publishing; 2008. p. 31–40.
47. Cappuccino A, Cornwall GB, Turner AW, Fogel GR, Duong HT, Kim KD, Brodke DS. Biomechanical analysis and review of lateral lumbar fusion constructs. Spine. 2010;35:S361–7.
48. Knight RQ, Schwaegler P, Hanscom D, Roh J. Direct lateral lumbar interbody fusion for degenerative conditions: early complication profile. J Spinal Disord Tech. 2009;22:34–7.
49. Cummock MD, Vanni S, Levi AD, Yu Y, Wang MY. An analysis of postoperative thigh symptoms after minimally invasive transpsoas lumbar interbody fusion. J Neurosurg Spine. 2011;15:11–8.
50. Pimenta L, Oliveira L, Schaffa T, Coutinho E, Marchi L. Lumbar total disc replacement from an extreme lateral approach: clinical experience with a minimum of 2 years' follow-up. J Neurosurg Spine. 2011;14:38–45.
51. Rodgers WB, Gerber EJ, Patterson J. Intraoperative and early postoperative complications in extreme lateral interbody fusion: an analysis of 600 cases. Spine. 2011;36:26–32.
52. Januszewski J, Keem SK, Smith W, Beckman JM, Kanter AS, Oskuian RJ, Taylor W, Uribe JS. The potentially fatal Ogilvie's syndrome in lateral transpsoas access surgery: a multi-institutional experience with 2930 patients. World Neurosurg 2016.
53. Maloney N, Vargas HD. Acute intestinal pseudo-obstruction (Ogilvie's syndrome). Clin Colon Rectal Surg. 2005;18:96–101.
54. Ponec RJ, Saunders MD, Kimmey MB. Neostigmine for the treatment of acute colonic pseudo-obstruction. N Engl J Med. 1999;341:137–41.
55. Vanek VW, Al-Salti M. Acute pseudo-obstruction of the colon (Ogilvie's syndrome). An analysis of 400 cases. Dis Colon Rectum. 1986;29:203–10.
56. Hooten KG, Oliveria SF, Larson SD, Pincus DW. Ogilvie's syndrome after pediatric spinal deformity surgery: successful treatment with neostigmine. J Neurosurg Pediatr. 2014;14:255–8.
57. Dua K, Kepler CK, Huang RC, Marchenko A. Vertebral body fracture after anterolateral instrumentation and interbody fusion in two osteoporotic patients. Spine J Off J North Am Spine Soc. 2010;10:e11–5.
58. Le TV, Smith DA, Greenberg MS, Dakwar E, Baaj AA, Uribe JS. Complications of lateral plating in the minimally invasive lateral transpsoas approach. J Neurosurg Spine. 2012;16:302–7.
59. Disch AC, Knop C, Schaser KD, Blauth M, Schmoelz W. Angular stable anterior plating following thoracolumbar corpectomy reveals superior segmental stabil-

ity compared to conventional polyaxial plate fixation. Spine. 2008;33:1429–37.
60. Kozak JA, Heilman AE, O'Brien JP. Anterior lumbar fusion options. Technique and graft materials. Clin Orthop Relat Res. 1994:45–51.
61. Le TV, Baaj AA, Dakwar E, Burkett CJ, Murray G, Smith DA, Uribe JS. Subsidence of polyetheretherketone intervertebral cages in minimally invasive lateral retroperitoneal transpsoas lumbar interbody fusion. Spine. 2012;37:1268–73.
62. Dakwar E, Rifkin SI, Volcan IJ, Goodrich JA, Uribe JS. Rhabdomyolysis and acute renal failure following minimally invasive spine surgery: report of 5 cases. J Neurosurg Spine. 2011;14:785–8.
63. Beckman JM, Vincent B, Park MS, Billys JB, Isaacs RE, Pimenta L, Uribe JS. Contralateral psoas hematoma after minimally invasive, lateral retroperitoneal transpsoas lumbar interbody fusion: a multicenter review of 3950 lumbar levels. J Neurosurg Spine. 2016:1–5.

Lumbar Disc Arthroplasty

27

Tyler Atkins, Domagoj Coric, James J. Yue, Benjamin J. Geddes, and Jason Toy

Introduction

Lumbar total disc replacement (L-TDR) is a motion-preserving treatment for patients with degenerative disc disease (DDD) and debilitating mechanical low back pain (LBP) refractory to nonsurgical management. L-TDR can be viewed as the latest evolution in the surgical treatment of DDD based on the logical progression of the pathophysiologic understanding of LBP. The goal of this chapter is to provide an overview of the topic of total disc replacement, with a particular focus on the operative technique utilized to insert these devices. Anecdotal pearls and pitfalls have also been included which should be helpful and educational for both the experienced and novice spine surgeon. As this technology becomes more widely accepted and utilized, it will be important for all spine surgeons to have at least a basic level of understanding of the procedure in order to appropriately educate patients on all available treatment modalities.

Low back pain is a significant challenge facing the modern healthcare system from an epidemiological, clinical, and economic standpoint. Approximately 80% of the population will have at least one episode of significant low back pain in their lives [1]. In a study by Carragee et al. in 2004, they found that low back pain cost the US healthcare system $50 billion a year and was the number one cause of disability in patients younger than 45 years old [2]. With the aging population, these numbers will likely continue to increase over time. Fortunately, the majority of pain remains minor and transient, often resolved over short periods of time with home management of rest, selected exercise, and over-the-counter analgesics prior to reaching medical attention. Even then, LBP is most often successfully managed by nonsurgical management including physical therapy, oral medications, or more invasive nonsurgical treatments such as epidural steroid injections [3].

As spinal imaging technologies have evolved and gained routine use in the evaluation of LBP, the list of potential pathological etiologies has grown. The identification of the degenerated disc on plain radiographs, computed tomography, and, most prominently, magnetic resonance imaging (MRI) in patients without other clear

T. Atkins • D. Coric
Carolina NeuroSurgery and Spine, Charlotte, NC, USA
e-mail: Domagoj.Coric@CNSA.com

J.J. Yue • B.J. Geddes • J. Toy (✉)
Department of Orthopedic Surgery, Yale University, 800 Howard Avenue, New Haven, CT 06519, USA
e-mail: james.yue@yale.edu; benjamin.geddes@yale.edu; jasontoy22@gmail.com

L.T. Holly, P.A. Anderson (eds.), *Essentials of Spinal Stabilization*, DOI 10.1007/978-3-319-59713-3_27

source of back pain has led to the concept of "discogenic back pain." Identification of degenerative disc disease on spinal imaging needs to be interpreted with caution as it has been shown that up to 30% of asymptomatic individuals have abnormal lumbar spine MRIs, with the majority of these revealing degenerative discs [4]. Even after careful diagnosis of discogenic back pain, the majority of such patients will not ultimately undergo surgical intervention, as most will still gain sufficient relief by conservative measures to avoid long-term disability and maintain a reasonable quality of life.

Discogenic back pain originates from the intervertebral discs and is defined by transverse low back pain that in some patients radiates to the sacroiliac region and may or may not be associated with lower extremity claudication and/or radicular symptoms. For those patients who fail a minimum of 6 months of nonsurgical therapy, surgery may be considered. Simple discectomy, indicated for neural decompression in treatment of radiculopathy and symptomatic spinal stenosis due to disc herniation, is not an effective treatment for primary discogenic back pain. Near-total removal of the disc and replacement with artificial materials (not necessarily with the goal of motion preservation) was utilized in early efforts to treat degenerative discs in the middle of the last century [5, 6]. Modern treatment strategies have focused primarily on arthrodesis of the motion segment to treat discogenic back pain that has failed appropriate nonsurgical therapy. This treatment strategy focuses on not only removal of the presumed pain generator (internal disc derangement with degenerative annulus) but also on stabilizing the motion segment (including both the disc and facet joints) preventing further painful degenerative change. With appropriate patient selection, lumbar arthrodesis has proven successful at decreasing pain and improving quality of life in select patients diagnosed with discogenic back pain [7, 8].

Lumbar arthrodesis is not without limitations however. Pseudarthrosis rates following lumbar fusion have decreased with the continued development of new instrumentation including more rigid constructs and interbody fusion techniques; however, the rate of this complication continues to be problematic and commonly leads to reoperation. Persistent back pain with or without pseudarthrosis, as well as reoperation rates, both at index and adjacent levels, has made the surgical treatment of DDD controversial and has triggered a larger public health debate about the effectiveness of fusion for treatment of LBP [9, 10]. Variable rates for adjacent segment pathology are reported in the literature depending on inconsistent use and definition by different authors of "adjacent segment degeneration," typically referring to a radiographic finding and "adjacent segment disease" which refers to the clinical symptoms requiring treatment of these changes. A systematic review by Harrop et al. reports a rate of adjacent segment disease of 14% across several studies including 1216 patients.[9]. In order to attempt to address these common sequelae, total disc replacements (TDR) were developed.

Modern L-TDR as an alternative to lumbar fusion for discogenic back pain began with the development of the Charite artificial disc in the 1980s and was subsequently followed by the ProDisc-L (Figs. 27.1a–c and 27.2a) [11, 12]. Numerous other artificial discs have been developed with an evolution of design and materials with the Activ-L device the latest to receive US FDA approval in 2015 and the M6-L gaining widespread usage in Europe (Fig. 27.2b). The primary theoretical advantage of L-TDR compared to fusion is the preservation of physiologic motion which may lead to less axial back pain as well as to decreased rates of adjacent segment disease and reoperation. Secondary advantages include potential shorter recovery times, as well as decreased local postoperative pain owing to the anterior retroperitoneal approach versus a more standard posterior fusion (this advantage of course is lost in comparison to anterior or lateral approaches to interbody fusion [10, 13, 14]). Two multicenter, randomized, controlled investigational device exemption trials in the United States of the Charite and ProDisc-L artificial disc vs lumbar fusion have demonstrated near-equivalent safety and preliminary efficacy in relief of back pain up to 2 years following surgery [15–17]. Furthermore, the theoretical advantage of motion

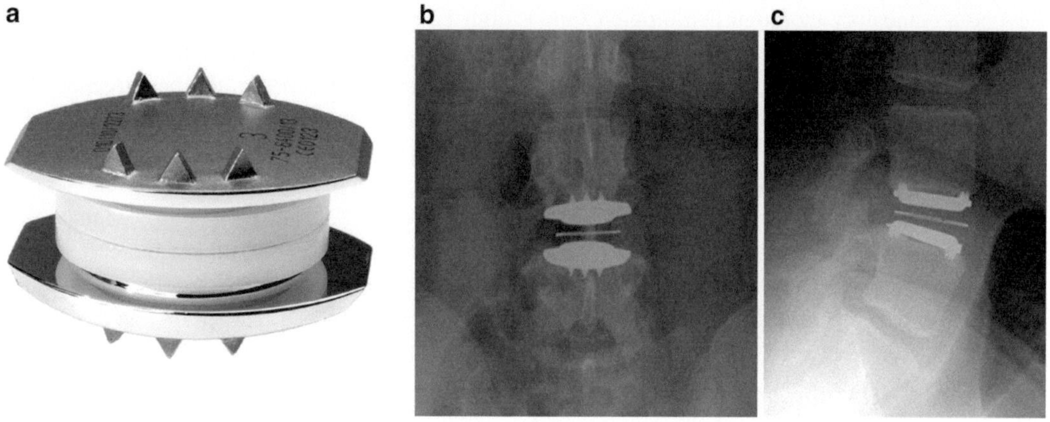

Fig. 27.1 (**a**) The Charite artificial disc. (**b**) Anteroposterior radiograph of Charitie disc placed at L4-L5. (**c**) Postoperative lateral radiograph at L4-L5 of Charitie artificial disc

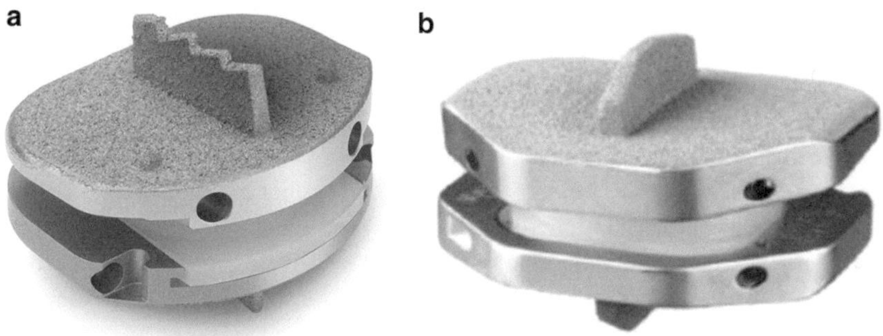

Fig. 27.2 (**a**) ProDisc-L artificial disc. (**b**) Activ-L artificial disc

preservation in the lumbar spine and limitation of adjacent segment degeneration (ASD) has been supported in the literature. The systematic review of ASD which demonstrated a rate of 14% in lumbar fusion revealed a rate of only 1% (7/595 patients across 4 studies) in TDR with an approximate average follow-up of 10 years [9].

There are currently only two FDA-approved lumbar artificial discs (ProDisc-L, DePuy Synthes; Activ-L, Aesculap) that are marketed and available in the United States. Lumbar TDR is used primarily to treat discogenic (i.e., axial, mechanical) LBP [8]. Given the controversy surrounding the surgical treatment of DDD in general, many insurance carriers do not provide coverage for fusion or L-TDR which has affected the utilization of lumbar arthroplasty devices [7, 18].

Indications and Patient Selection

The ideal indications for the treatment of DDD with L-TDR include relatively young patient (ideally age 18–60 years) suffering mechanical LBP (pain exacerbated by activity and somewhat relieved with rest) and imaging (generally MRI) revealing an isolated degenerative, desiccated, and spondylotic disc with little or no facet disease. The patient should have failed a minimum of 6 months of nonoperative treatment. Clinically, the evaluation and medical therapies utilized in working up a patient for consideration of L-TDR are similar to that of any other lumbar surgery. The surgeon must focus on the details of the pain itself (location, symmetry, timing, radiation, exacerbating and ameliorating factors, etc.).

Beyond a mandatory thorough neurologic exam, specific attention must be given to range of motion, posture, and gait [3, 7, 18, 19]. There has also been concern with using lumbar disc arthroplasty in multilevel disease. It has been the experience of these authors that multilevel patients can do well. In a study by Hannibal et al., they compared one-level and two-level ProDisc arthroplasty patients. They found no statistically significant difference in disability, functional, or satisfaction scores between the two groups [20].

There are two categories of contraindications: (1) painful conditions not corrected by the implant (central stenosis, facet arthropathy, +/− foraminal stenosis, herniated nucleus pulposus with radiculopathy) and (2) conditions that may destabilize the spine (scoliosis, spondylolisthesis, spondylolysis, compromise of the posterior elements, osteoporosis T-score < -1.0) [19]. Although facet disease is a strong relative contraindication for this surgery, many do not consider foraminal stenosis a contraindication. The disc space increases with the prosthesis which often causes indirect decompression of the foramen [19]. For patients with the aforementioned contraindications, fusion procedures remain the gold standard.

Preoperative Considerations and Contraindications

The evaluation of a patient with low back pain should be thorough and systematic. As with any musculoskeletal pathology, the evaluation should begin with a comprehensive history and physical exam. It is important to ask the patient when they experience the pain and what aggravates/alleviates the symptoms. Is the pain worse with flexing the low back or extending it? Are there radicular symptoms which radiate down the legs or is this isolated to the low back? What other therapies have they attempted? Many patients will have already tried exercise (yoga, home stretching, etc.) or even formal physical therapy.

It is important to assess the type of pain and the length of pain when assessing a new patient. Approximately 80–90% of low back pain resolves after 12 weeks with no invasive therapy required [21]. It was initially believed that resting and limiting range of motion was the best treatment of acute low back pain. Hagen et al. conducted a Cochrane review of all clinical trials comparing rest vs early active motion for the treatment of low back pain [22]. The review showed that there was a decreased level of pain and increased functional level in the early motion group. It is therefore advisable to begin flexibility and strength training in the acute period of low back pain.

Formal physical therapy which focuses on strengthening core muscle groups has been shown to improve discogenic back pain [23]. In addition to therapy, nonsteroidal anti-inflammatory medications have also been shown to help alleviate symptoms. Some patients have already tried corticosteroid injections, and it is important to understand where these were placed in the spine and what level of relief they provided. There are many other non-spine pathologies that can cause a similar type of pain. It is important to ask questions which would help rule out these other causes. Some of the more common conditions that can cause such pain include Crohn's disease, abdominal aortic aneurysm, nephrolithiasis, pancreatic disease, ovarian pathology, and tumors. In our practice patients also get evaluated by a rheumatologist to rule out inflammatory arthropathy such as rheumatoid arthritis, psoriatic arthritis, and Lyme arthritis. If the pain is not well explained by the spine, make sure your patient is receiving the appropriate work-up for these other conditions.

The next step in evaluating these patients is a physical exam. The initial examination should include inspection of the back to look for any obvious deformity or overlying skin conditions. A standard neurologic exam should be performed to assess for strength and sensation in all extremities. Unlike facet arthropathy which causes low back pain with extension, discogenic back pain typically causes pain with flexion. Also, in this population the straight leg raise is negative. In most patients, the pain is reproducible with low back palpation. They also frequently have decreased range of motion as well as an antalgic gait. It is vital to have the patients stand and point to the location of their pain. Waddell signs and other psychological overlay components of the history should also be defined.

Radiographic evaluation should include plain radiographs of the lumbar spine, with a strong recommendation to obtain standing scoliosis films, as well as CT of the lumbar spine. These will serve to help identify degenerative levels but more importantly will rule out other confounding pathologies such as spondylolisthesis, significant facet disease, ankylosing spondylitis, Baastrup syndrome, sagittal imbalance, or scoliotic deformity. These bony images will also help to identify patients that are likely to have osteoporosis who might warrant further investigation with DEXA scan. Lumbar MRI is the key imaging modality for identifying the pathology that is best suited for treatment with L-TDR. A degenerative disc (most frequently at L4-L5, L5-S1) can be identified by a loss of height relative to other disc levels, a loss of T2 hyperintense signal (desiccation of the nucleus pulposus), annular defects, and Modic changes in the surrounding endplates including endplate changes on T1/T2 and especially STIR signal changes. MRI will also allow the surgeon to rule out other pathologies not well suited to treatment by TDR including: disc herniations in areas difficult to assess via an anterior approach, facet arthropathy, clinically significant central and lateral recess stenosis, or less common pathologies such as neoplastic, infectious, or intradural processes [7, 19].

Despite the many advantages of advanced imaging described above, it is often difficult to assess if the pathology seen on imaging is truly symptomatic or if the main generator of pain is elsewhere. Boden obtained an MRI in a large cohort of subjects that had no back pain symptoms [4]. Of the patients <60 years old, 20% had pathology read by blinded neuroradiologists. In the 60+-year-old group, 57% were read as having spine pathology. Similarly, a study by Borenstein et al. showed that incidental spine pathology found on MRI in asymptomatic patients was not predictive of low back pain at 7-year follow-up [24].

Unfortunately, when it comes to the spine, often the severity of the pathology as seen on classical imaging (MRI, CT, etc.) does not correlate with the severity of symptoms. This is particularly true when it comes to discogenic pain. It would therefore be useful to have a way to assess the level of pain associated with the pathology seen on imaging.

Provocative discography is an example of functional imaging that has been used to help correlate prior imaging with symptoms but remains a controversial study in the diagnosis of symptomatic DDD [2, 25]. During discography individual discs are pressurized using a needle inserted under fluoroscopic guidance and a saline, radiopaque dye combination. If the low back pain is reproduced with this exam, then this may indicate that this particular disc is causing all or a portion of the low back symptoms. The utility of this modality is controversial. A study by Carragee et al. seeking to evaluate the validity of provocative discography in diagnosing true discogenic pain could only establish a positive predictive value of 50–60% and postulated that discography may actually accelerate degenerative changes in the disc [25]. In a prospective study Derby et al. performed discograms on a large cohort of patients with significant disc herniation (Grade III on the Dallas Discogram scale) [26]. One group had low back pain prior to the study and one group did not. In the group with no back pain prior to the study, 100% of the patients had a negative or pain-free response to discography. In the symptomatic group, 52% of patients had a negative discogram despite having clinical back pain. Interestingly, this study also showed that the positive discogram group had lower pain tolerance than the other groups which could certainly be a confounder. In addition, it has been shown in this study, as well as in prior studies, that there is less of a correlation between low back pain and lower grade tears (Grades 1 and 2) which is why only Grade 3 tears were ultimately considered. Despite the conflicting evidence on the utility of this diagnostic test, many surgeons still use it as part of a multifaceted approach to assessing low back pain.

Patients who have undergone prior discectomy at the pathologic level remain candidates for L-TDR; however, previous (failed) fusion at the level in question is a contraindication. Patients with inadequate bone quality (osteopenia with a DEXA T-score between −1.5 and −2.0 should be considered a relative contraindication, while a T-score less than −2.5 is an absolute contraindication) are at significant risk for implant subsidence or displacement. Similar to any anterior spinal approach, there are other relative contraindications related to practical or anatomic limitations often best left to the discretion of the approach surgeon. These include but are not limited to morbid obesity, pregnancy, multiple prior abdominal surgeries, certain abnormalities of the genitourinary system, and abdominal aortic or iliac aneurysm [3, 18, 19].

Surgical Technique

Appropriate patient preparation prior to surgery is imperative. The patient is given a prescription for two doses of magnesium citrate for bowel preparation 1.5 days prior to surgery. Thirty-six hours prior to surgery, the patient drinks the first dose and is started on a clear liquid diet. The second dose is taken 12 h prior to surgery. For male patients they are given the option of sperm donation prior to surgery.

Under general anesthesia the patient is positioned supine on a radiolucent operating table taking routine care to protect and pad all pressure points. A Foley catheter is required to decompress the urinary bladder to optimize the working corridor. Ureter stents are placed in patients with a history of prior abdominal surgery or in patients who have only one kidney for whatever reason. They are also routinely placed in patients undergoing replacements from L1 to L3 given the proximity of the ureters to the operative field. The surgeon should be careful not to position the patient in too much extension as this can lead to postoperative facet irritation syndrome.

Preoperatively, pulse oximeters are placed on bilateral great toes. If a discrepancy between these devices occurs during the surgery, the retractors are temporarily released allowing the left lower extremity to again be fully perfused. Neuromonitoring is not routinely used in our practice, but in more complex patients, it can be considered.

Anteroposterior (AP) and lateral fluoroscopy are utilized to identify the level of the replacement as well as the optimal angle of approach. The goal is for the spinous processes to be equidistant from the medial wall of each pedicle, in other words, eliminating all torsional rotation of the spine. Fine adjustments to the patient's position are made using rolled blue towels or inflatable pads.

The lateral view is then obtained to determine the appropriate vertebral levels aiding in the positioning of the incision. Once the positioning is complete and the level is determined, the abdominal and pelvic area are prepped and draped in the normal sterile fashion. We feel that the iliac wing should be prepped into the field so that, in the unlikely event that the arthroplasty must be abandoned, the iliac crest can be used as autologous bone graft for fusion.

In most circumstances, and certainly in upper lumbar or multilevel surgery, an access vascular surgery is used. This reduces operative time and reduces the amount of retraction time on the great vessels. The skin incision and approach are best decided by the approach surgeon (typically a general or vascular surgeon). Options include a midline or para-midline vertical incision for transperitoneal or anterior mini-open retroperitoneal approach (more common). For L5-S1 a transverse incision may be utilized. A left-sided approach is most common given the greater safety and ease in mobilizing the aorta as opposed to the inferior vena cava or iliac veins. However, right-sided approach may be considered for males when done at L5-S1 to avoid disruption of the superior hypogastric plexus and potential resultant retrograde ejaculation.

Because of the downward slope of the L5-S1 vertebra, a more distal incision is required to accommodate the necessary angle. In general the L4-L5 disc is within a few centimeters of the umbilicus. The incision is carried down to the rectus sheath. The left rectus sheath is incised in line with the incision exposing the medial aspect of the left rectus abdominal muscle. The edge of this muscle belly is lifted to expose the dorsal fascia and arcuate line being careful to preserve the inferior epigastric vessels. This layer is incised revealing the peritoneum. This is the plane that will be utilized for this surgery. Sweeping along this plane toward the left, retroperitoneal fat will be observed, and eventually the left psoas muscle will be identified (Fig. 27.3a). The genitofemoral nerve can be identified on the psoas lying just medial to the common iliac artery. The iliac vein is dorsal to the artery. All soft tissue structures should be retracted medially. The middle sacral veins should be ligated prior to addressing the disc space. If the level desired is proximal to the L5-S1 disc space, then the great vessels must be mobilized by bluntly developing a plane between the psoas and iliac vessels. In this approach the iliolumbar vein must be identified and ligated before mobilizing the great vessels.

Once the anterior spine has been reached, the adjacent visceral and vascular structures are safely mobilized and retracted (Fig. 27.3b). The correct spinal level is confirmed by lateral fluoroscopy. The midline must be meticulously identified by anatomic landmarks and AP fluoroscopy. The surgeon can either make a Bovie mark, or a small osteotome can be used to make a superficial indentation. A wide annulotomy is performed. This is followed by near-total discectomy using standard technique of curettes, pituitary, and Kerrison rongeurs (Fig. 27.3c). The discectomy is facilitated by interbody distractors to open the disc space as well as ultimate resection of the posterior annulus and posterior longitudinal ligament. Special attention is given to removal of the cartilaginous endplates while maintaining the integrity of the bony endplates. Any posterior osteophytes or extruded disc material should be removed. Following discectomy, only the lateral annulus should remain fully intact bilaterally. The posterior annulus should be resected to aid in disc space mobilization. The posterior longitudinal ligament does not need to be resected except in circumstances requiring removal of extruded disc material. Retained lateral disc material is at risk of displacement into the foramen with placement of the device and should be thoroughly removed.

Using AP and lateral fluoroscopy, as well as tactile feel, the disc space is measured for height,

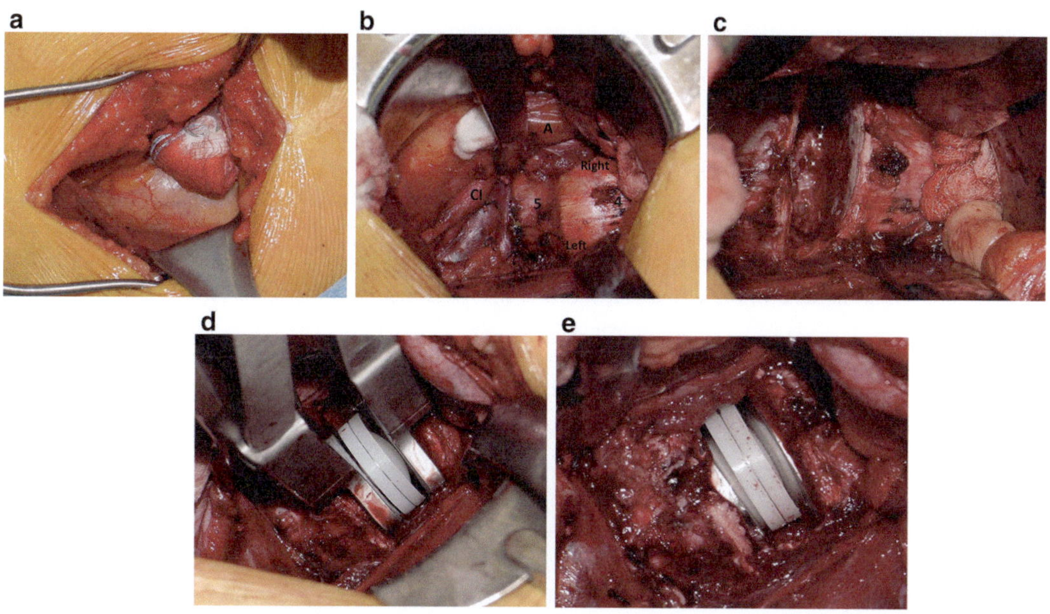

Fig. 27.3 (**a**) Intraoperative image showing mobilization of the retroperitoneal space below the umbilicus. (**b**) Exposure at the L4-L5 disc space. There is wide exposure from the left to right side. The aorta (*A*) and left common iliac vessel (*CI*) is protected. (**c**) Complete discectomy has been performed from left to right side. (**d**) Placement of a Charite artificial disc at L4-L5. (**e**) Final in situ position of the Charite artificial disc

degree of lordosis, and footprint (depending on the specifics of the device in use). Each device has its own nuanced surgical technique but typically involves the following steps. The disc space is sized and then trialed, followed by midline keel cutting (if necessary for the device in use) and ultimately placement of the device itself (Fig. 27.3d–e). Once the implants are impacted into place, the alignment of the spine should again be confirmed with intraoperative fluoroscopy. Again, strict adherence to midline placement is an absolute necessity for best device function. Ideal AP position of the device on lateral fluoroscopy places the device's center of rotation approximately 1–2 mm posterior to the sagittal midline of the vertebral body. The integrity of the vertebral bodies should be assessed as fractures can occur during insertion. If any fractures are observed or there are any other concerns regarding the stability of the implants or bony structures, then the implant should be removed and an interbody fusion should be performed.

For multilevel surgery, the most distal disc space is typically addressed first, and then one works proximally to allow for collinear alignment of the spine. In multilevel surgery, if there is concern that the implant may not be able to be placed after the adjacent levels are complete, then trial implants should be used first to assure the ability to place all implants. Once all levels are mobilized and trialed, the hardware can again be inserted starting most distally and working proximally to assure optimal alignment.

All soft tissue structures, including the sympathetic chain, great vessels, ureters, and retroperitoneal structures, should be thoroughly investigated for any signs of iatrogenic injury. All soft tissue bleeding should be controlled by electrocautery, and any bony bleeding should be controlled with bone wax. This is critically important to minimize the risk of postoperative retroperitoneal hematoma formation. Occasionally, epidural bleeding is induced, usually from distraction, and it should be controlled by applying a small amount of Surgiflo (Ethicon, Somerville, NJ USA) hemostatic agent or an equivalent product. The lower extremity pulses should be reevaluated immediately prior to the end of the case.

The wound is then irrigated thoroughly and closed in routine fashion. A Gore-Tex patch may be placed over the anterior annulotomy to provide a dissection plane for revision exposure if reoperation proves necessary.

Illustrative Cases

Case 1

History

The patient is a 45-year-old female who presents to the clinic for progressively severe mechanical lower back pain which is exacerbated by physical activity and relieved by rest. She has a history of right microdiscectomy at L5-S1 2 year prior to presentation. The patient has undergone maximal nonsurgical management including physical therapy, epidural steroid injections, and selective nerve root block. Despite this, her pain remains intolerable even on a regimen of chronic narcotic therapy centered on fentanyl patches.

Physical Examination

Physical examination reveals healthy-appearing female with appropriate appearance for age and a BMI of 26. Neurologic exam revealed normal motor, sensory, and reflexes of the lower extremity. Her gait is normal. She has slight restriction in forward flexion at the waist. Her lower back reveals a well-healed paramedian scar from her microdiscectomy and very mild tenderness to deep palpation of the lower back symmetrically just off midline.

Imaging

Imaging includes MRI of the lumbar spine without contrast which demonstrates her previous laminotomy defect, without any evidence of recurrent or residual disc herniation at L5-S1 (Fig. 27.4a). There is, however, a broad-based disc bulge at L4-L5 not resulting in any foraminal or central stenosis. Both L4-L5 and L5-S1 disc levels appear degenerative owing to mild loss of height as well as loss of T2 hyperintense signal within the nucleus pulposus. Provocative discography is performed reveal-

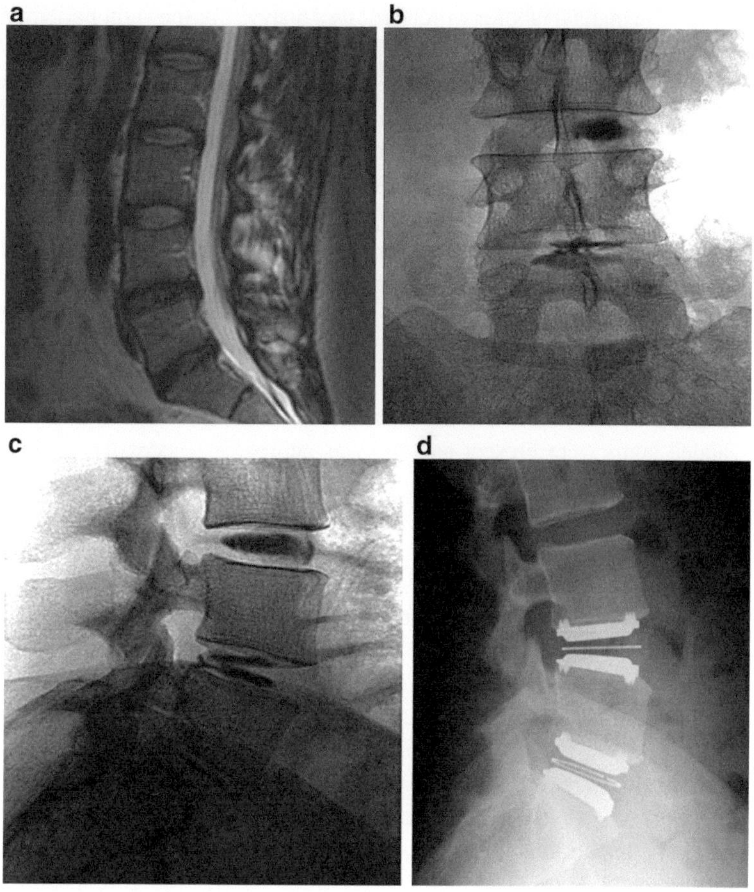

Fig. 27.4 (**a**) Sagittal T2 MRI showing no recurrent disc degeneration and disc degeneration at L4-L5 and L5-S1. (**b**) Anteroposterior discography at L4-L5 and L5-S1 revealing disc degeneration at L4-L5 and L5-S1. Provocative pain response was positive at both levels but negative at L3-L4 that served as a control level. (**c**) Lateral discography. L4-L5 and L5-S1 show abnormal degeneration, while L3-L4 has normal morphology. (**d**) Postoperative lateral radiograph following L4-L5 and L5-S1 Charite disc replacement

ing mild/moderate annular degeneration at L5-S1 and a posterior annular tear at L4-L5 (Fig. 27.4b, c). Reproduction of the patient's pain with injection is concordant at L4-L5 and L5-S1 with L3-L4 serving as a negative control (Fig. 27.4b, c).

Treatment

Following appropriate explanation of associated risks and benefits, the patient elects to proceed with (off-label indication) two-level Charite total disc replacement at L4-L5 and L5-S1 (Fig. 27.4d). Surgery is performed with the assistance of a vascular surgeon for anterior access. There are no intraoperative complications. Estimated blood loss is 150 mL. Total operating room time is 2 h and 55 min. The patient undergoes routine postoperative care on a neurosurgical floor and is discharged to home in good condition on postoperative day 4.

Outcome

The patient returns to the clinic for routine postoperative follow-up at 6 and 12 weeks, as well as 6, 12, and 24 months following her date of surgery. She reports an excellent functional recovery with significant diminution of pain. By 24 months she is off all narcotic medications and has increased her activity level. She reports that she is regularly jogging and lifting weights without limitation. Upright AP and lateral and flexion/extension radiographs at 24 months post-op show good disc placement with maintenance of normal lumbar vertebral motion (Fig. 27.4d).

Case 2

History

This patient was a 33-year-old female who first presented to the clinic with low back pain. She worked as a manual laborer which required heavy lifting and a significant amount of bending and twisting. Over the last several years, the pain had intensified such that it was becoming difficult to work. The pain was primarily in her lower back, but also was present in her buttock and upper thighs. She denied any weakness or difficulty with coordination in either lower extremity. She had failed physical therapy and epidural corticosteroid injection.

Physical Examination

The physical examination was unremarkable. No Waddell signs were present and she was neurologically intact.

Imaging

The MRI showed disc disease at L3-L4, L4-L5, and L5-S1 (Fig. 27.5a, b). In addition to the MRI, discography was performed to assess for the presence of discogenic pain. The exam was positive for pathology at L4-L5 and L5-S1.

Treatment

Ultimately, it is the combination of history, physical exam, and all imaging studies that drives the decision to operate and at what levels. Given this patient's overall picture, it was determined to perform a three-level lumbar TDR on L3-S1. The procedure proceeded with no intraoperative complications, and the implants were placed in good alignment (Fig. 27.5c, d). The patient tolerated the procedure well and was discharged home on postoperative day 3.

Outcome

Over the next several months, her incisions healed well and the incisional pain improved. She had significant improvement in her low back pain which was present preoperatively. After a period of activity restriction, she was able to get back to working which meant bending over to lift objects which she tolerated well. This operation not only provided pain relief and a stable mechanical solution to her problem, but it also allowed for the range of motion necessary for a young patient to get back to her physically demanding livelihood. This example case demonstrates that in the right patient, TDR in the lumbar spine can be highly efficacious and allows patients to return to an acceptable activity level.

Technical Pearls

- Be sure the patient's spine is in neutral position on the operative table at the start of the case. An inflatable pillow may be placed in the low lumbar region and utilized to gain better access to a collapsed disc space.
- True AP and lateral fluoroscopic views are a necessity as the midline and AP position of the replacement disc is more crucial to success than when using standard interbody fusion cages.
- Take special care to preserve autonomic nerves in dissection around L5-S1 to avoid the complication of retrograde ejaculation in male patients by minimizing use of Bovie electrocautery in the prevertebral space.
- Do not violate the bony endplates at the discectomy site; to do so increases the risk of device subsidence and ultimate failure.
- Be sure all lateral disc material except for a thin rim of annulus is removed prior to placing distractors, trials, or the graft in order to avoid displacing fragments into the foramina.
- Complete the near-total discectomy in a piecemeal fashion, checking for retained disc material in between each of the sizing/trialing/keel cutting steps.
- Resecting the posterior longitudinal ligament will allow for the best mobilizing of the disc space and creation of the anatomic height and lordotic curve. Parallel distractors help expedite this process.
- The lateral annulus should not be released for mobilization purposes.
- Proper sizing of the replacement disc which maximizes endplate coverage will benefit the maintenance of lordosis and proper vertebral motion, as well as minimize subsidence and may help avoid heterotopic ossification or off-midline placement.
- Avoid "overstuffing" the disc space with an oversized disc as this can limit motion. When

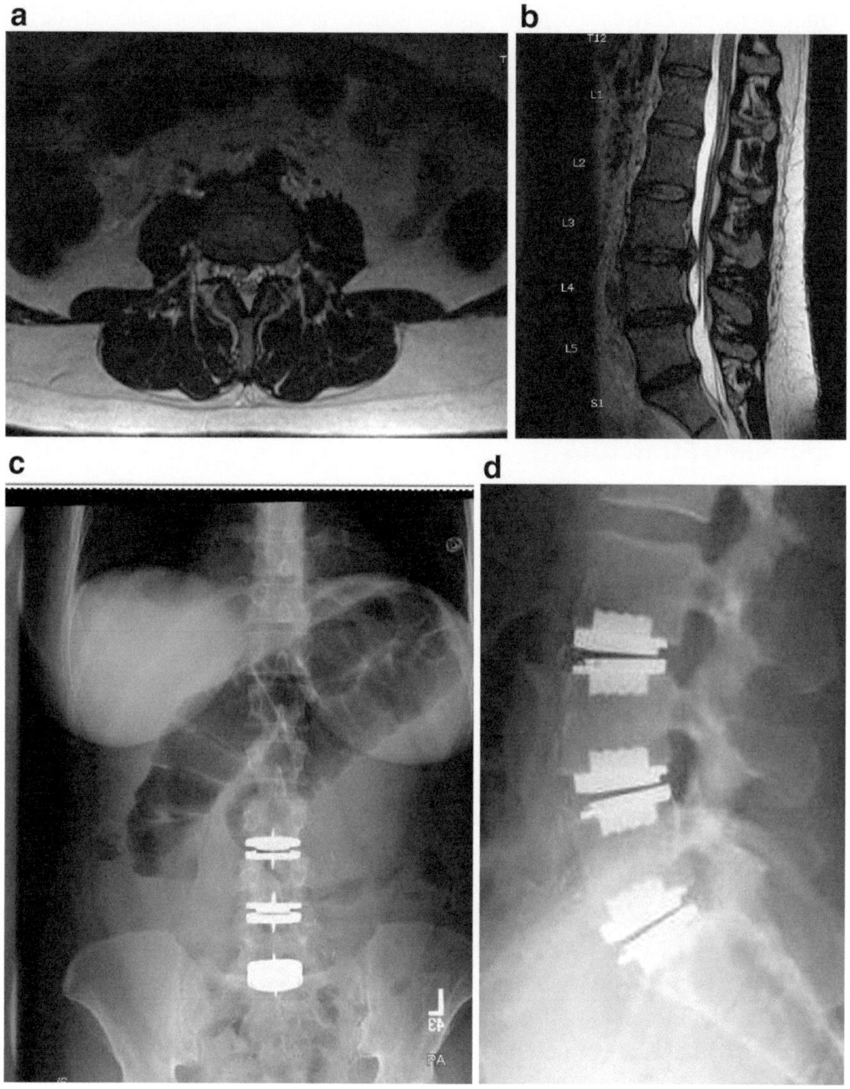

Fig. 27.5 (**a**) T1-weighted axial image from a preoperative MRI showing minimal central stenosis. (**b**) T2-weighted sagittal image from a preoperative MRI showing minimal disc herniation or canal stenosis at all levels being considered for TDR. (**c**) Postoperative anteroposterior radiograph following L3-L4, L4-L5, and L5-S1 ProDisc-L placement. The discs are well aligned in the midline and the overall coronal balance is excellent. (**d**) Postoperative lateral radiograph following L3-L4, L4-L5, and L5-S1 ProDisc-L placement showing good restoration of disc height and sagittal alignment

choosing between two heights, generally choose the smaller size.

In some cases, coronal realignment is required which can add a level of complexity to the case. For these situations we suggest the use of a 3.5 mm AO reconstruction plate (DePuy Synthes Spine, Raynham, Massachusetts). A ball-spike pusher can be used to manually obtain the appropriate coronal alignment, and the plate can be applied over the anterolateral vertebral bodies to secure the reduction. At this point, the endplates can be modified with a chisel in such a way to allow for appropriate alignment with the use of the implant alone. Through a process of trial and error using the trial implants, the bony anatomy can be modified to assure adequate coronal (and also sagittal) alignment. Once this is achieved, the final implant is inserted and the 3.5 mm plate is removed. Vertebral body pin distractors can also be used to achieve coronal and sagittal alignment. However, in our experience, these devices do not always reproduce anatomic alignment which is ultimately the goal. If these devices are to be used, caution should be taken to assure anatomic alignment with the help of intraoperative fluoroscopy.

Complications and Strategies for Avoidance

Generic complications of any spine operation also exist for L-TDR including neurologic injury, hematoma formation due to inadequate hemostasis, and postoperative infection. Furthermore, L-TDR entails the risks and complications unique to anterior spine approaches: postoperative ileus, abdominal visceral or vascular injury including injury to iliac vessels, and injury to the autonomic nerves of the superior hypogastric plexus which can result in retrograde ejaculation in males [3, 12]. The most feared and dangerous complications include major vascular injury. The risk of this complication is low, particularly if an experienced access surgeon is utilized. The ureters are also at risk with this exposure, so liberal use of ureter stents should be employed. The exposure becomes significantly more difficult in patients with a BMI of 35 or greater. In our own practice we do not offer TDR surgery to these patients. Surgery should not be performed on individuals with dermatological issues that affect the abdominal skin such as eczema, psoriasis, or intertrigo.

Intraoperative complications during discectomy and implant placement can be minimized by meticulous technique. Particular care should be take when placing and tensioning distractor devices in the interspace. Using parallel distractors with the largest surface area possible can help minimize this risk. Fluoroscopy can be helpful in preventing these iatrogenic problems. If they are encountered, the TDR should be abandoned and a fusion should be performed. Although rare, occasionally an intraoperative durotomy is encountered. Depending on the size and location, a primary repair can be attempted or a sealant can be utilized. Given our experience, we recommend not doing a primary repair in most cases. Usually the use of a sealant and the application of a fat or muscle patch is enough to control the leak, which will resolve over time. Normal durotomy care should be carried out postoperatively. Some patients have a significant concavity to their endplates. This is important to identify since keeled devices, even large keels, do not work. In these cases spiked implants can be utilized to overcome this problem.

Unique risks associated with L-TDR include subsidence of the disc replacement into the vertebral body, dislocation of the device from the disc space, or undesired ankylosis and fusion across the disc space (heterotopic ossification). The former two complications can be minimized with proper surgical technique. The primary means to avoid these complications include preservation of the bony endplates and proper sizing and positioning of the replacement disc. A disc that is too short risks dislocation, whereas a disc that has too small of a footprint risks either dislocation or subsidence. Additionally, the risk of subsidence increases significantly in patients with osteopenia or osteoporosis. In any patient in whom these conditions are suspected, such as female over the age of 50 or those with a positive family history, a preoperative DEXA scan is required. If subsidence occurs and the implant appears stable, then revision surgery is not always necessary. A brace to limit mobility should be worn for 6–8 weeks in these patients. If there is a fracture through the vertebral body or the implant is extruded anteriorly, then a revision surgery is usually indicated.

The complication of failure to maintain motion across the disc space due to fusion is largely an issue of patient selection. Patients at risk for undesired fusion or ankylosis are those older than 60 or those with more diffuse multilevel degenerative/spondylotic change in the lumbar spine.

The rare complication of wear debris reactions, such as granuloma or pseudotumor formation, is often unpredictable except in patients with known reaction or allergy to any of the materials utilized in the replacement disc. If this information is known, such patients are not candidates for L-TDR [3, 12, 14, 16, 27].

Careful surveillance for thromboembolic events is advisable as these patients are at particularly high risk because of the mobilization of the great vessels. Postoperative DVT chemical prophylaxis should be discussed with the access vascular surgeon. Infections are rare but if they do occur decompression and fusion procedures with or without removal of the hardware are often indicated.

Conclusion

Lumbar disc replacement surgery continues to evolve based on our expanding knowledge of lumbar segmental biomechanics and results of long-term Level 1 evidence-based clinical trials. Data from recent long-term multicenter prospective randomized trials as well as meta-analysis studies reveal superiority to fusion in both clinical and radiographic outcomes. Devices which permit controlled posterior translation of the superior articular facet processes in flexion and also limit the over-distraction of the disc interspace correlate with improved clinical outcomes. Careful patient selection, including facet joint assessment with appropriate imaging and diagnostic pain injections, is recommended especially at the L5-S1 level. Expanded indications include broad-based disc herniations with spinal stenosis, multilevel degenerative disc disease, and hybrid surgical indications. The principles of lumbar disc replacement surgery include careful patient preoperative evaluation and selection, meticulous and careful spine access, and appropriate implant selection based on vertebral body dimensions. Further assessment of endplate morphology needs to be considered to ensure optimal clinical and radiographic outcomes.

References

1. Allan DB, Waddell G. An historical perspective on low back pain and disability. Acta Orthop Scand Suppl. 1989;234:1–23.
2. Carragee EJ, Hannibal M. Diagnostic evaluation of low back pain. Orthop Clin North Am. 2004;35(1):7–16.
3. Yue JJ, Lawrence JP. Indications and contraindications for lumbar nonfusion surgery: patient selection. In: Yue JJ, Bertagnoli R, McAfee PC, An HS, editors. Motion preservation surgery of the spine. Philadelphia: Saunders Elsevier; 2008.
4. Boden SD, Davis DO, Dina TS, Patronas NJ, Wiesel SW. Abnormal magnetic-resonance scans of the lumbar spine in asymptomatic subjects. A prospective investigation. J Bone Joint Surg Am. 1990;72(3):403–8.
5. Fernstrom U. Arthroplasty with intercorporal endoprothesis in herniated disc and in painful disc. Acta Chir Scand Suppl. 1966;357:154–9.
6. Hamby WB, Glaser HT. Replacement of spinal intervertebral discs with locally polymerizing methyl methacrylate: experimental study of effects upon tissues and report of a small clinical series. J Neurosurg. 1959;16(3):311–3.
7. Buttner-Janz K, Guyer RD, Ohnmeiss DD. Indications for lumbar total disc replacement: selecting the right patient with the right indication for the right total disc. Int J Spine Surg. 2014;8
8. Garcia R Jr, Yue JJ, Blumenthal S, Coric D, Patel VV, Leary SP, et al. Lumbar total disc replacement for discogenic low back pain: two-year outcomes of the activL multicenter randomized controlled IDE clinical trial. Spine. 2015;40(24):1873–81.
9. Harrop JS, Youssef JA, Maltenfort M, Vorwald P, Jabbour P, Bono CM, et al. Lumbar adjacent segment degeneration and disease after arthrodesis and total disc arthroplasty. Spine. 2008;33(15):1701–7.
10. Freeman BJ, Davenport J. Total disc replacement in the lumbar spine: a systematic review of the literature. Eur Spine J Off Publ Eur Spine Soc Eur Spinal Deform Soc Eur Sect Cerv Spine Res Soc. 2006;15(Suppl 3):S439–47.
11. Guyer RD, Pettine K, Roh JS, Dimmig TA, Coric D, McAfee PC, et al. Comparison of 2 lumbar total disc replacements: results of a prospective, randomized, controlled, multicenter Food and Drug Administration trial with 24-month follow-up. Spine. 2014;39(12):925–31.
12. Coric D, Kim P. Lumbar arthroplasty: Total disk replacement and nucleus replacement technologies. In: Winn HR, editor. Youmans neurological surgery. 6th ed. Philadelphia: Saunders Elsevier; 2011.
13. Gamradt SC, Wang JC. Lumbar disc arthroplasty. Spine J Off J North Am Spine Soc. 2005;5(1):95–103.
14. Nie H, Chen G, Wang X, Zeng J. Comparison of total disc replacement with lumbar fusion: a meta-analysis

of randomized controlled trials. J Coll Physicians Surg Pak: JCPSP. 2015;25(1):60–7.
15. McAfee PC, Cunningham B, Holsapple G, Adams K, Blumenthal S, Guyer RD, et al. A prospective, randomized, multicenter Food and Drug Administration investigational device exemption study of lumbar total disc replacement with the CHARITE artificial disc versus lumbar fusion: part II: evaluation of radiographic outcomes and correlation of surgical technique accuracy with clinical outcomes. Spine. 2005;30(14):1576–83. discussion E388–90
16. Blumenthal S, McAfee PC, Guyer RD, Hochschuler SH, Geisler FH, Holt RT, et al. A prospective, randomized, multicenter Food and Drug Administration investigational device exemptions study of lumbar total disc replacement with the CHARITE artificial disc versus lumbar fusion: part I: evaluation of clinical outcomes. Spine. 2005;30(14):1565–75. discussion E387–91
17. Park SJ, Lee CS, Chung SS, Lee KH, Kim WS, Lee JY. Long-term outcomes following lumbar Total disc replacement using ProDisc-II: average 10-year follow-up at a single institute. Spine. 2016;41(11):971–7.
18. Zigler J, Garcia R. ISASS policy statement – lumbar artificial disc. Int J Spine Surg. 2015;9:7.
19. Huang RC, Lim MR, Girardi FP, Cammisa FP Jr. The prevalence of contraindications to total disc replacement in a cohort of lumbar surgical patients. Spine. 2004;29(22):2538–41.
20. Hannibal M, Thomas DJ, Low J, Hsu KY, Zucherman J. ProDisc-L total disc replacement: a comparison of 1-level versus 2-level arthroplasty patients with a minimum 2-year follow-up. Spine. 2007;32(21):2322–6.
21. Andersson GB. Epidemiological features of chronic low-back pain. Lancet (London, England). 1999;354(9178):581–5.
22. Hagen KB, Jamtvedt G, Hilde G, Winnem MF. The updated cochrane review of bed rest for low back pain and sciatica. Spine. 2005;30(5):542–6.
23. Oesch P, Kool J, Hagen KB, Bachmann S. Effectiveness of exercise on work disability in patients with non-acute non-specific low back pain: systematic review and meta-analysis of randomised controlled trials. J Rehabil Med. 2010;42(3):193–205.
24. Borenstein DG, O'Mara JW Jr, Boden SD, Lauerman WC, Jacobson A, Platenberg C, et al. The value of magnetic resonance imaging of the lumbar spine to predict low-back pain in asymptomatic subjects: a seven-year follow-up study. J Bone Joint Surg Am. 2001;83-A(9):1306–11.
25. Carragee EJ, Alamin TF. Discography. A review. Spine JOff J North Am Spine Soc. 2001;1(5):364–72.
26. Derby R, Kim BJ, Lee SH, Chen Y, Seo KS, Aprill C. Comparison of discographic findings in asymptomatic subject discs and the negative discs of chronic LBP patients: can discography distinguish asymptomatic discs among morphologically abnormal discs? Spine JOff J North Am Spine Soc. 2005;5(4):389–94.
27. Yue JK, Chan AK, Winkler EA, Upadhyayula PS, Readdy WJ, Dhall SS. A review and update on the guidelines for the acute management of cervical spinal cord injury – part II. J Neurosurg Sci. 2016;60(3):367–84.

Minimally Invasive Posterior Lumbar Fusion Techniques

28

Luis M. Tumialán

Abbreviations

ALIF	Anterior lumbar interbody fusion
AP	Anteroposterior
MIS	Minimally invasive surgery
MR	Magnetic resonance
TLIF	Transforaminal lumbar interbody fusion
VAS	Visual analog scale

Introduction

In 1997, Foley and Smith introduced a paramedian transmuscular approach to the lumbar spine to perform microdiscectomies through a cylindrical access port secured after dilatation of the paraspinal muscles [1]. Building on the familiarity of the transmuscular decompression techniques, surgeons combined well-established percutaneous techniques for instrumentation of the pedicles. The subsequent development of minimally invasive techniques to accomplish the goals of lumbar fusion followed a logical stepwise progression from that minimally invasive decompression platform.

From an anatomical standpoint, the paramedian transmuscular access to the lumbar segment lent itself especially well to transforaminal access to the disc space. In short order, the tenets of interbody fusion established by Cloward [2] were applied to the unilateral transforaminal corridor popularized by Harms and Jeszenszky [2, 3]. As spine surgeons synthesized percutaneous and minimally invasive techniques with experience in traditional midline open surgery, the minimally invasive transforaminal lumbar interbody fusion (MIS TLIF) arose as the leading procedure for the management of single-level lumbar degenerative disc disease.

Currently, three main approaches to the MIS TLIF reflect the evolution of the procedure: percutaneous microendoscopic, mini-open, and hybrid (percutaneous/mini-open) approaches. The first main approach that arose was instrumentation of the pedicle by a purely percutaneous technique with tubular access to the segment for decompression and interbody; this technique was popularized by groups led by Foley and Fessler [4, 5]. The percutaneous instrumentation of the pedicle reconciled the anatomical challenge of attempting to expose pedicle screw entry points through the same incision that also exposes the midline elements. A percutaneous approach spared the patient the lateral exposure needed from a midline approach, which was linked with extensive tis-

L.M. Tumialán, MD (✉)
Department of Neurosurgery, Barrow Neurological Institute, St. Joseph's Hospital and Medical Center, 350 W. Thomas Rd., Phoenix, AZ 85013, USA
e-mail: luis.tumialan@barrowbrainandspine.com

L.T. Holly, P.A. Anderson (eds.), *Essentials of Spinal Stabilization*,
DOI 10.1007/978-3-319-59713-3_28

sue trauma. Instead, the instrumentation of the pedicles was accomplished with direct cannulation of the pedicle through a distinct operative site, which was nothing more than a stab incision. With the percutaneous technique, there was no need to widely expose the anatomy, with the resultant disruption of the musculature and consequential decrease in blood flow because of the considerable muscle-retractor interface. The benefit of minimizing the extent of exposure translated into reduced postoperative discomfort, shorter hospitalizations, and a lower risk of infection [5–7].

Refinements to the minimal access ports prompted further evolution of the percutaneous form of the procedure. Instead of four stab incisions for the percutaneous pedicle fixation and the incision for the paramedian transmuscular decompression and interbody, an expandable minimal access port secured over the facet allowed for exposure of the entire transforaminal corridor in addition to access to the pedicle screw entry point. In this manner, a hybrid percutaneous mini-open procedure was described.

However, limitations to the percutaneous procedure prompted surgeons to consider the application of other minimally invasive techniques and other minimal access ports. The first limitation was the radiation exposure to the surgeon involved in percutaneous instrumentation of the lumbar spine [8]. The recent availability of computer-assisted navigation has minimized this concern. However, as MIS TLIF continues to be used more in an ambulatory surgery setting, it is unlikely that computer-assisted navigation will increase in this setting given its cost. The second limitation was the inability to perform a posterolateral fusion. While this inability may be of varying importance given the high reliability of interbody fusion, access to the transverse processes also provided access to the facet joint contralateral to the transforaminal approach. Having that access is becoming increasingly important to preserve, if not restore, segmental lordosis. In a comparison study of anterior lumbar interbody fusion (ALIF) and TLIF, Hsieh and colleagues [9] demonstrated a two-degree loss of lumbar lordosis and a loss in foraminal height in a TLIF cohort compared to an ALIF cohort.

To address these limitations, surgeons began to explore what has been labeled the mini-open TLIF. With this technique, expandable minimal access ports are used to directly visualize the pedicle screw entry points for instrumentation of the spine, and then that same exposure is simultaneously used to complete the decompression on one side and the posterolateral fusion and a modified Smith-Petersen osteotomy on the other [10].

The most important element of a minimally invasive procedure is that the result can be equivalent to its open counterpart. All surgeons should explore the various technologies available as they proceed through their learning curves to achieve the goals of decompression, stabilization, and successful long-term clinical outcomes. Throughout that process, a thoughtful analysis of the clinical and radiographic outcomes should guide each surgeon to the technique that works best in his or her hands. Among the radiographic criteria that should be scrutinized is the capacity to restore foraminal height and segmental lordosis in the short term and to achieve radiographic union and subsidence of the interbody in the long term. Additionally, an analysis of validated clinical outcomes measures should be used to carefully examine the patient's return to functional mobility and demonstrate improvements in visual analog scale (VAS) leg and VAS back scores. The thoughtful analysis of those outcomes, both clinical and radiographic, will lead surgeons to find the minimally invasive technique that offers the most reliable surgical intervention. In keeping with that spirit of refinement, the technique described in this chapter represents the technique that evolved during the author's learning curve while performing over 500 MIS TLIFs.

Indications and Patient Selection

The most common indications for the MIS TLIF are single-level and two-level lumbar degenerative pathologies that include spondylolisthesis, recurrent disc herniation (third recurrence), recurrent facet cyst, and advanced degenerative disc disease with radiculopathy [11]. In the author's experience, three-level lumbar degenerative disc disease may not be outside the realm of minimally invasive surgery, but it does tend to be outside the realm of the MIS TLIF. A three-level pathology may be best treated with a combination of other surgical approaches, such as transpsoas interbody approaches, minimally invasive decompressions, and percutaneous instrumentation.

The ability to proficiently select patients offers the greatest likelihood of clinical and radiographic success. Patients with elevated body mass indices should be encouraged to make every effort to move toward their ideal body mass index before surgery and to continue that trend after surgery. It has been the author's experience that instituting a core-strengthening program before surgery may further facilitate the weight-loss goal. Concern for osteoporosis in a patient should prompt a bone mineral density study; evidence of osteoporosis should prompt consideration of formal treatment for 3–6 months before surgery, but should not alter the decision to proceed with a minimally invasive approach.

Preoperative Considerations

After obtaining a history and performing a physical examination, anteroposterior (AP), lateral, and flexion-extension radiographs, along with magnetic resonance (MR) images, are obtained. The MR image can clearly demonstrate compression of the neural elements, which should correlate with the patient's neurological examination and subjective complaints. MR imaging may also adequately demonstrate alignment and allow for grading of spondylolisthesis. Patients may present with either unilateral symptoms or bilateral symptoms. Unilateral symptoms mandate a transforaminal approach from the symptomatic side. Bilateral symptoms, in the presence of bilateral foraminal stenosis, may mandate bilateral facetectomies. In the setting of bilateral facetectomies, bilateral access to the disc space may be considered; however, the author's preference is to perform a unilateral transforaminal interbody. Careful analysis of the T1-weighted parasagittal MR image is critical in assessing the neural foramen compromise, which may help in deciding whether facetectomy is needed. In the setting of central stenosis with symptoms of neurogenic claudication, severe foraminal stenosis on one side alone may prompt a transforaminal approach from that side.

Flexion and extension studies are helpful in determining the degree of stability of the segment. Extension studies are particularly helpful in determining how much reduction will be obtainable by positioning (Fig. 28.1).

The AP and lateral radiographs will be predictive of the type of imaging that can be obtained with fluoroscopy in surgery. It is valuable to appreciate a severe coronal imbalance before surgery, so that necessary adjustments can be made to the fluoroscope and incision. Figure 28.2 illustrates the capacity to adjust the fluoroscope based on preoperative imaging. In this patient with a severe coronal imbalance to the left, her symptomatic side, an AP preoperative radiograph prompted a preoperative AP fluoroscopic image to guide the angle for the fluoroscope and to guide the markings for the incisions.

Any concern for scoliosis on AP or lateral imaging should prompt standing 36-inch scoliosis films. It is important to recognize that there is an inherent limitation to the amount of lumbar lordosis that may be restored in a single-level MIS TLIF. In the author's experience, 12 degrees of lordosis is at the upper threshold that can reliably be achieved. Therefore, a significant mismatch in lumbar lordosis and pelvic incidence warrants careful consideration of the operative plan.

Surgical Technique

The operative goals of the MIS TLIF include instrumentation of the pedicles, decompression of the neural elements, and restoration of the disc height and segmental lordosis through interbody placement. The operating room, the scrub technician's back table, and a Mayo stand should all be set up to facilitate the flow of the operation to accomplish these goals. The MIS TLIF, which is

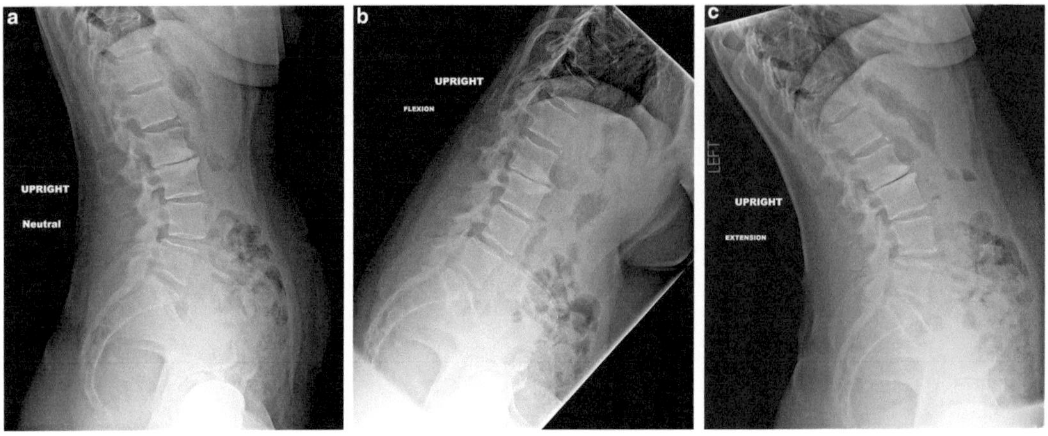

Fig. 28.1 Grade 1 spondylolisthesis. Standing lateral neutral, flexion, and extension radiographs demonstrating the mobility of Grade 1 spondylolisthesis. (**a**) Standing neutral radiograph revealing a subtle Grade 1 spondylolisthesis. (**b**) Flexion study clearly demonstrating anterior translation of the L4 vertebral body on L5. (**c**) Extension study demonstrating near anatomical reduction of the L4 vertebral body on L5. The extension study predicts how much reduction can be achieved just by positioning the patient on a Jackson table (Used with permission from Barrow Neurological Institute, Phoenix, Arizona)

performed through two paramedian incisions with instrumentation placed under direct visualization of the bony anatomy and minimal fluoroscopy, has a logical progression of three phases: instrumentation phase, decompression phase, and interbody phase. Creating these distinct phases of the operation allows the entire operative team to anticipate and thereby facilitate, if not expedite, each phase of the operation.

Operating Room Setup

The patient is positioned on a Jackson table that has the capacity to rotate, which will facilitate the decompression phase. Positioning the patient on the Jackson table will also optimize the capacity to restore segmental lordosis and minimize blood loss by decreasing intra-abdominal pressure. Hyperextension of the hips will also optimize capturing the maximum lumbar lordosis that can be achieved. An electrophysiologist connects the patient for neuromonitoring. The operating microscope is positioned on the side of the transforaminal approach. The fluoroscope is positioned with the image intensifier opposite the side of the microscope. It is the author's preference not to obtain fluoroscopic images at this point unless there is a significant coronal imbalance demonstrated on preoperative AP and lateral radiographs. Instead, the bony landmarks are palpated, and the L4–L5 level is approximated on the basis of the anterior superior iliac spine. However, it is commonplace in other institutions to obtain both preoperative AP and lateral fluoroscopic images before preparing and draping the patient. If the operative level is L3–L4, then the planned incisions are shifted upward; for L5–S1, the incisions are shifted downward. Two incisions 28 mm in length and 3.5–4 cm from the midline are marked (3.5 cm for patients with a low body mass index, 4 cm for a high body mass index). The patient is prepared and draped with the fluoroscope draped immediately into the field (Fig. 28.3).

Instrumentation Phase

Step One: Plan and Confirm Incisions At this point in the operation, because the incisions were planned with palpation of the bony landmarks, the level must be confirmed with fluoroscopy. A spinal needle is passed through the midpoint of the proposed incision and a fluoroscopic image taken. The incision is accordingly adjusted,

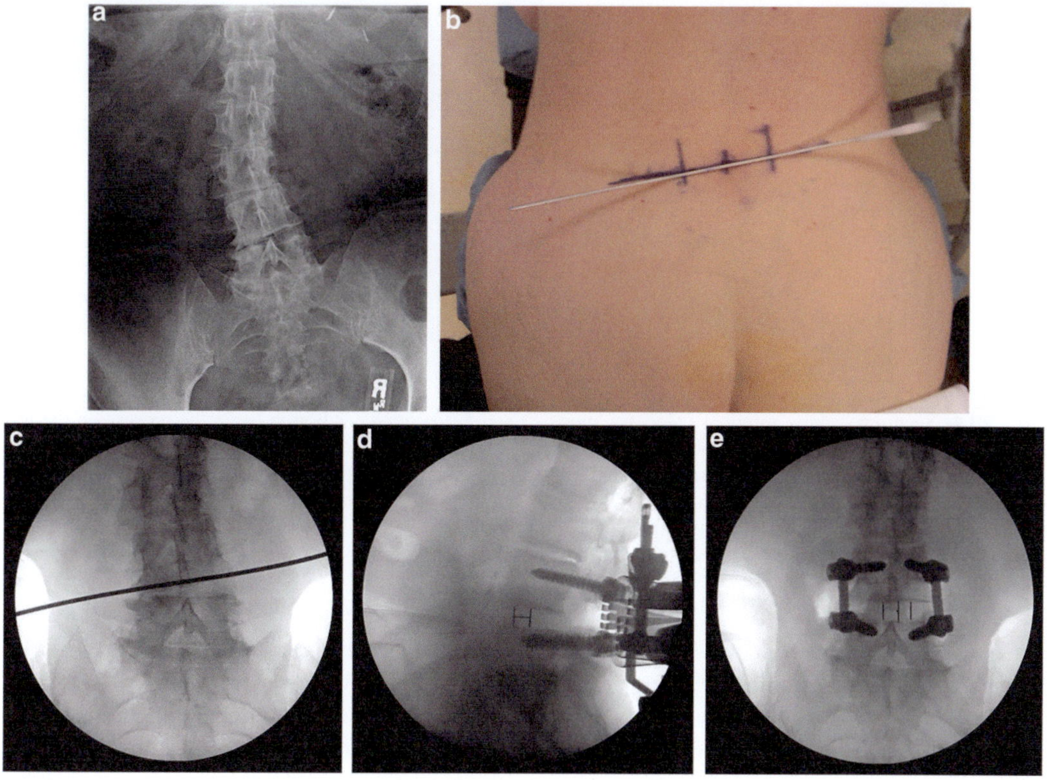

Fig. 28.2 Severe coronal imbalance requiring an L4–L5 MIS TLIF. (**a**) Anteroposterior (AP) radiograph demonstrating the severe coronal imbalance (image has been flipped to match fluoroscopic images taken at surgery). (**b**) Preoperative photograph shows a Steinmann pin placed over the operative segment to plan the incisions and adjust the fluoroscope. (**c**) AP fluoroscope image demonstrating a true lateral despite the coronal imbalance. Optimizing visualization of the pedicles with a true lateral facilitates instrumentation. (**d**) Lateral and (**e**) AP fluoroscopic images demonstrating placement of the interbody and the pedicle screws (Used with permission from Barrow Neurological Institute, Phoenix, Arizona)

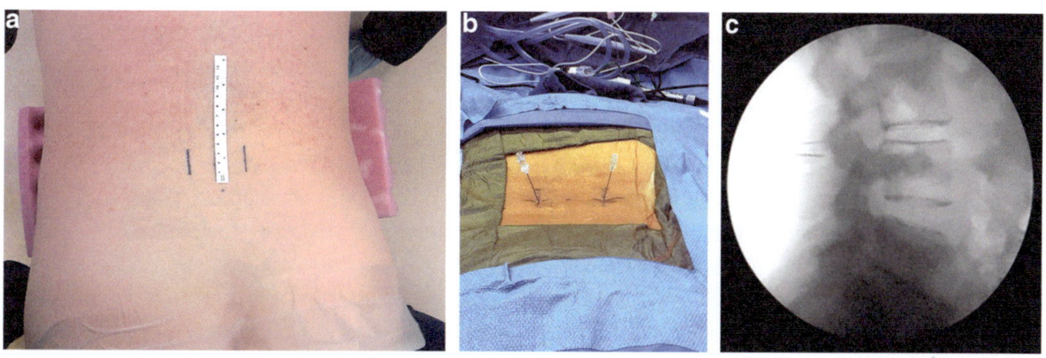

Fig. 28.3 Planning and confirmation phase of the MIS TLIF. Photographs of the planning and confirmation phase. (**a**) Photograph of the two 28-mm proposed incisions located 3.5 cm off the midline based on landmarks. (**b**) Spinal needles are docked onto the facet to confirm the level. (**c**) Lateral fluoroscopic image confirms the ideal placement of the incision parallel to the disc space (Used with permission from Barrow Neurological Institute, Phoenix, Arizona)

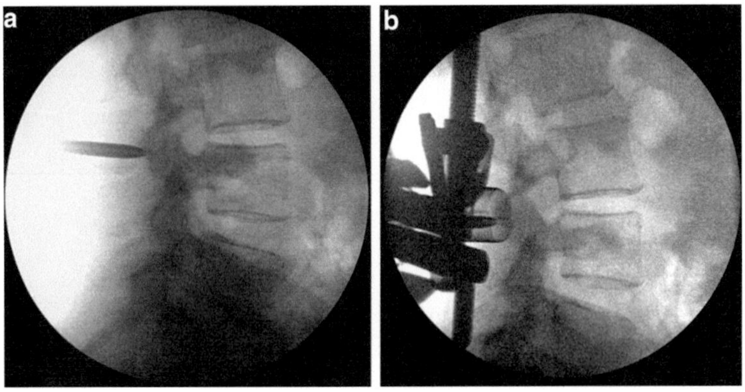

Fig. 28.4 Securing the minimal access ports. Fluoroscopic images demonstrating the securing of the minimal access ports. (**a**) Lateral fluoroscopic image demonstrating the initial dilator docked onto the L3–L4 facet joint. (**b**) Subsequent lateral fluoroscopic image with the right-sided expandable minimal access port in position and a dilator in position to begin the process on the left side. After the second minimal access port is secured, exposure of the pedicle screw entry points can begin (Used with permission from Barrow Neurological Institute, Phoenix, Arizona)

remarked, and infiltrated with a lidocaine/bupivacaine hydrochloride mixture to begin pain control. Two incisions 3.5–4 cm lateral to the midline and 28 mm long are made. Blunt dissection is used to dissect down to the fascia, which is then divided with cautery. The division of the fascia is slightly more medial than the skin incision, which will optimize a trajectory toward the pedicle. At L3–L4 and L4–L5, the fascial opening has to be more generous in the rostral direction to reach rostral pedicle screw entry points. At L5–S1, the fascial opening needs to be more generous in the caudal direction to reach the sacral pedicle screw entry point. Direct palpation of the facet and transverse processes should be easily performed before beginning the dilatation process.

Step Two: Secure Expandable Minimal Access Ports The first dilator is placed over the top of the facet on one side and confirmed with a fluoroscopic image. The ideal trajectory of the dilator is parallel to the disc space in the center of the facet (Fig. 28.4). Once the ideal position is captured, the first dilator is anchored into position and sequential dilators placed on top. As the dilators increase in diameter, they will reach a point where they will begin to engulf the entire facet. There is an unmistakable sensation of the final dilator encompassing the entire facet that does not allow for movement in any direction. There is little utility in subsequent fluoroscopic images after confirmation of the initial dilator unless the dilators are dislodged. The length of the retractor blades is determined by the measurements on the outside of the dilator and the expandable minimal access which has been secured in position. If two surgeons are operating, the process is repeated on the contralateral side. If one surgeon is operating, the exposure and the instrumentation is completed on one side before proceeding with the dilatation and exposure of the contralateral side. Upon completion of securing the minimal access ports, the fluoroscope is rolled to the foot of the bed and kept there until the exposure of the pedicle screw entry points is completed.

Step Three: Exposure of the Pedicle Screw Entry Points Any desire to open the minimal access port should be suppressed until the entire facet is exposed. Opening the blades of the minimal access port too soon can result in a compromised exposure from a wall of muscle collapsing over the anatomy. Under ideal circumstances, a thin veil of muscle is all that resides over the top of the facet; this muscle can be quickly painted away with cauterization. Once the entire facet can be visualized, exposure proceeds onto the inferior lateral aspect of the facet where the transverse process of the caudal segment will be quickly encountered. At this point, it is reasonable to begin to open the inferior blade of the expandable retractor to further visualize the pedicle screw entry point. Within the first few minutes of exposure, the caudal pedicle screw entry point should come into view.

Following the inferior articular process in the rostral direction will locate the pars interarticularis and more rostrally to the pedicle screw entry point. With exposure of the pars interarticularis, a gradual opening of the rostral blade will provide access to the transverse process and the rostral facet. It is essential to prevent any disruption of the facet capsule of the facet located above to mitigate the risk of adjacent segment degeneration. The focus for exposure of the rostral pedicle screw entry point should be the transverse process and the pars interarticularis first with the inferior lateral aspect of the facet last.

Fluoroscopy at this phase is of little utility; rather, it should not be used until the transverse process of the levels to be instrumented can be clearly visualized. The pedicle is reliably at the junction of the midpoint of the transverse process, lateral inferior facet, and pars interarticularis. When all four of these entry points can clearly be visualized, the fluoroscope is rolled back into position. The drill is then used to make a small opening at the junction of these three anatomical landmarks after confirmation with a lateral fluoroscopic image. A pedicle probe with 15–20 degrees of angulation (at L3 or L4) or 20–25 degrees of angulation (at L5 or S1) is then used to probe into the pedicle with the sagittal trajectory parallel to the superior endplate of the vertebral body.

Probing the pedicle is a purely tactile process. There is an unmistakable sensation of having the tip of the pedicle probe advance as it displaces the cancellous bone within the center of the pedicle. If significant resistance is met, it is likely that a cortical wall has been encountered. Forcing the probe at this point is a recipe for a breach. It is a worthwhile endeavor to remove the probe, evaluate the entry point, and consider an AP image. If the probe advances with a converging trajectory, it need not be advanced more than 30 mm. Most pedicle probes are graduated with markings every 5 or 10 mm. If electrophysiological monitoring is used, the pedicle probe may be stimulated to 20 mA. The generation of a compound motor action potential will mandate careful evaluation of the entry point, an AP image, and identification of the breach with a ball-tipped probe [12]. If no compound motor action potential is generated, the pedicle probe is removed, and the ball-tip probe confirms intact medial, lateral, superior, and inferior walls along with a bottom within the vertebral body. A tap is used to further prepare for the pedicle screw. Typically, the hole for the pedicle is undertapped by 1 mm (i.e., if the intention is to place a 7.5-mm-diameter screw, then a 6.5-mm tap is used). Knowing the length of the tap is also valuable in determining the length of the screw. Once the threads of the tap have been buried, a lateral fluoroscopic image can determine the ideal length of the pedicle screw to be placed (Fig. 28.5). The process described above is repeated for all pedicle screws. If two surgeons are operating, simultaneous confirmation of the pedicle screw entry points is a strategy to minimize fluoroscopy. After all the pedicles have been tapped, all four screws may be secured into position. More recent pedicle screw configurations allow for either headless screws or lower profile tulip heads, neither one of which interferes with the decompression phase. An alternative is to place guidewires to mark the pedicle screw holes.

Decompression Phase

Step One: Exposure of the Lamina and Pars Interarticularis After successful placement of the pedicle screws, the fluoroscope is now rolled to the head of the bed and the operating microscope placed into position. The base of the spinous process is exposed, along with the entire hemilamina extending out to the pars interarticularis. When all the bony anatomy can be clearly visualized from pedicle screw to pedicle screw and to the base of the spinous process, drilling of the osteotomy cuts may begin.

Step Two: Osteotomy Cuts The first osteotomy cut is a horizontal osteotomy made just below the rostral pedicle screw (Fig. 28.6). A drill is used to

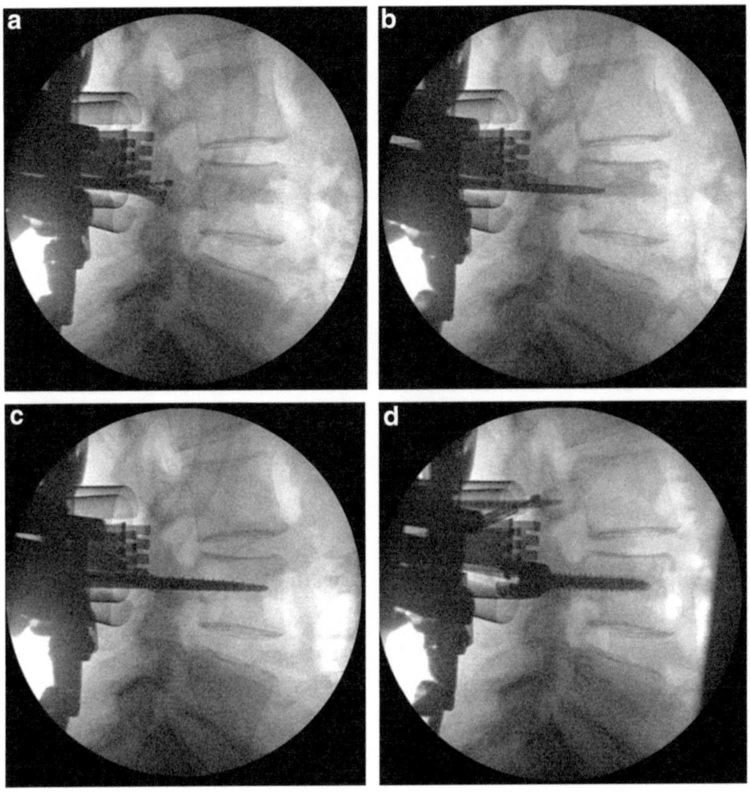

Fig. 28.5 Pedicle screw placement sequence. (**a**) Lateral fluoroscopic image with a drill at the junction of the mid-transverse process, inferior lateral facet, and pars interarticularis. (**b**) Pedicle probe with a converging trajectory of 15–20 degrees parallel to the endplate advances with the unmistakable tactile feel of displacing cancellous bone. (**c**) After the integrity of the pedicle is ensured with a ball-tipped probe, the pedicle is undertapped. The length of the tap threads determines the ideal length of the screw. (**d**) In this case, the 5.5-mm tap measured 37.5 mm and a 40-mm-long, 6.5-mm-diameter pedicle screw was placed (Used with permission from Barrow Neurological Institute, Phoenix, Arizona)

thin the bone down to the ligamentum flavum, extending the osteotomy medial into the lamina to the junction of the spinous process. The next osteotomy is a vertical osteotomy cut that undercuts the base of the spinous process so that the contralateral recess may be reached. Once again, drilling continues until the bone is thinned to the level of the ligamentum flavum. Completion of the osteotomy cuts allows for removal of the inferior articular process and lamina. Removal of this large segment of bone provides a large amount of autograft that can be milled and used for graft in the disc space. Access to the superior articular process and caudal lamina allows for an osteotomy of the superior articular process and the superior aspect of the rostral lamina. The caudal pedicle screw is a guide for the level of the osteotomy of the superior articular facet. Extending the bone work medially and caudally to the pedicle screw allows for a generous foraminotomy of the traversing root and the insertion of the ligamentum flavum for the segment.

Step Three: Resection of the Ligamentum Flavum After bony resection, the ligamentum flavum may be accessed from insertion point to insertion point. Rotating the operating table away from the surgeon is helpful in accessing the contralateral recess. A plane may be developed over the top of the thecal sac with a right-angle ball-tipped probe and a Kerrison punch used to resect the ligamentum flavum. A piecemeal approach is one way to complete the decompression. Another viable alternative is to identify the insertion

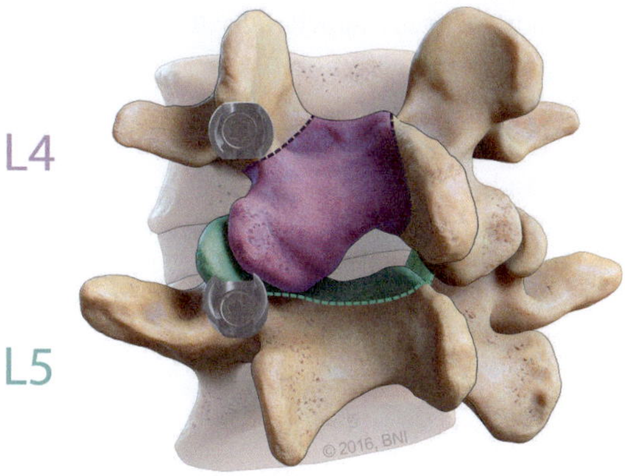

Fig. 28.6 Osteotomy cuts. Artist's illustration demonstrating the osteotomy cuts (*dashed lines*) made with the drill to disarticulate the inferior articulate process and the lamina of L4 (*purple shading*). The first osteotomy cut is made across the pars interarticularis just beneath the L4 pedicle screw. The second cut is made at the base of the spinous process, undercutting the spinous process and drilling the contralateral lamina. Upon completion of these two osteotomy cuts, the entire segment can be disarticulated. Then the superior articular process of L5 and the L5 lamina (*green shading*) is drilled and disarticulated, offering a generous transforaminal corridor into the disc space (Used with permission from Barrow Neurological Institute, Phoenix, Arizona)

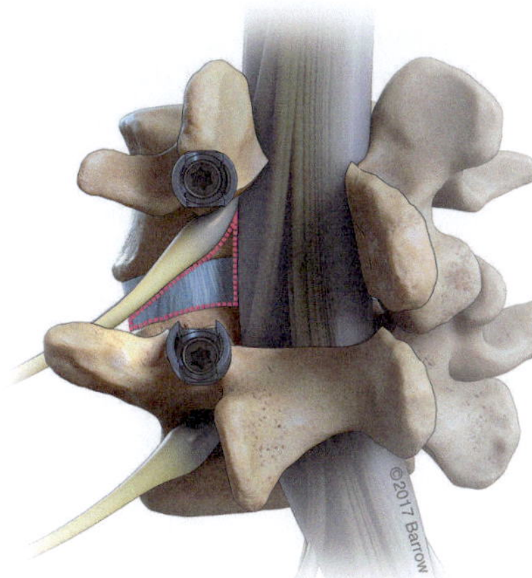

Fig. 28.7 Expanded Kambin's triangle for MIS TLIF. Artist's illustration depicts the triangle (*dashed line*) formed by the exiting root, the traversing root, and the superior endplate of the caudal vertebral body. Completion of the laminectomy and facetectomy creates the transforaminal corridor into the disc space. Kambin's triangle is classically defined by the boundaries of the superior endplate of the inferior vertebral body, the lateral aspect of the superior articulating facet, and the exiting superior nerve root (Used with permission from Barrow Neurological Institute, Phoenix, Arizona)

points of the ligamentum flavum and resect those insertion points with a Kerrison rongeur. An en bloc resection of the ligamentum flavum then becomes possible and ensures a widely decompressed thecal sac and nerve roots. Typically, some ligamentum remains over the exiting nerve root, which is resected to clearly visualize the location of the exiting nerve root. Completing that exposure ensures that the boundaries of an expanded Kambin's triangle may be clearly delineated (Fig. 28.7). The medial aspect of the Kambin's triangle (the height) is classically defined by the lateral aspect of the superior articular process [13]. However, in a transforaminal approach, the entire facet (along with the lamina and pars interarticularis) has been removed, which moves the medial aspect of Kambin's triangle to the lateral aspect of the dural edge and the traversing root. The expanded Kambin's triangle is a more relevant anatomical triangle to define the transforaminal corridor.

The resection of the ligamentum flavum allows for ready access to the disc space. Little, if any, retraction of the traversing or exiting nerve root is needed to access the disc space at this point. A complex venous network is typically found in the vicinity of the pedicle and overlying the disc space. It is worthwhile to cauterize that venous network before incising the disc space.

Step Four: Discectomy After completion of the preemptive cauterization of the epidural veins in the vicinity of the pedicle and disc space, a No. 11 blade on a bayoneted knife handle is used to perform a generous annulotomy. Large Kerrison rongeurs may be used to enlarge the annulotomy as far medial and as far lateral as the exposure will allow. A series of downward-angled curettes, straight curettes, and straight and forward-angled pituitary rongeurs are used to remove the disc material. In many cases, there is a far-lateral component to the disc extrusion that will require removal. Inspection around and under the exiting nerve root identifies disc material that may have migrated into the axilla or under the nerve root. Paddle distractors are inserted into the disc space and used to restore disc height, facilitating preparation of the endplates. The goals of the discectomy are to remove as much of the disc material as possible, to remove the cartilaginous endplate, and to prepare a bleeding cortical endplate without violating it. Concern about violating the cortical endplate has prompted the author to avoid cutting interbody paddles and to use only blunt paddles to restore height. It is important to note that this is the author's preference and that some surgeons routinely use shavers as part of their disc preparation.

After 15 min of dedicated disc removal and endplate preparation, a point of diminishing returns is reached. If less than that amount of time is spent, the surgeon may not have optimized the environment for fusion. Spending more than that amount of time may not offer any more advantage toward achieving arthrodesis.

Interbody Phase

Step One: Ensure a Complete Discectomy The operating microscope is rolled out, the fluoroscope is rolled back in, and the bed is rotated to the neutral position. Angled interbody curettes are then used to ensure that the disc space has been optimally prepared. These curettes are graduated and their placement within the interbody should easily reveal the capacity to reach 40 mm across the disc space, which is compatible with rotating a large interbody spacer into the disc space. If there is any resistance in passing the angled interbody curette to 40 mm, it is wise to continue to work within the disc space to prepare it. That additional investment in time will pay immediate dividends when the interbody spacer is placed.

Step Two: Interbody Trials The size of the last paddle distractor should be the size of the first interbody trial placed into the disc space. Typically, the dimensions of Kambin's triangle allow for the trial to be placed without the need for retraction of either the exiting or traversing root. The tip of the trial is placed into the annulotomy, and the trajectory is set by obtaining a lateral fluoroscopic image (Fig. 28.8). The interbody is then tapped into the disc space. Sizing the interbody space by tactile feel is purely subjective. The trialing should continue until the interbody trial wedges into the disc space and requires a slap hammer to remove. Such a fit will result in an ideally sized interbody spacer that has an exceedingly low likelihood of migration and high likelihood of achieving an arthrodesis. If the trial can be dislodged without a slap hammer, the interbody is too small, which may lead to pseudarthrosis or migration of the interbody.

Step Three: Placement of the Interbody With the size of the interbody selected, morcellized bone graft is packed into the disc space through a funnel. It is important not to overpack the disc space in a manner that will affect placement of the interbody. A down-sloping interbody curette can be used to distribute the graft into the anterior third of the disc space.

The preference of the author is to use a curved interbody spacer that is rotated into the disc space to occupy as much surface area as possible and engage the apophyseal ring. The largest interbody spacers currently available are 36 mm in length, which when rotated into the disc space will occupy that same dimension in width.

Similar to the trialing process, the tip of the interbody is placed into the annulotomy, and a lateral fluoroscopic image is taken to confirm an ideal trajectory into the disc space (Fig. 28.9). The interbody is inserted with an oblique trajectory across the disc space parallel to the endplates. Once the posterior aspect of the interbody has cleared the posterior margin of the disc space, the rotation of the interbody can begin. The interbody is rotated and advanced until it reaches the anterior half of the disc space. When a final AP fluoroscopic image demonstrates that the interbody is well centered in the disc space, the rods may be placed onto the tulip heads of the pedicle screws and the construct compressed. Once satisfied with the position of the implant and the lordosis, the set screws are tightened according to the manufacturer's recommendations (Fig. 28.9).

Compression of the pedicle screws on the rod achieves two key objectives: restoration of seg-

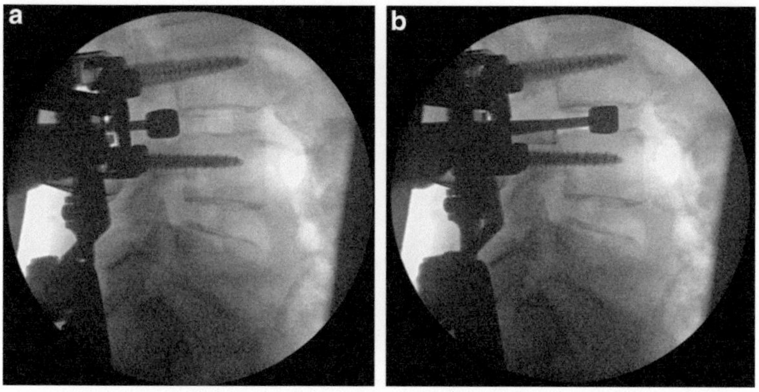

Fig. 28.8 Trialing the interbody. (**a**) Lateral fluoroscopic image demonstrating placement of the interbody into the annulotomy and establishing the ideal trajectory into the disc space. (**b**) The ideal-sized trial wedge, once it is moved into position, requires the use of a slap hammer to remove. When this criterion has been met, the interbody can be placed (Used with permission from Barrow Neurological Institute, Phoenix, Arizona)

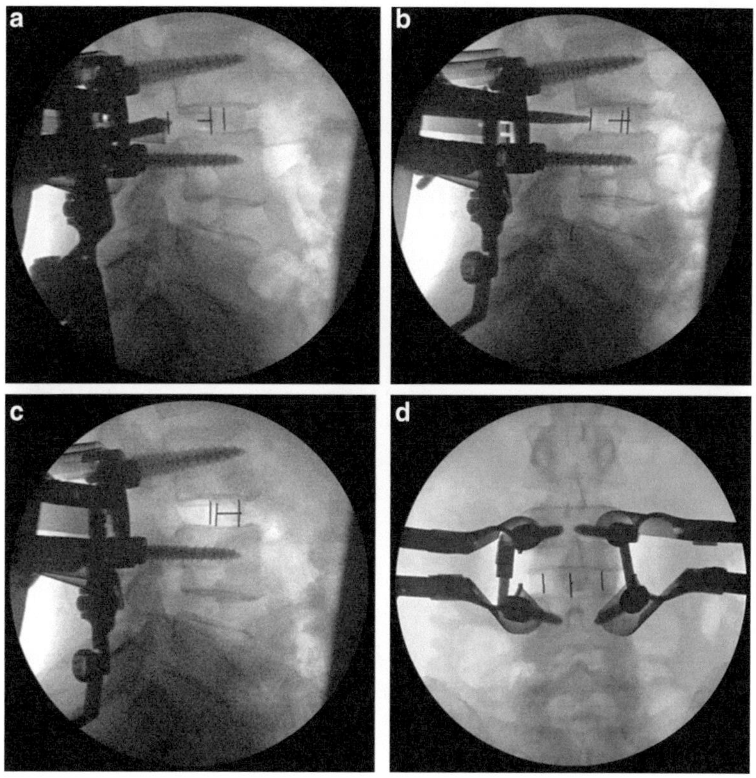

Fig. 28.9 Fluoroscopy sequence of curved interbody spacer placement. (**a**) Lateral fluoroscopic image demonstrating initial insertion of the interbody in an oblique trajectory into the disc space. (**b**) After the spacer has cleared the posterior margin of the disc space, rotation of the interbody begins. (**c**) The interbody is rotated into position to occupy the anterior half of the disc space. (**d**) AP image with the interbody in the geometric center of the disc space (Used with permission from Barrow Neurological Institute, Phoenix, Arizona)

mental lordosis and loading of the interbody spacer. It is important when performing TLIF to avoid loss of lumbar lordosis [9]. This is avoided by placing the largest interbody that is appropriate for the interbody space in the anterior half of the disc space under compression preventing the loss of lordosis identified in the literature. Also, compression loads the interbody spacer, reducing the risk of migration. Migration of the interbody is a complication that is often described in the literature; it is prevented by optimizing the interbody graft endplate interface [14]. Compression

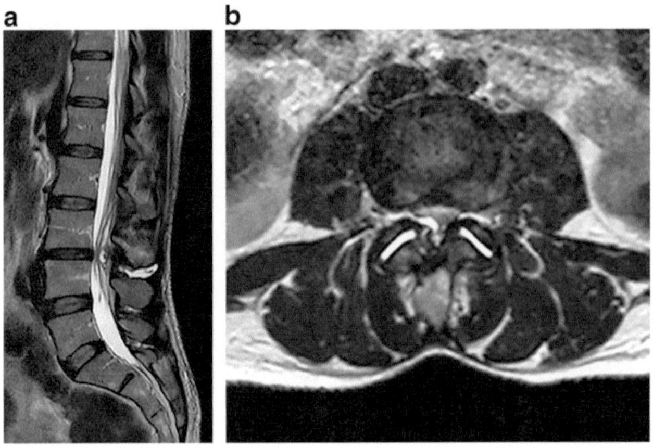

Fig. 28.10 L3–L4 facet cyst and degenerative disc disease. (**a**) Sagittal T2-weighted MR image demonstrating disruption of the interspinous process ligament. The increased signal intensity between the spinous processes suggests instability of the segment that would be confirmed on flexion-extension studies. The facet cyst causing central stenosis can be seen. (**b**) Axial T2-weighted MR image revealing the facet cyst to the right, resulting in compression of the traversing nerve root of L4. There is increased signal within the facet joints bilaterally (Used with permission from Barrow Neurological Institute, Phoenix, Arizona)

loads the bone graft against the endplates, thereby optimizing an environment for fusion by embracing the principles of Wolff's law.

Illustrative Case

History

A 48-year-old woman presented with progressive, worsening axial back pain and radicular right-leg pain.

Physical Examination

On examination, the patient demonstrated absence of a right patellar reflex and 4−/5 strength of the right quadriceps.

Radiographic Imaging

MR imaging of the lumbar spine demonstrated disruption of the interspinous process ligament, widened facets, and a facet cyst compressing the traversing nerve root of L4 (Fig. 28.10). Flexion-extension studies revealed instability of the segment (Fig. 28.11). At the time of presentation, her Oswestry Disability Index score was 43, her VAS pain score for the leg was 8, and her VAS pain score for the back was 5.

Treatment

The patient was taken for an L3–L4 MIS TLIF with a right transforaminal approach. With the patient positioned on a Jackson table, two incisions were planned 3.5 cm from midline over the L3–L4 segment. After the level was confirmed with a lateral fluoroscopic image, the incisions were made, and cautery was used to divide the fascia. Sequential dilatation was performed over the L3–L4 facets on the left and right sides. Pedicle screw entry points were directly exposed, and the pedicles were instrumented as described above. Under the operating microscope, a drill was used to undercut the spinous process at the junction of the lamina and spinous process. Another osteotomy cut was made just inferior to the L3 pedicle screw, extending to the base of the spinous process. After both of these osteotomy cuts, the inferior articular process and lamina were dissected from the ligamentum flavum and removed. The superior articular process of L4 was then removed. The L4 nerve root and thecal sac were decompressed completely with resection of

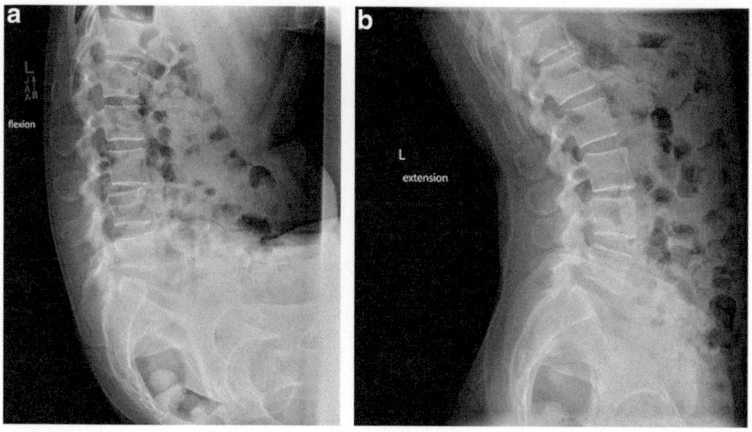

Fig. 28.11 Flexion and extension radiographs. (**a**) The lateral flexion study demonstrates not only the anterior translation of the L3 vertebral body on L4 but also bone-on-bone contact of the inferior aspect of the L3 on the superior aspect of L4 at the anterior aspect of the disc space. (**b**) The lateral extension study demonstrates anatomical alignment of the L3 and L4 vertebral bodies. Degeneration of the disc space is demonstrated by the degree of collapse relative to the segments above and below (Used with permission from Barrow Neurological Institute, Phoenix, Arizona)

the ligamentum flavum and the facet cyst. The L3 nerve root was then exposed with resection of the lateral ligamentum flavum.

A complete discectomy was performed, the cartilaginous endplate was removed, and the cortical endplate was prepared. A 12 × 36-mm interbody spacer with autograft and allograft was rotated into the midline of the disc space, and rods were placed atop the tulip heads of the pedicle screws. Compression restored the segmental lordosis and the set screws were tightened. The access ports were removed and the incisions closed.

Outcome

The patient was discharged the following morning with some incisional discomfort, but with complete resolution of her right radicular leg pain. After 1 month, the patient returned to work and was off all narcotic pain medication with a weight-carrying restriction of 25 pounds. By the second postoperative month, she was at work without restrictions or limitations. At her 6-month postoperative follow-up, her Oswestry Disability Index score was 11, and her postoperative VAS pain scores for leg and back were 0 and 2, respectively. At 1-year follow-up, the patient demonstrated radiographic evidence of interbody fusion (Fig. 28.12).

Technical Pearls

Instrumentation Phase

- Fluoroscopy: You may feel tempted to rely more on fluoroscopy than on direct visualization to determine a pedicle screw entry point. Such reliance will increase radiation exposure during this procedure without increasing the accuracy of pedicle screw placement. The advantage of a mini-open approach is that it allows direct visualization of the pedicle screw entry point. Percutaneous placement of pedicle screws mandates fluoroscopy at every step. Direct visualization of the anatomy does not. The mentality for fluoroscopy in a mini-open approach should be to confirm the entry point that you have already determined to be ideal for a pedicle screw. After the junction of the pars interarticularis, inferior lateral facet, and transverse process has been unequivocally visualized, the use of fluoroscopy should be reserved only for con-

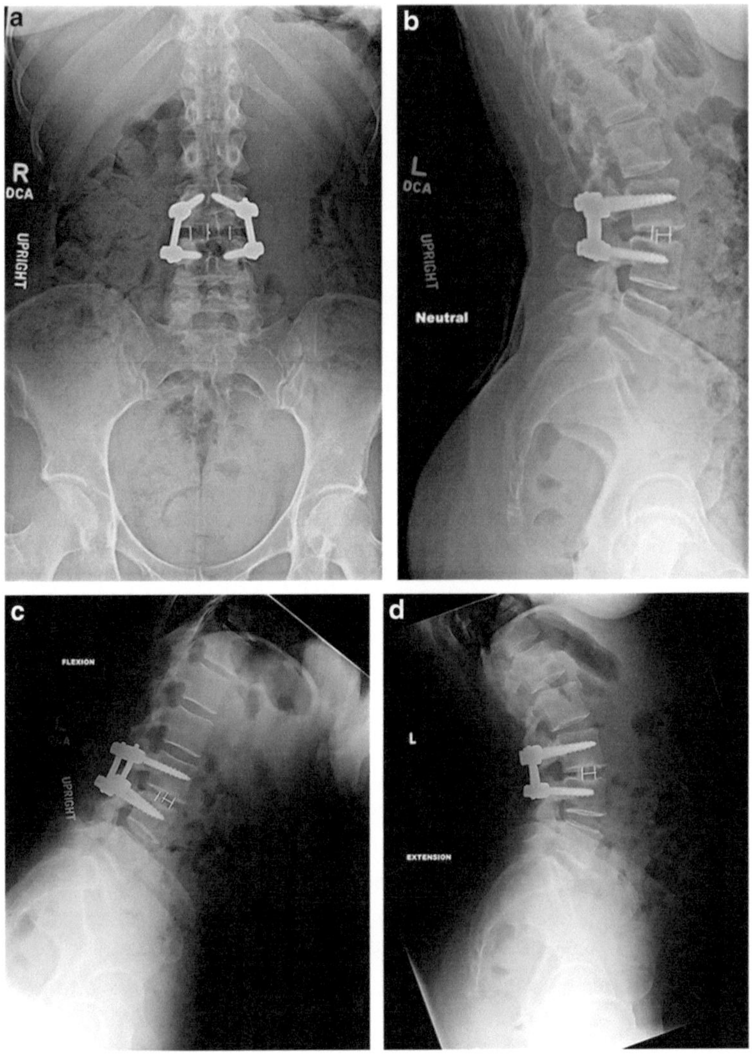

Fig. 28.12 Postoperative radiographs at 1-year follow-up. (**a**) AP radiograph demonstrating a well-centered interbody spacer and converging pedicle screws. (**b**) Lateral neutral radiograph demonstrating restoration of the lumbar lordosis and disc height compared to preoperative studies. Lateral radiographs (**c**, flexion; **d**, extension) demonstrating the absence of motion of the vertebral bodies and the stability of the segment. Arthrodesis can be appreciated immediately behind the interbody spacer and within the spacer (Used with permission from Barrow Neurological Institute, Phoenix, Arizona)

firming the entry point itself. The emphasis should be on exposing the anatomy.

- Pedicle probing: Probing the pedicle is a purely tactile feedback process. Use of a mallet completely eliminates that feedback loop. A mallet will easily force the tip of the pedicle probe through a cortical wall, resulting in a breach. Resist any urge to ask for a mallet when encountering resistance while probing a pedicle. Instead, when resistance is encountered, begin softly probing less medially or more medially until the tip of the pedicle probe finds its way into the unmistakable trove of cancellous bone.
- Tapping and placing pedicle screws: Use the minimal access port as a reference point; specifically, register the position of the pedicle probe within the port. That position will be the same for the tap and the pedicle screw. Incorporating the relative position within the port will further decrease the need for fluoroscopy and will increase the efficiency of the procedure.

Decompression Phase

- Maintain the ligamentum flavum intact for as long as possible. Instead of a piecemeal resection, strive for an en bloc resection. Such an approach mitigates the risk of a cerebrospinal fluid leak and minimizes the action of the Kerrison rongeur.

- Extending the bone work caudally to the caudal pedicle screw into the lamina below achieves comprehensive foraminotomy and exposes the insertion of the ligamentum flavum.
- Conjoined root: Removal of the facet, lamina, and ligamentum flavum reveals an unmistakable continuation of the dura between the exiting and traversing root. The dura drapes over the entire disc space. When such an anatomical circumstance is encountered, it is no longer feasible to access the disc space, and placement of an interbody through that corridor is not an option. Such an anatomical circumstance is not common, but it is important to recognize. The author has encountered this situation on only three occasions in more than 500 TLIFs. At this point, there are two options. The first is to proceed to the contralateral facet and expose the disc space on that side to determine whether a viable transforaminal corridor will allow access to the disc space. The second option is to proceed with a posterolateral fusion. In reality, the access and visibility for a posterolateral fusion are far superior with a paramedian mini-open approach. The absence of an interbody means that the arthrodesis will rely entirely on the posterolateral fusion. Meticulous bilateral exposure of the entire transverse process of the rostral and caudal vertebrae, along with decortication of the entire posterior face of the transverse process with generous amounts of morcellized bone graft spanning from transverse process to transverse process, will optimize an environment for arthrodesis, despite the absence of an interbody.

Interbody Phase

- Always create the most generous annulotomy that the Kambin's triangle will allow before beginning the trialing process. Opening the annulotomy with a 4-mm Kerrison rongeur medially up to the lateral aspect of the thecal sac and laterally at least to the midpedicular line will vastly facilitate access to the disc space and placement of the interbody.
- Removing the posterior scallop of the disc space with either a box-cutting chisel or a standard osteotome will facilitate placement of the ideal interbody that will address the mismatch in height at the center of the disc space and the posterior margin of the disc space. A No. 4 Kerrison rongeur can also be used to level out the scallop.

Complications and Strategies for Avoidance

Complications may arise at three distinct intervals in this type of operation: surgical phase, early postoperative phase, and late postoperative phase.

Surgical

Cerebrospinal fluid leak, errant placement of instrumentation, and suboptimal decompression are the three leading complications that can occur during surgery. The risk of a cerebrospinal fluid leak can be mitigated by performing the instrumentation first, which prevents the need for wielding sharp instruments, such as a tap, with the neural elements exposed. When instrumentation is performed before the decompression, the neural elements are kept safe by the bony elements. Furthermore, accomplishing as much of the bone work as possible while keeping the ligamentum flavum intact prevents an errant pass of an instrument or drill. In that manner, the neural elements are protected by the ligamentum flavum until it becomes time for the decompression with the resection of the ligamentum. Every effort should be made to complete all drilling before exposure of the neural elements.

A suboptimal decompression results in a symptomatic patient immediately after surgery. It is rarely necessary to perform bilateral decompression, to include bilateral facetectomies, in order to adequately address the extent of compression of the neural elements. However, bilateral decompression may be necessary in patients who have bilateral facet arthropathy resulting in bilateral severe foraminal narrowing. Such a complication may be avoided by detailed history taking, examination, and careful review of the T1-weighted parasagittal MR images.

Early Postoperative Phase

The most common early postoperative phase complication is migration of the interbody graft [14], which may occur for two reasons. First, an undersized graft may have been placed at the time of surgery; second, violation of the cortical endplate may have occurred. It is vital to sense a firm placement of the interbody trial. As noted previously, it should require a slap hammer to dislodge the trial from its position before considering the height to be appropriate. A curved interbody rotated into position is much less likely to migrate, especially under compression. The action of compression further engages the graft endplate interface. Bullet-shaped grafts may extrude along the same path they were inserted. A curved graft rotated into position is much less likely to do so.

Late Postoperative Phase

Pseudarthrosis and adjacent-level degeneration are late complications of this procedure. Pseudarthrosis and migration of the graft go hand in hand. Thus, the measures to mitigate the risk of graft migration or extrusion are the same measures needed to prevent pseudarthrosis. However, pseudarthrosis may occur in a well-positioned interbody graft that has not migrated. In those circumstances, the cartilaginous endplate was likely not completely removed from either the inferior or superior endplate or both. In that case, the interbody is wedged between two sheets of cartilaginous endplate that will reliably block bone growth. The preparation of the endplate is done by tactile feel, but it also has a visual component. Although direct visualization of the endplate is difficult, in the process of removing the disc material and preparing the endplate, you may appreciate entire sheets of the cartilaginous endplates coming out of the disc space. With regard to the tactile feel, you should have the unmistakable feel of rasping against cortical endplate as compared to cartilaginous endplate. The endplate preparation phase should never be rushed. Time invested in this phase of the operation will mitigate the risk of this late complication.

Finally, adjacent segment degeneration may be difficult to avoid altogether because it is an element of the natural history of lumbar disc degeneration. However, certain measures can be taken to mitigate that risk. Minimizing the extent of exposure is the first measure. The advantage of a minimally invasive approach is the capacity to perform a procedure without the wide exposures that weaken muscle and cause inadvertent injury to surrounding structures. The second measure is respecting the integrity of the facet capsule at the rostral level. While it is essential to expose the inferior and lateral aspects of the rostral facet to visualize the pedicle screw entry point, that exposure does not require violating the facet capsule. Beginning on the transverse process and working laterally to medially are the surest ways to prevent inadvertent disruption of the facet capsule.

Conclusion

The capacity to reliably and efficiently perform an MIS TLIF results from the culmination of skills developed through minimally invasive microdiscectomies and laminectomies. It is a difficult operation to embark upon without that minimally invasive skill set. However, once facility has been achieved with bayoneted instruments and minimally invasive techniques, the paramedian approach is actually more efficient. The direct approach to the facet allows for easier access to the anatomy for instrumentation and decompression, with less blood loss, less postoperative discomfort, and shorter hospital stays. The investment in overcoming the learning curve pays immediate dividends in the management of degenerative processes of the lumbar spine.

References

1. Foley KT, Smith MM. Microendoscopic discectomy. Tech. Neurosurg. 1997;3(4): 301–7
2. Cloward RB. The degenerated lumbar disc: treatment by vertebral body fusion. J Int Coll Surg. 1954;22(4 Sect. 1):375–86. Epub 1954/10/01
3. Harms J, Jeszenszky D. The unilateral, transforaminal approach for posterior lumbar interbody fusion. Orhtopaedics and Traumatology. 1998;6(2):88–99.
4. Foley KT, Holly LT, Schwender JD. Minimally invasive lumbar fusion. Spine. 2003;28(15 Suppl):S26–35. Epub 2003/08/05
5. Isaacs RE, Podichetty VK, Santiago P, Sandhu FA, Spears J, Kelly K, et al. Minimally invasive microendoscopy-assisted transforaminal lumbar interbody fusion with instrumentation. J Neurosurg Spine. 2005;3(2):98–105. Epub 2005/12/24
6. Holly LT, Schwender JD, Rouben DP, Foley KT. Minimally invasive transforaminal lumbar interbody fusion: indications, technique, and complications. Neurosurg Focus. 2006;20(3):E6. Epub 2006/04/08
7. O'Toole JE, Eichholz KM, Fessler RG. Surgical site infection rates after minimally invasive spinal surgery. J Neurosurg Spine. 2009;11(4):471–6. Epub 2009/11/26
8. Rampersaud YR, Foley KT, Shen AC, Williams S, Solomito M. Radiation exposure to the spine surgeon during fluoroscopically assisted pedicle screw insertion. Spine. 2000;25(20):2637–45. Epub 2000/10/18
9. Hsieh PC, Koski TR, O'Shaughnessy BA, Sugrue P, Salehi S, Ondra S, et al. Anterior lumbar interbody fusion in comparison with transforaminal lumbar interbody fusion: implications for the restoration of foraminal height, local disc angle, lumbar lordosis, and sagittal balance. J Neurosurg Spine. 2007;7(4):379–86. Epub 2007/10/16
10. Mummaneni PV, Rodts GE Jr. The mini-open transforaminal lumbar interbody fusion. Neurosurgery. 2005;57(4 Suppl):256–61. discussion -61. Epub 2005/10/20
11. Wong AP, Smith ZA, Nixon AT, Lawton CD, Dahdaleh NS, Wong RH, et al. Intraoperative and perioperative complications in minimally invasive transforaminal lumbar interbody fusion: a review of 513 patients. J Neurosurg Spine. 2015;22(5):487–95. Epub 2015/02/24
12. Raynor BL, Lenke LG, Bridwell KH, Taylor BA, Padberg AM. Correlation between low triggered electromyographic thresholds and lumbar pedicle screw malposition: analysis of 4857 screws. Spine. 2007;32(24):2673–8. Epub 2007/11/17
13. Hoshide R, Feldman E, Taylor W. Cadaveric analysis of the Kambin's triangle. Cureus. 2016;8(2):e475. Epub 2016/03/24
14. Bakhsheshian J, Khanna R, Choy W, Lawton CD, Nixon AT, Wong AP, et al. Incidence of graft extrusion following minimally invasive transforaminal lumbar interbody fusion. J Clin Neurosci. 2016;24:88–93. Epub 2015/11/19

Cortical Bone Screw Fixation

29

Mark Benjamin Frenkel, J.J. Renfrow, and Charles L. Branch Jr.

Introduction

The cortical bone trajectory (CBT) for lumbar pedicle screws was first reported in 2009 by Santoni et al. [1] as an alternative to traditional, medially directed pedicle screws. Screws placed using this trajectory, which has a starting point in the pars interarticularis and is more laterally and cranially oriented than traditional trajectory pedicle screws (TTS) (Fig. 29.1), have come to be referred to as cortical bone trajectory screws or cortical screws (CS). There are numerous benefits to cortical screws compared to pedicle screws, including less muscle dissection, stronger pullout strength, and less risk to neural elements. In this chapter, we discuss the available clinical and biomechanical literature pertaining to cortical screws and indications for their use and review the surgical technique of placing cortical screws in the setting of a midline lumbar fusion.

As a result of the more medial starting point of the cortical screw trajectory, the tulip head of the screw is more medially seated than pedicle screws. This more medially seated head requires less lateral exposure for placement than pedicle screws and thus can be performed through a smaller midline incision with less muscular dissection (Fig. 29.2). One radiographic study compared the fat infiltration ratio, which correlates with muscle damage, of the multifidus muscles at 18-month follow-up in 16 patients who underwent posterior lumbar interbody fusion (PLIF) with cortical screws compared with patients who underwent PLIF with pedicle screws. Hung found that the smaller dissection afforded by the cortical screws induced significantly less multifidus muscle damage which could theoretically help to prevent the development of adjacent-level disease [2]. The less invasive properties of cortical screws could theoretically decrease postoperative pain, shorten operative duration, and minimize blood loss, and these outcome measures remain ripe for future study.

In both healthy and osteoporotic patients, the subcortical and cortical bone of the pedicle is more dense than the trabecular bone of the vertebral body with the greatest fixation being more dependent on its purchase in this denser bone [3]. The cortical bone trajectory was specifically designed to maximally purchase the higher density cortical bone of the pedicle [1] (Fig. 29.3). A radiographic study examining the density of bone along cortical screws and pedicle screws pathways in 180 randomly selected patients found that the cortical screw pathway had a statistically significantly greater bone density at fixation points compared to those along a traditional trajectory [4].

M.B. Frenkel • J.J. Renfrow • C.L. Branch Jr. (✉)
Department of Neurosurgery, Wake Forest Baptist Medical Center, One Medical Center Blvd, Winston Salem, NC 27157, USA
e-mail: mfrenkel@wakehealth.edu; jrenfrow@wakehealth.edu; cbranch@wakehealth.edu

L.T. Holly, P.A. Anderson (eds.), *Essentials of Spinal Stabilization*,
DOI 10.1007/978-3-319-59713-3_29

Numerous biomechanical studies have demonstrated benefits of this enhanced cortical purchase. Several investigators have instrumented cadaveric lumbar vertebrae with pedicle screws in one pedicle and cortical screws in the contralateral pedicle before subjecting both screws to biomechanical testing. Santoni found that cortical screws had a 30% increase in uniaxial yield pullout load and no significant difference in construct stiffness compared to traditional pedicle screws [1]. İnceoğlu found a statistically significant increase in pullout strength of cortical screws compared with pedicle screws; however, cortical screws had less tangential stiffness compared to the pedicle screws [5]. Cyclical toggling of the screws at increasing physiologic loads has demonstrated significantly increased resistance to toggling for the cortical screw [6]. It has been proposed that this high toggling resistance may be attributable to the angle of the cortical screw providing purchase of the thick cortical bone of both the inferior and superior pedicle isthmus [7]. In regard to multilevel constructs, Cheng in one cadaveric study demonstrated equivalence of cortical screws with pedicle screws in stabilization of multilevel low-grade spondylolisthesis models [7].

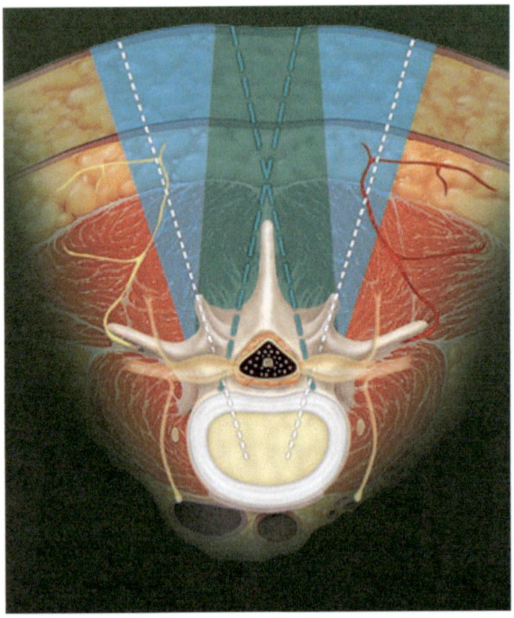

Fig. 29.1 Width of exposure needed for placement of cortical trajectory screws (*green tissue*) compared to traditional trajectory pedicle screws (*blue tissue*). *Dashed blue lines* represent the approach trajectory for cortical screws, while *dashed white lines* represent the same for traditional trajectory pedicle screws (Courtesy Medtronic)

Another cadaveric study compared pedicle screws and cortical screw rod fixation in specimens with intact intervertebral disc, transforaminal lumbar interbody fusion (TLIF) support, or direct lateral interbody fusion (DLIF) support. The authors found that the cortical screw group had comparable stability in flexion/extension and lateral bending when an intact disc was present but the pedicle screw group was stiffer during axial rotation. There was no difference in stability with DLIF. In the TLIF group, they found that the pedicle screw fixation was stiffer than cortical screw fixation during lateral bending [8]. A separate finite element analysis also reported similar results, with cortical screws having greater pullout strength and superior resistance to flexion/extension loading but inferior resistance to lateral

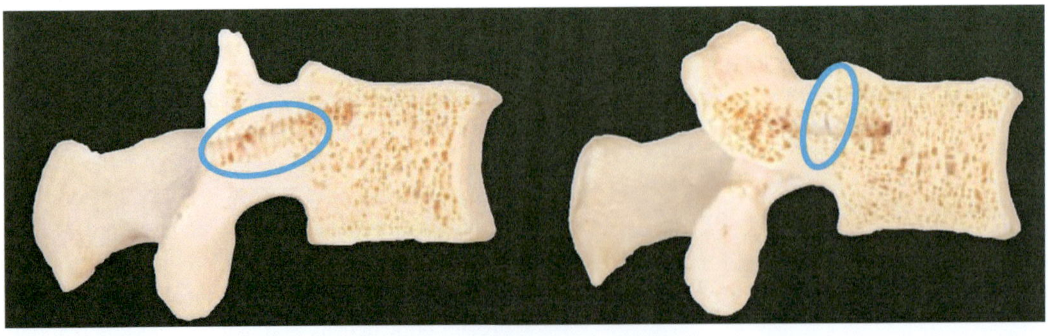

Fig. 29.2 Cross sections of cadaveric vertebrae previously instrumented with cortical trajectory screws (*left*) and traditional trajectory pedicle screws (*right*). The *blue circle* indicates the amount of cortical bone encountered along each trajectory (Courtesy Medtronic)

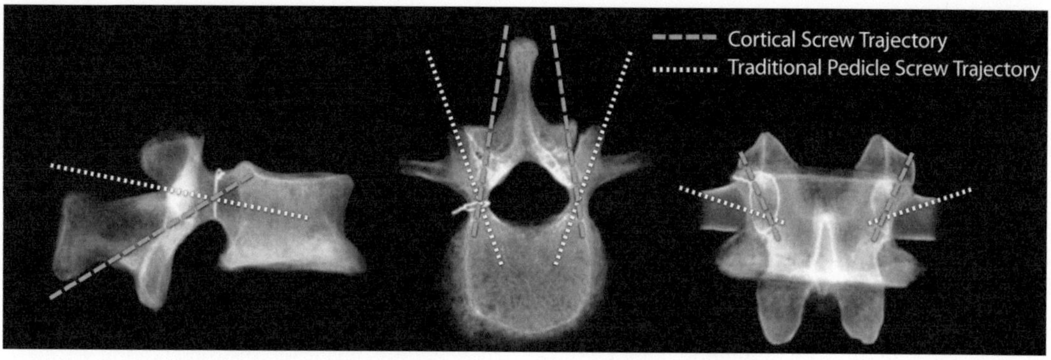

Fig. 29.3 Lateral (*left*), superoinferior (*middle*), and anteroposterior (*right*) fluoroscopic views of a cadaveric lumbar vertebra with the trajectories of cortical (*green line*) and traditional pedicle screws (*dashed white line*) overlaid. Note that the trajectory of the cortical screws has a more medial insertion point compared to the traditional pedicle screw trajectory, as well as a medial to lateral and caudal to rostral trajectory (Courtesy Medtronic)

bending and axial rotation compared to pedicle screws [9].

In addition, an in vivo biomechanical study comparing pedicle screws and cortical screws was performed by measuring the insertional torque during screw placement in 48 consecutive patients. Matsukawa found that the insertional torque of cortical screws was about 1.7 times higher than pedicle screws [10].

Aside from increased cortical purchase, several other benefits of the medial to lateral and caudal to cephalad cortical screw trajectory have been reported. A retrospective study of 202 patients who underwent cortical screw placement found the incidence of adjacent cranial facet joint violation by the screw, a phenomenon which can contribute to the development of adjacent level disease, to be lower than or comparable to most historical reports of open or percutaneous pedicle screw placement [11]. Matsukawa et al. have suggested that this unique trajectory may result in a lower rate of damage to neural elements, as a misplaced screw would be less likely to breach medially or inferiorly and injure the thecal sac or exiting nerve root [12].

With regard to clinical outcomes, the largest published series of patients who underwent lumbar fusion with cortical screws included 79 patients at a single institution with mean follow-up of 13 months. Snyder reported only one case of screw loosening, two cases of pseudoarthrosis, and one case of graft migration in the entire population. They had no complications caused by misplaced screws in any patients [13]. A retrospective study of ten TLIFs performed with cortical screws reported less intraoperative blood loss compared with similar cohorts of patients who underwent TLIFs with pedicle screws placed either via the Wiltse or percutaneous approach. Kasukawa also reported good outcomes at a mean follow-up of 11.4 months with no evidence of hardware loosening and fusion rates comparable to the other groups [14]. Lee performed the first prospective randomized trial comparing 40 cortical screw patients to 39 pedicle screw patients in single-level PLIF patients who had minimum 12-month follow-up. The authors found similar fusion rates and improvement in pain and functional status between the two groups. They also observed shorter operative time, incision length, and less blood loss in the cortical screw group [15]. These findings are also consistent with a number of other published case reports [16–18].

One early report of clinical outcomes had less than desirable results, with five of eight patients demonstrating evidence of screw loosening and two requiring revision within 1 year [19]. More recently, Cheng experienced a unique intraoperative pars fracture while placing cortical screws in 2 of 22 patients, one of which was not discovered until the patient subsequently developed complications from screw loosening. The fracture spanned from the screw insertion point on the lateral border of the pars through the superior facet and into the lateral aspect of the pedicle. The authors performed a cadaveric study and attempted to reproduce the fracture while video recording their screw insertion. They were successful and discovered that during final screw placement, the head of the screw impinged medially against the lamina and base of the spinous process, suddenly deviating the screw trajectory. The authors attributed the prior group's high rate of loosening to this phenomenon and recommended leaving the screw proud to avoid hubbing, as well as performing laminectomy before final screw insertion to attempt to avoid this phenomenon [20]. Similar concerns over the head of the screw resting on the junction of the spinous process and lamina were voiced by Akpolat et al. [21] who were unable to fully insert some screws because of fear of damage to the lamina or pars.

As a consequence of the shorter trajectory and increased cortical purchase of cortical screws compared to pedicle screws, specialized screws have been developed for use along this trajectory. These cortical bone screws (CBS) differ from traditional pedicle screws in that they have a shorter distance between threads (narrower pitch) and smaller ratio of inner to outer diameter [5]. A cadaveric study investigated the differences in pullout strength in both a traditional and cortical bone trajectory when using two screws which were similar except for thread pitch. They found that while the narrower pitch screws provided a small increase in pullout strength with both trajectories, it was actually the cortical screw trajectory which had the most significant impact on pullout strength [22]. Wray had similar results and also determined that their findings remained true in both high- and low-density bone groups, suggesting benefits of cortical screws in osteoporotic patients [23].

Indications and Patient Selection

The indications for cortical screws appear to be the same as those for traditional pedicle screws for degenerative lumbar pathology with segmental instability. These include both degenerative and in some circumstances lytic spondylolisthesis, lumbar stenosis with instability, recurrent disc herniation, adjacent level degeneration, and pseudoarthrosis. There are a number of situations in which cortical screws may be preferred over pedicle screws. The shorter length and more vertical trajectory of cortical screws relative to pedicle screws are less likely to interfere with anterior vertebral body screws and thus may be preferred when adding posterior instrumentation to these patients [13].

As previously discussed, there is biomechanical evidence supporting the use of cortical screws in osteoporotic patients, and cortical screws may be preferred over pedicle screws in this population. Ueno has described a "double-trajectory" technique in which pedicle screws and cortical screws were placed together in all pedicles in a severely osteoporotic patient requiring L1–S1 fusion and correction for degenerative scoliosis. They reported good results at 14-month follow-up with no hardware complications [24].

The use of cortical screws for "rescue" of a failed pedicle screw has also been examined in a cadaveric biomechanical study. Calvert et al. stressed pedicle screws to failure in an instrumented lumbar spine model and then replaced them with cortical screws. They found that in addition to retaining 60% of the original pedicle screw pullout strength, the rescue cortical screw provided similar stiffness to that of the primary pedicle screw in flexion/extension and axial rotation. The authors also found similar results when testing a pedicle for replacement of a failed cortical screw [25].

Rodriguez et al. reported [16] the use of cortical screws in pedicles already instrumented with pedicle screws for treatment of adjacent-segment lumbar disease (ASLD) (Fig. 29.4). This method allowed for the treatment of ASLD through a minimally invasive approach without the need for exposure or removal of old hardware. At least one group has reported a hybrid technique in which they use cortical screws cranially and pedicle screws caudally in single-level fusions [26].

Contraindications to using cortical screws include cases where competent pedicles are

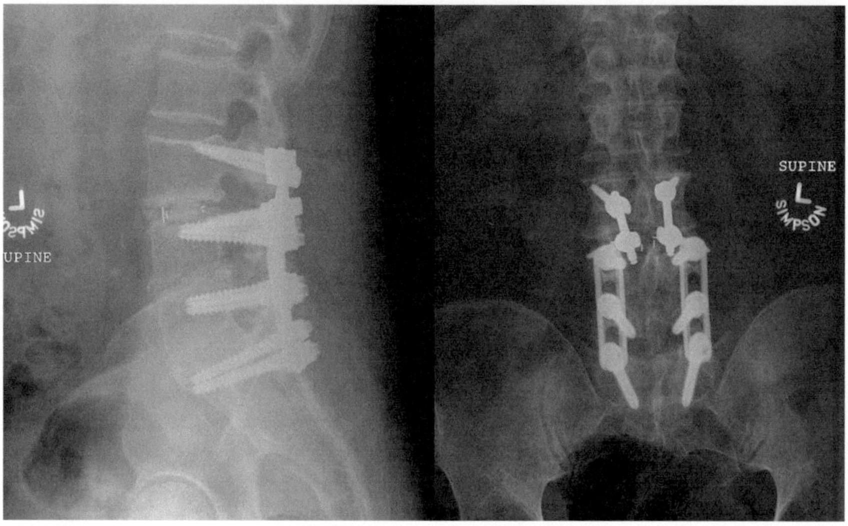

Fig. 29.4 Postoperative anteroposterior (*left*) and lateral (*right*) fluoroscopic imaging of a L3–L4 cortical screw construct added above a prior L4–S1 traditional pedicle screw construct. Note that cortical screws were added to the L4 vertebrae without disrupting the existing traditional pedicle screws

lacking, such as in the case of fractured pedicles or pedicles affected by a neoplastic or infectious process. It may be more difficult to place cortical screws when the screw starting point at the junction of pars and transverse process is absent from prior decompression.

The use of cortical screws may be less optimal in spondylolytic vertebrae as a finite element study demonstrated lower fixation strength in all planes of motion compared with a pedicle screw construct. One explanation for these findings is that pedicle screw relies mainly on the trabecular bone within the pedicle for its fixation strength, while the cortical screw relies largely on the pars and adjacent lamina which is lacking in spondylolytic vertebrae [27].

Cortical screws can be used both with or without additional interbody support. A previously mentioned cadaveric study [9] demonstrated that cortical screws have similar overall stability compared to pedicle screws in specimens with intact intervertebral discs, specimens with TLIF support, and specimens with DLIF support. It is at the surgeon's discretion whether or not to use interbody support with cortical screws, but based on this evidence, the decision-making process should mirror that of pedicle screws.

Preoperative Considerations

When planning fixation, the surgeon must always keep placement of the more medial head of the cortical screw in mind. In a number of scenarios, such as extending upward from an old construct with pedicle screws or mixing pedicle screws and cortical screws in the same construct, the surgeon may have difficulty lining up rods between cortical screw and pedicle screw heads. In this circumstance, the rod would be oriented obliquely instead of vertically as it angles from the more lateral caudal screw heads.

We perform our cortical screw placement with the use of intraoperative fluoroscopy. In the past, we have reported [16] the use of intraoperative navigation for placement of these screws, and we recommend its use when placing a cortical screw in a pedicle which is already instrumented with a pedicle screw. We have also had good early experience with the use of an intraoperative robot for placement of cortical screws. This represents a potential advance which provides the benefit of preoperatively planning the exact screw trajectory.

Finally, the surgeon should ensure the availability of appropriate cortical bone screws. As previously discussed, screws with a narrower pitch provide increased pullout strength over conventional cancellous thread patterns, and we recommend their use. In general, we use 5.0 mm diameter by 30–35 mm in length screws.

Surgical Technique

After the induction of general anesthesia, we position the patient prone on two chest rolls on a conventional surgical table. We do not typically perform any additional manipulation at this stage to increase lordosis as we accomplish this primarily through the use of lordotic interbody grafts and compression of the screws during final tightening. The correct operative level is identified using fluoroscopy, and a midline incision is marked before prepping and draping in a sterile fashion. We do not the routinely use intraoperative monitoring for cortical screw procedures which are generally one or two level procedures. For single-level operations, we make an incision roughly 30–40 mm in length, but this is elongated for multilevel procedures. Once incision is made, it is extended down through the fascia over the paraspinal muscles in the midline. We use the minimal access spinal technologies (MAST) midline lumbar fusion (MIDLF) system (Medtronic, Minneapolis, MN) for retraction. Muscle from the spinous process and lamina of the operative levels are bluntly dissected with the speculum retractor. This speculum retractor has a ruler which is then used to determine the appropriate MAST retractor blade length. The speculum retractor is rotated 90° and opened so that the MAST retractor blade may be inserted between the blades of the speculum retractor over the operative disc space. The other MAST retractor blade is inserted on the contralateral side in the same manner. These MAST blades are then attached to the retractor device which is then used to angle them outward laterally, maximizing the operative field visible through the incision. The retractor is then opened, exposing the operative corridor. The surgeon may then either attach the light source to the retractor and continue the operation using loupes or use the operative microscope.

Prior to screw insertion, bilateral PLIF or TLIF is performed but can be done unilaterally if the surgeon desires. The inferior facets of the superior vertebral level to be fused are amputated using an osteotome and mallet. This exposes the superior facet of the inferior vertebra to be fused which is then removed with a Kerrison rongeur. This bone is then ground for use as autograft later in the case. Some authors have reported that spinous processes must be removed in order to reach a necessary angle for the medial to lateral trajectomy [20], and this may be performed now as well. The yellow ligament and soft tissues are also removed with the Kerrison rongeur to expose the dura and disc space and to achieve central and lateral recess decompression. The borders of the pedicle at the inferior level are identified with a Woodson elevator or angled curette.

The dura is gently retracted and annulotomy is performed. The disc material is removed with pituitary rongeurs and down-pushing curettes. Sequential dilators are used to gradually restore the disc space to its normal height, and a template is used to determine an appropriate interbody device size. Morselized autograft, which may be combined with a biologic extender material, is inserted into the central disc space and the implants. The interbody devices are inserted with caution to avoid injury to traversing or exiting nerve roots.

Once interbody fusion is completed, attention is turned to screw placement. The starting point for the cortical screw is approximately 1 mm inferior to the transverse process, 4 mm medial to the lateral aspect of the pars interarticularis. If the inferior articular process is disrupted due to the patient's pathology or previous surgery, locating an insertion point for the screw may be difficult. In these cases, a starting point 4 mm medial to the lateral aspect of the pars may be used as a horizontal starting point with a vertical starting point at the level of the superior margin of the intervertebral foramen as seen on lateral fluoroscopy [28]. Relative to an anteroposterior view of the pedicle, the optimal screw insertion point can be imagined projecting from a starting point at the 5 o'clock orientation in the left pedicle and 7 o'clock orientation in the right pedicle [12].

The trajectory of the screws is caudocephalad and mediolateral. Matsukawa used in vivo measurements of insertional torque to determine an ideal trajectory for placement of cortical screws and found it to be 25–30 degrees cranially and 10 degrees laterally along the inferior border of the pedicle [29].

The entry point and trajectory are confirmed prior to and during pilot hole drilling using the C-arm for fluoroscopic imaging. The entry point is made using a high-speed drill with a routing bit measuring approximately 2 mm at the tip. During drilling, we frequently pause to confirm the tip remains in cortical bone by tapping the bit against the bottom of the hole. AP and lateral fluoroscopy can be used to verify the correct screw trajectory. The tip of the drill is slowly advanced to approximately 30 mm. We inspect the tract to ensure no breach has occurred before tapping with the 5.0 or 5.5 mm cortical thread tap. The hole is reinspected for a breach after tapping and the screw is then inserted. This is repeated for the remaining cortical screws to be placed (Fig. 29.5).

For screws placed at S1, we modify our technique slightly. At this level, we identify the medial and superior borders of the S1 pedicle during the decompression. The routing drill bit is then used to drill a tract with a "straight-in" trajectory into the S1 pedicle. We also place a larger diameter screw at this level, usually 7.5 mm.

The rods are inserted and secured with set screws tightened under compression to help secure segmental lordosis. We then close fascia and skin in a usual fashion and cover the incision with a topical skin adhesive.

Illustrative Case

History

A 74-year-old female presented with complaints of radicular pain in the right lower extremity as well as midline axial back pain. The pain had been present for more than 10 years but had been gradually worsening and had recently progressed to include numbness and weakness with standing. She had undergone multiple epidural steroid injections which helped at first but were no longer providing her any relief. She endorsed some relief when lying flat, but her pain was refractory to pain medication. She had also tried physical therapy with no relief.

Physical Exam

On examination, the patient was noted to have an antalgic gait. Patellar and Achilles deep tendon reflexes were present but decreased in amplitude. She endorsed hypoesthesia to light touch in the lateral and posterior left lower extremity. She had significant pain with straight leg raise on the left. All lower extremity muscle groups appeared full strength, and she had no signs of myelopathy.

Radiographical Imaging

Magnetic resonance imaging of the patient's lumbar spine revealed a Grade 1 degenerative spondylolisthesis at L5–S1 with disc collapse and foraminal stenosis (Fig. 29.6). Dynamic radiographs of her lumbar spine demonstrated a 9 mm anterolisthesis of L5 on S1 which worsened with flexion.

Treatment

She was taken to the operating suite where a MAST bilateral L5–S1 PLIF was performed with cortical screws at L5 as previously discussed. The described "straight-in" trajectory was used for the S1 screws. Her hospital course was uneventful, and she was discharged home on the second postoperative day.

Outcome

Lumbar radiographs obtained immediately post-op and at 1-month, 3-month (Fig. 29.7), and 12-month follow-up showed good hardware placement with no evidence of screw back out or loosening. At her 1-month postoperative visit, she

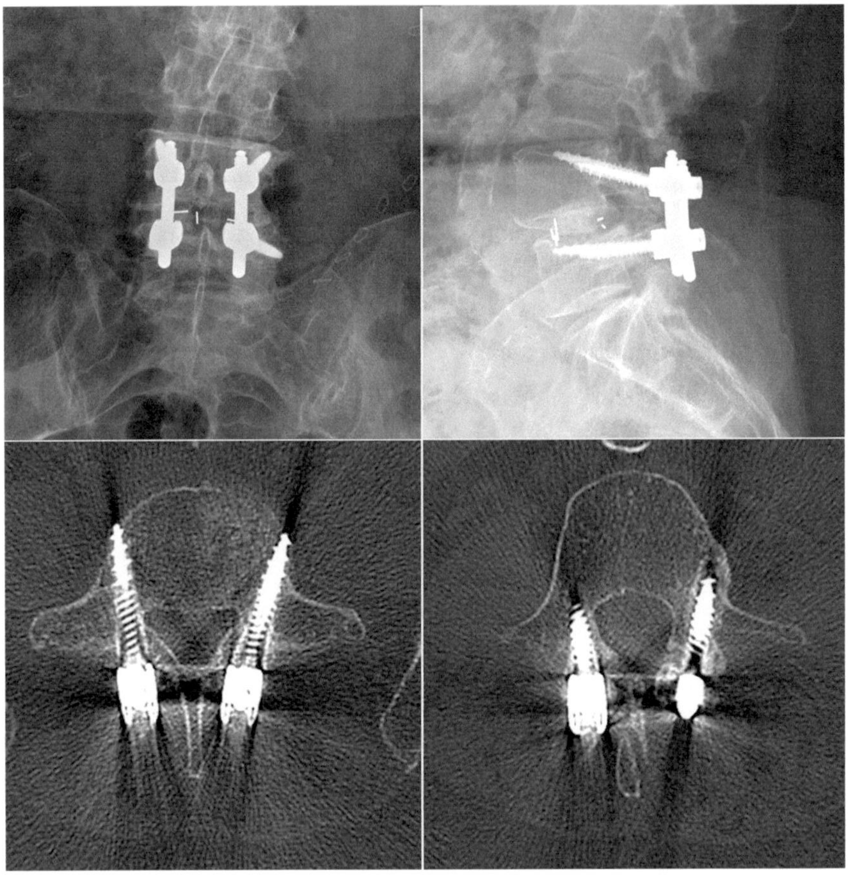

Fig. 29.5 Postoperative AP (*top left*) and lateral (*top right*) radiographs demonstrating cortical screw fixation of L4 and L5 vertebral bodies. Axial CT imaging in the same patient demonstrating screw trajectory in both L5 (*bottom left*) and L4 (*bottom right*)

reported an improvement in her leg numbness and a resolution of her radicular pain. Twelve months postoperatively, she reported a complete resolution of all her symptoms and noted that she had lost 20 lbs through an exercise program she had previously been unable to participate in.

Technical Pearls

- Surgeons may initially use CT-guided navigation or both AP and lateral fluoroscopy while gaining familiarity with the trajectory to help avoid pedicle breach and optimize bone screw fixation.
- Given the medial trajectory starting point for CBT, the technique can be easily incorporated with midline minimally invasive systems.
- Visually confirm the lateral pars and transverse process junction before initial pilot drilling. Occasionally contours in the lamina pars junction may be misleading and lead to a medial screw placement.
- The length of the drill bit must equate to the proposed length of the screw. Inadequate drill depth may lead to fracture of the lateral cortical wall.
- Should the lateral pars fracture upon insertion of the screw, this is easily converted to a

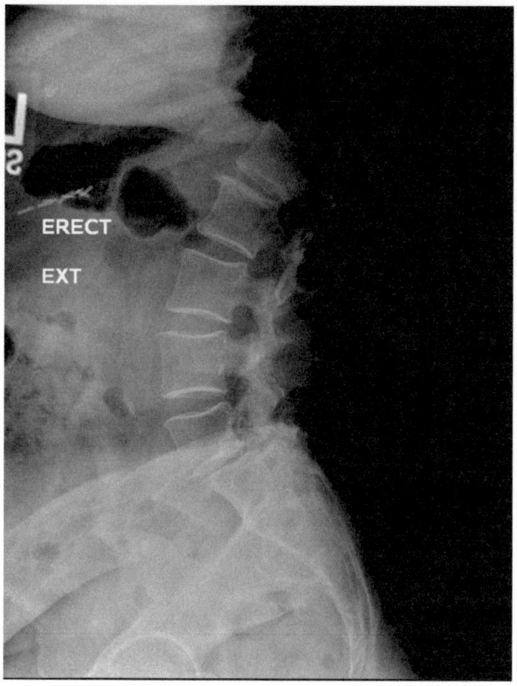

Fig. 29.6 Preoperative lateral fluoroscopic imaging demonstrating a Grade 1 spondylolisthesis at L5–S1

traditional pedicle screw approach as a salvage technique without requisite addition of the adjacent level.

Complications and Strategies for Avoidance

Placement of the screw in S1 requires a slightly modified technique. At this level, an alar cortical screw trajectory can lead to damage of the traversing L5 roots. In our early experience, 2 of 21 patients who underwent CBT sacral fixation with an attempted alar trajectory required subsequent revision due to impingement of the L5 nerve roots. We now use shorter screws with a "straight-in" trajectory at S1. The tips of these screws terminate within the sacrum. Other authors have described a similar trajectory with the tip of the screw penetrating the S1 superior end plate [30]. Caution should be taken with placement of cortical screws at this level, and the surgeon may want to consider

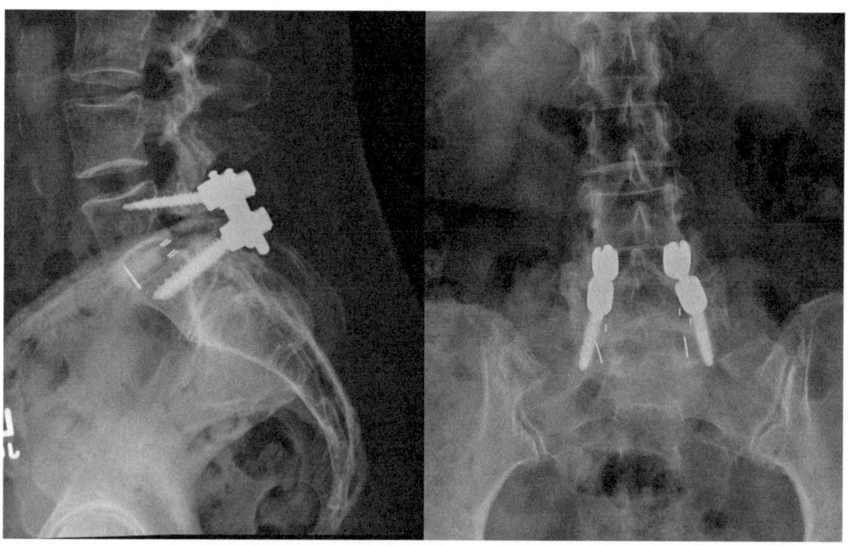

Fig. 29.7 Postoperative anteroposterior (*right*) and lateral (*left*) fluoroscopic imaging demonstrating the posterior lumbar interbody fusion performed at L5–S1 using cortical screws in the L5 vertebral body

an intraoperative O-arm CT after placement of these screws if CT-guided navigation is not used.

Salvage of a pedicle fracture during insertion of a cortical screw with a pedicle screw has been described in the literature [14] and may be of benefit in this situation.

Conclusion

Cortical bone trajectory screws are an exciting new addition to the armamentarium of spinal techniques. Their more medial insertion point provides for a faster, less invasive exposure than traditional trajectory pedicle screws while still maintaining similar biomechanical strength.

References

1. Santoni BG, Hynes RA, McGilvray KC, et al. Cortical bone trajectory for lumbar pedicle screws. Spine J. 2009;9(5):366–73.
2. Hung C-W, Wu M-F, Hong R-T, Weng M-J, Yu G-F, Kao C-H. Comparison of multifidus muscle atrophy after posterior lumbar interbody fusion with conventional and cortical bone trajectory. Clin Neurol Neurosurg. 2016;145:41–5.
3. Hirano T, Hasegawa K, Takahashi HE, et al. Structural characteristics of the pedicle and its role in screw stability. Spine. 1997;22(21):2504–9–discussion 2510.
4. Mai HT, Mitchell SM, Hashmi SZ, Jenkins TJ, Patel AA, Hsu WK. Differences in bone mineral density of fixation points between lumbar cortical and traditional pedicle screws. Spine J. 2015;16(7):835–41.
5. İnceoğlu S, Montgomery WH, St Clair S, McLain RF. Pedicle screw insertion angle and pullout strength: comparison of 2 proposed strategies. J Neurosurg Spine. 2011;14(5):670–6.
6. Baluch DA, Patel AA, Lullo B, et al. Effect of physiological loads on cortical and traditional pedicle screw fixation. Spine. 2014;39(22):E1297–302.
7. Cheng WK, İnceoğlu S. Cortical and standard trajectory pedicle screw fixation techniques in stabilizing multisegment lumbar spine with low grade spondylolisthesis. Int J Spine Surg. 2015;9:46.
8. Perez-Orribo L, Kalb S, Reyes PM, Chang SW, Crawford NR. Biomechanics of lumbar cortical screw-rod fixation versus pedicle screw-rod fixation with and without interbody support. Spine. 2013;38(8):635–41.
9. Matsukawa K, Yato Y, Imabayashi H, Hosogane N, Asazuma T, Nemoto K. Biomechanical evaluation of the fixation strength of lumbar pedicle screws using cortical bone trajectory: a finite element study. J Neurosurg Spine. 2015;23(4):471–8.
10. Matsukawa K, Yato Y, Kato T, Imabayashi H, Asazuma T, Nemoto K. In vivo analysis of insertional torque during pedicle screwing using cortical bone trajectory technique. Spine. 2014;39(4):E240–5.
11. Matsukawa K, Kato T, Yato Y, et al. Incidence and risk factors of adjacent cranial facet joint violation following pedicle screw insertion using cortical bone trajectory technique. Spine. 2016;41(14):E851–6.
12. Matsukawa K, Yato Y, Nemoto O, Imabayashi H, Asazuma T, Nemoto K. Morphometric measurement of cortical bone trajectory for lumbar pedicle screw insertion using computed tomography. J Spinal Disord Tech. 2013;26(6):E248–53.
13. Snyder LA, Martinez-Del-Campo E, Neal MT, et al. Lumbar spinal fixation with cortical bone trajectory pedicle screws in 79 patients with degenerative disease: perioperative outcomes and complications. World Neurosurg. 2016;88:205–13.
14. Kasukawa Y, Miyakoshi N, Hongo M, Ishikawa Y, Kudo D, Shimada Y. Short-term results of transforaminal lumbar interbody fusion using pedicle screw with cortical bone trajectory compared with conventional trajectory. Asian Spine J. 2015;9(3):440–8.
15. Lee GW, Son J-H, Ahn M-W, Kim H-J, Yeom JS. The comparison of pedicle screw and cortical screw in posterior lumbar interbody fusion: a prospective randomized noninferiority trial. Spine J. 2015;15(7):1519–26.
16. Rodriguez A, Neal MT, Liu A, Somasundaram A, Hsu W, Branch CL. Novel placement of cortical bone trajectory screws in previously instrumented pedicles for adjacent-segment lumbar disease using CT image-guided navigation. Neurosurg Focus. 2014;36(3):E9.
17. Berjano P, Damilano M, Ismael M, Formica C, Garbossa D. Erratum to: Minimally invasive PLIF with divergent, cortical trajectory pedicle screws. Eur Spine J. 2015;24(5):654–5.
18. Ninomiya K, Iwatsuki K, Ohnishi Y-I, Ohkawa T, Yoshimine T. Clear zone formation around screws in the early postoperative stages after posterior lumbar fusion using the cortical bone trajectory technique. Asian Spine J. 2015;9(6):884–8.
19. Glennie RA, Dea N, Kwon BK, Street JT. Early clinical results with cortically based pedicle screw trajectory for fusion of the degenerative lumbar spine. J Clin Neurosci. 2015;22(6):972–5.
20. Cheng WK, Akpolat YT, İnceoğlu S, Patel S, Danisa OA. Pars and pedicle fracture and screw loosening associated with cortical bone trajectory: a case series and proposed mechanism through a cadaveric study. Spine J. 2016;16(2):e59–65.
21. Akpolat YT, İnceoğlu S, Kinne N, Hunt D, Cheng WK. Fatigue performance of cortical bone trajectory screw compared with standard trajectory pedicle screw. Spine. 2016;41(6):E335–41.
22. Ueno M, Sakai R, Tanaka K, et al. Should we use cortical bone screws for cortical bone trajectory? J Neurosurg Spine. 2015;22(4):416–21.
23. Wray S, Mimran R, Vadapalli S, Shetye SS, McGilvray KC, Puttlitz CM. Pedicle screw placement in the lumbar spine: effect of trajectory and screw

design on acute biomechanical purchase. J Neurosurg Spine. 2015;22(5):503–10.

24. Ueno M, Imura T, Inoue G, Takaso M. Posterior corrective fusion using a double-trajectory technique (cortical bone trajectory combined with traditional trajectory) for degenerative lumbar scoliosis with osteoporosis: technical note. J Neurosurg Spine. 2013;19(5):600–7.
25. Calvert GC, Lawrence BD, Abtahi AM, Bachus KN, Brodke DS. Cortical screws used to rescue failed lumbar pedicle screw construct: a biomechanical analysis. J Neurosurg Spine. 2015;22(2):166–72.
26. Takata Y, Matsuura T, Higashino K, et al. Hybrid technique of cortical bone trajectory and pedicle screwing for minimally invasive spine reconstruction surgery: a technical note. J Med Investig. 2014;61(3–4):388–92.
27. Matsukawa K, Yato Y, Imabayashi H, Hosogane N, Asazuma T, Chiba K. Biomechanical evaluation of lumbar pedicle screws in spondylolytic vertebrae: comparison of fixation strength between the traditional trajectory and a cortical bone trajectory. J Neurosurg Spine. 2016;24(6):1–6.
28. Iwatsuki K, Yoshimine T, Ohnishi Y-I, Ninomiya K, Ohkawa T. Isthmus-guided cortical bone trajectory for pedicle screw insertion. Orthop Surg. 2014;6(3):244–8.
29. Matsukawa K, Taguchi E, Yato Y, et al. Evaluation of the fixation strength of pedicle screws using cortical bone trajectory: what is the ideal trajectory for optimal fixation? Spine. 2015;40(15):E873–8.
30. Matsukawa K, Yato Y, Kato T, Imabayashi H, Asazuma T, Nemoto K. Cortical bone trajectory for lumbosacral fixation: penetrating S-1 endplate screw technique: technical note. J Neurosurg Spine. 2014;21(2):203–9.

Lumbosacral and Pelvic Fixation Techniques

30

Osama N. Kashlan, Kevin S. Chen,
and Frank La Marca

Introduction

The lumbosacral region is important for the alignment and movement of the lumbar spine, with the L5–S1 segment shown to provide the greatest amount of flexion/extension in the lumbar spine [1–3]. Due to the considerable motion at that segment, long-segment fusions to the sacrum have high pseudarthrosis rates at L5–S1. Also this may explain the difficulty in achieving bony fusion at the lumbosacral segment. In addition, the high rate of instrumentation failure at the lumbosacral junction is related to pseudoarthrosis, poor bone quality of the sacrum, the complex anatomy, and the substantial biomechanical forces at the lumbosacral junction [4].

Pelvic fixation was developed and is used to help solve this problem. The first use of pelvic fixation was described in the 1980s with development of the Galveston technique [5, 6]. In this technique, pelvic anchors were inserted at the posterior superior iliac spine (PSIS) between the inner and outer tables of the pelvis (Fig. 30.1). The Galveston technique was a major advancement in addressing the problem of lumbosacral pseudarthrosis and set the stage for development of the modern pelvic fixation techniques described elsewhere in this chapter [4].

Anatomy

The sacrum and ilium constitute the posterior aspect of the pelvic ring and articulate through the sacroiliac joint (Fig. 30.2). Although not fused, this joint is composed of an irregular yet complementary bony cartilaginous surface that interlocks the ilium to the sacrum. The sacroiliac joint is stabilized by the anterior sacroiliac ligament and the posterior sacroiliac ligament (Fig. 30.3). Other ligaments that serve as reinforcements include the iliolumbar ligament which links the L4 and L5 transverse processes to the iliac crest, the sacrospinous ligament which connects the ischial spine to the lateral edge of the sacrum, and the sacrotuberous ligament which connects the whole lateral edge of the sacrum and PSIS to the ischial tuberosity [7]. The posterior sacroiliac ligament is commonly encountered during surgical preparation of the iliac crest for a bone harvest or iliac screw placement. Ligaments of the sacropelvis are also important in transmission of axial loads through

O.N. Kashlan, MD • K.S. Chen, MD
F. La Marca, MD (✉)
Department of Neurosurgery, University of Michigan, 1500 E. Medical Center Drive, Room 3552 TCx, Ann Arbor, MI 48109-5338, USA
e-mail: okashlan@med.umich.edu; kechen@med.umich.edu; Frank.LaMarca@allegiancehealth.org

L.T. Holly, P.A. Anderson (eds.), *Essentials of Spinal Stabilization*,
DOI 10.1007/978-3-319-59713-3_30

the first sacral segment and through the iliac wings to the acetabulum bilaterally by permitting a certain degree of shock force absorbance [8, 9].

In addition to having knowledge of the anatomy, it is also important for a surgeon instrumenting the pelvis to be familiar with how to correlate radiographs to anatomic landmarks. Lateral fluoroscopy is the most common view utilized in our practice as shown in Fig. 30.4A. The most important landmarks to note in this view are the greater sciatic notch, the femoral heads with the associated acetabulum, and the anterior inferior iliac spine. The greater sciatic notch contains the sciatic nerve and superior gluteal artery. The pelvic inlet view is a fluoroscopic trajectory parallel to the sacrum and is important in visualizing the main pelvic ring (Fig. 30.4B). The pelvic outlet view is a fluoroscopic trajectory perpendicular to the sacrum and can be used in visualizing the sacral foramina (Fig. 30.4C). Obturator oblique imaging of the pelvis, also named as obturator outlet views, can be used to visualize the "teardrop" of the ilium. The teardrop signifies the safe zone within the iliac bony cortices in which fixation can be placed (Fig. 30.5).

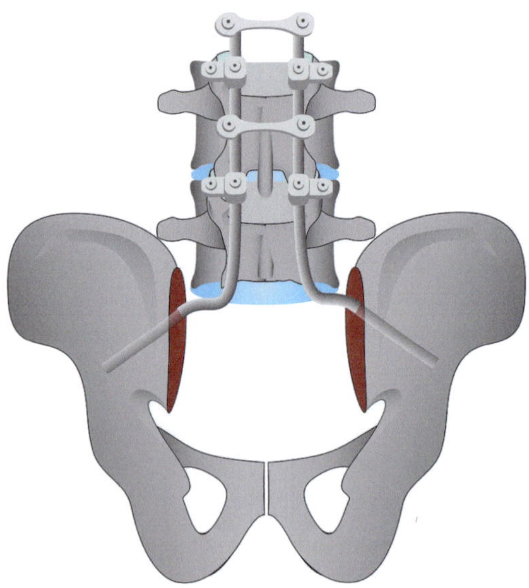

Fig. 30.1 Galveston rods, one of the first successful techniques for pelvic fixation, visualized via posterior approach

Indications and Patient Selection

There are no absolute indications for when to instrument the pelvis or whether to stop at the sacrum when performing a long-segment construct. Until there is more robust data in the literature, most of this decision-making is left to surgeon preference and comfort level. The benefits of pelvic fixation include securing distal fixation, protecting sacral screws, adding pelvic derotation, and protecting/overriding the sacroiliac joint. Disadvantages include the extra surgical time it

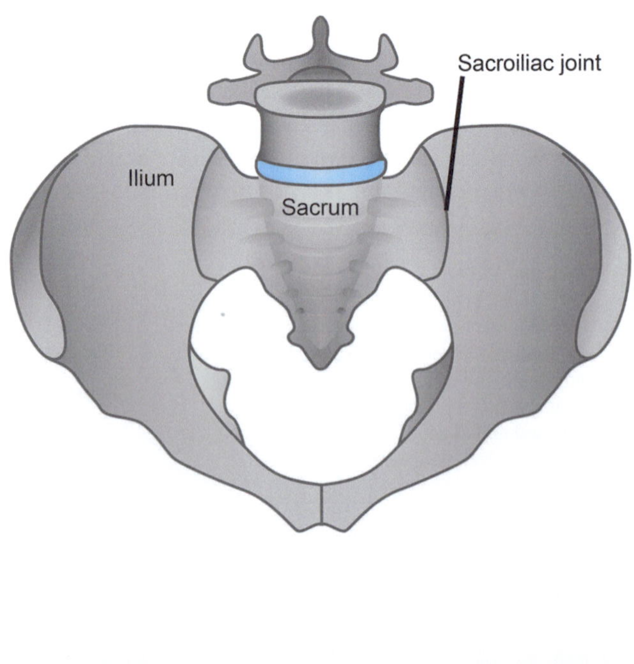

Fig. 30.2 Illustration of the articulation between sacrum and ilium

takes to place the pelvic hardware, the technical difficulty in placement via a minimally invasive approach, the added risk of greater sciatic notch violation of important neurovascular structures within, and the possible high profile of the hardware causing pain and ultimately requiring removal.

Even with the lack of absolute indications, the relative indications for pelvic fixation [1, 4, 5, 10–13] include:

- High-grade spondylolisthesis (Meyerding Grade 3 or higher)
- Unstable sacral fractures
- Sacral tumors requiring sacrectomy
- Long construct with proximal end around or past thoracolumbar junction
- Osteoporosis and/or poor sacral fixation
- Lumbar deformity and pelvic obliquity correction, especially in children with neuromuscular deformity
- Three-column osteotomy at the lumbosacral junction
- Sacral insufficiency fractures

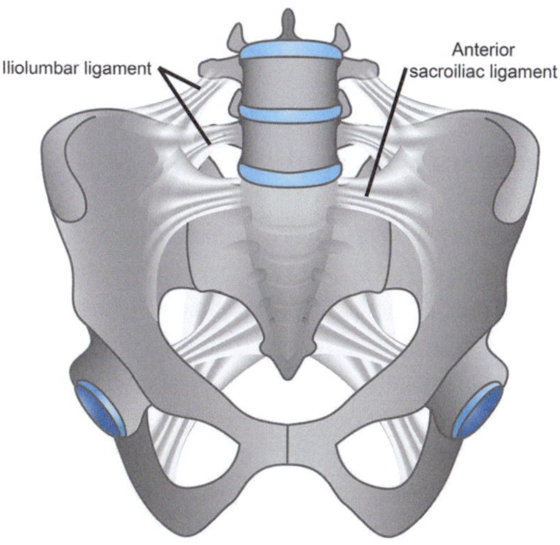

Fig. 30.3 Important ligaments of the sacrum including the anterior sacroiliac ligament, posterior sacroiliac ligament (not shown), and iliolumbar ligament

Sacral insufficiency fractures can also be an indication for lumbopelvic fixation [1, 14, 15]. These fractures occur in osteoporotic patients, in patients with metabolic derangements, and in patients with a history of lumbosacral fixation. From all the etiologies listed, the most common indication is management of long constructs in adult deformity patients [1].

There is controversy over what constitutes a long construct. A recent review article defines a long arthrodesis requiring pelvic fixation as one involving five or more levels [5, 16]. Another biomechanical study showed that constructs extending above L3 should have the sacral screws protected by pelvic instrumentation [5, 17]. With the lack of guidelines, the final decision rests with the surgeon and should depend on specific patient characteristics, including patient body

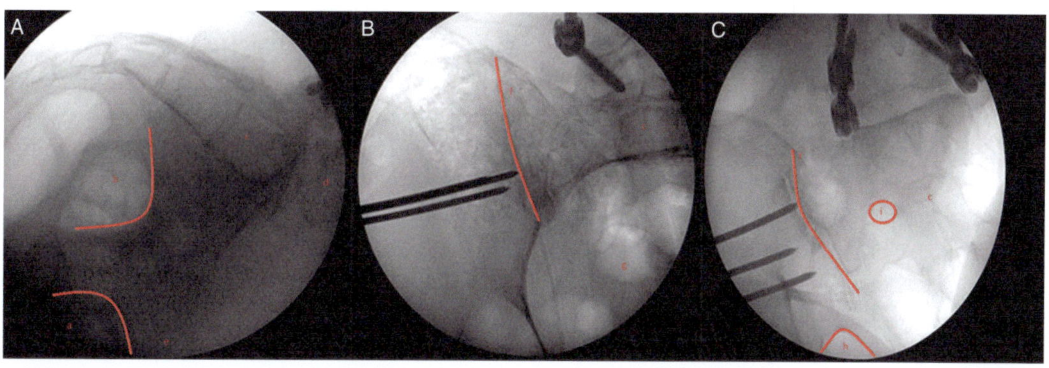

Fig. 30.4 Important pelvic landmarks on lateral fluoroscopy (**A**), pelvic inlet view (**B**), and pelvic outlet view (**C**) on a patient undergoing a minimally invasive sacroiliac fusion (technique not discussed in this chapter). Structures labeled are femoral heads (*a*), greater sciatic notch (*b*), sacrum (*c*), L5 (*d*), anterior inferior iliac spine (*e*), sacroiliac join (*f*), main pelvic ring (*g*), obturator foramen (*h*), and sacral foramen (*i*)

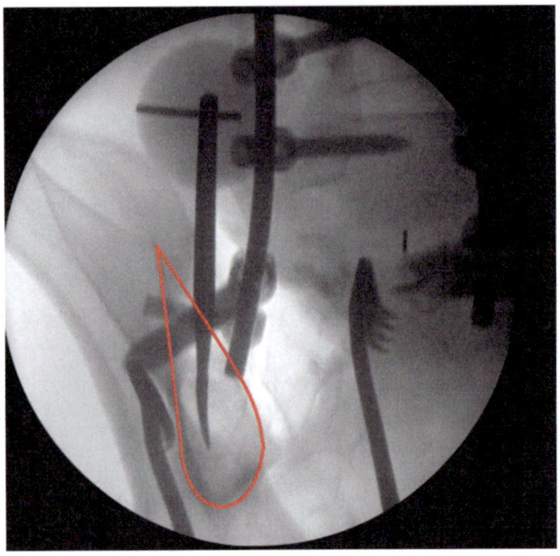

Fig. 30.5 Obturator outlet view of a salvage procedure to replace a misplaced iliac bolt. The misplaced iliac bolt laterally breaches the "teardrop." The Lenke probe visualized demonstrates adequate trajectory within confines of "teardrop" for placement of a new iliac screw

mass index (BMI), nutritional status, bone mineral density, and medical comorbidities.

Relative contraindications to placement of pelvic instrumentation include patients with poor anatomy or previous surgery precluding safe placement of hardware [1]. A history of an iliac bone harvest does not inhibit the ability to place pelvic fixation; however, it is important to determine if an iliac crest bone harvest was performed, as this will affect tactile feedback during placement of hardware as discussed later in this chapter.

Preoperative Considerations

As described above, an important preoperative decision is whether pelvic fixation is definitely needed at the end of a construct or not. This decision should be based on multiple factors including patient bone quality, BMI, medical comorbidities, and goals of surgery. In our practice, we are more likely to plan placement of pelvic instrumentation in patients requiring a long construct that also have a history of osteoporosis, smoking, high BMI, and diabetes, or in patients with sacral tumors requiring a sacrectomy. In contrast, in patients with terminal cancer with involvement of the lower lumbar spine requiring a corpectomy, we are more likely to limit instrumentation to the sacrum, as the patient's lifespan likely is shorter than the time it would take for pseudarthrosis at the lumbosacral segment to occur. In this situation, placement of pelvic fixation can have risks that outweigh any potential benefits. In reality, the decision to place pelvic instrumentation is made intraoperatively after evaluating the quality of sacral fixation. Specific preoperative considerations for each type of instrumentation that can be used are discussed below. In some cases, such as after iliac crest bone grafting, pelvis CT is useful to plan surgical technique and to assess adequacy of bone stock.

Sacral Instrumentation

S1 Pedicle Screw The S1 pedicles are wide with less cortical bone to allow for screw purchase. Therefore, S1 screws at the end of long constructs can be prone to failure [1]. In terms of pedicle screw length, the average length of an S1 pedicle is 46.9 mm in women and 49.7 mm in men [4, 18]. Tricortical fixation with S1 screws breaching anteriorly through the promontory improves biomechanical stability and should be the goal [1, 19]. However, even with that improved strength, long fusions ending at the sacrum can have failure rates as high as 44% [4, 20, 21].

S2 Pedicle Screw S2 pedicle screws are not used in our practice. They are technically demanding due to a narrow safe zone and have not been shown to increase construct stiffness [1, 22, 23]. Because the S2 pedicles are dorsal to the biomechanical pivot point, they offer very little additional strength for resisting pullout and flexion forces [4, 23, 24].

S1 Alar Screw Alar screws, which are screws that start at S1 and are aimed laterally into the ala, also have a narrow safe zone and have not been shown to significantly reduce pseudarthrosis rates clinically [1, 23]. In fact, despite being resistant to higher pullout forces, long fusion to the sacrum using these techniques has been associated with poor clinical results in addition to high pseudarthrosis rates [4, 20, 23].

Dual S1 Pedicle/S1 Alar Screws There are devices available that allow for insertion of both an S1 pedicle screw and an S1 alar screw, which allows for triangulation of these two screws. These devices allow for greater construct stability when compared to an S1 pedicle screw in isolation [25]. However, these devices also have disadvantages, including increased muscle dissection, decreased bone surface available for fusion, and mechanical inferiority to iliac screws [4, 26].

Pelvic Instrumentation

Iliac Screw (Iliac Bolt) Iliac screws (also called iliac bolts) have an attractive biomechanical profile when compared to sacral screws for two reasons: they are divergent from the proximal fixation points in the coronal plane, and they are longer screws enabling placement anterior to the axis of pelvic rotation [1]. Both attributes make them better able to prevent pseudarthrosis and hardware failure at the distal end of the construct. In our practice, bilateral screws are placed whenever feasible. Unilateral iliac screw fixation has the potential to improve clinical outcomes without compromising biomechanical stability, but long-term studies are needed to determine equivalence between unilateral and bilateral iliac screw pseudarthrosis rates [1, 27].

S2 Alar-Iliac (S2AI) Screw The S2AI screw has the benefit over traditional iliac screws in that it minimizes the prominent screws present when the PSIS is used as a starting point and also makes it easier to attach these screws to the rest of the construct (Fig. 30.6). This is due to their starting point being more in line with the pedicle screws used in the rest of the construct. Not having to use an offset connector theoretically takes away the additional point where loosening of the construct may occur. The S2AI screw is also noted to have greater cortical purchase than the traditional iliac screw as it crosses over the cortical bone at the sacroiliac joint [28]. The drawback of this technique is that this screw traverses the sacroiliac joint. In a study of 51 adult patients with S2AI screws, there was no evidence of sacroiliac joint arthritis or fusion at 2 years or 5 years radiographically [5]. However, the effect of this trajectory on sacroiliac joint arthritis and sacroiliac pain continues to be debated.

Galveston Technique The Galveston technique has a low pseudarthrosis rate but is associated with a high incidence of loosening secondary to micromotion at the rod tips within the ilium, despite achieving a fusion at the lumbosacral junction [4]. When loosening occurs, there is the potential for pain and the need for implant removal [4]. This technique has been replaced by the use of iliac screws (whose pullout strength has been shown to be three times greater) and S2AI screws [4, 29].

Other fixation techniques that are used rarely or mostly have historic significance include the sacral sublaminar wires and hooks, the iliosacral screws, the Jackson intrasacral rods, and the Kostuik transiliac bar [4, 5]. These techniques will not be discussed in this chapter.

Comparison of Iliac Screws to S2AI Screws There are mixed results regarding which method (sacral screws vs. S2AI screws) has a lower complication rate. Sponseller et al. found a statistically significant improvement in pelvic obliquity but no difference in postoperative complications, including infection, dehiscence, and hardware loosening, in pediatric patients [30]. However, a more recent study retrospectively reviewed the pelvic fixation techniques used in 120 consecutive cases of adult and pediatric deformity and showed that there is a clear difference between the two techniques [31]. The S2AI pelvic fixation technique was associated with a statistically significant decrease in implant loosening, acute wound infections, delayed wound problems, need for revision surgery, and the incidence of persistent posterior pelvic pain >3 months after surgery [31]. The reason for the decrease in infections was theorized to be lack of

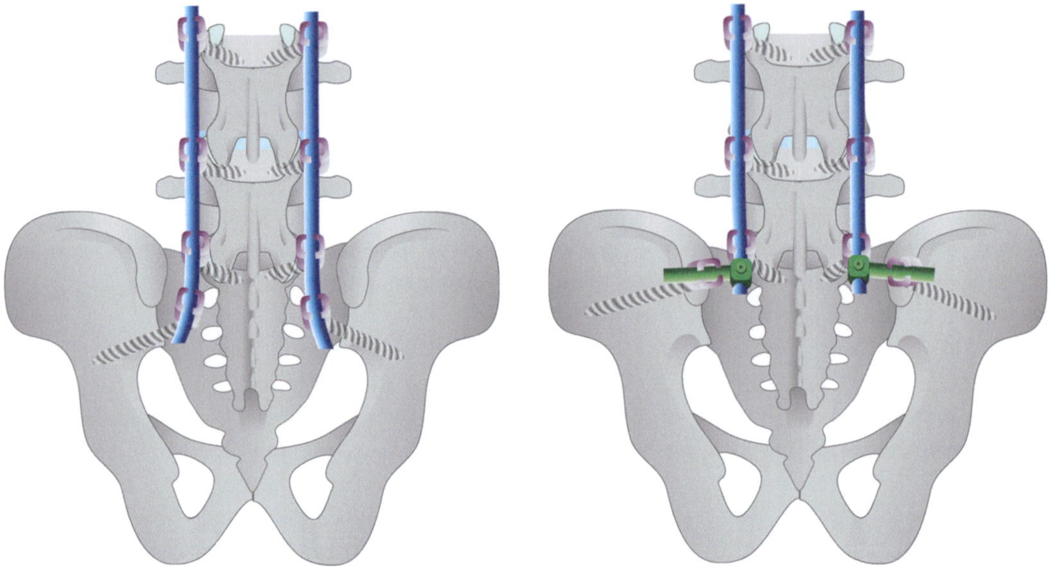

Fig. 30.6 Anteroposterior views of S2AI screws (*left*) versus iliac screws (*right*)

the need for tissue dissection over the PSIS, as is required during an iliac screw placement. However, more prospective studies are needed before determining if there is a difference in complication rate of either method.

Surgical Technique

Sacral Instrumentation

The S1 screw starting point is inferior and slightly lateral to the midpoint of the L5–S1 facet joint. A pilot hole is drilled at that position. Utilizing fluoroscopy or CT image guidance, a trajectory pointing toward the sacral promontory is undertaken. A Lenke probe is advanced by hand until the promontory point of the anterior sacral cortical bone is reached. At that point, a mallet is used to break through the cortical bone. A pedicle screw sized to reach slightly anterior to this point is placed. Tapping of the far cortex is useful to prevent screw stripping during insertion if it does not penetrate the pilot hole. S1 screws can be placed via a minimally invasive approach. A novel proposed method to place lumbosacral screws in a medial-to-lateral trajectory has been shown to be a safe alternative to the usual lateral-to-medial trajectory described above [32]. The potential benefits of these cortical bone trajectory pedicle screws include less lateral muscle dissection, decreased potential for pain, and reduced chance of a medial breach resulting in nerve root injury.

Pelvic Instrumentation

Iliac Screw In our practice, a separate fascial opening is utilized which is more lateral to the midline fascial opening used in the placement of lumbosacral pedicle screws. The starting point for an iliac screw is found by exposing the PSIS. In an attempt to deeply insert the screw head to decrease the chance of prominent hardware causing discomfort to the patient, the entry point is below (ventral to) the PSIS along the medial aspect of the ilium just above the sacrum. After the muscle/ligamentous attachments are cleared, the starting point is marked with a burr or rongeur. The trajectory is from the PSIS to the anterior inferior iliac spine and is highly variable, but typically angled 20–45 degrees caudal and 30–45 degrees lateral [1, 5]. Utilizing an iliac probe and gently advancing by hand allow for the trajectory to stay between the inner and outer tables of the ilium. The screw should be positioned just above the sciatic notch. Obturator outlet views that show the "teardrop" of the ilium and position of the probe or screw within the teardrop can be helpful.

In cases where two ipsilateral iliac screws are necessary, care must be taken when passing the first screw so as to leave enough room for the second screw. Either fluoroscopy or CT guidance can be used to place these screws. A lateral radiographic view can be utilized to guide the screw approximately 1 cm above the greater sciatic notch in the supra-acetabular region where the thickest part of the ilium allows for optimum screw purchase [1]. Screws of up to 100 mm in length can be used with this technique. Obturator oblique views and iliac oblique views can also be utilized to better visualize the thick column of the bone just above the greater sciatic notch, also known as the "teardrop" and the greater sciatic notch, respectively [1]. Iliac screws can also be placed in a minimally invasive manner [33, 34].

S2AI Screw The S2AI screw technique involves fixation along a pathway between the second sacral segment and the anterior inferior iliac spine [5]. The starting point for S2AI screws is 2–4 mm lateral and 2–8 mm inferior to the S1 foramen. This point aligns on the dorsal aspect of the sacral ala, at the midpoint of a line that connects the lateral aspect of the S1 and S2 dorsal foramina. The screw trajectory is directed toward the anterior inferior iliac spine [1, 4, 5]. Feeling the greater trochanter is a palpable landmark for this trajectory [5]. After a starting point is found and a pilot hole formed using a drill or awl, a 2.5-mm drill is pointed 40 degrees lateral and 20–30 degrees caudal [4]. Using anteroposterior fluoroscopy to visualize the pelvis and sciatic notch, the drill is advanced slightly past the sacroiliac joint. The path of the drill should be within 20 mm proximal to the greater sciatic notch and aimed toward the anteroinferior iliac spine [4]. Past the sacroiliac joint, a 3.2-mm drill is used to protect against breaking the smaller drill bit in the ilium [4]. At this point, obtaining an obturator oblique fluoroscopy view with a 30-degree caudal and 30-degree lateral beam visualizing the "teardrop" can help avoid a cortical breach [4, 5]. The most common screw size is 9 × 90 mm [5]. S2AI screw insertion can be also performed via a minimally invasive approach, or utilizing image guidance [35].

Galveston Technique The Galveston technique allows for incorporation of the ilium via insertion of rods between the inner and outer tables of cortical bone. The transverse portions of the rods are inserted submuscularly and enter the ilium at the PSIS [4]. The rods are oriented 30–35 degrees caudally and 20–25 degrees laterally [4]. The rods cross the sacroiliac joint and contouring can be difficult [4, 36]. This technique is used much less frequently than the iliac screw or the S2AI screw.

Illustrative Case

History

A 62-year-old male with no significant history presented with progressive difficulty with balance, sexual dysfunction, and bladder dysfunction over the course of a year. He also had pain involving his left buttock and hip radiating down the posterior aspect of his thigh and calf and stopping at his ankle. The patient noted difficulty with ankle plantar flexion over the past 2 years.

Physical Exam

On physical examination, the patient had full strength throughout. His reflexes were normal and symmetric. His sensory examination was normal.

Radiographical Imaging

CT scan demonstrated a large destructive lesion involving the lower lumbar and upper sacral spine on the left (Fig. 30.7). Sagittal T2-weighted MRI shows the amount of involvement of the sacrum and spinal canal (Fig. 30.8); the significant extension of this mass into the pelvis is not shown.

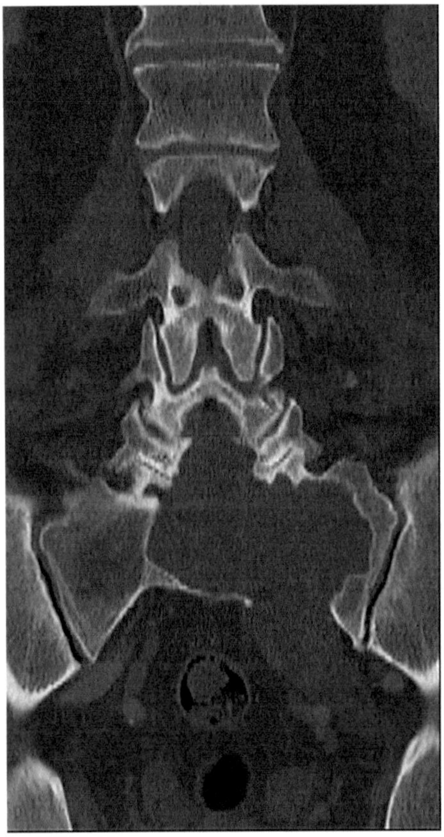

Fig. 30.7 Coronal CT of lumbosacral spine demonstrating a destructive bony lesion at the lower lumbar and upper sacral spine. Pathology was consistent with neurofibroma

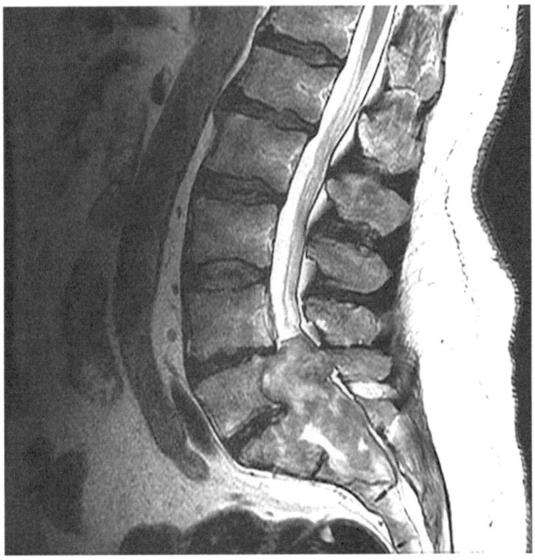

Fig. 30.8 Sagittal T2-weighted MRI demonstrating extension of the destructive mass into spinal canal. Not shown is extension into left hemipelvis

Treatment

CT-guided biopsy of the mass was consistent with neurofibroma. The patient was then offered surgical debulking of the mass for symptom control. Because of the bony destruction seen at L5 and the sacrum, the decision was made preoperatively to place iliac screws to achieve fusion across the lumbosacral junction. In the operating room, the patient was positioned prone and a midline incision utilized. Subperiosteal dissection was carried out with exposure of the posterior elements from L3 to the midsacrum. After bilateral L4 pedicle screws were inserted, attention was then directed to placement of iliac screws. Using suprafascial dissection, the PSIS was digitally palpated. The fascia was opened and the PSIS exposed. Using an osteotome, a bony defect was created. Under direct and fluoroscopic visualization, the Lenke probe was passed along the trajectory to cannulate the iliac wing. The trajectory was probed and found to be without bony breach. Iliac bolts of the appropriate length and diameter were placed. Dissecting superiorly from the primary iliac bolt, entry points were selected. Under direct and fluoroscopic visualization, a drill was used to create pilot holes. The Lenke probe was then passed in an appropriate trajectory to create solid bone on palpation. Double iliac bolts of the appropriate length and diameter were inserted. L4 through S1 laminectomies were performed, and the lesion, which was partially extradural and partially intradural, was debulked. Adequate arthrodesis was performed. Autograft and allograft materials were used to spur bony fusion.

Outcome

The patient did well postoperatively with improvement in his left-sided radicular symptoms. His postoperative radiographs demonstrated normal sagittal balance, restoration of lumbar lordosis, and adequate hardware placement (Fig. 30.9).

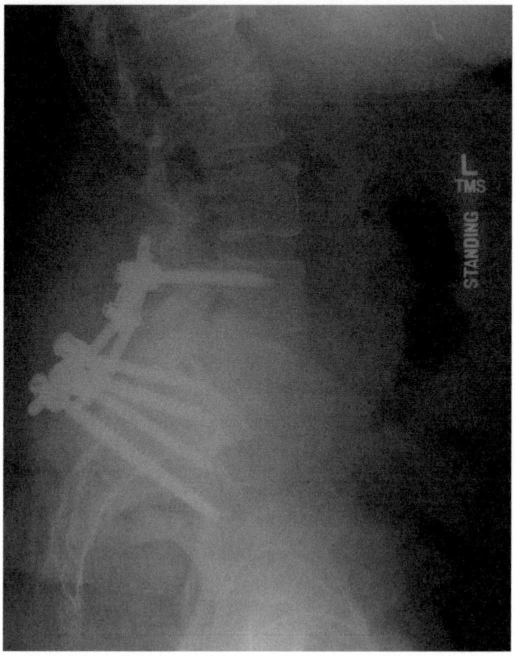

Fig. 30.9 Sagittal standing postoperative radiograph demonstrating L4-ilium fusion with no sign of hardware malposition or failure

Technical Pearls

- In cases where both an S1 pedicle screw and an iliac bolt are to be used, having the starting point of the iliac screw more inferior than the sacral screw is crucial in order to make connection to the rod easier. In our practice, a medial-lateral connector is used. However, if this is not desired, then a more dramatic lordotic bend in the rod combined with leaving the S1 screw head slightly more lateral and prominent can help with this connection [1].
- When a minimally invasive approach is undertaken to place an iliac screw, contouring the rod and connecting the iliac screw to the proximal hardware present a challenge. To solve this problem, a hyperacute lordotic bend of 30–40 degrees at the distal 2–3 cm of the rod enables easier connection [33]. This connection is even more difficult in the presence of an S1 screw due to the shorter rod segment requiring contouring in two planes to link the iliac screw and the S1 screw [33]. As such, an option for consideration would be to not place an S1 screw when pelvic fixation is enough to sustain functional demand and maintain hardware integrity until bone fusion occurs [33].
- During placement of S2AI screws, difficulty advancing through the cancellous bone of the ilium is commonly caused by abutting the lateral cortex of the ilium [5]. To overcome this issue, start more lateral with a more vertical trajectory, closely abutting the notch [5].
- Loosening of iliac screws and S2AI screws is not an uncommon phenomenon. As long as a patient is not having pain due to prominent hardware and there is no evidence of pseudarthrosis across the lumbosacral junction, these patients should be followed with serial imaging rather than taken for reoperation.

Complications and Strategies for Avoidance

Prominent Implants

A common complication associated with iliac screws is prominent, painful implants, with a prevalence of up to 20% postoperatively [1, 26, 35]. Another study showed that 22% of patients needed to have the screws removed at 2 years [4, 37]. The strategy to avoid this complication includes starting the iliac screw deep to the PSIS and removing enough bone at the entry site for the screw head to sit comfortably without protruding above the outer margin of the iliac crest. Alternatively, if patient anatomy does not allow for placement of a non-prominent iliac screw, an S2AI screw can be utilized instead. Having non-prominent implants can also theoretically help with wound healing as it takes pressure off the incision. This fact is especially important in trauma cases where wound healing can be an issue. Options to utilize in high-risk wounds include negative-pressure wound therapy and vancomycin powder.

Potential Need for Interbody Fusion

In adult deformity patients, there is an 11% major failure rate when pelvic fixation is used, including rod breakage between L4 and S1, failure of S1 screws, and prominent iliac screws requiring removal [1]. The most important goal in pelvic fixation is achieving a fusion at the lumbosacral junction. However, if a bony fusion does not occur in a timely manner, fixation failure is bound to happen, either from implant breakage or loosening [4]. As such, many authors advocate anterior column support through interbody cage placement at L4–L5 and/or L5–S1, as this greatly improves solid fusion [4, 38–40]. However, this point is controversial, as some studies did not demonstrate any change in pseudarthrosis rates with interbody cage placement when pelvic fixation and/or recombinant human bone morphogenetic protein is used [28, 41]. Even though not proven to be of benefit, this should be considered in long fusion constructs that extend to the upper thoracic spine to remove some of the stresses from posterior implants and allow for early bony fusion [4].

Greater Sciatic Notch Breach

During placement of pelvic instrumentation, there is potential for injury to the sciatic nerve or superior gluteal artery if the sciatic notch is breached. To protect against this complication, it is of utmost importance to follow the cancellous bone as the iliac probe is advanced by hand. If a cortical rim is felt, redirection of the probe should be entertained. Fluoroscopy or image guidance can be used to decrease the risk of breaching the greater sciatic notch. More importantly, this complication can be avoided by familiarization with sacropelvic anatomy, which can be accomplished with the use of cadavers [4]. Moreover, in cases where a patient has a history of an iliac bone graft harvest, it is important to utilize the different fluoroscopic views or place the screw with CT guidance as the tactile feedback from feeling for the cancellous bone in the ilium will be altered drastically. In these instances, both cancellous and cortical bones are hard, and a breach into the greater sciatic notch is more likely.

Problems with Rod Fracture

Even though newer titanium alloy metals along with the use of cobalt chrome or stainless steel have reduced the chance of rod fracture, it has not been eliminated entirely. In cases of rod failure, a 4-rod technique can be used where differing insertion angles of pedicle screws allow for placement of two rods on each side of the construct [42]. In this method, only a subset of pedicle screws on each side are joined by one rod, while another joins the rest. This is repeated on the other side. Another alternate method of placing four rods is by utilizing a side-to-side connector with all pedicle screws being joined by one of the rods on each side.

Pelvic Screw Fracture

In a review of 51 adults treated for spinal deformity with S2AI screws and a minimum 5-year follow-up, there were 6 broken screws in 4 patients [5]. In a similar study of 80 children with a minimum follow-up of 2 years, 9 patients had fractured S2AI screws, and 3 had pseudarthrosis at L5–S1 requiring revision surgery [5]. None of the adult patients were symptomatic and therefore required no revision [5]. All screws in both groups that fractured were 7 mm or less in diameter with the exception of 38-mm screws that broke in the pediatric population [5]. Therefore, it is advised to use at least 8-mm screws when utilizing this technique [5]. Another group demonstrated that adult patients with S2AI screws underwent fewer unplanned reoperations for symptomatic instrumentation failure, wound breakdown, or removal of pelvic fixation because of painful prominence than those who received iliac screws [28].

Conclusion

Pelvic fixation was developed to solve the problem of achieving adequate fusion at the mobile L5–S1 segment. There are no absolute indications for situations for when to instrument the pelvis, but relative indications do exist. As such, much of this decision-making is left with the surgeon who utilizes preoperative patient characteristics and intraoperative findings including quality of sacral fixation and the amount of stress placed on the construct in making the decision to instrument the pelvis. The two most common methods for pelvic fixation are iliac screws and S2 alar-iliac (S2AI) screws. Spine surgeons should be comfortable with both methods as there are benefits and risks for each method that could be individualized to a specific patient.

References

1. Shen FH, Mason JR, Shimer AL, Arlet VM. Pelvic fixation for adult scoliosis. Eur Spine J. 2013;22(Suppl 2):S265–75.
2. Tsuchiya K, Bridwell KH, Kuklo TR, Lenke LG, Baldus C. Minimum 5-year analysis of L5-S1 fusion using sacropelvic fixation (bilateral S1 and iliac screws) for spinal deformity. Spine (Phila Pa 1976). 2006;31(3):303–8.
3. White AA 3rd, Panjabi MM. The basic kinematics of the human spine. A review of past and current knowledge. Spine (Phila Pa 1976). 1978;3(1):12–20.
4. Kebaish KM. Sacropelvic fixation: techniques and complications. Spine (Phila Pa 1976). 2010;35(25):2245–51.
5. Jain A, Hassanzadeh H, Strike SA, Menga EN, Sponseller PD, Kebaish KM. Pelvic fixation in adult and pediatric spine surgery: historical perspective, indications, and techniques: AAOS exhibit selection. J Bone Joint Surg Am. 2015;97(18):1521–8.
6. Allen BL Jr, Ferguson RL. The Galveston experience with L-rod instrumentation for adolescent idiopathic scoliosis. Clin Orthop Relat Res. 1988;229:59–69.
7. Pascal-Moussellard H, Hirsch C, Bonaccorsi R. Osteosynthesis in sacral fracture and lumbosacral dislocation. Orthop Traumatol Surg Res. 2016;102(1 Suppl):S45–57.
8. Pohlemann T, Angst M, Schneider E, Ganz R, Tscherne H. Fixation of transforaminal sacrum fractures: a biomechanical study. J Orthop Trauma. 1993;7(2):107–17.
9. Mehta S, Auerbach JD, Born CT, Chin KR. Sacral fractures. J Am Acad Orthop Surg. 2006;14(12):656–65.
10. Gau YL, Lonstein JE, Winter RB, Koop S, Denis F. Luque-Galveston procedure for correction and stabilization of neuromuscular scoliosis and pelvic obliquity: a review of 68 patients. J Spinal Disord. 1991;4(4):399–410.
11. Gitelman A, Joseph SA Jr, Carrion W, Stephen M. Results and morbidity in a consecutive series of patients undergoing spinal fusion with iliac screws for neuromuscular scoliosis. Orthopedics. 2008;31(12):1–5.
12. Myung KS, Lee C, Skaggs DL. Early pelvic fixation failure in neuromuscular scoliosis. J Pediatr Orthop. 2015;35(3):258–65.
13. Phillips JH, Gutheil JP, Knapp DR Jr. Iliac screw fixation in neuromuscular scoliosis. Spine (Phila Pa 1976). 2007;32(14):1566–70.
14. Dasgupta B, Shah N, Brown H, Gordon TE, Tanqueray AB, Mellor JA. Sacral insufficiency fractures: an unsuspected cause of low back pain. Br J Rheumatol. 1998;37(7):789–93.
15. Gotis-Graham I, McGuigan L, Diamond T, Portek I, Quinn R, Sturgess A, et al. Sacral insufficiency fractures in the elderly. J Bone Joint Surg Br. 1994;76(6):882–6.
16. Perra JH. Techniques of instrumentation in long fusions to the sacrum. Orthop Clin North Am. 1994;25(2):287–99.
17. Cunningham BW, Sefter JC, Hu N, Kim SW, Bridwell KH, McAfee PC. Biomechanical comparison of iliac screws versus interbody femoral ring allograft on lumbosacral kinematics and sacral screw strain. Spine (Phila Pa 1976). 2010;35(6):E198–205.
18. Asher MA, Strippgen WE. Anthropometric studies of the human sacrum relating to dorsal transsacral implant designs. Clin Orthop Relat Res. 1986;203:58–62.
19. Lehman RA Jr, Kuklo TR, Belmont PJ Jr, Andersen RC, Polly DW Jr. Advantage of pedicle screw fixation directed into the apex of the sacral promontory over bicortical fixation: a biomechanical analysis. Spine (Phila Pa 1976). 2002;27(8):806–11.
20. Devlin VJ, Boachie-Adjei O, Bradford DS, Ogilvie JW, Transfeldt EE. Treatment of adult spinal deformity with fusion to the sacrum using CD instrumentation. J Spinal Disord. 1991;4(1):1–14.
21. Camp JF, Caudle R, Ashmun RD, Roach J. Immediate complications of Cotrel-Dubousset instrumentation to the sacro-pelvis. A clinical and biomechanical study. Spine (Phila Pa 1976). 1990;15(9):932–41.
22. Lebwohl NH, Cunningham BW, Dmitriev A, Shimamoto N, Gooch L, Devlin V, et al. Biomechanical comparison of lumbosacral fixation techniques in a calf spine model. Spine (Phila Pa 1976). 2002;27(21):2312–20.
23. Zindrick MR, Wiltse LL, Widell EH, Thomas JC, Holland WR, Field BT, et al. A biomechanical study of intrapeduncular screw fixation in the lumbosacral spine. Clin Orthop Relat Res. 1986;203:99–112.
24. McCord DH, Cunningham BW, Shono Y, Myers JJ, McAfee PC. Biomechanical analysis of lumbo-

sacral fixation. Spine (Phila Pa 1976). 1992;17(8 Suppl):S235–43.
25. Mayer M, Stephan D, Resch H, Augat P, Auffarth A, Blocher M, et al. Biomechanical comparison of sacral fixation characteristics of standard S1-pedicle screw fixation versus a novel constrained S1-dual-screw anchorage in the S1-pedicle and S1-alar bone. Spine (Phila Pa 1976). 2015;40(24):1890–7.
26. Kuklo TR, Bridwell KH, Lewis SJ, Baldus C, Blanke K, Iffrig TM, et al. Minimum 2-year analysis of sacropelvic fixation and L5-S1 fusion using S1 and iliac screws. Spine (Phila Pa 1976). 2001;26(18):1976–83.
27. Garant M. Sacroplasty: a new treatment for sacral insufficiency fracture. J Vasc Interv Radiol. 2002;13(12):1265–7.
28. Mazur MD, Ravindra VM, Schmidt MH, Brodke DS, Lawrence BD, Riva-Cambrin J, et al. Unplanned reoperation after lumbopelvic fixation with S-2 alar-iliac screws or iliac bolts. J Neurosurg Spine. 2015;23(1):67–76.
29. Schwend RM, Sluyters R, Najdzionek J. The pylon concept of pelvic anchorage for spinal instrumentation in the human cadaver. Spine (Phila Pa 1976). 2003;28(6):542–7.
30. Sponseller PD, Zimmerman RM, Ko PS, Pull Ter Gunne AF, Mohamed AS, Chang TL, et al. Low profile pelvic fixation with the sacral alar iliac technique in the pediatric population improves results at two-year minimum follow-up. Spine (Phila Pa 1976). 2010;35(20):1887–92.
31. Ilyas H, Place H, Puryear A. A comparison of early clinical and radiographic complications of iliac screw fixation versus S2 alar iliac (S2AI) fixation in the adult and pediatric populations. J Spinal Disord Tech. 2015;28(4):E199–205.
32. Snyder LA, Martinez-Del-Campo E, Neal MT, Zaidi HA, Awad AW, Bina R, et al. Lumbar spinal fixation with cortical bone trajectory pedicle screws in 79 patients with degenerative disease: perioperative outcomes and complications. World Neurosurg. 2016;88:205–13.
33. Liu G, Hasan MY, Wong HK. Minimally invasive iliac screw fixation in treating painful metastatic lumbosacral deformity: a technique description and clinical results. Eur Spine J. 2016;25(12):4043–51.
34. Wang MY, Ludwig SC, Anderson DG, Mummaneni PV. Percutaneous iliac screw placement: description of a new minimally invasive technique. Neurosurg Focus. 2008;25(2):E17.
35. O'Brien JR, Matteini L, Yu WD, Kebaish KM. Feasibility of minimally invasive sacropelvic fixation: percutaneous S2 alar iliac fixation. Spine (Phila Pa 1976). 2010;35(4):460–4.
36. Allen BL Jr, Ferguson RL. The Galveston technique of pelvic fixation with L-rod instrumentation of the spine. Spine (Phila Pa 1976). 1984;9(4):388–94.
37. Emami A, Deviren V, Berven S, Smith JA, Hu SS, Bradford DS. Outcome and complications of long fusions to the sacrum in adult spine deformity: luque-galveston, combined iliac and sacral screws, and sacral fixation. Spine (Phila Pa 1976). 2002;27(7):776–86.
38. Kostuik JP. Treatment of scoliosis in the adult thoracolumbar spine with special reference to fusion to the sacrum. Orthop Clin North Am. 1988;19(2):371–81.
39. Kostuik JP, Hall BB. Spinal fusions to the sacrum in adults with scoliosis. Spine (Phila Pa 1976). 1983;8(5):489–500.
40. Ogilvie JW, Schendel M. Comparison of lumbosacral fixation devices. Clin Orthop Relat Res. 1986;203:120–5.
41. Annis P, Brodke DS, Spiker WR, Daubs MD, Lawrence BD. The fate of L5-S1 with low-dose BMP-2 and pelvic fixation, with or without interbody fusion, in adult deformity surgery. Spine (Phila Pa 1976). 2015;40(11):E634–9.
42. Shen FH, Harper M, Foster WC, Marks I, Arlet V. A novel "four-rod technique" for lumbo-pelvic reconstruction: theory and technical considerations. Spine (Phila Pa 1976). 2006;31(12):1395–401.

Trans-sacral Lumbar Interbody Fusion

31

Gohar Majeed and Farbod Asgarzadie

Introduction

Minimally invasive techniques used for arthrodesis at the L5–S1 disc space offer advantages over the traditional open approaches by allowing relatively easy access to the intended spinal level using a smaller incision and less tissue disruption. This allows for increased biomechanical stability secondary to minimal disruption of the muscles, ligaments, and posterior elements. These procedures also offer the added advantages of minimal blood loss, decreased postoperative pain, and shorter hospital stays. The most widely used MIS approaches for fusion of the lumbosacral spine are the posterior lumbar interbody fusion (PLIF), transforaminal lumbar interbody fusion (TLIF), and anterior lumbar interbody fusion (ALIF). These techniques employ either a posterior, anterior, or lateral approach to perform interbody fusion at the intended level. However, all of these approaches have certain pitfalls associated with them making them less suitable in certain cases [1, 2].

The ALIF procedure employs a retroperitoneal approach to gain access to the lumbar disc spaces. It allows release of the anterior longitudinal ligament (ALL) and restoration of sagittal balance using a lordotic graft with a large footprint [1]. However, the ALIF procedure is associated with disadvantages including muscular disruption of the abdominal wall, retraction of the iliac vessels, and the need for a vascular or general surgeon for exposure. Retraction of the great vessels and hypogastric plexus can also cause increased rates of deep venous thrombosis and retrograde ejaculation in male patients. Resection of the ALL and disruption of the annulus can also lead to increased graft and biomechanical instability. Burks et al. reported a 9.3% incidence of exposure complications in a study of 279 patients who underwent the ALIF procedure. This included a 7.9% rate of vascular complications and a 1.4% rate of retrograde ejaculation [3].

The PLIF procedure provides a posterior route of entry to the L5–S1 disc space. However, bilateral dural sac and nerve root retraction can result in increased incidence of CSF leak, nerve root injury, epidural fibrosis, and dysesthetic nerve root pain syndromes [2].

The TLIF procedure provides exposure to the intended disc space through an ipsilateral and/or bilateral foraminal approach. It allows for lower

G. Majeed, DO, MSc (✉)
Neurosurgery Resident, Riverside University Health System Medical Center, Moreno Valley, CA, USA
e-mail: gmajeed@gmail.com

F. Asgarzadie, MD
Department of Neurosurgery, Kaiser Permanente Hospital, Fontana, CA, USA

L.T. Holly, P.A. Anderson (eds.), *Essentials of Spinal Stabilization*,
DOI 10.1007/978-3-319-59713-3_31

rates of exposure complications compared to the PLIF [2]. However, it can still be associated with dysesthetic nerve root pain syndromes and CSF leak. The posterior approaches can also lead to lower rates of arthrodesis secondary to the use of grafts with smaller footprints, due to the limited amount of space available for placement [1].

The trans-sacral approach described first by Cragg et al. [4] in 2004 has become a viable option for fusion across the lumbosacral spine. This approach utilizes a retroperitoneal presacral corridor for fusion across the L5–S1 disc space. It offers clear advantages over other MIS techniques by minimizing disruption of musculature and minimizing injury to vital neurovascular, abdominal, and pelvic structures. It also increases implant and biomechanical stability due to complete preservation of the annulus and the anterior longitudinal ligament [5, 6].

The differential thread pitch of the implant provides disc height restoration upon implantation. Thus, the trans-sacral approach for lumbosacral fusion provides increased stability and indirect decompression with added distraction [2].

Outcome analysis of patients undergoing the trans-sacral approach has shown promising results with improvement in both radiographic and clinical outcome measures. Patil et al. [7] showed that in patients who underwent an L5–S1 fusion through the trans-sacral approach at a single institution, long-term follow-up ODI scores were reduced from 46 to 22 and VAS scores were lowered from 8.1 to 3.6. Of the 49 patients with post-operative radiographs, 47 (96%) achieved a solid fusion. Bohinski et al. [1] showed that at 1-year follow-up there was an improvement of 46% and 50% in the visual analog scale and the Oswestry Disability Index, respectively. Overall, the trans-sacral approach has demonstrated high fusion rates, significant improvements in pain and function, low complication rates, and short hospitalization stays [8].

The trans-sacral approach offers an alternative method of fusion across the lumbosacral spine for certain indications which will be described in greater detail below. Our goal is to provide the reader with an introduction to this approach and provide an overview of the surgical technique, technical nuances, and strategies to avoid complications.

Biomechanical Evaluation

The lumbosacral junction experiences high amounts of compressive forces resisted mainly by the intervertebral disc. It also experiences a great amount of shear resisted by the intervertebral disc and posterior elements. The anterior column supports 80% of the axial loading of the lumbosacral spine. Due to a high amount of shear across the anterior column, the rates of pseudoarthrosis are relatively increased when only posterior stabilization is performed. The addition of an anterior load-sharing interbody construct along with posterior stabilization is warranted to effectively minimize the range of motion across this level and restore the normal load-sharing properties in some cases [5, 9–12, 21].

Akensen et al. [9] showed that in biomechanical testing, the stand-alone trans-sacral approach reduced the range of motion by 55% in axial torsion, 41% in lateral bending, and 45% in flexion-extension compared to intact specimens. These statistically significant values were further increased when posterior fixation was applied in combination with trans-sacral fixation. On average, the combination of trans-sacral fixation and facet screws decreased range of motion by 70%, 80%, and 90% in axial torsion, lateral bending, and flexion-extension, respectively. When used in combination with pedicle screws, the range of motion was found to be decreased by 73%, 87%, and 88% in axial torsion, lateral bending, and flexion-extension, respectively.

Thus the device decreases the amount of shear stress across the lumbosacral junction. Biomechanical stability is further increased by preservation of the facet joints and other ligamentous structures [5].

The approach is especially useful in the case of low-grade spondylolisthesis where an axial construct can reduce the amount of shear transfer across the already compromised posterior elements during normal range of motion. Fleischer et al. [5, 12] performed range of motion testing across a destabilized L5–S1 spondylolytic spondylolisthesis cadaveric model using a posterior pedicle screw fixation combined with either a transforaminal or trans-sacral fusion. It showed that a posterior fixation with pedicle screws combined with anterior fusion using the trans-sacral approach showed statistically significant reduction in range of motion in flexion, lateral bending, and axial torsion when compared to stand-alone posterior fixation and/or a combination of pedicle screws plus transforaminal lumbar interbody fusion.

The rate of pseudoarthrosis at the L5–S1 level is directly proportional to the number of levels fused. The trans-sacral approach can be used to decrease nonunion rates in long posteriorly instrumented constructs by providing an anterior load-sharing construct. This decreases the amount of S1 screw strain and increases the surface area available for fusion. Fleischer et al. [12] showed that the amount of S1 screw strain was significantly reduced in the pedicle screw plus trans-sacral group versus the pedicle screw plus TLIF group with differences in strain reduction of 50% in extension, 29% in lateral bending, and 24% in axial torsion.

Indications and Patient Selection

- Indications are similar to other fusion approaches and include the following:
  - Lumbosacral pseudoarthrosis (in the absence of a previously placed interbody device)
  - Anterior lumbosacral fixation in the setting of a long construct ending at the sacrum
  - Spondylolisthesis Grade 1–2 (isthmic or degenerative)
  - Degenerative disc disease defined as back pain of discogenic origin with degeneration of the disc confirmed by history and radiographic studies [4, 6, 11, 13]

Contraindications

The trans-sacral approach is contraindicated in patients who have comorbidities or previous surgery that may compromise the access route through the pre-sacral space or cause adhesions of the bowel to the sacrum such as Crohn's disease, ulcerative colitis, or previous pelvic or bowel surgery. It is also contraindicated in patients who are pregnant and have scoliosis that extends to the treated level(s), sacral agenesis, severe spondylolisthesis (> Grade 2), tumor, prior radiation treatment to the sacral or pre-sacral anatomy, trauma, or coagulopathy [1, 8].

Preoperative Considerations

Preoperative imaging such as an MRI, flexion/extension films, and/or CT scan of the lumbosacral spine should be available to determine the patient's suitability for surgery. It is important that these imaging modalities include the tip of the coccyx as a detailed anatomical overview of the pre-sacral area is important to avoid any possible damage to the surrounding neurovascular, abdominopelvic, and urogenital structures. It also helps with assessing the desired trajectory. An MRI allows great visualization of the pre-sacral space. A surgeon is able to preoperatively determine the thickness of the pre-sacral fat pad and visualize any potential areas of pre-sacral scarring and rectal adherence to the sacrum and accurately assess the height of the intended disc space. If there is any suspicion of bowel adherence, some authors recommend a preoperative CT scan with rectal contrast to clearly delineate the boundaries of the bowel/rectum and rule out any preexisting perforations [6, 13].

Careful considerations should be paid to the paired vascular structures in this region because subtle anatomical variations could lead to potential intraoperative vascular injury. If a vascular anomaly is suspected, consider a CT angiogram preoperatively to avoid any potential injury to the neurovascular structures [14].

The MRI of a patient being evaluated for a possible trans-sacral fusion at L5–S1 is shown (Fig. 31.1). The patient was deemed to be an

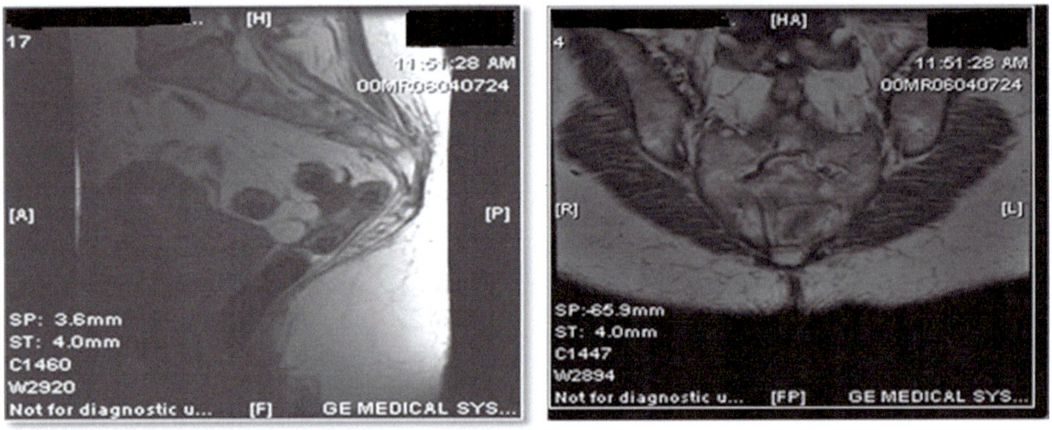

Fig. 31.1 (**a**, **b**) An MRI of a patient undergoing preoperative planning for a trans-sacral approach

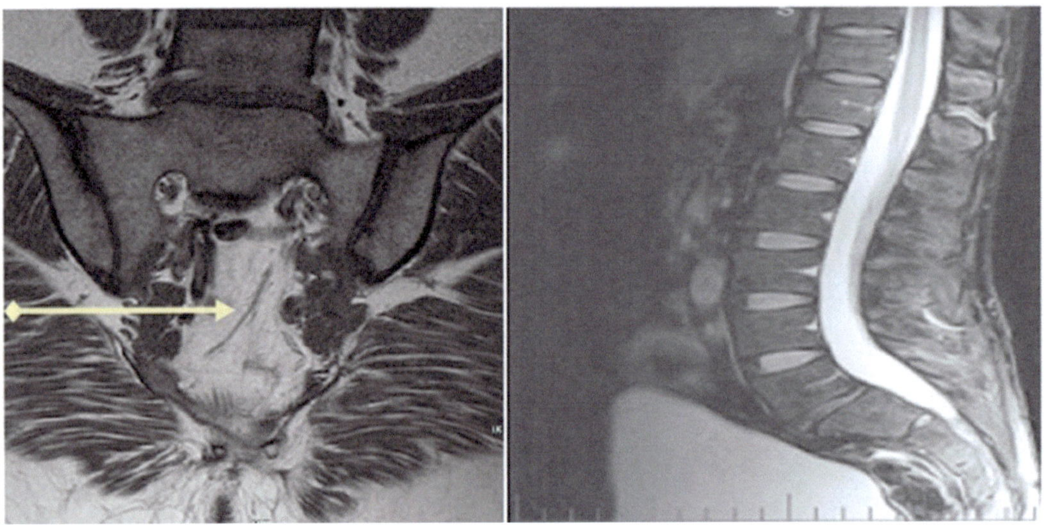

Fig. 31.2 (**a**, **b**) A pre-op MRI of a patient that was not a candidate for the trans-sacral approach. (**a**) A midline pre-sacral vessel; (**b**) Significant amount of pre-sacral scarring

unsuitable candidate due to his history of previous bowel surgery which caused bowel adherence to the sacrum. In addition to this, the MRI demonstrates a poor trajectory to the intended disc space and a pre-sacral vessel traversing across midline at S3.

Identifying the midline is highly important for this approach. This is considered the safest corridor as it is normally away from any major neurovascular structure. Preoperative imaging should be reviewed to identify this, and this should be confirmed intraoperatively using biplanar fluoroscopy. The pre-op MRI of a patient undergoing the trans-sacral approach demonstrates a midline pre-sacral vessel and significant amount of pre-sacral scarring (Fig. 31.2).

As with any other surgery that involves instrumentation, implantation should be avoided in the setting of an active infection. Preoperative antibiotics should be administered. Although there is a less than 1% risk of bowel injury with this approach [6], it is recommended that antibiotics

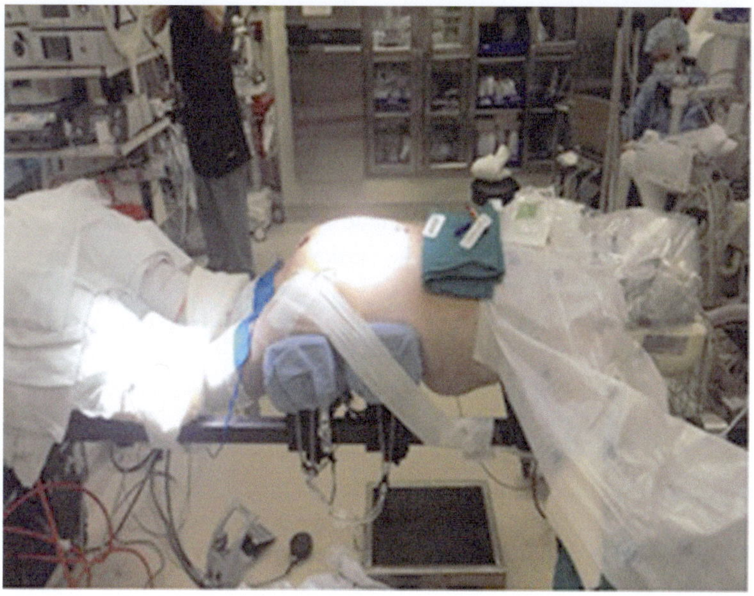

Fig. 31.3 Patient positioning for the trans-sacral approach

with appropriate gram-negative and anaerobic coverage be administered.

Preoperatively the patient should undergo a full bowel preparation the day before surgery. This aids in increasing the pre-sacral working space, thus facilitating dissection and mobilization of the rectum. It also minimizes the risk of any bowel injury and minimizes fecal contamination in case of intraoperative bowel perforation [14]. Miralax and Golytely are some of the common bowel preps used. One should also keep in mind that some of these patients have chronic pain and are long-term opioid users making them constipated and more susceptible to fecal impaction [1, 6].

Surgical Technique

The patient is prone on the Jackson table. Ideally the table should be radiolucent; however, a Wilson Frame may be used as a substitute. Bolsters are placed under the hips and shoulders. A pillow is normally placed underneath the pelvis to elevate the sacrum and achieve appropriate lumbar lordosis. Thighs should be spread apart by placing a pillow between the legs. This allows one to drop the hand during the initial approach, thus keeping the blunt dissector in contact with the sacrum (Fig. 31.3) [1, 2, 4, 14, 18, 20].

A thorough skin prep using chlorhexidine-/alcohol-based skin prep (Chloraprep) is an important aspect of the procedure. Proper technique can minimize infections and subsequent complications. After proper positioning, the patient's skin should be prepped down to the anus. 10x10 drapes with mastisol or benzoin can be used to cordon off the desired area and exclude the anus. If a combined approach is to be utilized, the two procedures should be considered separate with two sterile areas, changing gloves and utilizing new instruments for each of them [2, 14].

External landmarks are identified and palpated before skin incision is made. These include the tip of the coccyx in the midline and the ligamentous arch more laterally. Lateral fluoroscopy can be used to accurately identify the tip of coccyx especially in heavier patients. A point 1 cm lateral to the tip of the coccyx is the base of the incision. The ligamentous arch is then palpated and the incision can be extended toward it. Care should be taken to stay slightly inferior to the ligamentous arch. Orientation of the incision is surgeon dependent and can be either horizontal or vertical. Each type of incision offers its pros and cons. The horizontal incision may allow for lower risk of wound dehiscence and decrease scar tissue formation due to the direction of the Langer lines. It could also potentially allow for more horizontal trajectory correction. However, its major drawback is relatively limited anterior-posterior trajectory correction. The vertical incision on the other hand allows for more A/P trajectory correction and is more widely used for this approach [4, 6, 13, 14].

(a) A paramedian incision (approximately 1 cm off of midline) just caudal to transverse process of the first coccygeal or occasionally the second coccygeal level is made. The incision is then extended caudally 2–3 cm (Fig. 31.4). (b) A small Weitlaner Retractor is then inserted.

This can be retracted medially to be on top of the bony coccyx (Fig. 31.5). This allows one to use the coccyx as a rigid backstop, thus minimizing the risk of direct bowel injury with the incision. We also recommend to incise only the skin and to refrain from "hubbing" the skin knife. The soft tissue dissection should be continued until the dorsal surface of the coccyx is exposed. The dissection is then continued laterally and ventrally along the coccyx using cautery and/or a periosteal elevator with palpation of the bony landmarks along the way (Fig. 31.6) [13].

This is the point of entry to the pre-sacral space and should be in the narrow bony part of the coccyx inferior to transverse process. After the initial incision is made, a 8"curved Kelly clamp is used to bluntly dissect down to the parietal fascia. The dissection is then continued through the fascial layer which extends laterally from the ventral surface of the coccyx. Penetration of the fascial layer is necessary to gain access to the retroperitoneal space which lies on the anterior face of the sacrum. The finger sweep method increases the pre-sacral workspace in an effective and safe manner. The operator's finger is used to bluntly dissect tissues away from the ventral surface of the sacrum while pushing the rectum anteriorly. This allows creation of a midline pathway to the docking site. A decompressed bowel and rectal vault due to the bowel prep aids in the mobilization process. [13].

At this point a bowel retractor system can be inserted to aid in further mobilization and retraction of the bowel. It is a low-profile polyurethane balloon which is inserted after the pre-sacral space has carefully been dissected by the curved dissector. Prior to deploying the bowel retractor system, care should be taken to insert the proper amount of contrast. We recommend using 30 cc of diluted contrast solution, premixed in a 2:1 contrast and saline ratio, respectively. It should

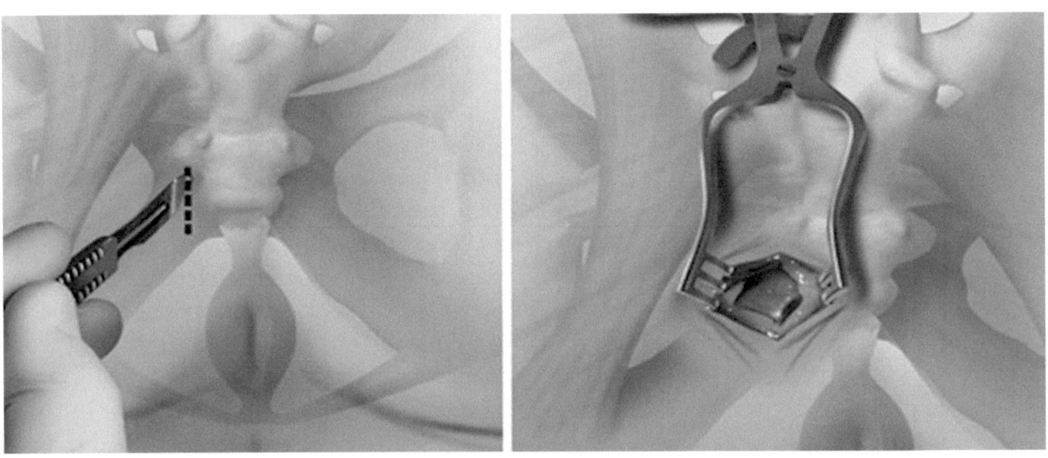

Fig. 31.4 (**a**) A paramedian incision (approximately 1 cm off of midline) just caudal (distal) to transverse process of the first coccygeal or occasionally the second coccygeal level is made. The incision is then extended caudally 2–3 cm. (**b**) A small Weitlaner Retractor is then inserted

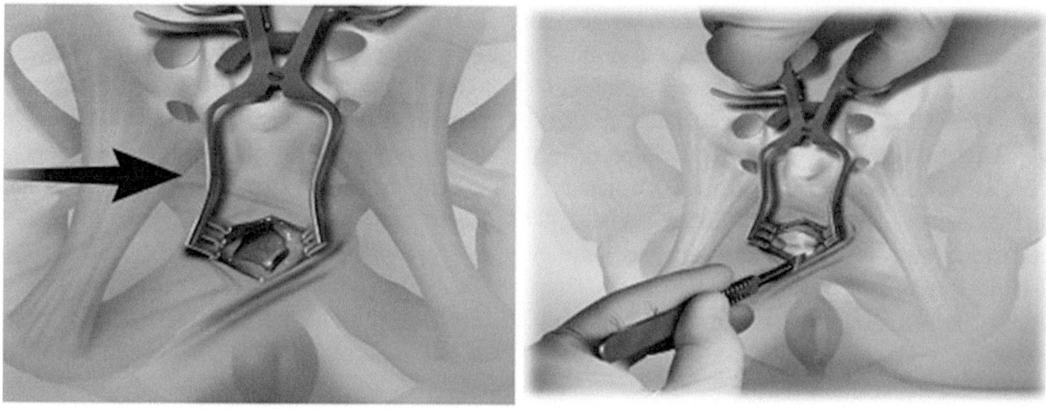

Fig. 31.5 The retractor is medialized to be on top of the underlying coccyx by either the operating surgeon or assitant during further dissection

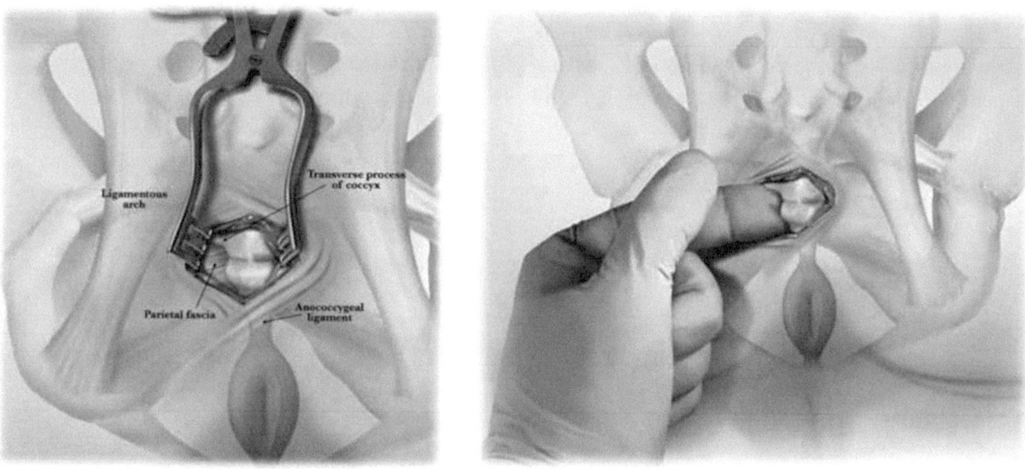

Fig. 31.6 (**a**) Exposure of the underlying dorsal surface of the coccyx with surrounding ligamentous structures. (**b**) Insertion of a finger to conduct blunt dissection of the pre-sacral point of entry

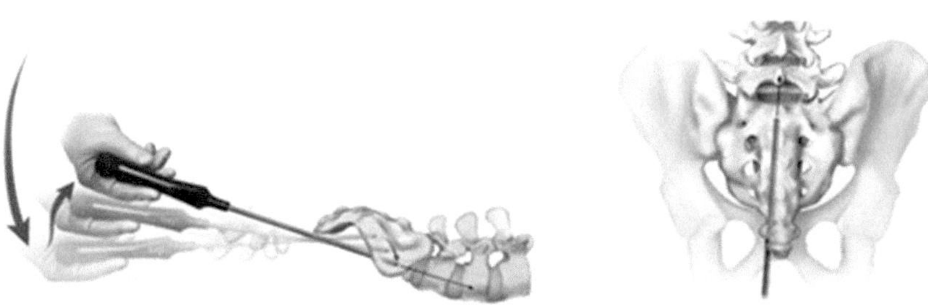

Fig. 31.7 Insertion of the guide pin

be noted that overinflation can cause the bowel retractor to burst and underinflation can cause inadequate retraction. The retractor system can be adjusted as necessary. The inserter is then removed, leaving the bowel retractor in place.

The blunt dissecting tool is then used to continue the dissection. It is advanced cephalad in a midline trajectory, always keeping the tip engaged on the anterior surface of the sacrum to approximately the S1/S2 junction. We recommend using biplanar fluoroscopy to maintain a midline trajectory and keeping the dissecting tool in the pre-sacral "safe zone." This is accomplished with "fingertip" control on the handle of the dissecting tool and fluoroscopic guidance in both A/P and lateral planes.

Once the proper trajectory is established, the blunt stylet is exchanged for the beveled guide pin (Fig. 31.8). The tip of the bevel must be aligned with the thumbscrew on the handle. The beveled guide pin is then docked into the sacrum by gently tapping it with a mallet. Under A/P and lateral fluoroscopy guidance, the beveled guide pin can be tapped through the sacrum and 1–2 mm into the L5 vertebral body.

The next step involves removal of the guide pin handle and attachment of the guide pin extension. This is followed by careful removal of the dissecting tool over the beveled guide pin using the extension attached previously.

A series of dilators are then used to create a wider working channel (Fig. 31.9). The 6 mm dilator is slid over the beveled guide pin. Use the slap hammer to advance the dilator into the sacrum approximately halfway to the disc space. Remove the 6 mm dilator, leaving the beveled guide pin in place, and repeat with the 8 mm dilator. Remove the 8 mm dilator and repeat with the 10 mm dilator assembly. The 10 mm dilator is assembled together with the 10 mm dilator sheath, which slides over the 10 mm dilator body and engages with a pin and slot configuration. Advance the 10 mm dilator

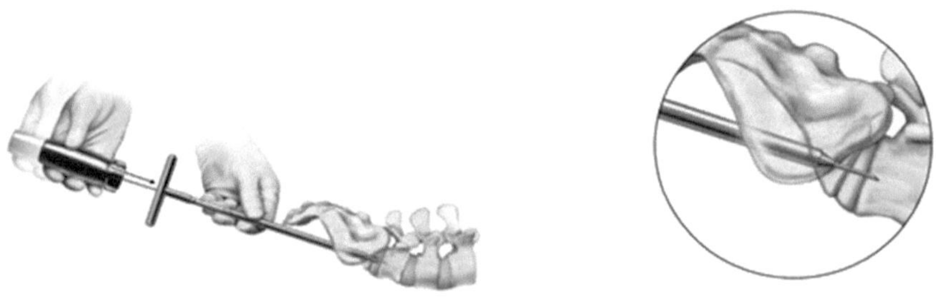

Fig. 31.8 Attachment of the guide pin handle

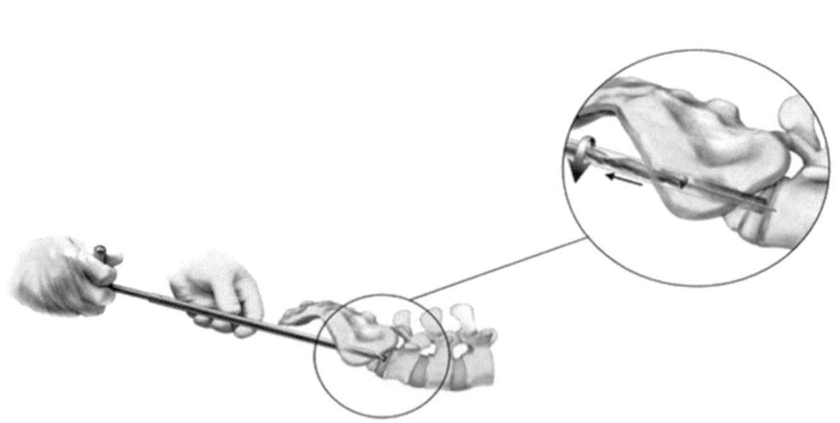

Fig. 31.9 Series of dilators are used to create a wide working channel

far enough into the sacrum to ensure the outer diameter of the 10 mm dilator sheath is placed completely within the sacral cortex. Once the 10 mm dilator with sheath is docked into the sacrum, its body is carefully removed, leaving the dilator sheath behind.

A 9 mm cannulated drill is then inserted over the guide pin to create a channel within the L5–S1 disc space by rotating the drill in a clockwise direction (Fig. 31.10). Biplanar fluoroscopy should be used at all times while drilling [6, 13].

The discectomy is performed using a variety of disc cutters of different configurations and sizes. The loop cutters are designed to debulk the nucleus pulposus and lightly abrade the end plates. Tight disc cutters are designed to debulk the nucleus and lightly abrade end plates in tight disc spaces (less than 2.5 mm). Multiple tissue extractors are used to remove the disc material. In addition, end plate rasps are available to scrape the remaining tissue and cartilage off the vertebral end plates. They provide aggressive end plate preparation, increasing blood supply and providing the necessary fusion bed, similar to a curette. A trigger system on the loop cutters allows tip angle adjustment to match the angle of the end plate.

The discectomy can be thought of as a two-step process, utilizing cutters for the first step and end plate rasps for the second step. We recommend starting with the L5 portion of the disc and using small radial cutters and then moving up to large radial cutters for the center of the disc space. This should be followed by small and large radial down cutters for the S1 portion of the disc space. We recommend using small cutters in the direction of least constraint first (Fig. 31.11) [4, 13].

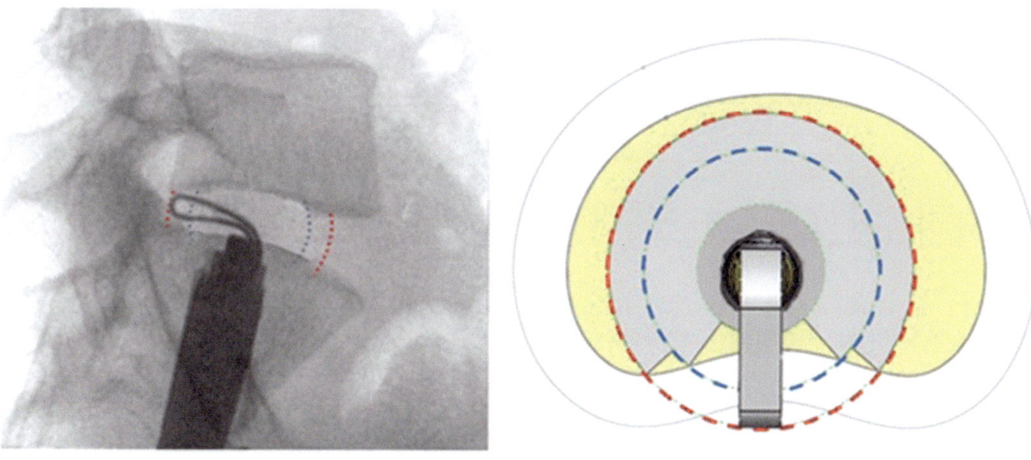

Fig. 31.10 The use of the 9 mm cannulated drill

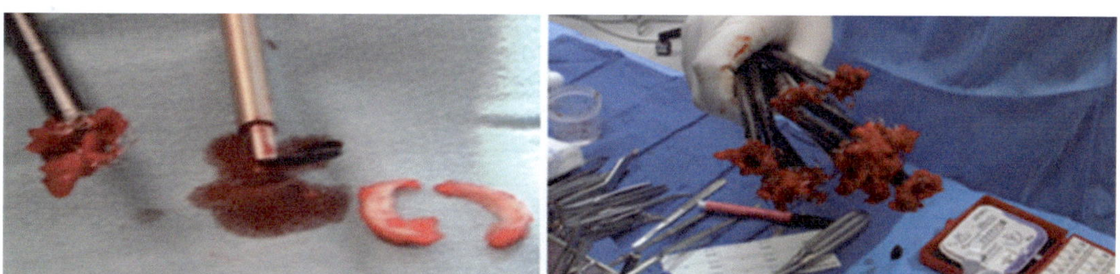

Fig. 31.11 (**a**) The use of fluoroscopy to confirm accurate position of the disc cutters prior to beginning the discectomy. (**b**) The circular area of discectomy with avoidance of the annulus

Each cutter should be utilized twice. Use the first pass to remove the nucleus pulposus and the second pass to prepare the end plates. Several tissue extractors should be used to remove the loosened disc material (Fig. 31.12). This sequence should be continued until the tissue extractors come out clean. The disc space should be irrigated and suctioned prior to bone grafting.

Bone grafting is performed before drilling into the L5 vertebral body to avoid packing the defect with bone graft material (Fig. 31.13). A beveled bone graft inserter is advanced through the working cannula into the intended disc space. Approximately 2–3 cc of bone graft per tube is inserted into the distal end of the inserter. The bone graft material is then slowly pushed into the disc space with the plunger. Care should be taken not to advance the beveled edge of the tube into the L5 vertebral body. The beveled tip allows for rotational delivery. One should be careful not to deliver bone graft material directly posterior in patients who have had a prior discectomy at the same level [1, 4].

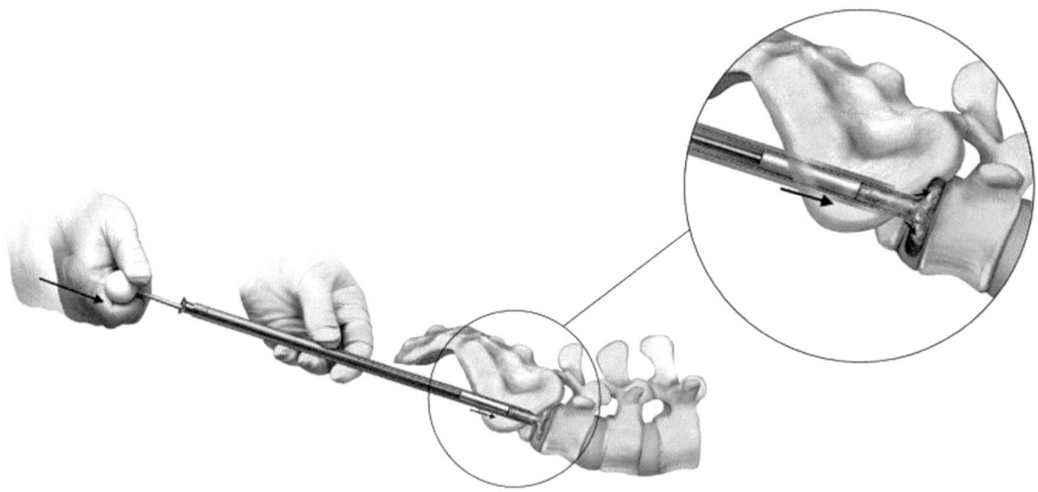

Fig. 31.12 (**a**) A tissue extractor and a disc cutter with extracted disc material placed on the surgical field. (**b**) The use of several disc extractors to remove loosened disc material

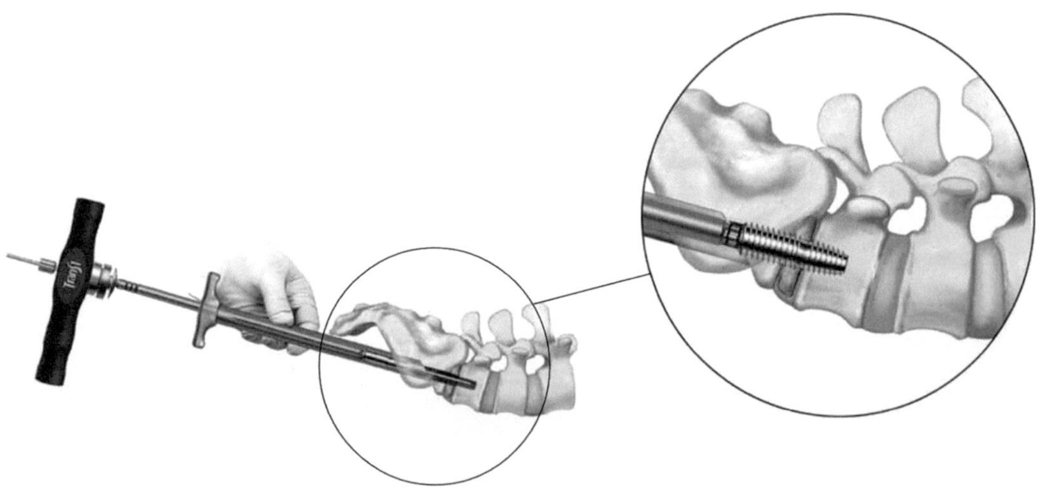

Fig. 31.13 Bone grafting performed through the beveled bone graft inserter

For improved bony fusion, the graft material should have osteoconductive, osteoinductive, and osteogenic properties. Several options are available. The bone recovered during the creation of the intervertebral tract can be mixed with osteoconductive matrices (bone graft extenders) with or without osteoinductive properties. Iliac crest autograft can also be obtained minimally invasively and combined with other agents. Approximately 5–8 cc of graft is used. Bone marrow aspirate is also a valid option. This is normally harvested from the iliac crest or the vertebral body. The aspirate should then be combined with matrix, ceramic, or allograft chips. Using the appropriate bone graft material is imperative for good bony fusion and long-term stability [1, 8, 9, 13, 15, 22].

After insertion of the bone graft material, the beveled guide pin is reinserted. The 10 mm dilator sheath is removed. A 12 mm dilator with sheath is passed over the guide pin. The 12 mm dilator is subsequently removed, leaving the sheath in place. A 10.5 mm drill is then used to drill past the S1 end plate. Care should be taken not to remove any of the bone graft material during removal of the drill.

The beveled guide pin is reinserted and tapped into the inferior end plate of L5. A 12 mm dilator tamp is then used to advance the 12 mm dilator tamp and sheath into the L5 vertebral body so that sheath is flushed against the end plate of L5.

The 10.5 mm drill is then used to drill 10–15 mm into the L5 vertebral body. Fluoroscopy should be used to verify depth at all times. A dilator trial is then used to select the appropriate size implant.

At this point a conformable tip tubular retractor can be inserted and docked into place. It is a lightweight option which offers rigidity due to its inner metal liner and conformability due to its radiopaque silicone tip. The outside liner which is a continuation of the silicone tip offers proper lubrication due to its hydrophilic coating. The conformable tip tubular retractor has been demonstrated to minimize bowel perforations near the promontory.

The assembled implant construct consisting of the appropriately sized S1 anchor, distraction rod, and L5 anchor is inserted into the conformable tip tubular retractor until the superior end is engaged with the sacrum. At this point, clockwise rotation is applied to insert the implant into the L5 and S1 vertebral body (Fig. 31.14). Please note that the waist section between the anchors should be in the L5/S1 disc space to allow for distraction.

The distraction driver is then used to obtain the desired amount of distraction as deemed necessary. The varying diameter allows the rod to have two different thread pitches. This allows for dynamic axial distraction upon implantation with restoration of disc height and the potential for indirect decompression of the neural foramen [6].

The final step involves insertion of the fixation rod. We recommend using fluoroscopy to ensure that the L5 anchor does not advance during this step. Proper fixation can be confirmed using fluoroscopy as the tip of the fixation rod will be seen protruding from the superior end of the L5 anchor.

The next step involves insertion of the fixation rod (Fig. 31.14). This brings the entire construct together and provides bending stability at the L5–S1 section of the implant [13]. Upon completion, the retractor is removed. The wound should be thoroughly irrigated followed by a layered closure.

Posterior instrumentation can be applied either before or after the trans-sacral approach. The type of approach used is based solely upon the surgeon's preference.

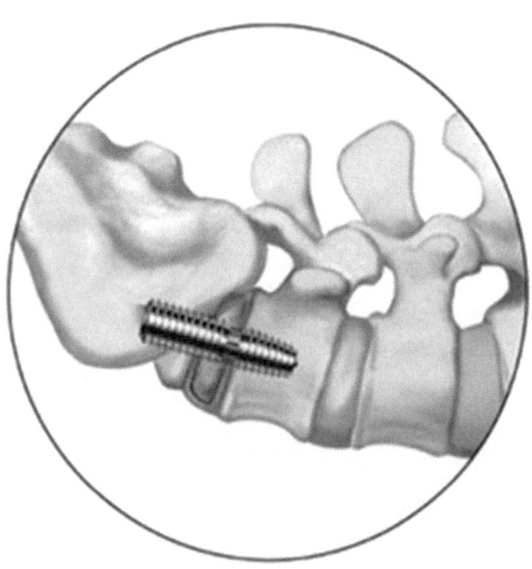

Fig. 31.14 Insertion of the fixation rod

Illustrative Case

History

A 45-year-old female who presented with low back pain and bilateral S1 radiculopathy for 2 years. Worsening of radicular symptoms noted with movement. No saddle anesthesia, bowel/bladder dysfunction noted. No reported history of trauma noted.

Physical Exam

General: NAD, overweight

GCS 15, alert and oriented

Muscle strength: 5/5 muscle strength noted except in B/L planar flexor 4+/5

Sensation: mildly diminished to light touch Left > Right S1 dermatomal distribution

Rectal tone: Intact, + perianal sensation to pinprick noted

Imaging

Flexion/extension lumbar spine radiographs: Grade 2 isthmic spondylolisthesis at L5–S1 noted (Fig. 31.15a)

Treatment

The patient was deemed suitable for the trans-sacral approach and underwent L5–S1 pedicle screw placement through a minimally invasive approach with subsequent reduction of the spondylolisthesis followed by trans-sacral rod implantation to "lock" the reduction in place. The postoperative films clearly illustrate satisfactory placement of the trans-sacral implant along with restoration of disc height post-distraction (Fig. 31.15b).

Outcome

She had a benign postoperative course and serial postoperative imaging revealed excellent bony fusion.

Technical Pearls

- A preoperative MRI visualizing the most caudal point of the coccyx or a CT scan with rectal contrast improves the accuracy of the operative trajectory and allows the surgeon to avoid important neurovascular structures [13, 14].

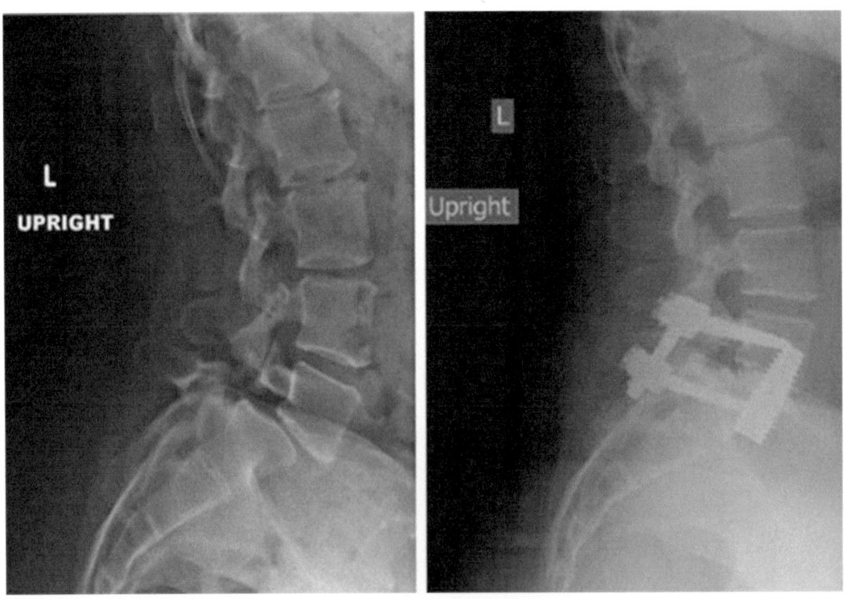

Fig. 31.15 (**a**, **b**) Pre- and postoperative films after L5–S1 trans-sacral fusion and pedicle screw fixation

- Preoperative imaging should be carefully reviewed to identify any neurovascular anomalies in the midline safe zone.
- The preoperative imaging should also be used to check for rectal adherence to the sacrum and accurately assess the height of the disc space [13, 14, 16].
- Proper patient positioning is extremely important for the success of this procedure. The appropriate amount of lumbar lordosis should be achieved preoperatively by placing pillows under the hips to elevate the sacrum prop with pads under the hips to elevate the sacrum and the patient's legs apart.
- Complete bowel prep prior to surgery gives the additional benefit of the bowel being empty and flexible, so it moves forward easily and helps to decrease the risk of bowel injury.
- If a bowel retractor is used, proper dissection with the curved dissector is critical to its successful deployment.
- When deploying the retractor system, be mindful of the amount of contrast injected as too much contrast could result in overinflation and eventual rupture of the retractor system.
- Proper lumbar lordosis should be ensured prior to draping and confirmed by fluoroscopy if needed.
- During patient positioning the thighs can be spread apart by placing pillows between the legs to allow enough working room to drop the hand during initial access to keep the tip of the blunt dissecting tool in contact with the anterior surface of the sacrum.
- To minimize the risk of incision-related bowel injury, the coccyx can be used as a rigid backstop. Direct bowel injury with the incision can also be avoided by incising the skin only and never "hubbing" the skin knife.
- The trajectory and placement of the beveled guide pin should be confirmed with fluoroscopy. If the guide pin is improperly positioned, it should be removed completely and repositioned again under fluoroscopic guidance until the proper trajectory is achieved.
- When removing the dissecting tool back over the guide pin, careful attention should be paid not to disengage the guide pin inadvertently. This can be avoided by using an extension attachment prior to removal of the dissecting tool.
- When removing the drill, continue rotating it in a clockwise direction. This allows bone pieces to remain in the flutes of the drill during removal. These pieces can be later used as part of the bone graft.
- Fluoroscopy should be used to confirm accurate position of the disc cutters prior to beginning the discectomy. It should be ensured that the cutters are not going too far anterior or posterior to ensure the integrity of the annulus.
- The flexible blade of the radial cutter should be retracted into the cutter sleeve prior to insertion and removal from the disc space.
- In patients with a history of discectomy, the bevel of the bone graft inserter should be aimed anteriorly and laterally to avoid accidental spillage into the spinal canal.

Complications

According to a large retrospective study, the trans-sacral approach had an overall complication rate of 1.3%.

Some of the complications associated with this procedure are the following: infection, bleeding complications, bowel/rectal perforation, vascular injury, neurological injury, hardware failure, and osseous fracture.

The most serious complication associated with this approach is injury to the rectum or other surrounding abdominal structures. The rate of bowel perforation with the trans-sacral approach has been reported to be between 0.4% and 2.9%. Lindley et al. [6] showed that in their study of 68 patients who underwent a trans-sacral fusion, rectal perforation occurred in 2% of the study population. It is important to note that one of the patients who developed rectal injury in the previously mentioned study had preexisting risk factors (prior abdominal surgeries, pelvic inflammatory disease, and undisclosed diverticulitis) making her susceptible to bowel injury.

Strategies for Avoidance of Complications

Detailed preoperative evaluation should be performed on all patients being considered for the trans-sacral approach. Preexisting risk factors that may compromise the access route through the pre-sacral space or cause adhesions of the bowel to the sacrum such as Crohn's disease, ulcerative colitis, and previous pelvic or bowel surgery, prior radiation treatment to the sacral and/or pre-sacral contents should be identified.

A midline sacral trajectory should be identified which would allow for a relatively clear pathway toward the L5–S1 disc space avoiding intra-abdominal and neurovascular structures. Preoperative MRI of the lumbosacral spine with images that include the tip of the coccyx should be carefully evaluated to determine the patient's suitability for surgery. While advancing the dissecting tool, AP and lateral fluoroscopy should constantly be utilized to ensure proper midline trajectory.

Conclusion

We believe that the trans-sacral approach is a viable option for fusion across the lumbosacral spine and is especially useful for patients with lumbosacral pseudoarthrosis as well as Grade 1 or 2 spondylolisthesis. In conjunction with posterior stabilization techniques, the trans-sacral approach offers a muscle-sparing circumferential fusion construct at L5–S1 and effectively decreases range of motion in axial torsion, lateral bending, and flexion-extension. Patient selection and perioperative planning are extremely important for the success of this surgery and for minimizing the risk of complications.

References

1. Bohinski RJ, Jain VV, Tobler WD. Presacral retroperitoneal approach to axial lumbar interbody fusion: a new, minimally invasive technique at L5-S1: clinical outcomes, complications, and fusion rates in 50 patients at 1-year follow up. SAS J. 2010;4(2):54–62. doi:10.1016/j.esas.2010.03.003.
2. Issack PS, Boachie-Adjei O. Axial lumbosacral interbody fusion appears safe as a method to obtain lumbosacral arthrodesis distal to long fusion. HSS J. 2012;8(2):116–21. doi:10.1007/s11420-0119227-y.
3. Burkus JK, Gornet MF, Dickman CA, Zdeblick TA. Anterior lumbar interbody fusion using rhBMP-2 with tapered interbody cages. J Spinal Disord Tech. 2002;15:337–49.
4. Cragg A, Carl A, Casteneda F, Dickman C, Guterman L, Oliveira C. New percutaneous access method for minimally invasive anterior lumbosacral surgery. J Spinal Disord Tech. 2004;17(1):21–8.
5. Fleischer GD, Hart D, Ferrara LA, Freeman AL, Avidano EE. Biomechanical effect of transforaminal lumbar interbody fusion and axial interbody threaded rod on range of motion and S1 screw loading in a destabilized L5-S1 spondylolisthesis model. Spine (Phila Pa 1976). 2014;39(2):E82–8. doi:10.1097/BRS.0000000000000077.
6. Lindley EM, McCullough MA, Burger EL, Brown CW, Patel VV. Complications of axial lumbar interbody fusion. J Neurosurg Spine. 2011;15(3):273–9. doi:10.3171/2011.3.SPINE10373.
7. Patil SS, Lindley EM, Patel VV, Burger EL. Clinical and radiological outcomes of axial lumbar interbody fusion. Orthopedics. 2010;33(12):883. doi:10.3928/01477447-20101021-05.
8. Rapp SM, Miller LE, Block JE. AxiaLIF system: minimally invasive device for presacral lumbar interbody spinal fusion. Med Devices (Auckl). 2011;4:125–31. doi:10.2147/MDER.S23606.
9. Akesen B, Wu C, Mehbod AA, Transfeldt EE. Biomechanical evaluation of paracoccygeal transsacral fixation. J Spinal Disord Tech. 2008;21(1):39–44. doi:10.1097/BSD.0b013e3180577242.
10. Anand N, Baron EM, Khandehroo B. Does minimally invasive transsacral fixation provide anterior column support in adult scoliosis? Clin Orthop Relat Res. 2014;472(6):1769–75. doi:10.1007/s11999-0133335-6.
11. Erkan S, Wu C, Mehbod AA, Hsu B, Pahl DW, Transfeldt EE. Biomechanical evaluation of a new axialif technique for two-level lumbar fusion. Eur Spine J. 2009;18(6):807–14. doi:10.1007/s00586-0090953-5.
12. Fleischer GD, Kim YJ, Ferrara LA, Freeman AL, Boachie-Adjei O. Biomechanical analysis of sacral screw strain and range of motion in long posterior spinal fixation constructs: effects of lumbosacral fixation strategies in reducing sacral screw strains. Spine (Phila Pa 1976). 2012;37(3):E163–9. doi:10.1097/BRS.0b013e31822ce9a7.
13. TranS1. L5-S1 fusion surgical technique. http://www.trans1.com/wp-content/uploads/2015/07/AxiaLIF-Surgical-Technique.pdf.
14. Perez-Cruet MJ, Khoo LT, Fessler RG. Percutaneous axial lumbar spine surgery. In: An anatomic approach to minimally invasive spine surgery. St. Louis: Quality Medical Pub; 2006. p. 653–70.

15. Whang PG, Sasso RC, Patel VV, Ali RM, Fischgrund JS. Comparison of axial and anterior interbody fusions of the L5-S1 segment: a retrospective cohort analysis. J Spinal Disord Tech. 2013;26(8):437–43. doi:10.1097/BSD.0b013e318292aad7.
16. Gundanna MI, Miller LE, Block JE. Complications with axial presacral lumbar interbody fusion: a 5-year postmarketing surveillance experience. SAS J. 2011;5(3):90–4. doi:10.1016/j.esas.2011.03.002.
17. Guvencer M, Dalbayrak S, Tayefi H, et al. Surgical anatomy of the presacral area. Surg Radiol Anat. 2009;31(4):251–7. doi:10.1007/s00276-008-0435-1.
18. Li X, Zhang Y, Hou Z, Wu T, Ding Z. The relevant anatomy of the approach for axial lumbar interbody fusion. Spine (Phila Pa 1976). 2012;37(4):266–71. doi:10.1097/BRS.0b013e31821b8f6d.
19. Yan N, Zhang HL, Gu GF, et al. Magnetic resonance imaging analysis of surgical trans-sacral axial L5/S1 interbody fusion. Chin Med J. 2011;124(18):2911–291.
20. Schroeder GD, Kepler CK, Vaccaro AR. Axial interbody arthrodesis of the L5-S1 segment: a systematic review of the literature. J Neurosurg Spine. 2015;23(3):314–9. doi:10.3171/2015.1.SPINE14900.
21. Tobler WD, Ferrara LA. The presacral retroperitoneal approach for axial lumbar interbody fusion: a prospective study of clinical outcomes, complications and fusion rates at a follow-up of two years in 26 patients. J Bone Joint Surg Br. 2011;93(7):955–60. doi:10.1302/0301-620X.93B7.25188.
22. Aryan HE, Newman CB, Gold JJ, Acosta FL, Coover C, Ames C. Percutaneous axial lumbar interbody fusion (axialif) of the L5-S1 segment: initial clinical and radiographic experience. Minim Invasive Neurosurg. 2008;51(4):225–30. doi:10.1055/s-2008-1080915.

Sacroiliac Joint Fusion

32

Sharon C. Yson, Jonathan N. Sembrano, and David W. Polly Jr.

Introduction

The sacroiliac joint (SIJ) is a complex joint that is mobile and innervated and transmits significant loads and degenerates with aging. Its range of motion is reportedly small with just 2.5° of rotation and less than a millimeter of translation [1]. The exact pattern of innervation is debated. Hilton's law suggests that any nerve crossing a joint may innervate that joint. In the case of the SIJ, there are many possibilities, both dorsal and ventral. There are pain receptors within the joint as well [2–4]. Load transmission from the trunk to the lower extremity occurs through the sacroiliac joint. As with all other diarthrodial joints, the SIJ can and does develop degenerative joint changes that may or may not be symptomatic.

Approximately 15% of low back pain can be attributed to SIJ pathology [5]. There is a wide spectrum of treatment available. This ranges from benign neglect to active physical therapy, passive manual therapy, use of a sacroiliac belt, injections, radiofrequency ablation, and surgical fusion. The role of imaging to diagnose SIJ pain is unclear. Typically it is used to rule out tumors or infections and, perhaps more importantly, to rule out spinal or hip problems. There is great overlap in pain perception between the sacroiliac joint, hip, and lumbar spine [5] (Fig. 32.1). Therefore, lumbar spine and hip imaging should be strongly considered prior to committing to a diagnosis of SIJ pain. MRI may be useful in the workup for inflammatory arthritides (e.g., ankylosing spondylitis) [6].

The burden of disease for SIJ pain is high, perhaps even more disabling than hip and knee osteoarthritis requiring total joint replacement, spinal stenosis requiring decompression, and degenerative spondylolisthesis requiring surgical treatment [7]. In addition, chronic nonsurgical management is likewise expensive. There is no compelling data that if left untreated, SIJ pain and disability will resolve. The purpose of this chapter is to review the diagnostic protocol to determine when patients have symptomatic SIJ disease, specific indications for surgery, and technical points regarding surgical options and how to reduce complications.

Indications and Patient Selection

The best algorithm to determine if the SIJ is a pain generator involves physical exam and diagnostic injections. There are six provocative tests commonly used. Reproduction of usual pain is a

S.C. Yson, MD (✉) • J.N. Sembrano, MD
D.W. Polly Jr., MD
Department of Orthopaedic Surgery, University of Minnesota, 2450 Riverside Ave S R200, Minneapolis, MN 55454, USA
e-mail: scyson@umn.edu; sembr001@umn.edu; pollydw@umn.edu

L.T. Holly, P.A. Anderson (eds.), *Essentials of Spinal Stabilization*,
DOI 10.1007/978-3-319-59713-3_32

positive sign. On applicable tests, these should be done on both sides: (1) distraction test, (2) compression test, (3) flexion abduction external rotation (FABER) test, (4) thigh thrust test, (5) sacral thrust test, and (6) Gaenslen's test (see Figs. 32.2, 32.3, 32.4, 32.5, 32.6, and 32.7).

Multiple studies have shown that if three or more of these provocative maneuvers are positive, there is an 82–94% probability that pain is coming from the SIJ [8–10]. Additional useful tests include the Fortin finger sign (if pain is localized enough that patient can point to it with a finger and if this area is at or around the posterior superior iliac spine [PSIS]) and tenderness over the PSIS.

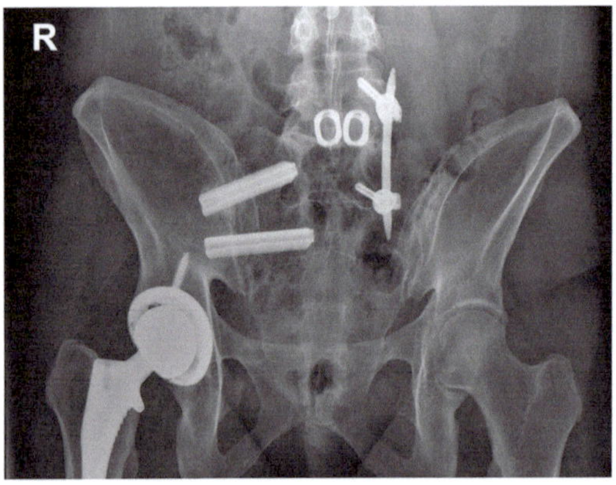

Fig. 32.1 A pelvis Ferguson view of a patient who initially complained of low back pain. She eventually underwent lumbosacral fusion, sacroiliac joint fusion, and hip arthroplasty. This highlights the difficulty of determining the pain generator for some patients who come to clinic for low back pain

Intra-articular sacroiliac injection with an anesthetic agent is the currently accepted gold standard for confirming a diagnosis of SIJ pain if suspected based on physical exam. Based on recent studies, it is generally accepted that >50% reduction of pain after a local anesthetic injection is indicative of sacroiliac joint dysfunction [11, 12]. Cases with obvious spinal or hip joint etiology of their pain based on examination and imaging studies do not need to undergo an SIJ injection. Furthermore, those with pain localization above the anatomic L5 level, pinpoint midline pain (e.g., tailbone pain), diffuse body pain, or zero positive provocative test results likewise are not recommended to undergo an injection, as the likelihood of SIJ pain is very low, and a false-positive injection response may only lead to unnecessary and unsuccessful interventions. If surgery is contemplated, a second or confirmatory injection may be considered, especially if there is still some doubt as to the diagnosis or if the first injection response was not convincingly positive. The authors generally aim for at least two positive injections prior to recommending surgery.

Fig. 32.2 Distraction (gapping) test. This is performed with the patient supine while the examiner, with arms crossed, places hands over ASIS. Force is applied laterally and posteriorly over both contact areas

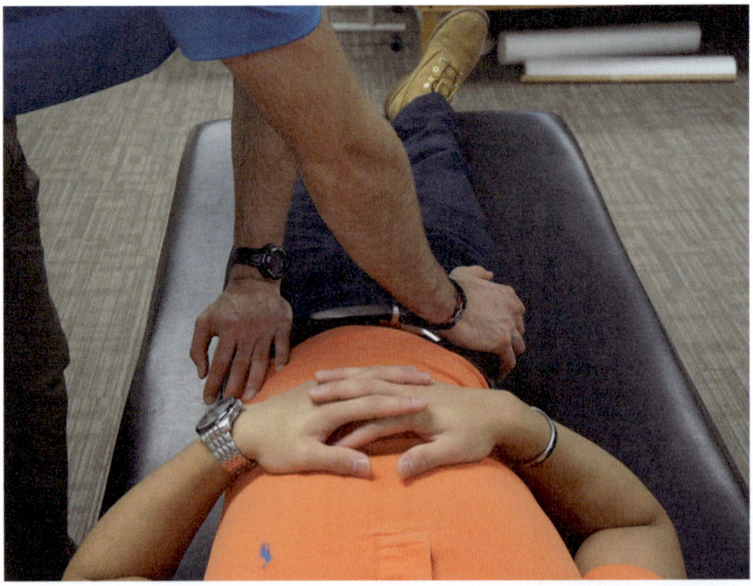

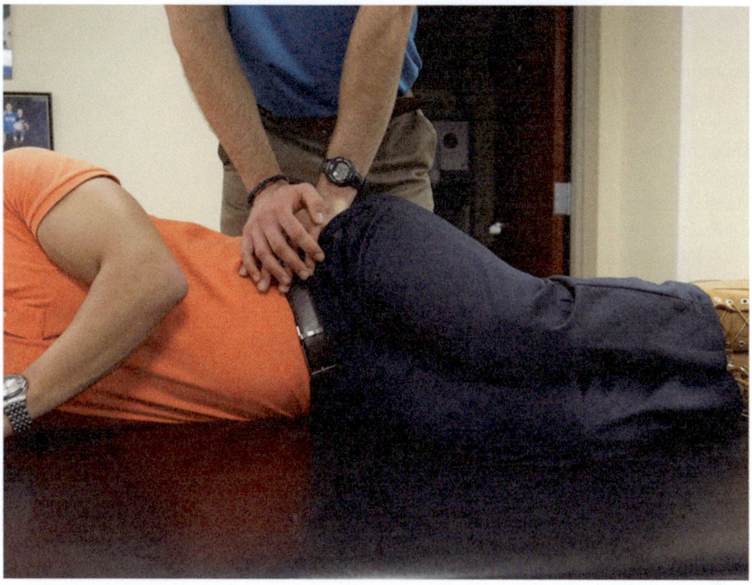

Fig. 32.3 Compression (approximation) test. Best done with patient on side-lying position with the affected joint up. Examiner stands behind the patient, puts both hands over the iliac crest, and applies a downward force to stress the posterior sacroiliac ligaments

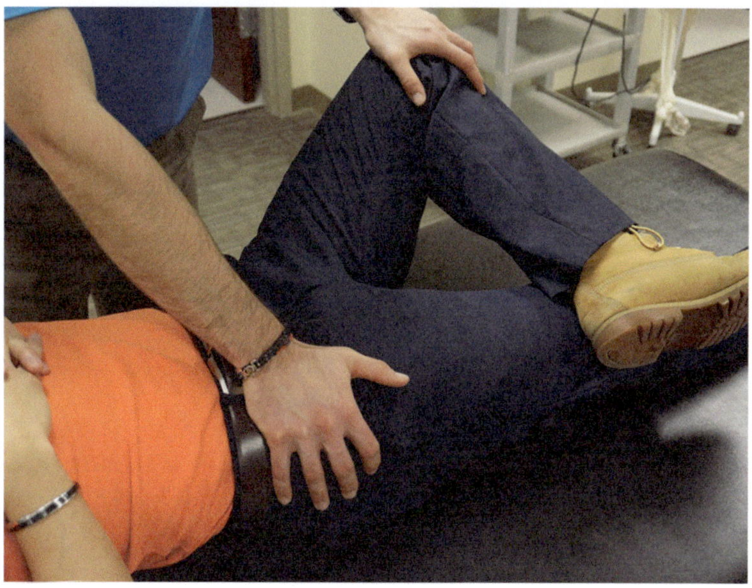

Fig. 32.4 Flexion abduction external rotation (FABER) test. Patient is positioned supine while examiner flexes, abducts, and externally rotates the hip to bring the foot over the contralateral knee. Examiner then exerts a downward force on medial ipsilateral knee

An important step when evaluating SIJ pain is to evaluate other potentially painful structures. Ruling out the hip joint is done by physical exam and imaging. The most sensitive physical exam maneuver is probably loaded internal rotation. Although hip pain is usually felt anteriorly in the groin, a small number of hip patients will present with primary buttock pain which can be confused with SIJ-mediated pain. Femoroacetabular impingement (FAI) may be reproduced by passive flexion, adduction, and internal rotation (hip impingement sign) and may be helpful to identify labral tears or bony impingement. Groin pain on resisted active hip flexion (Stinchfield test) may signal intra-articular hip pathology. Clear radiographic joint loss or findings suggestive of bony impingement (i.e., pistol grip deformity of proximal femur, crossover sign of acetabulum) on a pelvis AP radiograph also are suggestive. The definitive test to rule out hip pathology is an

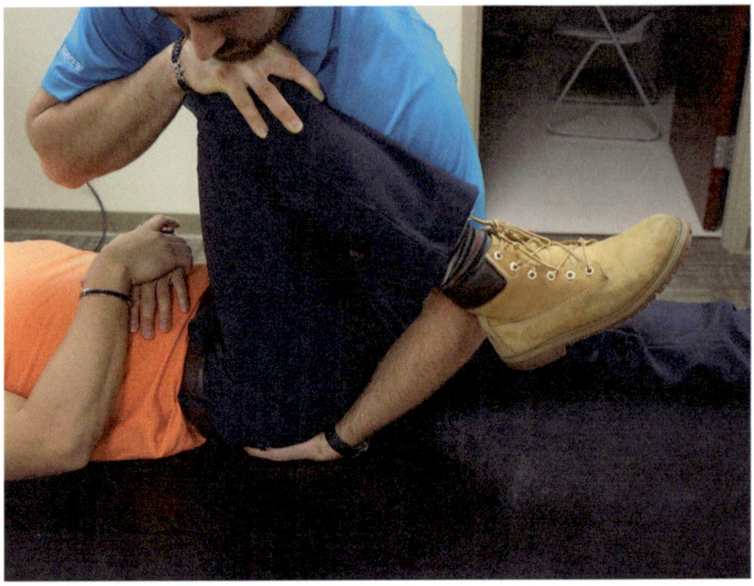

Fig. 32.5 Thigh thrust test. Also called posterior/femoral shear test because a shearing pressure is applied to the sacroiliac joint. Patient lies supine and examiner stands on the contralateral side of symptomatic joint. The hip and knee at the affected side are flexed to 90°. Examiner puts the right hand behind the sacrum to stabilize it and uses the left hand to push down on the flexed knee to exert a posterior force

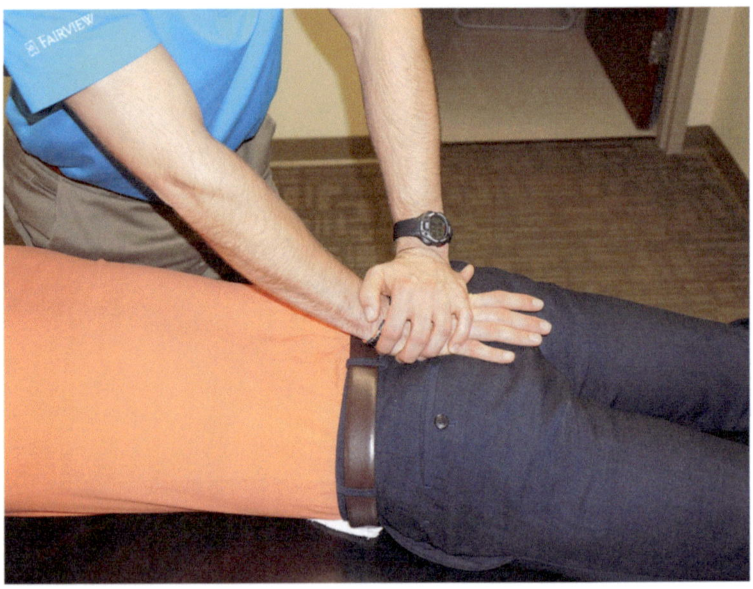

Fig. 32.6 Sacral thrust test. The purpose of this test is to apply an anteriorly directed shear force to the sacroiliac joint. With the patient prone, the examiner puts hands over the sacrum and applies a downward force. Hands are positioned as if doing cardiac compression during a cardiopulmonary resuscitation

intra-articular local anesthetic injection [13]. Relief of the pain by the local anesthetic strongly points to the hip as the source of pain. Advance imaging (MRI, MR arthrogram) may also be beneficial in some cases.

Diagnosing symptomatic spine pathology may be straightforward or difficult. When clear radiculopathy that correlates with imaging is relieved by a selective nerve root block or by a targeted transforaminal epidural steroid injection, then confidence is high about the spine diagnosis. Radicular pain can be generated by the sacroiliac joint, perhaps from cytokine presence near the traversing lumbosacral plexus [14]. Facet loading and diagnostic facet blocks can also be helpful. Differentiation of axial discogenic pain is much more challenging. MRI with Modic end plate changes can be suggestive. Discography was more commonly used previously but is currently a source of significant controversy.

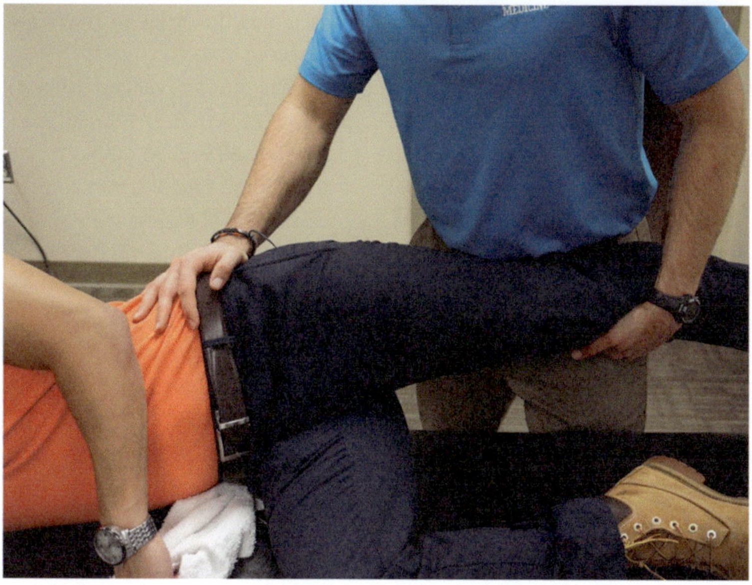

Fig. 32.7 Pelvic torsion test. Popularly known as Gaenslen's test. Typically performed with the patient supine with the leg of symptomatic side dangling on the side edge of examining table. Patient is requested to hold the contralateral knee as close to the chest as possible. Examiner pushes the thigh of symptomatic side down, hyperextending the hip. This maneuver can also be performed with the patient lying on the side with the symptomatic side up. This modification is helpful in patients who are at higher risk of falling off the table in the supine dangling position (e.g., obese patients)

If the physical exam, imaging studies and diagnostic injections are all consistent with sacroiliac joint pathology and rule out other pain generators, then the presumptive diagnosis is established. Prior to considering surgery, patients should have had a reasonable trial of nonsurgical management. At a minimum this should involve evaluation and treatment by a skilled physical therapist with expertise in the sacroiliac joint and spine. Therapeutic steroid injections and radiofrequency ablations are both commonly used nonoperative treatment methods. Lastly, addressing non-spinal factors, including medical and mental health problems, obesity, osteoporosis/osteopenia, smoking, opioid dependence, secondary gain issues, etc., can never be overemphasized.

Surgical Technique

When a trial of nonsurgical management has failed, surgery can be considered. More recently with the approval of multiple devices, minimally invasive techniques have been predominantly applied. New devices are regularly being introduced and it is not possible to cover all the nuances of each system. Interested surgeons are thus advised to reach out to manufacturers to avail themselves of individual surgical technique guides and videos specific to each system. Needless to say, before attempting MIS SIJ fusion, the surgeon has to thoroughly study the SIJ anatomy and the system he/she is planning to use and go through recommended/mandatory training offered by manufacturers, including performing the procedure on a cadaver or model.

The authors have utilized two different systems – one utilizing triangular plasma-sprayed titanium rods relying on bony ingrowth to the rod at both sides of the joint and a screw-based system that allows for joint decortication and bone graft placement in a circular area around the screw. While both systems are more commonly used with C-arm fluoroscopic imaging, the authors have extensive experience in placing them using computer navigation with intraoperative 3-D imaging.

1. C-Arm Fluoroscopy

   Both screw- and rod-based systems utilize transgluteal transiliac sacral fixation. The authors prefer to position the patient prone, as for most spine surgeries. However, patient may also be positioned supine, depending on surgeon preference. Generally, three intraoperative views are useful – inlet, outlet, and lateral. An inlet view is taken with the AP beam angled cephalad ~30–45°, corresponds to a true axial view of the sacrum, and is helpful in assessing for screw violation through the anterior sacral cortex or into spinal canal. An outlet view is taken with the AP beam angled caudad ~30–45°, corresponds to a true AP view of the sacrum, and is helpful in assessing whether the screw/pin has crossed the joint and its relationship with the sacral foramina. The lateral view is taken along the true lateral plane of the body and is helpful for identifying. These correspond to an axial view, a true AP view, and a lateral view of the sacrum, respectively.

   Both systems initially require placement of a guide pin (Steinmann) on the desired bony starting point for each screw/rod. This is best localized on a lateral image (Fig. 32.8). The two systems that the authors use have different suggested pin starting points and trajectories; thus, there is no one perfect starting point. However, it is important to avoid placing a pin above the sacral ala, which is usually seen as a faint oblique line coursing below or sometimes crossing the S1 endplate; violation of the sacral alar cortex may result in L5 nerve root injury. It might initially seem counterintuitive, but the sacroiliac joint projected on the lateral image extends far anterior to the anterior sacral margin; in fact, the true synovial portion of the joint is its anterior region. Thus, it is certainly acceptable and even preferable to have a starting point anterior to the anterior sacral cortex. However, when doing so, the pin should be directed posteriorly and should be assessed on an inlet view prior to advancing the pin across the joint, in order to prevent injury to pelvic viscera/vessels.

   The pin is advanced using a mallet or power drill. Once in the ilium, inlet and outlet images can be utilized to adjust or confirm the pin's trajectory. Once acceptable pin trajectory is confirmed on inlet view, pin advancement is performed while taking regular outlet view images. This is to ensure that the pins either stay short of or avoid the sacral foramina. Driving the pins deeper than the medial foraminal border increases the risk of canal violation and is probably unnecessary in most cases.

   The steps are repeated for each implant (2 or 3, depending on surgeon's preference). Drilling, broaching, and implant placement can be performed over the guide pin (Figs. 32.9 and 32.10). Final inlet, outlet, and lateral C-arm images are taken to confirm satisfactory placement of all implants prior to wound closure (Fig. 32.11).
2. Computer Navigation with 3-D Intraoperative Imaging

At the authors' institution, SIJ fusion is generally performed using an intraoperative 3-D imaging system (O-arm) paired with a navigation system (Stealth) which allows for automated image registration. The O-arm is likewise utilized for 2-D fluoroscopic imaging, including the requisite inlet, outlet, and lateral images. At the beginning of the procedure, a reference frame or fiducial marker is attached to a fixed bony landmark, typically the contralateral PSIS. A 3-D scan is then taken. Navigation is utilized for identifying skin entry points, placing the guide pins, and selecting implant length. Guide pins are inserted through a navigated drill guide. Since the images shown on the navigation screen are virtual images, these may not correspond to the actual guide pin position; thus, it is imperative that pin position still be checked with inlet, outlet, and lateral images prior to drilling/broaching/implant placement. These latter steps are carried out in similar fashion to a non-navigated procedure.

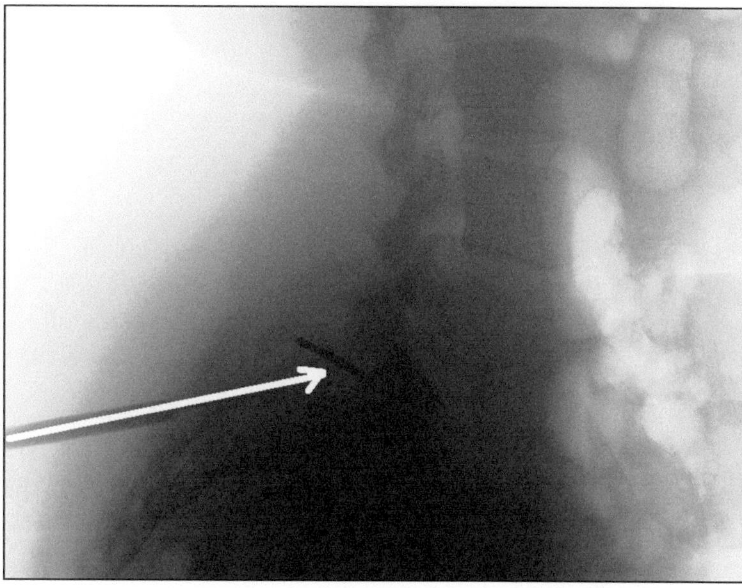

Fig. 32.8 Lateral view of the pelvis taken with the C-arm. Bony starting point using Steinmann pin (*white arrow*) is best localized using this view

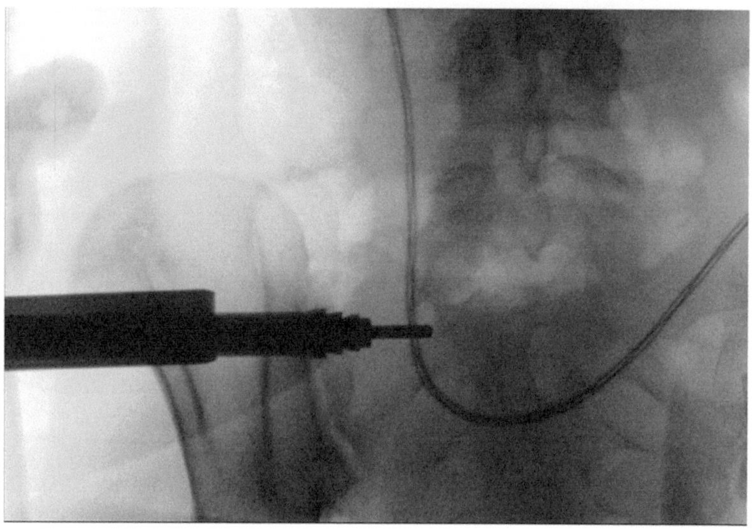

Fig. 32.9 Intraoperative Ferguson view showing a broach being driven over a guide pin

Postoperative Care

Patients are advised early on that they should observe 50% partial weight bearing on the affected extremity with bilateral axillary crutches or walker ambulation for 6 weeks postoperative. No lifting greater than 10 lbs., avoid excessive bending or twisting activities. Patient is taught by the physical therapist regarding ambulation and transfer techniques either preoperatively or before going home after surgery. Most patients stay outpatient overnight (23 h stay), although some go home the same day and some stay longer for pain control issues, particularly those who are opioid tolerant/dependent. At the 6-week visit, repeat radiographs (pelvis inlet-outlet-lateral) are taken; if stable and doing well, patient is advanced to full weight bearing. Formal postoperative physical therapy may be initiated at this point, consisting of pelvic stabilization and transversus abdominis strengthening program, similar to nonoperative SIJ-focused PT program.

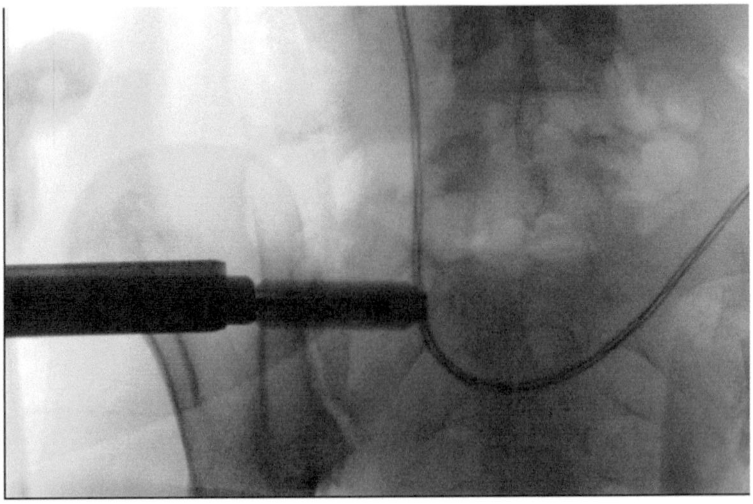

Fig. 32.10 Intraoperative Ferguson view showing a titanium rod being driven over a guide pin

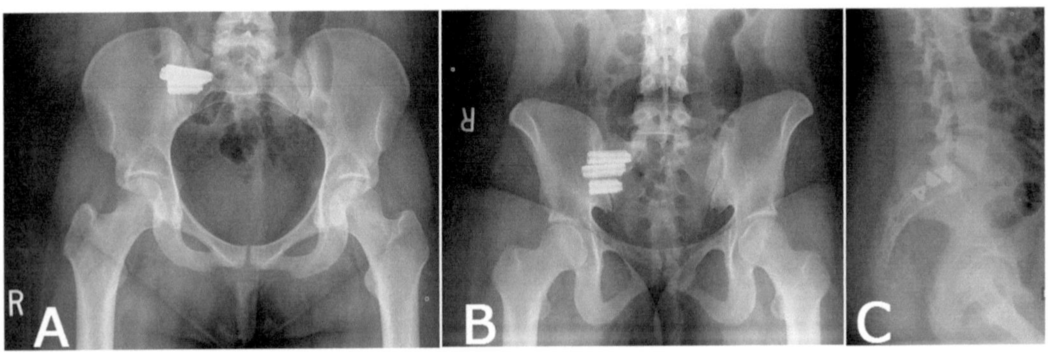

Fig. 32.11 Inlet (**a**), outlet (**b**), and lateral (**c**) views of the pelvis showing proper implant placement

Case Example

History

This is the case of a 58-year-old housewife who presented with a 2-year history of right-sided back pain. She was initially managed by a physiatrist. Her symptoms were initially attributed to her spine for which L3–L4 facet injections and radiofrequency ablations were performed and subsequently her right hip for which she received diagnostic hip injections. She reported no relief from the aforementioned procedures. Her Oswestry Disability Index (ODI) was 64. Her back pain was 8/10 and right leg pain was 2/10.

Physical Examination

She walks with an antalgic gait and localizes her pain at the PSIS (Fortin finger sign). Her pain was reproduced by the following provocative maneuvers: FABER, thigh thrust, and Gaenslen's. The following exams were negative: sacral thrust, pelvic gapping, and compression maneuvers. Motor and sensory examinations are normal.

Imaging

Pelvic inlet, outlet, and lateral views showed mild osteophytic spurring and subchondral sclerosis seen on both sides of the sacroiliac joints.

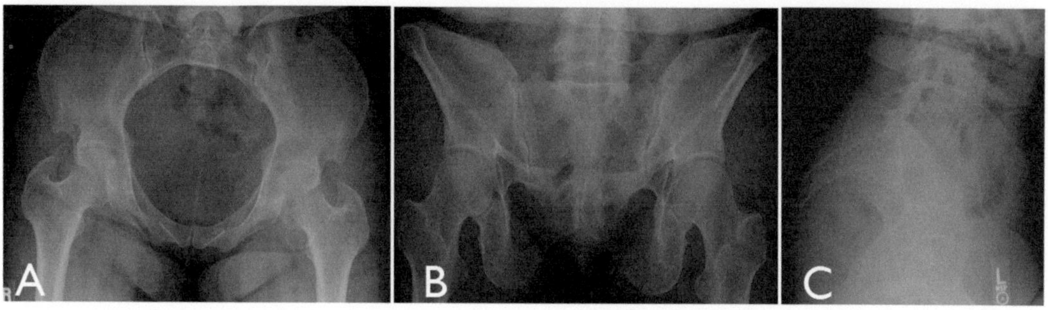

Fig. 32.12 Pelvic inlet (**a**), outlet (**b**), and lateral (**c**) views of a 58-year-old woman diagnosed with sacroiliac joint dysfunction. Mild degenerative changes are seen on both sides of the joint

No lesions, fracture, and gross malalignment were evident (Fig. 32.12).

Management and Treatment

The patient underwent a diagnostic (anesthetic) injection of the right SIJ which provided complete relief for several hours. She subsequently received steroid injection which provided significant but temporary relief. She then underwent a comprehensive physical therapy for 6 months which reportedly did not provide substantial improvement. Eventually she underwent minimally invasive SIJ fusion.

Outcome

At 1 and a half year postsurgery, she reports an ODI of 4 and no back or leg pain.

Technical Pearls

- Evaluate preoperative pelvis inlet-outlet and lateral x-rays for sacral dysmorphism [15]. Although different terms have been used to describe anatomic variations along the same spectrum (e.g., sacropelvic dysmorphism, lumbosacral transitional segmentation, lumbarized S1, sacralized L5, etc.), the bottom-line is that the anatomy in the region is different from what is considered typical or normal, which may likely require modifications to implant starting points/trajectories. While an anatomic variation does not affect diagnosis of the patient's pain generator one way or another, it may have profound implications on implant placement (Fig. 32.13). The lateral sacrum or ala can be vacuous bone and provide limited fixation. The best bones within the sacrum are the cortices and the subchondral regions. Optimizing fixation in these regions is best for fixation but also carries risk of injury to neural, vascular, and visceral structures.
- Positioning and draping are key. Authors prefer to use a radiolucent, carbon fiber, four-poster table; this allows for optimal intraoperative imaging. Care must be taken so that the pads do not preclude access to the surgical site. Prep and drape must be done with care in order to not drape oneself out of the necessary entry site. If using O-arm, arm boards must be positioned close to the table to allow the O-arm gantry to slide cephalad and away from the surgical site.
- When using C-arm, the lateral view is critical. Ensure that the superior margins of the right and left sacral alae and the right and left sciatic notches are superimposed as much as possible, thus giving a true lateral image. Failure to do so may lead to implant malposition.
- When using navigation, working in the sacrum could be challenging as the anatomy is very different as compared to when using navigation to place pedicle screws. There are several imaging windows available for viewing.

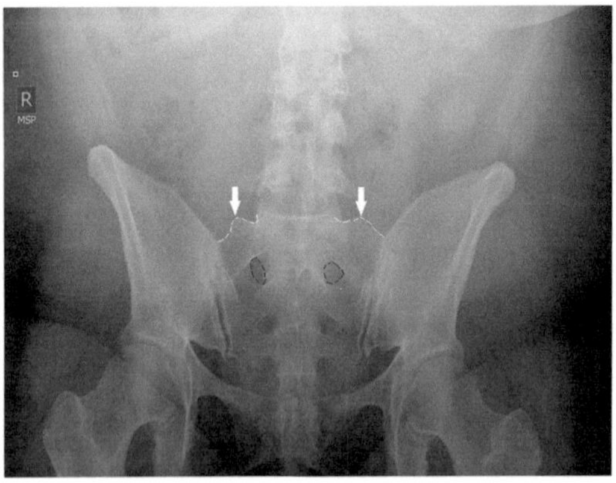

Fig. 32.13 Ferguson view of the pelvis showing a dysmorphic sacrum: upsloping sacral ala (*broken white lines*), prominent mammillary processes (*white arrow*), and noncircular S1 foramen (*broken black lines*)

While each surgeon may develop his/her own preference, the authors have found it useful to use three windows simultaneously: (1) a synthetic true AP of the sacrum or outlet view, (2) axial window, and (3) coronal window. As with navigated pedicle screw placement, it is recommended to adjust the instrument trajectory one plane at a time in order to not lose orientation.

- Some systems come with a pin placement guide that allows identification of subsequent bony starting points on the outer iliac cortex after the first pin had been placed. Although its use is optional, this may help ensure that implants at minimum do not hit each other and promote separation. Emerging biomechanical data suggests that greater implant separation and being in a nonlinear pattern appear to achieve greater initial stability.

Complications and Strategies for Avoidance

Implant malposition is a key complication to be avoided. This requires appropriate preoperative anatomic analysis and adequate intraoperative imaging and image interpretation. Large patients or low-resolution imaging equipment are typical causes. If it is not possible to adequately discern the anatomic landmarks, the case should be aborted. With the use of advanced intraoperative imaging, this is less likely to be a problem. Typical problems include entry into the sacral neural canal, rarely to the sacral spinal canal, and anterior or posterior cortical perforation. With passage of instruments over the guide pins, inadvertent pin advancement may occur; this may be avoided/mitigated by switching to a blunt guide pin. Likewise, guide pins may inadvertently come out with the instrument. Using a second guide pin held by an assistant to gently push the guide pin while the drill or broach is being backed out helps avoid this problem.

The use of local anesthetic in the surgical field helps to lessen the postoperative pain. Enhanced recovery after surgery (ERAS) strategy for spine surgery population is an emerging concept. The authors have no experience on it but the concept is promising. This strategy typically uses preemptive multi-pharmaceutical strategy to minimize pain [16].

Surgical Outcomes

Multiple prospective studies have shown that minimally invasive SIJ fusion is a viable treatment option for SIJ pain [11, 17, 18]. Compared to nonoperative treatment, SIJ fusion has been demonstrated to reduce pain and improve quality of life [11, 17]. Long-term retrospective studies seem to suggest that favorable outcomes are maintained for up to 5 years [19]. Of note, most of these outcome studies mainly refer to transiliac fixation devices, whether triangular titanium rods or hollow anchorage screws [20, 21].

Conclusion

In summary, the diagnosis of sacroiliac joint pain cannot not be easily distinguished from pain coming from other sources based on history or imaging alone. No single physical examination test has been shown to be pathognomonic for sacroiliac pain. Performing a composite of tests adds to the validity of results (e.g., more positive tests lead to a higher likelihood of pain coming from the sacroiliac joint). Fluoroscopic- or CT-guided intra-articular injection is currently the accepted reference standard for confirming the diagnosis of a painful sacroiliac joint. Once diagnosis is confirmed, a trial of nonoperative management should be done prior to considering surgery. Minimally invasive fusion procedures are now available, making surgery less morbid. As with other elective surgical procedures, careful planning is essential to avoiding intra- and postoperative complications.

References

1. Sturesson B, Selvik G, Uden A. Movements of the sacroiliac joints. A roentgen stereophotogrammetric analysis. Spine (Phila Pa 1976). 1989;14(2):162–5.
2. Fortin JD, et al. Sacroiliac joint: pain referral maps upon applying a new injection/arthrography technique. Part II: clinical evaluation. Spine (Phila Pa 1976). 1994;19(13):1483–9.
3. Fortin JD, et al. Sacroiliac joint: pain referral maps upon applying a new injection/arthrography technique. Part I: asymptomatic volunteers. Spine (Phila Pa 1976). 1994;19(13):1475–82.
4. Vilensky JA, et al. Histologic analysis of neural elements in the human sacroiliac joint. Spine (Phila Pa 1976). 2002;27(11):1202–7.
5. Sembrano JN, Polly DW Jr. How often is low back pain not coming from the back? Spine (Phila Pa 1976). 2009;34(1):E27–32.
6. Kang KY, et al. Positive correlation between inflammation on sacroiliac joint MRI and serum C-terminal telopeptide of type-I collagen in ankylosing spondylitis but not in non-radiographic axial spondyloarthritis. Clin Exp Rheumatol. 2017;35(3):415–22. Epub 2016 Dec 14
7. Cher D, Polly D, Berven S. Sacroiliac joint pain: burden of disease. Med Devices (Auckl). 2014;7:73–81.
8. van der Wurff P, Buijs EJ, Groen GJ. A multitest regimen of pain provocation tests as an aid to reduce unnecessary minimally invasive sacroiliac joint procedures. Arch Phys Med Rehabil. 2006;87(1):10–4.
9. Stanford G, Burnham RS. Is it useful to repeat sacroiliac joint provocative tests post-block? Pain Med. 2010;11(12):1774–6.
10. Laslett M, et al. Diagnosis of sacroiliac joint pain: validity of individual provocation tests and composites of tests. Man Ther. 2005;10(3):207–18.
11. Polly DW, et al. Two-year outcomes from a randomized controlled trial of minimally invasive sacroiliac joint fusion vs non-surgical Management for Sacroiliac Joint Dysfunction. Int J Spine Surg. 2016;10:28.
12. Polly D, et al. Does level of response to SI joint block predict response to SI joint fusion? Int J Spine Surg. 2016;10:4.
13. Illgen RL 2nd, et al. The diagnostic and predictive value of hip anesthetic arthrograms in selected patients before total hip arthroplasty. J Arthroplast. 2006;21(5):724–30.
14. Fortin JD, Washington WJ, Falco FJ. Three pathways between the sacroiliac joint and neural structures. AJNR Am J Neuroradiol. 1999;20(8):1429–34.
15. Miller AN, Routt ML Jr. Variations in sacral morphology and implications for iliosacral screw fixation. J Am Acad Orthop Surg. 2012;20(1):8–16.
16. Wainwright TW, Immins T, Middleton RG. Enhanced recovery after surgery (ERAS) and its applicability for major spine surgery. Best Pract Res Clin Anaesthesiol. 2016;30(1):91–102.
17. Sturesson B, et al. Six-month outcomes from a randomized controlled trial of minimally invasive SI joint fusion with triangular titanium implants vs conservative management. Eur Spine J. 2016;26(3):708–19.
18. Duhon BS, et al. Triangular titanium implants for minimally invasive sacroiliac joint fusion: 2-year follow-up from a prospective Multicenter trial. Int J Spine Surg. 2016;10:13.
19. Rudolf L, Capobianco R. Five-year clinical and radiographic outcomes after minimally invasive sacroiliac joint fusion using triangular implants. Open Orthop J. 2014;8:375–83.
20. Mason LW, Chopra I, Mohanty K. The percutaneous stabilisation of the sacroiliac joint with hollow modular anchorage screws: a prospective outcome study. Eur Spine J. 2013;22(10):2325–31.
21. Khurana A, et al. Percutaneous fusion of the sacroiliac joint with hollow modular anchorage screws: clinical and radiological outcome. J Bone Joint Surg Br. 2009;91(5):627–31.

Biomechanical Principles of Spine Stabilization

33

Alvin Y. Chan, Jeffrey P. Mullin, Emily Bennett, Karin Swartz, and Edward C. Benzel

Introduction

An understanding of biomechanical principles is crucial to making appropriate decisions with respect to proper spine stabilization. Surgeons have more methods than ever at their disposal to stabilize the spine, and each option has its own specific nuances, complications, and advantages; thus, understanding the fundamental biomechanical principles that lie at the core of each intervention is crucial to matching the patient's specific requirements to the most suitable construct. This chapter lays the foundation on which proper spine stabilization is established and hopefully encourages the reader to consider the pertinent biomechanical principles to optimize patient outcome.

A.Y. Chan, BS • K. Swartz, MD
Department of Neurosurgery, Froedtert Hospital and the Medical College of Wisconsin, 8701 W Watertown Plank Rd., Milwaukee, WI 53226, USA

J.P. Mullin, MD • E. Bennett, MD
E.C. Benzel, MD (✉)
Department of Neurosurgery, Cleveland Clinic, Neurological Institute, 9500 Euclid Avenue, Cleveland, OH 44195, USA
e-mail: benzele@ccf.org

Basic Principles of Spine Biomechanics

Biomechanically Relevant Spinal Anatomy

The main structural element of the spine is the vertebral body (VB) which provides the main resistance against axial loading. The following terms should be defined: (1) the "width" of the VB is measured from the right-left direction, (2) the "depth" is measured in anteroposterior planes, and (3) the "height" is measured craniocaudally. The VB is generally cylindrical in shape, where the depth and width measurements are typically greater than the height. The VB has a rim of cortical bone, an interior of cancellous bone, and is flanked craniocaudally by two end plates. Furthermore, the width and depth of the VB increase as you move caudally down the spine, leading to a larger cross-sectional area to accommodate for the increased axial loading at the base of the spine. An exception to this generalization is the L5 VB, which tends to be narrower in depth than the L4 VB (Fig. 33.1).

Two adjacent vertebral bodies combine with the intervening intervertebral disc and adjoining ligaments to compose a functional spinal unit (FSU) or motion segment. The intervertebral disc serves as a "shock absorber" and a primary stabilizing structure of the FSU [1]. Although the disc

L.T. Holly, P.A. Anderson (eds.), *Essentials of Spinal Stabilization*, DOI 10.1007/978-3-319-59713-3_33

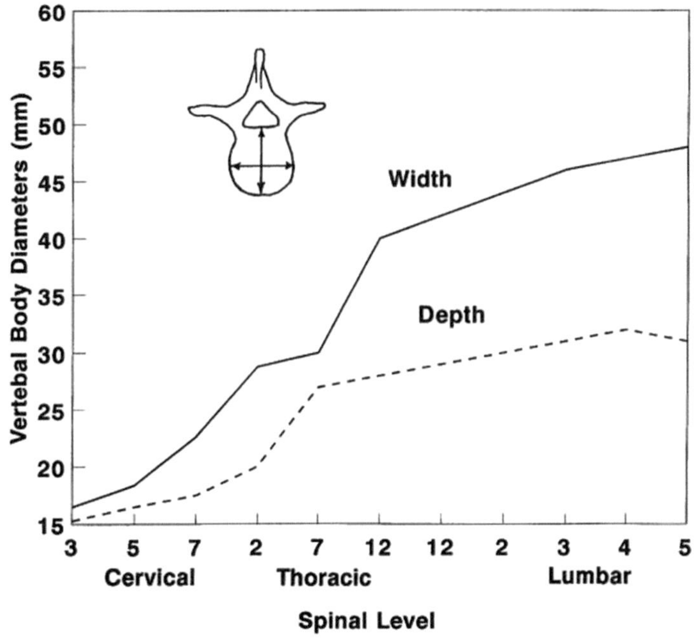

Fig. 33.1 Vertebral body diameter versus spinal level. The width (*solid line*) and depth (*dashed line*) of the vertebral bodies are depicted separately (Fig. 1.1 in Biomechanics of spine stabilization, Benzel E, ed. Printed with permission from Thieme Medical Publishing)

is vaguely similar in outline to the VB in depth and width, the composition is vastly different. It consists of the nucleus pulposus (proteoglycans suspended in a loose collagenous network) located posterocentrally and is surrounded by the annulus fibrosus (a fibrocartilaginous ring). Similar to the VB, the intervertebral discs increase in cross-sectional area in the caudal direction, allowing the lower region of the spine (e.g., lumbar) to sustain higher axial loading [2].

Moreover, the type of loading influences how the disc responds. For example, concentric axial loading creates an equally distributed force within the disc, while an eccentric axial load will bulge the annulus fibrosis on the ipsilateral side and displace the nucleus pulposus to the contralateral side. The sharply angulated fibers of the annulus fibrosus provides the disc's main resistance to shearing and rotational forces which allows for increased force during a broad range of activities. For example, during normal walking, the compressive axial loading on the discs in the lumbar region can be up to 2.5 times the body weight. When lifting 14–27 kg objects, the axial load can increase further to nearly ten times the body weight [3, 4]. Increasing activity requires the discs to undergo significant and repetitive forces without failure.

Between motion segments of the spine, the facet joint is the main load-bearer and stabilizer. The orientation of the facet joints differs depending on the spinal level (e.g., cervical, thoracic, lumbar), and these differences allow for contrasting degrees of motion and resistance among them. Generally, the pattern of flexibility decreases in the cranial to caudal direction. Specifically, the facet joint articulations in the cervical spine lie in the coronal plane which allows for high degrees of motion in flexion, extension, and rotation, whereas the lumbar facet joint articulations lie in the sagittal plane preserving flexion and extension but allowing for less rotation than in the cervical spine. The thoracic facet joint articulations lie in between the coronal and sagittal planes and therefore provide an "intermediate" range of motion (Fig. 33.2). The rib cage also stabilizes the thoracic region by acting as a barrel attached to the spine. Stress, extension, and ventrally directed forces "load" the facets, while flexion and dorsally directed forces "unload" the facets. Facet joints take on additional load-bearing responsibilities when other

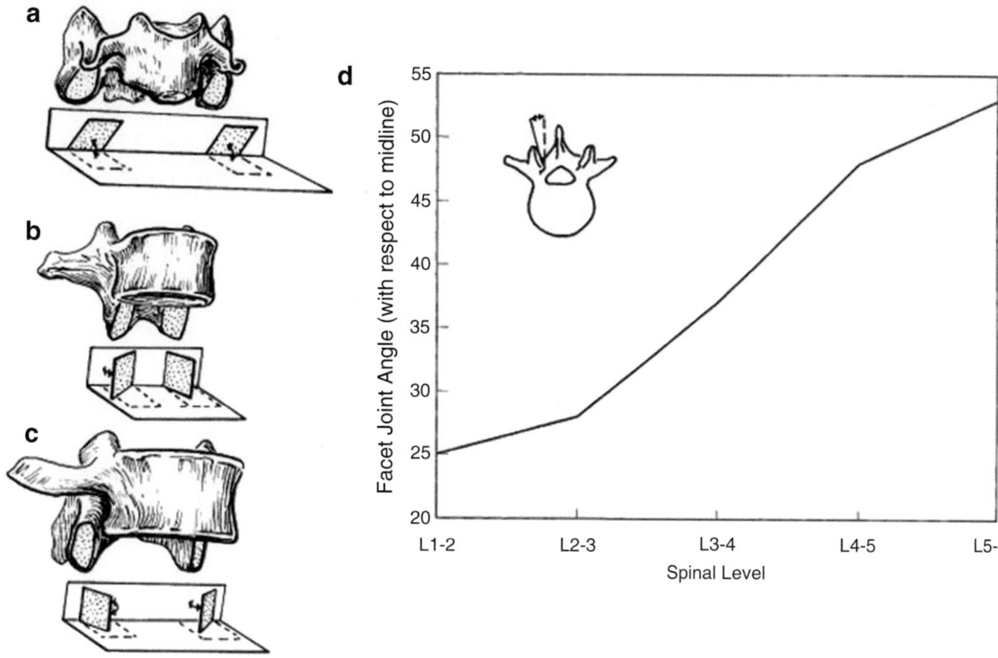

Fig. 33.2 Facet joint orientation. The relative coronal plane orientation in the cervical region (**a**), the intermediate orientation in the thoracic region (**b**), and the relative sagittal orientation in the lumbar region (**c**). The facet joint orientation changes substantially in the lumbar region; here the facet joint angle (with respect to midline) is depicted versus spinal level (**d**) (Fig. 1.6 in Biomechanics of spine stabilization, Benzel E, ed. Printed with permission from Thieme Medical Publishing)

load-bearing structures of the spine (e.g., intervertebral discs) fail as well.

Spinal ligaments also provide important stabilization. Each ligament confers differing strength, but together they act as a tension band along the length of the spine to resist translational forces. This tension band effect is derived from the overall tensile strength of the ligaments. Lastly, a destabilizing force can result from an imbalance in the aggregate musculature which will accentuate strain on the other stabilizing components of the spine. The most important musculature is the paraspinal muscles and its multiple attachments spanning several segments.

Biomechanical Physical Principles and Kinematics

Any force applied to the spine can be deconstructed into three component vectors that exist within a three-dimensional Cartesian coordinate system and have fixed orientations. Each force can act either directly on the spine or as a lever arm that can rotate around an instantaneous axis of rotation (IAR) (i.e., a moment arm), which creates a bending moment when a force is applied perpendicularly. To rephrase, the effect of the force on the spine is relative to an IAR that acts as a fulcrum and is dependent on where the force is applied. The IAR is not a singular, permanent entity or property of the spine; rather, the IAR is dynamic, changing with every spinal segment over the time interval of a movement (i.e., the IAR migrates with motion).

The healthy spine allows physiological movement in the ventral-dorsal, right-left, and cranial-caudal axes with either a translational or rotational component resulting in six distinct potential movements that are referred to as degrees of freedom (Fig. 33.3). Physiologic range of motion is contextual and depends on the spinal region (i.e., cervical versus lumbar) and is dependent on the orientation and properties of structural components.

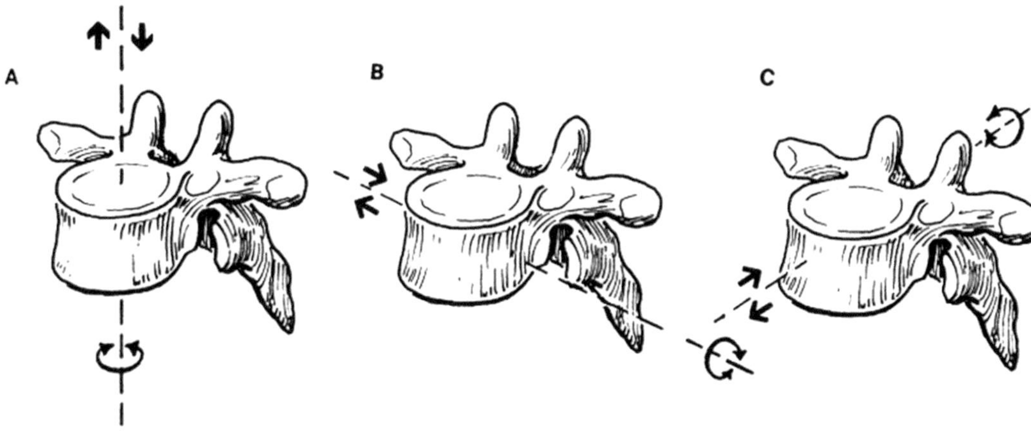

Fig. 33.3 The six fundamental segmental movements, or types of deformation, of the spine along or about the IAR are (1) rotation or translation about the long axis of the spine (**a**), (2) rotation or translation about the coronal axis of the spine (**b**), (3) rotation or translation about the sagittal axis of the spine (**c**), (4) translation along the long axis of the spine (**a**), (5) translation along the coronal axis of the spine (**b**), and (6) translation along the sagittal axis of the spine (**c**) (Fig. 6.1 in Biomechanics of spine stabilization, Benzel E, ed. Printed with permission from Thieme Medical Publishing)

Therefore, normal physiologic motion of one region of the spine can be considered pathologic in another.

External forces can change the physical characteristics of the spine. In theory, the magnitude of strain (i.e., the deforming force) of an ideal object is directly proportional to the stress applied to it (i.e., Hooke's Law). Biological tissues can deviate to make the relationship between strain and stress segmented and nonlinear; this can be described by the load-deformation curve (Fig. 33.4). First, there exists a neutral zone where there is high flexibility at low levels of stress which is essential for normal physiologic motion. Second, there is a point where enough stress is applied to the tissue to cause permanent distortion known as the "elastic limit." If additional stress is applied beyond the elastic limit, it causes a disproportionate amount of strain that eventually leads to failure of the tissue. Also important to these concepts is section modulus and moment of inertia.

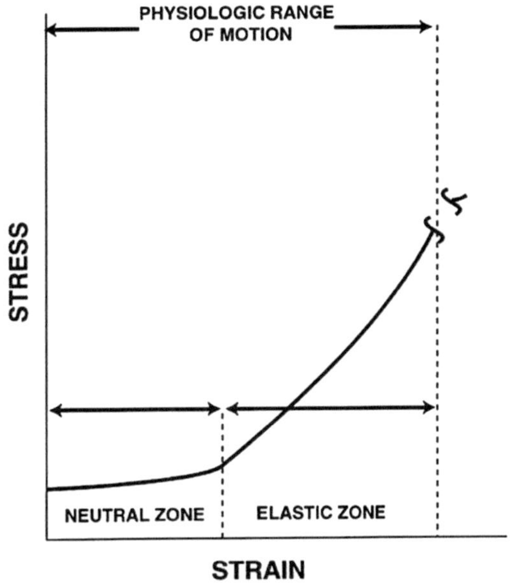

Fig. 33.4 A typical load-deformation curve depicting the neutral and elastic zones (deformation or strain versus load or stress) (Fig. 1.20 in Biomechanics of spine stabilization, Benzel E, ed. Printed with permission from Thieme Medical Publishing)

The section modulus is an indicator of the object's strength and therefore reflects the ability to resist failure (flexion or yield point of the tissue), whereas the moment of inertia portrays stiffness against angular rotation around a rotational axis (i.e., torque) and thus measures the object's distribution of mass around its center.

Spinal Stability Versus Instability

Clinical stability of the spine is equated to the ability of the spine to limit patterns of displacement under physiologic loads to prevent debilitating deformation or pain [5]. The goal of stabilization is to create an architecture of the vertebral column to allow fusion or healing (e.g., percutaneous screw fusionless constructs) to occur and to protect the neural elements. This stability is maintained by an active subsystem (i.e., the musculature), a passive subsystem (i.e., the vertebral column), and a neural-derived component.

Destabilization of the spine occurs when the spine is unable to resist loads or abnormal spinal movements. Instability should be thought of as a spectrum that ranges from "stable" to "grossly unstable" rather than an all-or-nothing phenomenon. Thus, defining a standard cutoff for "excessive" is difficult and may vary based on many factors including bone integrity, structural anatomy, forces applied, etc.

Furthermore, instability can be categorized as acute or chronic. Acute instability is described as being either overt or limited and associated with conditions such as trauma, iatrogenia, infection, or malignancy. Overt instability is when the spine loses integrity in both the ventral and dorsal elements, resulting in loss of sufficient support during physiologic activities. In other words, circumferentially vertebral column integrity is lost which prevents the ability to resist sudden development of a spinal deformity. Overt instability should almost always be treated surgically.

In contrast, limited instability is integrity lost in only the ventral or dorsal component of the vertebral column. It should be noted that limited instability usually confers enough support to allow most physiologic motions and that it is often treated without surgical intervention.

Overt and occasionally limited acute instability can progress to a chronic form if left untreated, but such can also be the result of degenerative changes without an inciting acute event (e.g., infection or trauma). Chronic instability can be categorized, including glacial instability or dysfunctional segment motion. Glacial instability is when the instability progresses slowly and steadily, likened to the movement of a glacier. Dysfunctional segment motion may contribute to the pain experienced without progression of instability but lacks precise consensus definitions.

Spinal Column Pathology

The spine can undergo pathological changes due to a variety of factors. For example, the spine degenerates over the individual's life due to combinations of genetics, health, and life events. Degeneration is an expected part of aging. The end result is the spine becomes less flexible with a lower range of motion as it ages [6–9]. The cervical spine in particular may be most vulnerable to these changes because it exhibits the highest degree of motion and complexity in certain aspects of its anatomy [6]. Another example of potential pathology is infection. Vertebral osteomyelitis can have devastating consequences like paralysis or death [10] and thus must be managed quickly and appropriately. Conversely, the intervertebral disc space can become infected and can present as a complication following surgery [11], though it has been shown to be spontaneous as well [12]. Further, the pathogen responsible for hematogenous pyogenic infections is often *Staphylococcus aureus* [13]. Ultimately, pathological changes in general can affect the biomechanical properties of the spine.

Spinal Alignment

The alignment of the spine may change due to age or pathology which leads to an altered stress distribution within the apophyseal joints and intervertebral discs. The spine has a conformation that maximizes tolerance of concentric and eccentric loads, allowing for flexibility of physiologic motions. Specifically, the cervical and lumbar regions are lordotic in curvature and the thoracic curvature is kyphotic; the curves are, ideally, of equal summative magnitude, which results in a balanced distribution that allows for bipedal upright posture. When lumbar lordosis decreases (or thoracic kyphosis increases), the moment arm lengthens for each vertebral segment which results in a greater bending moment when a force acts on the spine. Deformities in the coronal plane (e.g., scoliosis) occur by the same mechanism.

Spinal Fusions

Stabilization of the spine is ultimately achieved by bony fusion. A spinal implant will fail, eventually, unless bony fusion occurs prior to fatigue of the implant (Fig. 33.5). The structural integrities of the implant and affected bone have contrasting courses: the implant is strongest immediately and gradually weakens over time (i.e., implant failure), while the bone is weakest initially and strengthens over time (i.e., arthrodesis begets fusion). Thus, a proverbial "race" exists between implant failure and fusion of the bone, and bone graft should be utilized in most instances of internal fixation [1].

Ventral Fusion

The position of where a ventral bone graft is placed matters, especially in the sagittal plane. A ventral interbody graft has the advantage of lying in the weight-bearing region of the spine and is usually at the IAR within the sagittal plane. This maximizes axial loading resistance and thus stabilizes the torso. Moreover, the optimal graft is also placed within its neutral axis or the location that is displaced the least during flexion and extension. The position of the ventral graft at the IAR in the sagittal plane and neutral axis is most optimal if the dorsal spinal stability is not intact. However, if the dorsal elements are intact, an interbody graft may be positioned more ventrally, as the axial loading would be evenly distributed between the graft and the dorsal elements [5]. Lastly, even distribution of axial loads by placing a ventral interbody graft prevents kyphotic deformation in the region of the fusion [14].

Ideally, the consistency and integrity of a ventral bone graft should be similar to that of the vertebral bodies. This prevents graft penetration into the adjacent vertebral body or nonunion to occur from either a too strong or too weak interbody bone graft, respectively (Fig. 33.6). Specifically, the vertebral body end plate is weaker toward the center and strongest in the periphery; thus, interbody devices should account for this strength gradient and concentrate loading on the periphery to produce the best outcomes.

Posterior Fusion

In contrast to ventral fusions, posterior fusions do not contribute as much to axial load resistance which is intuitive since the ventral anatomy of the spine provides almost all of the resistance to axial

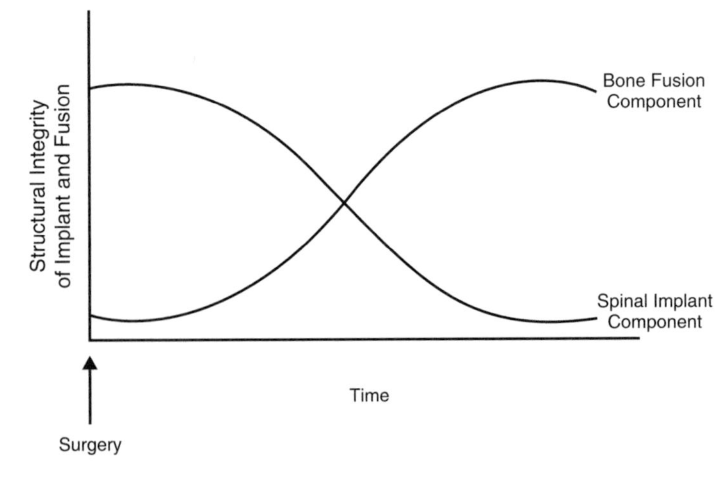

Fig. 33.5 After surgery, the relationship between bone fusion acquisition and spinal implant integrity changes over time (Fig. 10.1 in Biomechanics of spine stabilization, Benzel E, ed. Printed with permission from Thieme Medical Publishing)

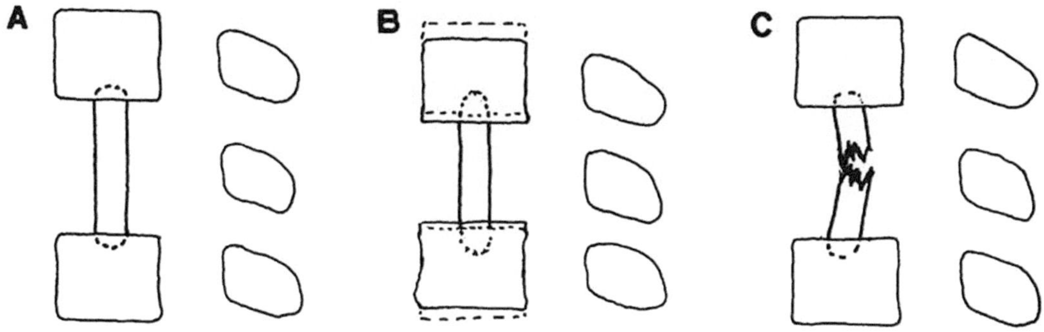

Fig. 33.6 The importance of matching the integrity of the bone graft bed (the vertebral body) and that of the bone graft with ventral interbody fusions cannot be overemphasized. If a bone graft that is denser than the vertebral body is used, the tendency of the graft to "knife" its way through the vertebral body (piston) is significant (**a** and **b**). Conversely, if the bone graft is less dense and weaker than the vertebral body, the bone graft may fail (**c**). Therefore, a bone graft that is of similar density, integrity, and modulus of elasticity to the vertebral body is optimal. It is neither the weakest nor the strongest link in the "stability linkage system" (Fig. 10.5 in Biomechanics of spine stabilization, Benzel E, ed. Printed with permission from Thieme Medical Publishing)

loading. Therefore, ventral fusions with higher compression on the graft confers a faster healing rate [15] compared to the fusion rate for a posterior fusion which is under tensile forces which have a less stimulatory effects on osteoblast function. However, the graft resists flexion well due to a flexion-resisting moment arm created by the distance between the graft and the IAR.

Fusion with Bone Graft Alone

One of the decisions made in spinal fusions is whether an implant is necessary. In some circumstances, the bone graft can act alone as a spinal instrument by providing structural support without deformation in response to applied forces. Allograft or autograft structural bone implants are stiff and resist unidirectional forces (mainly axial loading) immediately postoperatively, but they are contingent on intact tension bands (i.e., adequate ligament integrity or supplemental instrumentation). Furthermore, the integrity of bone grafts is affected by the ratio of cortical to medullary bone; the strength of the bone increases as the cortex to medulla ratio rises [16]. However, stand-alone ventral grafts may provide some translational resistance if the graft is placed in adequately carved mortise with proper depth. Still, the translational resistance is relatively weak even with a properly crafted mortise, and thus stand-alone grafts between vertebral bodies may not resist translational and rotational forces adequately.

Principles of Construct Design

Many spinal constructs provide stability by functioning as a tension band that has adequate strength to convert tension into a compressive force and provide resistance to bending moments. Specifically, a construct attached above and below a spinal segment will convert the tension into a compressive force that acts on the segment. This principle implies the spinal segment can withstand additional compressive force. The resulting compressive force may help encourage fusion. A posterior single-level fixation with cervical hook plates or posterior wire fixation is an example of a tension band.

When a weight-bearing component of the vertebral column cannot resist compressive forces temporarily (e.g., burst fracture), a construct can be used to span the entire length of the damaged spinal segment to provide support, as well as maintain alignment and proper length. This is known as bridge fixation and it allows for load sharing. The placement of dorsal pedicle screws and rods to treat a burst fracture is an example.

An implant can act as a buttress for a weak point and ideally is implemented on the side of the load application where the spine requires additional support for stability. A specific example is an anterior cervical locking plate system because it prevents axial deformity while providing some resistance against shearing or compressing.

In a cantilever system, the moment arm can be either fixed or non-fixed. When the moment arm is fixed, it is perpendicular to the screw, but when the moment arm is not fixed, the screw will experience a three-point moment force that is greatest at the fulcrum. In either case, the screw will fracture where the force is greatest.

Construct Failure

A construct fails when it stops providing the support necessary to maintain stability. A construct undergoes millions of loading cycles and failures can occur when inappropriate constructs are used. The amount or frequency of stress may have been underestimated, the construct poorly designed, or improper patient selection may have occurred.

Construct failure depends on both the intrinsic material property of the device and the amount of exposure to stress. Instrumentation will fail when the ratio of the applied bending moment and section modulus is highest which is the maximum stress that can be applied whether this arises from an instantaneous or cyclic overload. "Fatigue failure" describes the breakage of a construct following repeated bouts of sustained excessive force. Technical aspects of the procedure can also contribute to failure. For example, manipulating the shape of instrumentation (e.g., contouring or bending a rod or plate) can create structural weakness by altering the point where stress is concentrated.

Finally, significant vulnerability of the construct occurs at the implant attachment points. The bone may not be sturdy enough to resist the loading forces of the construct causing screws to loosen or pull out of the bone. The screwhead may even fracture from the screw shaft if excess force is applied. Multi-segmental constructs with long and rigid fixed moment arms may load the caudal screws more than the cranial ones and thus are associated with a high rate of failure of the caudal screws.

Avoiding Iatrogenic Spinal Destabilization

Unintentional destabilization during exposure and decompression of the spine, regardless of approach, is important as this may impact ultimate outcomes. Preserving load-resisting structures such as facet joints, interspinous ligaments, and muscular attachments minimize the risk of destabilization during a dorsal decompression. Resecting roughly one-third to one-half of the facet joint is tolerated without development of instability, though removing any of the facet joint may transfer forces to other areas of the spine (e.g., annulus and longitudinal ligaments). This may accelerate degeneration over time [17]. Further, avoiding excessive resection of the pars interarticularis can help preserve lumbar facet integrity during laminectomy. Lastly, the interspinous ligament is relatively weak but should be preserved during dorsal decompression if possible because its long moment arm stabilizes the spine.

Some parts of the ventral spine may be sacrificed, at least partially. In a corpectomy, for example, the amount of bone spared in the ventral part of the VB is directly related to the strength it can provide. For instance, removing the middle and/or dorsal part of the VB may not result in instability if the ventral part remains intact. Ligamentous disruption can also reduce the intrinsic stability of the spine. The anterior longitudinal ligament (ALL) and the posterior longitudinal ligament strength vary throughout the spine (Fig. 33.7). These ligaments are typically removed in certain procedures, but if it is unnecessary to remove a ligament, then it should be kept in place.

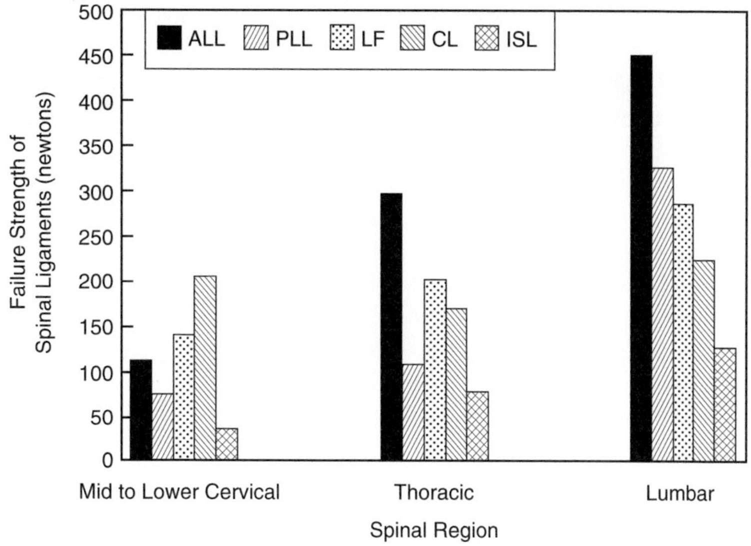

Fig. 33.7 Failure strength of spinal ligaments versus spinal regional (*ALL* anterior longitudinal ligament, *PLL* posterior longitudinal ligament, *LF* ligamentum flavum, *CL* capsular ligament, *ISL*, interspinous ligament) (Fig. 1.17 in Biomechanics of spine stabilization, Benzel E, ed. Printed with permission from Thieme Medical Publishing)

Biomechanics of Non-fusion Implants

There are currently three major categories of non-fusion implants: nuclear implants, total disc replacement (TDR), and posterior stabilization devices.

Nuclear Implants

Nuclear implants replace an injured nucleus pulposus, theoretically restoring viscoelastic disc function, proper tension within the annulus fibrosus, and thus biomechanically relevant load-bearing capabilities [18]. The VB in contact with the nuclear implant undergoes an adaptive remodeling that is probably caused by a shift in load concentration. To maximize the outcome, the material of the implant should be relatively pliable and have a high area of contact with the flanking VBs. Nuclear implants are still relatively new and additional research is needed to determine how they are best utilized. Their failure mode has been expulsion through entry point.

Total Disc Replacement (TDR)

For optimal function, total disc replacement should restore normal kinematics to the functional spinal unit. This will minimize stress on the implant and on adjacent load-bearing structures. If the replacement disc is not ideal, then loading in the anteroposterior or lateral translational direction could transfer to the facet joints which may accelerate their deterioration. Biomechanical constraints of the TDR design that restrict motion in these directions will ameliorate some of this concern and put more of the load on the implant and the implant-bone interface [18].

Ideally, a TDR will have a similar IAR as the original disc, meaning that a relatively posterior IAR will result in a better range of motion since this accurately mimics the normal physiologic IAR [19]. Additionally, the ratio of rotational to translational movement with a disc replacement is governed by the radius of curvature which is determined by the distance between the IAR and the surface of the implant. Essentially, a smaller radius confers more rotational movement, while a larger radius confers more translational.

Posterior Stabilization Devices

Posterior stabilization devices that are currently available restrict specific motions, alter load transferring, and unload the disc and/or facets. Normally these devices maintain a normal or slight focal kyphosis of the facet joints because it transfers the load from the anterior part of the disc to the posterior annulus as well as the facets. Another result is that the IAR is altered, causing the posterior portion of the disc to become more of a fulcrum between the tensile forces derived from the disc and the compressive forces that exist within the disc itself.

Technical Pearls

- The end plates of vertebral bodies are weakest in the center; optimize placement of interbody devices and constructs by focusing the load of the spinal column on the edges instead.
- Whether the bone graft fits into the mortise is crucial. The surgeon should take care to properly fashion the mortise and the bone graft to ensure a tight fit.
- The amount of surface contact between the graft and the vertebral body determines how much the graft will subside; i.e., the more surface contact will result in less subsidence because the loading is more evenly distributed.

Conclusion

Understanding the biomechanical principles of the spine is crucial to properly treating spine pathology that alters its normal properties. This chapter briefly describes the more basic principles that should be considered and contextualized when surgical treatment is appropriate. Importantly, surgery is not always appropriate; an old adage states that surgery can always be done, but never undone [1]. Therefore, meticulous and proper planning for every procedure is crucial. The biomechanical principles of the spine lie at the foundation of this planning, and understanding them will help in avoiding some mistakes that cannot be "undone."

References

1. Benzel EC. Biomechanics of spine stabilization. 3rd ed. New York: Thieme Medical Publishers; 2015.
2. Natarajan RN, Andersson GBJ. The influence of lumbar disc height and cross-sectional area on the mechanical response of the disc to physiological loading. Spine. 1999;24:1873.
3. Granata KP, Marras WS, Davis KG. Variation in spinal load and trunk dynamics during repeated lifting exertions. Clin Biomech (Bristol, Avon). 1999;14:367.
4. Cappozzo A. Compressive loads in the lumbar vertebral column during normal level walking. J Orthop Res. 1984;1:292.
5. White AA, Panjabi MM. Clinical biomechanics of the spine. 2nd ed. Philadelphia: JB Lippincott; 1990. p. 30–342.
6. Board D, Stemper BD, Yoganandan N, Pintar FA, Shender B, Paskoff G. Biomechanics of the aging spine. Biomed Sci Instrum. 2006;42:1.
7. Pintar FA, Yoganandan N, Voo L. Effect of age and loading rate on human cervical spine injury threshold. Spine. 1998;23:1957.
8. Kumaresan S, Yoganandan N, Pintar FA, Maiman DJ, Goel VK. Contribution of disc degeneration to osteophyte formation in the cervical spine: a biomechanical investigation. J Orthop Res. 2001;19:977.
9. Ng HW, Teo EC, Zhang Q. Influence of cervical disc degeneration after posterior surgical techniques in combined flexion-extension—a nonlinear analytical study. J Biomech Eng. 2005;127:186.
10. McHenry MC, Easley KA, Locker GA. Vertebral osteomyelitis: long-term outcome for 253 patients from 7 Cleveland-area hospitals. Clin Infect Dis. 2002;34:1342–50.
11. Rawlings CE, Wilkins RH, Gallas HA, Goldner LJ, Francis R. Postoperative intervertebral disc space infection. Neurosurgery. 1983;13:371–6.
12. Friedman JA, Maher CO, Quast LM, McClelland RL, Ebersold MJ. Spontaneous disc space infections in adults. Surg Neurol. 2002;57:81–6.
13. Hadjipavlou AG, Mader JT, Necessary JT, Muffoletto AJ. Hematogenous pyogenic spinal infections and their surgical management. Spine. 2000;25:1668–79.
14 Whang PG, Wang JC. Bone graft substitutes for spinal fusion. J Spine. 2003;3:155–65.
15 White AA, Panjabi MM, Thomas CL. The clinical biomechanics of kyphotic deformities. Clin Orthop Relat Res. 1977;128:8–17.

16 Mirvosky Y, Neuwirth MG. Comparison between the outer table and intracortical methods of obtaining autogenous bone graft from the iliac crest. Spine. 2000;25:1722–5.
17 Haher TR, O'Brien M, Dryer J, Nucci R, Zipnick R, Leone DJ. The role of the lumbar facet joints in spinal stability: identification of alternative paths of loading. Spine. 1994;19:2667–70.
18 Huang RC, Wright TM, Panjabi MM, Lipman JD. Biomechanics of nonfusion implants. Orthop Clin N Am. 2005;36:271–80.
19 Dooris AP, Goel VK, Grosland NM, Gilbertson LG, Wilder DG. Load-sharing between anterior and posterior elements in a lumbar motion segment implanted with an artificial disc. Spine. 2001;26: E122–9.

Bone Grafting and Spinal Fusion Options

34

Zorica Buser, Andre Jakoi, Bhavesh Katbamna, Rahul Basho, and Jeffrey C. Wang

Introduction

Low back pain and neck pain are the top contributors to high disability rates worldwide [1] with the annual costs for spine care in the United States averaging around $90 billion. When conservative treatments fail, spinal fusion is often a treatment of choice for various conditions including deformity, trauma, and degenerative disc disease. Bone healing and new bone formation are key components of spine fusion and are influenced by the local bone environment and graft materials. Initial stability in the fusion area is achieved with spine instrumentation, while bone grafts provide a foundation for bone healing and remodeling that happens over a longer period of time. While advancements in the fusion technique and bone biology have improved fusion success, nonunion (pseudarthrosis) remains a main procedural complication. Studies have shown that, depending on the approach, number of levels, and the type of grafting material, nonunion rates in the lumbar and cervical spine can range from several percent for single level to up to 60% for multilevel cervical procedures [2–4]. Patients with non-fused or partially fused segments often have poor clinical outcomes and require another surgery. The need for a revision surgery and further care contributes to extensive medical expenditures.

An ideal graft material has all three essential characteristics: it is osteogenic (contains mature osteoblasts and progenitor stem cells that will drive new bone formation), osteoinductive (growth factors facilitating stem cell recruitment and differentiation), and osteoconductive (mechanically stable scaffold with pore sizes that promote neovascularization and bone ingrowth). Grafting materials used in spine surgery can be divided into two major groups: autografts (have all the desired properties) and allografts (have some of the ideal graft characteristics). Allografts can be further stratified based on their function when coupled with autograft: graft extenders (reducing the amount of autograft needed), substitutes (fully replacing the autograft), or enhancers (combined with autograft to enhance fusion). Although allograft bone substitutes lack some of the properties of autograft, they have demonstrated

Z. Buser, PhD (✉) • A. Jakoi, MD • J.C. Wang, MD
Department of Orthopaedic Surgery, Keck School of Medicine, University of Southern California, Los Angeles, CA 90033, USA
e-mail: zbuser@usc.edu; ajakoi22@gmail.com; jeffrey.wang@med.usc.edu

B. Katbamna, BS
Medical College of Wisconsin, Milwaukee, WI, USA
e-mail: bhaveshkatbamna@gmail.com

R. Basho, MD
Department of Orthopaedic Surgery, Hannibal Regional Hospital, Hannibal, MO, USA
e-mail: rahulbasho@gmail.com

L.T. Holly, P.A. Anderson (eds.), *Essentials of Spinal Stabilization*, DOI 10.1007/978-3-319-59713-3_34

Table 34.1 Bone grafts used for spine fusions

	Properties		
Grafts	Osteoconductive	Osteoinductive	Osteogenic
Autograft	+	+	+
Allograft	+	+/–	–
DMB	+	+/–	–
Ceramics	+	–	–
Platelet gels	–	–	+
BMA	–	+	+
BMP	–	–	+

DBM demineralized bone matrix, *BMP* bone morphogenetic proteins, *BMA* bone marrow aspirate

similar fusion rates in both preclinical animal models and clinical studies. Commonly used grafting materials and their properties are summarized in Table 34.1.

Autograft

Autograft is considered the gold standard among graft materials in spinal fusion. It is the only material which possesses all three of the necessary elements for bone formation: osteogenic cells, an osteoconductive matrix, and osteoinductive factors [5, 6]. Based on the harvest site, autograft can be divided into two main categories: iliac bone crest graft (ICBG) and local bone. Local bone is commonly harvested during decompression from the lamina, facets, or processes. With no extra harvest procedure, local bone has advantage over ICBG when it comes to harvest morbidities and complications. Local bone is a cortical graft which provides immediate mechanical stability; however, due to the small pore size, cell migration is impaired. This leads to lower rates of bone remodeling and long-term instability. On the other hand, the iliac crest is the most common and frequently used source because it has the ability to provide sufficient quantities of unicortical, bicortical, tricortical, and cancellous bone [7–9]. In addition, the iliac crest is easily accessible; during posterior spinal fusion procedures, a separate incision is not required [9]. Despite being regarded as the gold standard, autograft is associated with several disadvantages. Donor site morbidity and complications such as deep infections, fracture, abdominal hernia, retroperitoneal hemorrhage, cutaneous nerve damage, blood loss, and vascular injury are well documented. In several studies, the aforementioned complications have been reported in up to 10% of cases [5, 7, 9–12]. Minor complications, such as superficial infections, superficial seromas, and minor hematomas, were reported in 10–21% of patients [9, 12]. Graft volume is also a concern, with studies showing the average volume harvested from the anterior iliac crest being 13 cm^3 and the posterior iliac crest 30 cm^3 [9]. The adequacy of these depends on the type of procedure and the number of levels included [5, 9]. Despite these limitations, autograft continues to remain the gold standard due to its availability and proven track record. Surgeons must thoroughly understand the types of autograft, their indications, and harvesting techniques.

Autologous Cancellous Bone

Cancellous bone has a high osteogenic potential due to the abundance of osteoblastic stem cells and osteoprogenitor cells. The trabecular structure and large surface area of cancellous bone are favorable, as they provide increased osteoconduction and promote vascular ingrowth [5, 9, 13]. Immediately after graft implantation, hemorrhage and inflammation occur [13]. This causes the graft site to become rich in inflammatory cells and mesenchymal stem cells. Within 48 h of the surgical procedure, these cells produce fibrous granulation tissue. While this is occurring, macrophages are recruited in order to remove the necrotic graft tissue [14]. Most of the graft cells do not survive; however, surface osteoblasts survive and begin to produce new bone. As soon as 48 h after the surgery, host vessels along with osteoblastic and osteoclastic precursors infiltrate the trabecular surfaces of the cancellous graft. While new blood vessels begin to form throughout the graft, osteoclasts begin to resorb it. As the vascular ingrowth progresses, osteoblasts line the dead trabecular surfaces and produce osteoid. Through remodeling, which lasts several months, necrotic bone is resorbed by osteoclasts while osteoblasts form new bone [9, 13]. Thus, the incorporation of cancellous autograft occurs through simultaneous bone formation and resorption [14]. Over the next 6–12 months following the grafting, newly formed osteoid is mineralized into bone and becomes fully integrated with the surrounding host bone. Integration is typically complete 1 year after the surgery [9, 13, 14].

Cancellous bone graft has been thoroughly studied to determine its clinical success. Throughout several historical studies, the rate of pseudarthrosis when using autogenous cancellous bone ranges from 5 to 44% [6, 7]. Herkowitz and Kurz studied the differences in clinical and radiographic results between decompressive laminectomy and decompressive laminectomy with intertransverse-process arthrodesis. The arthrodesis was performed with corticocancellous and cancellous bone grafts obtained from the iliac crest. Good to excellent results were found in 96% of the arthrodesis group and in 44% of the decompressive laminectomy group. Pseudarthrosis was found in 36% of the patients in the arthrodesis group, but the clinical results were significantly better in the arthrodesis group [15]. Fischgrund et al. performed a randomized study comparing posterolateral fusion with or without instrumentation with autogenous iliac crest bone graft [16]. At a 2-year follow-up, arthrodesis was successful in 82% of patients with instrumentation and 45% of the patients without instrumentation. However, the findings suggested that there were no significant differences in the clinical outcomes [16]. Kornblum et al. followed up on patients from the previous two studies in order to determine the long-term effects of pseudarthrosis and successful fusion. The clinical outcomes were good to excellent in 86% of the solid fusion group and in 56% of the pseudarthrosis group. Upon evaluating residual back and leg pain, the authors found that patients in the solid fusion group reported significantly lower pain scores in both areas as compared to the pseudarthrosis group [17]. The use of cancellous autograft has also shown improved fusion rates and clinical outcomes in cervical spine. Song et al. studied the efficacy of a three-level anterior cervical arthrodesis with cancellous bone, polyether ether ketone (PEEK) cages, and plate fixation in 21 patients [18]. Solid arthrodesis, which occurred 10–14 weeks after surgery, was found in all 21 patients. Although graft site morbidity was not evaluated, SF-36 and NDI improved after surgery and at final follow-up.

Non-vascularized Autologous Cortical Bone

In comparison to cancellous autograft, cortical autograft is less osteogenic and less biologically active [5, 7, 9]. It is also compact and resistant to remodeling and vascular invasion [7, 9]. Furthermore, cortical bone has a lower surface area which reduces the potential for new bone formation. In spite of its drawbacks, it has greater mechanical strength than cancellous bone and is therefore used to provide structural support [7, 9, 13, 19]. Resorption of the graft by osteoclasts then occurs to allow vascular ingrowth [13, 20]. In order for the cortical bone to become fully incorporated, creeping substitution occurs. During this process, which can continue over the next 6 months following the surgery, osteoclasts resorb the graft at a high rate, while osteoblasts replace it with new bone [5, 9, 14, 21]. During creeping substitution, the graft can sustain a 75% reduction in strength, and the risk of graft collapse is highest [5, 14, 19]. Structural strength is regained within 12–24 months [5, 9], and once healed, there is little to no remaining weakness [14, 21].

In several studies the rates of fusion for the cortical autograft in anterior cervical fusions were 89% or greater [7, 22–25]. Zdeblick and Ducker found that the use of tricortical autograft in anterior cervical fusions had an 8% nonunion after 1 year. Graft collapse was observed in 5% of patients as well [25]. Furthermore, Wright and Eisenstein assessed 97 patients 1 year after anterior cervical discectomy and fusion (ACDF) with tricortical iliac crest bone graft. The study noted that pseudarthrosis was found in 11% of patients who had one-level fusions and 28% of patients who had two-level fusions [26]. Samartzis et al. performed a radiographic and clinical study comparing the fusion rates between allograft and autograft in two- and three-level ACDF with anterior plate fixation [27]. Out of 80 patients in the study, 45 received autogenous tricortical iliac crest graft along with anterior plate fixation. Successful bone fusion was achieved in 100% of the autograft group and in 94% of the allograft group. Within the autograft group, approximately 94% of patients with two-level fusions had good to excellent results, while 64% of patients with three-level fusions had good to excellent results [27].

Allograft

Allografts are harvested from cadaveric bone and are often used as bone graft extenders or substitutes in lumbar and cervical fusions. Allografts have good osteoconductive, very minimal osteoinductive, and no osteogenic properties. Growth factors and cells are removed during graft processing to minimize their antigenicity. Commonly used forms of allografts are chips, strips, or demineralized bone matrix (DBM). Allografts of cortical origin provide good structural stability and are often used for interbody fusion, but the bone remodeling is slow and graft resorption is increased. Corticocancellous allografts provide minimal mechanical support at the start, but have large surface area that allows for better bone remodeling and graft resorption [28]. Based on the preparation, allografts can be fresh frozen or freeze-dried. Freeze-drying reduces immunogenicity more than the freezing procedure; however, freeze-dried grafting materials have inferior mechanical properties [29].

The main concern with the use of cadaver tissues is disease transmission, even though the preparation process is extensive. Standards for handling and preparation of bone allograft have been developed by the American Association Tissue Banking. Several cases of human immunodeficiency virus (HIV) and hepatitis transmission with the use of frozen allograft have been reported [30]. In all of the cases, donors and tissues were not adequately tested. Furthermore, Mroz and colleagues reported that 96.5% of musculoskeletal allografts between 1994 and 2007 were recalled due to the poor donor screening, graft contamination, and recipient infection [31]. Additional challenges with allografts are donor age and comorbidities, in particular osteoporosis, all of which can significantly diminish the mechanical properties of the graft and contribute to lower fusion rates.

Structural allografts have been extensively used for several decades in single-level anterior cervical discectomy and fusion (ACDF) showing similar fusion rates to autograft alone [32–34]. However, for multilevel ACDFs, there are mixed reports on the benefits of allograft substitutes vs. autograft [25, 27, 35]. Lumbar spine studies have reported excellent outcomes with the use of freeze-dried allografts in anterior fusion approaches [36, 37]. Furthermore, Butterman and coauthors found that the femoral ring allograft produced similar fusion rates as iliac crest bone graft (ICBG) and better overall outcomes than ICBG when used in anterior-posterior lumbar surgery [38]. Figure 34.1 demonstrates a successful lumbar posterior lateral fusion with autologous bone chips, cancellous allograft bone chips, and bone marrow aspirate.While autografts have shown superior performance in posterior fusions, allograft graft extenders have demonstrated promising results in spine deformity surgeries. Combination of freeze-dried allograft and autograft demonstrated high fusion rates (92.7%–97.3%) and up to 5.9 degrees loss of correction in patients undergoing a fusion procedure for the treatment of idiopathic scoliosis

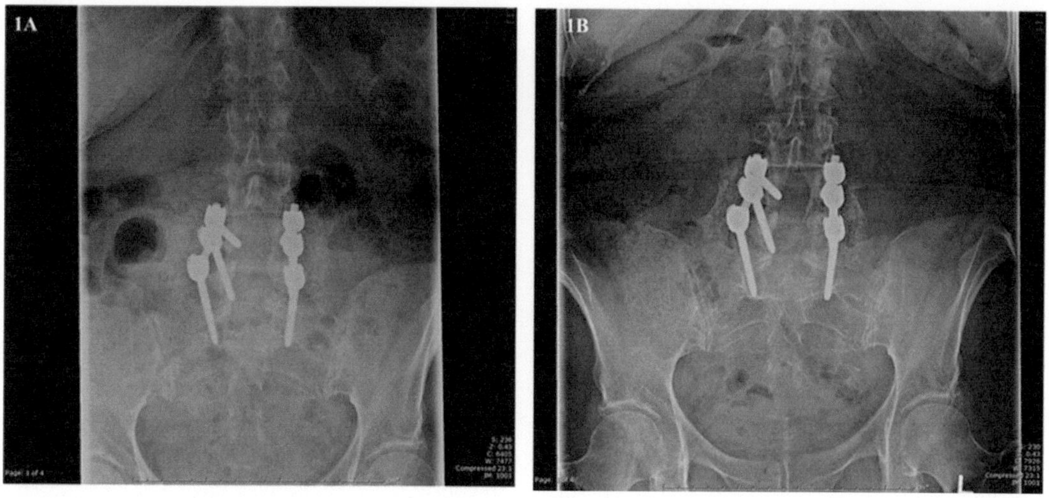

Fig. 34.1 (**a**) Patient 3 weeks postoperatively from a posterior lateral fusion with autologous bone chips and cancellous allograft bone chips, as well as the use of bone marrow aspirate. (**b**) Postoperative image of the same patient 8 months after surgery. Note the solid bony fusion in the lateral margins of the construct involving the transverse processes

[39, 40]. Most common complications with the use of structural allografts include nonunion and fracture due to the nature of graft material and slower rates of incorporation.

Ceramics

Ceramics are osteoconductive bone substitutes without cells and growth factors and limited mechanical stability [41]. Although they have a brittle structure and reduced shear strength, ceramic grafts have very desirable characteristics: biodegradable, unlimited supply, non-immunogenic, and no disease transmission. Mechanical instability is compensated for with the use of internal fixation which helps with the load force resistance in the initial period after the procedure. Most commonly used ceramic scaffolds for spinal fusion are calcium phosphates (hydroxyapatite (HA) and β-tricalcium phosphate (β-TCP)), calcium sulfates, or a combination of these materials. Both hydroxyapatite and β-TCP have pore sizes similar to cancellous bone and have prolonged resorption times. Hydroxyapatite is retained in vivo for up to a year, whereas the more porous β-TCP typically biodegrades in about 6 weeks [42]. When implanted within the fusion space ceramic, scaffolds support vascular ingrowth and cell migration leading to new bone formation.

Hydroxyapatite and β-TCP have been used as bone graft extenders for both lumbar and cervical spine fusion [43]. In a prospective non-randomized cohort study, patients underwent posterior lumbar fusion with HA + local bone or ICBG [44]. At 1-year follow-up, both groups had similar fusion rates, with the average fusion mass volume being greater in the group with hydroxyapatite chips. Similar results were reported by a few other cohort studies. On the other hand, Hsu et al. found that HA + local bone achieved only 57% fusion compared to the autograft group [45]. Acharya and coauthors compared hydroxyapatite-bioactive glass ceramic as a substitute for autograft and found almost no fusion in the hydroxyapatite group at 1-year follow-up [46]. Several studies explored the viability of HA as a graft extender or substitute in cervical fusion [43]. Both a randomized controlled trial and cohort studies reported similar fusion rates in HA group (alone or with local bone) compared to autograft. However, graft fragmentation, graft settling, and instrumentation-related problems were observed more in the HA groups [43]. On the other hand, Yoshii T et al. reported similar fusion rates between HA + local and autograft in ACDF with less blood loss and no graft fragmentation in the HA + local bone groups [47].

As hydroxyapatite, β-TCP has also been used as graft extender in lumbar posterior fusion and ACDF. Studies focusing on posterior lumbar fusion found that combining β-TCP and local bone led to similar fusion rates, outcomes, revision rates, and complications as autograft group [48–51]. In patients who underwent ACDF with a combination of β-TCP and HA, fusion rates were significantly lower in the first 5 months compared to ICBG, reaching solid fusion at 6 months postoperatively [52]. In addition, the ceramic group had shorter operative time, shorter hospital stay, and less blood loss. It is important to note that most of the studies lacked blinded assessment of fusion and patient randomization (various spinal conditions and comorbidities).

Calcium sulfate is another ceramic graft occasionally used in spine fusion in combination with local bone or bone marrow aspirate. In a posterolateral lumbar fusion study, patients who received calcium sulfate pellets mixed with local bone achieved 88% fusion rates at 1 year, compared to 100% fusion rates in the ICBG group [53]. Similarly, Chen et al. found that in single- and two-level posterolateral lumbar fusion, a mix of calcium sulfate and local bone produced similar fusion rates and bone mass compared to autogenous bone at 30–34 months follow-up [54]. However, when calcium sulfate was combined with bone marrow aspirate (BMA), fusion rates were significantly lower than in the ICBG group (46% vs. 91%, respectively) [55].

Silicate-substituted calcium phosphate (SiCaP) is another form of ceramic grafting material that has been shown to contain some osteogenic properties. Two studies evaluated the potential of SiCaP in spine fusion; however, their results were contradictory. In a randomized clinical trial (RCT), Licina et al. observed 100% fusion rates in patients undergoing posterior lumbar interbody fusion (PLIF) with SiCaP compared to 89% rate in patients who received recombinant human bone morphogenetic protein 2 (rhBMP-2) [56]. On the other hand, Nandyala and colleagues reported lower fusion rates (65%) with SiCaP when compared to rhBMP-2 (92%) in minimally invasive transforaminal lumbar interbody fusion [57].

Demineralized Bone Matrix (DBM)

In spine fusion, demineralized bone matrix (DBM) is used as graft extender or filler. DBM is produced from human cadaver allograft bone by removing the mineralized component, cells, and antigenic markers. DBMs have osteoconductive and some osteoinductive properties. The osteoconductive matrix consists of type I collagen, glycoproteins, calcium sulfate, and debris. The osteoinductive properties of DBMs come from several growth factors that are preserved during the processing. Those growth factors include bone sialoprotein, osteopontin, and tumor growth factor beta (TGF-β) family [58]. The bone morphogenetic proteins (BMPs) are the most important osteogenic factors that carry out progenitor cell differentiation toward the mature osteoblast. It has been shown that with aging the levels of BMPs decrease; however, several other growth factors including TGF-β are not affected and can further extend the bone formation cascades and interactions with BMPs [59]. DBMs are produced in powder form and are mixed with carriers (calcium sulfate, glycerol, gelatin, etc.) for easier delivery. Based on the carrier and the ratio, they come in different forms such as putty, gels, powder, and chips. Demineralized bone matrix has been extensively used in preclinical animal models and clinical trials. Rat spine fusion models have demonstrated great osteoinductive variability in commercially available DBMs which may reflect differences in the BMP content due to the donor variability and age [60–62]. In an athymic rat posterolateral fusion model, Wang and coworkers demonstrated that Osteofil DBM paste had the highest fusion rates (77.8%) overall and also at the early time point, 4 weeks [62]. However, DynaGraft DBM putty did not produce any fusion within the experimental time period. Although the donor variability is a main drawback, several other posterolateral spinal fusion animal studies have demonstrated good results with DBMs alone or in conjunction with autograft [63–65].

Early clinical studies on DBM as bone graft extenders for posterolateral spinal fusion reported similar fusion rates to the ICBG group as well as bone mineralization [66–68]. All of the studies concluded that DBM can be a successful graft extender reducing significantly the amounts of autograft needed to achieve solid fusion. It has also been found that DBM putty enriched with bone marrow is a good graft substitute for posterior spinal fusion with the fusion rates being comparable to DBM + autograft or autograft alone [69]. Conversely, An and colleagues [70] prospectively compared the fusion rates of freeze-dried allograft-DBM composite and autograft in ACDF and found that the allograft-DBM construct resulted in a higher rate of pseudarthrosis (33% in DBM vs. 22% in autograft). Furthermore, the allograft-DBM group had a higher rate of graft collapse (≥2 mm and ≥3 mm) than the autograft alone. Several studies prospectively evaluated DBM with or without autograft packed into polyether ether ketone (PEEK) cages [71, 72]. Park et al. observed 97% fusion rates in ACDF patients with DBM and local autograft packed in PEEK cages, while Moon and colleagues reported fusion in 77.8% patients at 25.5 months follow-up (mean). However, in the study by Moon et al., 84% of the patients had some subsidence influencing regional and global alignment [72].

Apart from bone extenders, DBM was used as a delivery vehicle for growth factors and cells. In a rat posterolateral fusion (PLF) model, DBM matrix with adenovirus carrying a Nell-1 gene or LacZ (control) was implanted at L4-L5 level, and at 6 weeks postoperatively, microCT demonstrated 70% fusion rates in DBM + Nell-1 group compared to 20% in DBM + LacZ control group [73].

Autologous Platelet Gel

Autologous platelet gels are created by concentrating platelet-rich plasma, and they can be combined with autograft or allograft. They consist of platelets, platelet-derived growth factor (PDGF), and TGF-β which promote chemotaxis and proliferation of mesenchymal stem cells and osteoblasts. Although the animal studies demonstrated promising results with platelet gels in spine fusion, clinical data is inconclusive. Two retrospective cohort studies looked at the effects of platelet gels on fusion rates in posterolateral spinal approach [74, 75]. Both studies found that when platelet gel was combined with autograft it failed to enhance fusion and it had lower fusion rates than autograft alone. In a transforaminal lumbar interbody fusion (TLIF) study done by Hee and colleagues, platelet gels promoted faster bone remodeling; however, there was no increase in the overall fusion rates [76]. On the other hand, Jenis et al. found similar fusion rates between (85%) and autograft supplemented with AGF (89%) in one- or two-level PLIF [77]. Autologous platelet gels have several disadvantages including blood draw and gel preparation, longer surgery time, and higher costs.

Bone Marrow Aspirates (BMAs)

Unfractionated bone marrow aspirate (BMA) has osteoinductive and some osteogenic characteristics. Due to the lack of osteoconductivity, BMA is always combined with a collagen or DBM carrier. Several studies have evaluated the amount of osteoprogenitor cells in aspirated bone marrow samples. The colony-forming units that produce alkaline phosphatase (CFU-AP) are used to determine the number of osteoblastic progenitors [78, 79]. Muschler et al. found that the prevalence of CFU-AP was 55 per million nucleated cells. The authors also studied changes in the prevalence of osteoblastic progenitors in relation to age and gender. In women, there was a significant decrease in the number of osteoblastic progenitors with age. On the other hand, men showed a slight increase or no change in the number of osteoblastic progenitors with age [78]. In a subsequent study, Muschler et al. determined the change in osteoblastic progenitors in relation to volume of aspirated bone marrow. As the volume of bone marrow aspirated increases, the number of osteoblastic progenitors also increases. Due to the increase in volume, however, the sample becomes increasingly contaminated by peripheral blood. The authors noted a 50% decrease in the concentration of osteoblast progenitor cells when the aspirate is increased from 1 to 4 milliliters [79]. Taghavi and colleagues retrospectively reviewed a cohort of patients undergoing instrumented revision PLF with autograft only, BMA and autograft, and rhBMP-2 on collagen sponge [80]. In single-level fusion, all groups achieved solid fusion, but in the multilevel the BMA group had a 63.6% fusion rate, while the other two groups had 100%. Niu and coauthors compared the efficacy of BMA with different carriers in promoting fusion in single-level PLF study [55]. They found that combination of BMA and autogenous graft had similar fusion rates to ICBG alone (85.7% vs. 90.5%, respectively). However, the calcium sulfate and BMA group achieved only 45.5% fusion compared to 90.9% with ICBG on the control side [55]. In a systematic review, Khashan et al. reported several PLF studies which had similar fusion rates between BMA with a carrier and ICBG group, but the overall level of evidence was weak [81].

Bone Morphogenetic Proteins (BMPs)

In 1965, Dr. Marshall Urist performed a landmark study in which demineralized bone implanted into the muscle of a rabbit induced bone growth in surrounding tissues [82]. Because this bone-forming activity could be extracted from the organic component of the bone, Dr. Urist theorized that some type of protein or proteins were responsible for these phenomena and gave it the name "bone morphogenetic protein." With the advances in recombinant DNA and protein purification techniques, isolates of the various BMPs were procured and studied for their ability to induce bone formation. They were categorized into the transforming growth factor beta (TGF-B or TGF-β) superfamily based on their primary amino acid sequence [83]. Unlike the other members of the family, the BMPs are differentiation factors, inducing mesenchymal stem cells to differentiate into bone-forming and cartilage-forming cells. The effects of BMPs occur through ligand-specific receptors found on the cell membrane. These receptors are complexes of type I and type II serine-threonine protein kinases. Upon ligand binding to the type II receptor, transphosphorylation occurs in the type I receptor. This then leads to phosphorylation of intracellular proteins known as Smads, with eventual activation of target genes [84]. The most extensively studied BMP is the recombinant human bone morphogenetic protein 2 (rhBMP-2). Validation studies of rhBMP-2 use in the spine showed excellent results with essentially zero complications [85, 86]. Based on these studies, BMP2 was FDA-approved for anterior lumbar interbody fusions with the use of a specific type of threaded cage (LT cages, Medtronic). Initial positive results led to widespread off-label use. The use of rhBMP-2 in the United States increased from 0.7% of all fusions in 2002 to more than 50% of primary ALIFs, 43% of PLIF/TLIFs, and 30% of PLFs in 2007 [87]. It became known as the "most successful medical device in history," garnering 40% of the bone graft market with annual sales approaching $900 million dollars in 2011 [88].

With widespread use, several complications were reported including radiculitis, cyst formation, seroma formation, endplate resorption, retrograde ejaculation, and ectopic bone formation. Because of well-documented reports of adverse events occurring with its use in ventral cervical spine surgery, the FDA issued a Public Health Notification in July of 2008, underscoring "life-threatening complications of rhBMP-2 in cervical spine surgery" [89]. A systematic review in 2010 by Mroz et al. evaluated the available literature regarding site- and procedure-specific complication rates with rhBMP-2 [90]. They found a high percentage of resorption (44%), graft subsidence (25%), and cage migration (27%) in the lumbar spine. Similar results were seen in the cervical spine with resorption (43%), but higher graft subsidence (43%) was seen. The incidence of dysphagia/neck swelling and respiratory difficulties were found to be approximately 6%. This systematic review concluded that the complications associated with the use of BMP could be "substantial." In 2011 Carragee et al. published an article questioning the veracity and reporting bias of the initial validation studies for rhBMP-2 [91]. They found that the rate of complications was 10–50 times higher than what was reported in the validation studies, critical methodological flaws within the studies themselves, and serious deficiencies within the peer review process that evaluated these studies. Faced with controversy and questions, Medtronic turned over all data to the Yale Open Data Analysis (YODA) Project. YODA was created as a new model to evaluate industry-sponsored clinical trials, with the goal of increasing transparency, disseminating data, and increasing the benefit with mitigation of risk to patients. YODA selected two different sites to the review the data, the Oregon Health and Science University and University of York in the United Kingdom. At the Oregon Health Sciences University, Fu et al. [92] reviewed 13 randomized control trials, 31 other cohort studies, 47 intervention series, and 34 case series and reports. Simmonds et al. at the York University reviewed 11 randomized control trials and 43 other publications [93]. Both papers commented on the methodological flaws in the validation studies, namely, a lack of blinding among physicians and patients. At the same time, both studies agreed that there were no significant differences in clinical outcomes between ICBG and rhBMP-2, a significantly higher risk with its use in anterior cervical fusions, and increased relative risk that did not reach significance with its use in both anterior and posterior lumbar fusions. There was a significantly increased risk of back and leg pain in the immediate postsurgical period when rhBMP-2 was used in posterolateral fusions. Fu et al. concluded that they could see no clear indication for the use of rhBMP-2 as there was no significant benefit in measured clinical outcomes. They also stated that though the overall rates of cancer were low, there was an increased risk of cancer with rhBMP-2 at 24 months; however, at 48 months these differences were no longer significant. Simmons et al. concluded the use of rhBMP-2 resulted in increased fusion rates that did not translate into improved clinical outcomes and increased back and leg pain with its use during the first 6 months. They found trends toward increases in cancer, but no significance in this regard [93]. Their differing conclusions indicate that the results are highly dependent on study selection; that if there is an increased risk of cancer with the use of rhBMP-2, it is likely small, that rhBMP-2 should be used in caution with patients that have a history of cancer; and that future analysis incorporating more of the data can help draw more definitive conclusions.

Cell-Based Therapies

Cell-based approaches have primarily focused on the use of mesenchymal stem cells (MSCs), exploiting their potential for differentiation into various lineages and their low immunogenicity. MSCs have been tested in various animal models for spine fusion together with a carrier or as a vehicle for the delivery of growth factors [94–100]. Bone marrow stem cells (BMSCs) in particular have shown a great potential in promoting osteogenesis and have been extensively used in in vitro and in vivo models [94, 95, 97–100]. However, the disadvantages of BMSC lie in their low numbers and the harvest morbidity. Because of that, the use of adipose stem cells has gained popularity, due to their fairly easy isolation, higher numbers of stem cells, and prolonged osteogenic potential [96, 98, 100]. Miyazaki et al. compared the potential of human bone marrow and adipose-derived stem cells transfected with BMP2 in inducing fusion in a posterolateral rat model. They found that at 8 weeks postoperatively animals that have received stem cells (either adipose or bone marrow) with BMP showed fusion that in most of the cases bridged the adjacent levels. Animals with stem cells alone however did not form new bone. These results are in agreement with other studies showing that predifferentiated stem cells had a higher osteogenic potential than naïve cells. Nakajima and coauthors reported that the successful fusion was the highest in animals that received scaffolds with osteogenic stem cells (80%), followed by autografts (66.7%) and non-differentiated stem cells (33.3%) [99]. The clinical use of stem cells for spine fusion is being investigated in several clinical trials. Khashan et al. conducted a systematic review evaluating the efficacy of MSC or BMA in conjunction with graft extenders for cervical and thoracolumbar fusions and how they compare to autograft [81]. Their review found that eligible studies had a low level of evidence and there was no clinical evidence on the use of MSC as graft extender or substitute [81]. While stem cells show great potential to be a powerful tool in spine fusions, there are also several limitations, starting with a decline in the number and quality of stem with age, metabolic diseases, or comorbidities such as smoking. Other obstacles are missing cell expansion protocols that will maintain a stable phenotype under GMP conditions and the potential for contaminations and complications.

Modulus of Elasticity

In the early stages of spine fusion, the mechanical loading is the key element which balances new bone formation and resorption. Various implants and instrumentation are used to lend initial mechanical support to the fusion site. To be considered suitable, those materials have to have mechanical properties similar to the host tissue (Table 34.2) [101, 102], have the right pore size for cell migration and blood vessel ingrowth, be biocompatible, and tolerate sterilization. Polyether ether ketone (PEEK), titanium (Ti), and its alloys are the most commonly used materials in spine fusions. PEEK cages are biocompatible and radiolucent and their elasticity modulus is lower than the cortical bone (Table 34.2). Fusion success with PEEK cages has been demonstrated in various studies; however, osteogenic cell migration and adhesion were reduced compared to Ti [101, 102]. Studies have shown that the addition of hydroxyapatite to PEEK increased osseointegration and the elasticity modulus (up to 10.6 GPa). Ti and its alloys are biocompatible, have great resistances to corrosion, have low density, and have been used in the spine field for decades [101, 102]. In contrast to PEEK, titanium has a very high elasticity modulus (Table 34.2) that is six- to sevenfold higher than the cortical bone which can contribute to subsidence and implant failure. Furthermore, Ti and its alloys are not radiolucent and have low osseointegration potential in their unmodified form. Various modifications have been used to improve the elasticity modulus and the in- and on-growth of osteoblasts. The most common modifications include creation of surface microscale roughness, thermal or chemical treatments, and HA coating [101, 102]. HA coating of Ti in particular has shown good results in bone formation, providing good mechanical stability, and osseointegration properties.

Other materials such as tantalum, polymethyl methacrylate (PMMA), and stainless steel have been used for spine implants. However, their elasticity modulus is very different from the autograft (Table 34.2) which can compromise the mechanical stability of the fusion site. The mechanical properties of the implant are not only important within the fusion site but also influence the adjacent, unfused segments and the progression of intervertebral disc degeneration.

Table 34.2 Modulus of elasticity

Tissue or implant material	Modulus (GPa)
Cortical bone	12.8–17.7
Cancellous bone	0.4
Stainless steel	190
Ti-alloy	116
PEEK	8.3
HA-PEEK	9.6–10.6
PMMA	2.6
HA	95

Values adopted from Ramakrishna et al. [102]

Surgical Technique Autologous Iliac Crest Harvesting

Anterior

The anterior approach to the iliac crest is used for anterior reconstructive procedures. Cancellous or corticocancellous grafts can be obtained with this method. This approach may be preferable during a procedure in which the patient is already supine, but a disadvantage is the lower volume of obtainable bone. Harvesting from the anterior iliac crest should be used only if less than 20–30 cc of the bone is required. The patient is positioned supine with a bump under the ipsilateral gluteal region to accentuate the anterior superior iliac spine (ASIS). The incision is made parallel to the hip and a wide area should be sterilely draped. At least 3 cm of the ASIS needs to be kept intact to avoid injury to the insertion of the sartorius muscle and inguinal ligament. The lateral femoral cutaneous nerve may have an anomalous course in this region and should be avoided. The integrity of the ASIS should not be compromised, or a stress fracture can result from the forces of the sartorius and rectus femoris musculature.

A 3–6 cm curved incision is placed 3–4 cm lateral to the ASIS. The incision, which runs superiorly and posteriorly, is made over or just below the crest to minimize postoperative pain. The fascia should be opened carefully to facilitate proper closure at the end of the procedure. Inadequate fascial closure increases the risk of hernia. The periosteum is incised and elevated from the ilium, thus exposing cortical bone which can be perforated with a Rongeur or osteotome. The iliac tubercle, located 5 cm posteriorly from the ASIS, contains a large amount of cancellous bone for harvesting. Once the cortex at the brim of the ilium has been violated, curettes are used to remove the inner graft material. An osteotome is used to enter the iliac crest obliquely, thus separating the inner and outer tables from a central graft, which provides a block of bone up to 10 by 8 cm in size. The muscle and periosteum are left attached to the outer ridge of the iliac crest. Wire or sutures are used to reapproximate the inner and outer ilium. Tricortical grafts require more dissection. A 6 cm incision is followed by subperiosteal dissection of the inner and outer tables of the ilium. Bone graft is harvested at least 3 cm posteriorly from the ASIS by using parallel saw blades to enter the tables of the ilium. An oscillating saw is preferable to an osteotome because of weakening of the remaining iliac crest that may occur with osteotomes. The peritoneal cavity, which lies medially, should not be violated. Careless dissection of the iliacus from the inner wall can injure the iliohypogastric and ilioinguinal nerves, femoral nerve, deep circumflex iliac artery, and iliolumbar arteries. Once the iliac crest is fully exposed, the size of the graft should be measured carefully in all three dimensions. The graft is fashioned with a reciprocating sagittal saw. Final removal of the bone may require the use of osteotomies to free the bone from attachments in the inferomedial region. Hemostasis of the exposed bony surfaces may be achieved using several techniques which include bone wax or other hemostatic agents. If necessary, a drain may be left in place to avoid formation of a seroma.

Posterior

For posterior procedures, onlay graft material may be needed to supplement the fusion construct. Dorsal spinal surgeries do not require structural graft because dorsal instrumentation is typically implanted. The advantage of dorsal iliac crest grafts is the large volume of available bone. Two approaches are available: the bone can either be harvested through the midline lumbar incision that has been made for the current spinal decompression, or a separate incision can be made lateral to the surgical site. If graft is to be harvested from the midline lumbar incision, a fascial incision is made approximately 6 cm laterally from the site of decompression. Dissection risks injury to the superior cluneal nerves, which exit from the lumbodorsal fascia and course as close as 6 cm lateral to the PSIS. The fascia over the PSIS is incised and elevated from the ilium with electrocautery and a Cobb elevator. Dissection should be at least 4 cm lateral to the PSIS to avoid iatrogenic injury to the sacroiliac joint and neurovascular structures exiting from the greater sciatic notch. Externally, the sciatic nerve, superior gluteal nerve, and branches of the superior gluteal artery travel cephalad after exiting the greater sciatic notch. Internally, the superior gluteal artery and the ureter are of concern. An opening in the cortical surface, directed caudally, is made with an osteotome. Cancellous bone can be obtained using curettes or gouges. Bone bleeding is controlled by packing the area with sponges and applying bone wax or hemostatic agents. The defect can be filled with allograft.

If a separate incision is required for bone graft harvesting, a vertical incision is made over the posterior superior iliac spine (PSIS) with the patient in the prone position. The alternative transverse incision, if used, should be made cautiously so as to avoid laceration of the cluneal nerves. Dissection through the fascia and graft removal occurs as described above.

To obtain a corticocancellous graft, a longer exposure is used. The incision for the exposure of the posterior iliac crest should not exceed 8 cm from the PSIS to avoid injury to the superior cluneal nerves, which course over the crest. The fascia over the crest is exposed and opened. The musculature is elevated using subperiosteal technique. The dissection should not extend too inferiorly to avoid jeopardizing the structures in the region of the sciatic notch.

The subcrestal approach is an alternative method for obtaining bicortical and cancellous graft. An incision 1 cm lateral to the PSIS allows exposure as described above. Instead of simply perforating the surface of the cortex, however, a unicortical window can be cut with osteotomes or a saw. Additional cancellous bone can then be harvested through the same opening. Care should be exerted during closure of the fascial layer to avoid damage to the gluteal musculature. With meticulous hemostasis, a postoperative drain is unnecessary.

Illustrative Case

History

Patient is 59-year-old, right-hand dominant female with a history of bilateral shoulder blade pain, worse on the left. She also has complaints of burning in the bilateral T1 distribution. She states that the pain is 80% in her shoulder blades, 10% down her arms in the T1 distribution, and 10% in her neck. She has had these symptoms for approximately 6 months.

Conservative Treatments

She has had physical therapy which was of no significant help. She underwent two epidural steroid injections; the first was at C5-C6 which gave her complete relief of shoulder blade pain for 2 days. The second was at C7-T1 and it helped the burning in her arms for approximately a week.

Physical Exam

Her exam is normal except for diminished sensation in the bilateral C7 and T1 distributions.

Imaging

Preoperative lateral radiograph shows multilevel spondylosis with disc space collapse from C5 to T1 (Fig. 34.2). MRI confirms spinal stenosis due to broad-based disc bulges from C5 to T1 (Fig. 34.3). There is disc extrusion at C7-T1 with caudal migration also noted.

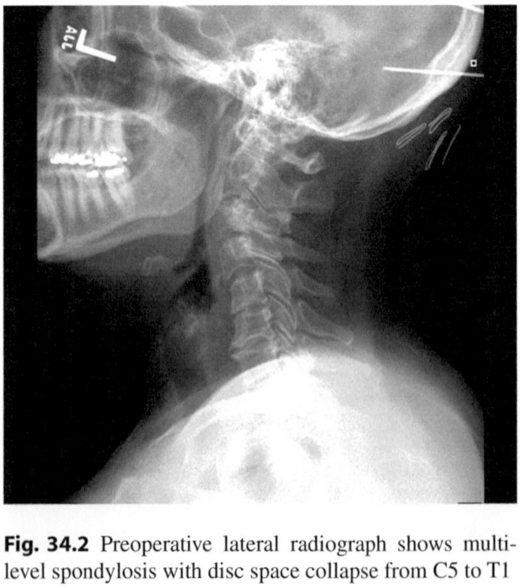

Fig. 34.2 Preoperative lateral radiograph shows multilevel spondylosis with disc space collapse from C5 to T1

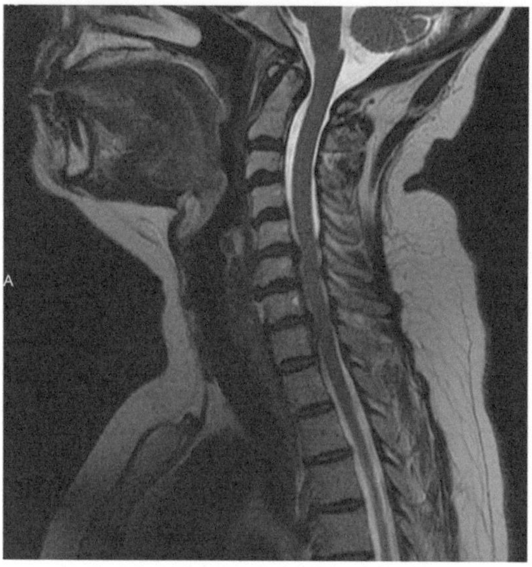

Fig. 34.3 Pre-op MRI shows stenosis due to broad-based disc bulges from C7 to T1. There is disc extrusion at C7-T1 with caudal migration also noted

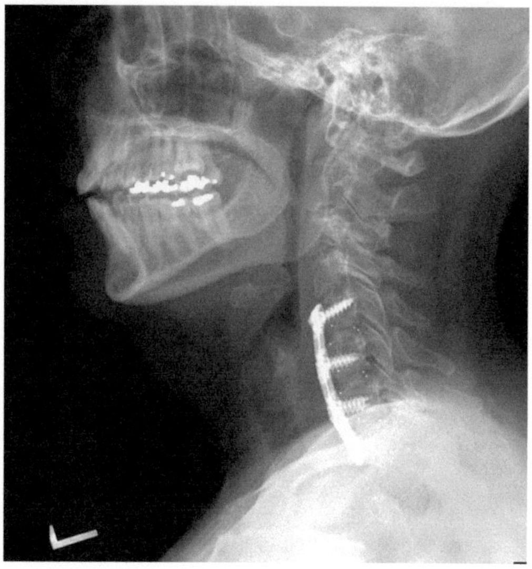

Fig. 34.4 Two-week postoperative radiograph showing cancellous bone within the PEEK interbody cages

Surgical Treatment

Due to the severity of her symptoms and failure of conservative management, the patient opted for surgical intervention. The planned procedure was a C5-T1 anterior cervical discectomy and fusion with harvesting of iliac crest autograft. The autograft was harvested through a small incision, and the cancellous bone was packed into PEEK interbody cages (Figs. 34.4 and 34.5).

Outcome

She had immediate improvement in pain and gradual improvement in hand sensation. Her fusion progressed and appeared healed on 6- and 12-month radio-graphs (Figs. 34.6 and 34.7).

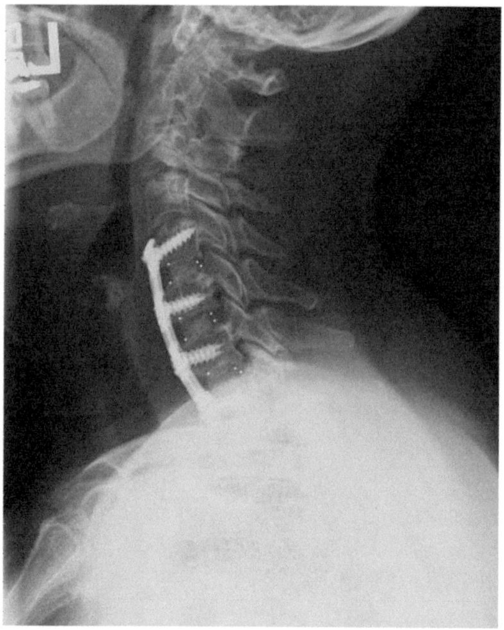

Fig. 34.5 At 6 weeks postoperative radiograph showed early maturation of the autograft

Technical Pearls

- Autologous bone graft (commonly harvested from the iliac crest) is the only graft that has all the three characteristics needed for bone formation: osteoconduction, osteoinduction, and osteogenicity.
- Bone grafts can function as graft substitutes, graft extenders, or graft enhancers.
- Allograft materials can be fresh, fresh frozen, or freeze-dried depending on the harvest and preparation.

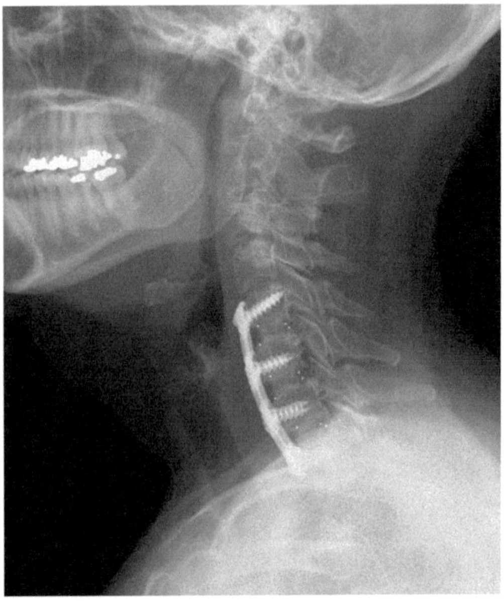

Fig. 34.6 Six-month postoperative radiograph showing continue maturation of graft

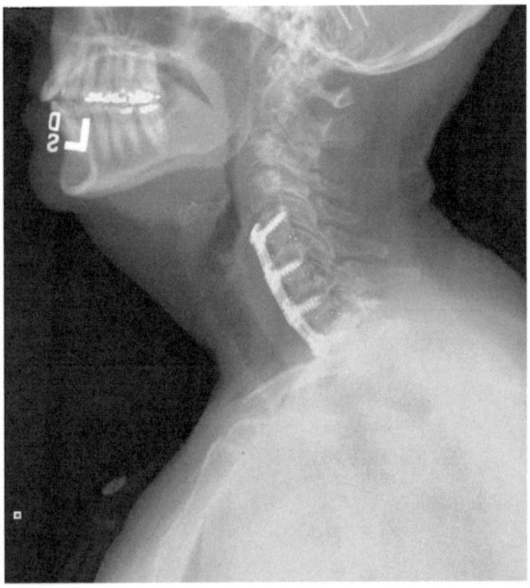

Fig. 34.7 One-year postoperative radiograph showing solid interbody fusion from C5 to T1

- Ceramics are easily obtainable in large amounts with appropriate pore size for cell and blood vessel ingrowth; however, they lack mechanical stability.
- Bone marrow aspirates contain cells and growth factors, but the quality varies with donor age and medical history.
- Irrigate before decorticating so you leave all bone dust and fragments in the area to promote bone healing. No need to wash away those small graft particles.
- Decorticate only the dorsal cortex off the structure. Expose the cancellous bone which promotes bone attachment. No need to decorticate the good cancellous bone away. Don't over-decorticate this cancellous bone which you want to leave in place.
- Expose as much of this cancellous bone as you can. Decorticate the cortical bone as much as possible to create as much surface area for new bone to heal. Expose not just the transverse processes but the facet joints and as much surface area as possible.
- Place the bone graft as much as you can on top of the decorticated bone. Don't leave it suspended in the paraspinal muscles, but instead put the graft right on top of where the bone needs to attach. Don't make it harder for the bone to bridge the gap.
- Remove soft tissues from local bone graft. The soft tissues attached to the graft particles will inhibit bone formation.
- Put your best material right on decorticated graft bed.
- Be very careful to examine the evidence supporting the efficacy of the particular product you are considering. Often the supporting evidence is poor, or it has in vitro data that does not convey any real significant support for efficacy.

Conclusion

A wide array of bone grafting materials has been used in spinal fusions in combination with autograft or as a graft substitute. Despite the existing literature on each of those graft substitutes, a strong level of preclinical and clinical research is missing. Understanding the biology of each bone allograft is critical for achieving successful spinal fusion. One must be cautious when choosing the grafting material and consider all factors such as patient's age, comorbidities, surgery type, and number of levels.

References

1. Global Burden of Disease Study 2013 Collaborators. Global, regional, and national incidence, prevalence, and years lived with disability for 301 acute and chronic diseases and injuries in 188 countries, 1990–2013: a systematic analysis for the Global Burden of Disease Study 2013. Lancet. 2015;386(9995):743–800.
2. Chun DS, Baker KC, Hsu WK. Lumbar pseudarthrosis: a review of current diagnosis and treatment. Neurosurg Focus. 2015;39(4):E10.
3. McAnany SJ, Baird EO, Overley SC, Kim JS, Qureshi SA, Anderson PA. A meta-analysis of the clinical and fusion results following treatment of symptomatic cervical pseudarthrosis. Global Spine J. 2015;5(2):148–55.
4. Raizman NM, O'Brien JR, Poehling-Monaghan KL, Yu WD. Pseudarthrosis of the spine. J Am Acad Orthop Surg. 2009;17(8):494–503.
5. Muschler GF, Takigami H, Nakamoto C. Principles of bone fusion. In: Herkowitz HN, Garfin SR, Eismont FJ, Bell GR, Balderston RA, editors. Rothman-Simeone the spine. 5th ed. Philadelphia: Elsevier Saunders; 2006. p. 385–98.
6. Miyazaki M, Tsumura H, Wang JC, Alanay A. An update on bone substitutes for spinal fusion. Eur Spine J. 2009;18(6):783–99.
7. Sandhu HS, Grewal HS, Parvataneni H. Bone grafting for spinal fusion. Orthop Clin North Am. 1999;30(4):685–98.
8. Zermatten P, Wettstein M. Iliac wing fracture following graft harvesting from the anterior iliac crest: literature review based on case report. Orthop Traumatol Surg Res. 2012;98(1):114–7.
9. Myeroff C, Archdeacon M. Autogenous bone graft: donor sites and techniques. J Bone Joint Surg Am. 2011;93(23):2227–36.
10. Arrington ED, Smith WJ, Chambers HG, Bucknell AL, Davino NA. Complications of the iliac crest bone graft harvesting. Clin Orthop Relat Res. 1996;329:300–9.
11. Goulet JA, Senunas LE, DeSilva GL, Greenfield ML. Autogenous iliac crest bone graft. Complications and functional assessment. Clin Orthop Relat Res. 1997;339:76–81.
12. Younger EM, Chapman MW. Morbidity at bone graft donor sites. J Orthop Trauma. 1989;3(3):192–5.
13. Stevenson S. Biology of bone grafts. Orthop Clin North Am. 1999;30(4):543–52.
14. Roberts TT, Rosenbaum AJ. Bone grafts, bone substitutes and orthobiologics: the bridge between basic science and clinical advancements in fracture healing. Organogenesis. 2012;8(4):114–24.
15. Herkowitz HN, Kurz LT. Degenerative lumbar spondylolisthesis with spinal stenosis. A prospective study comparing decompression with decompression and intertransverse process arthrodesis. J Bone Joint Surg Am. 1991;73(6):802–8.
16. Fischgrund JS, Mackay M, Herkowitz HN, Brower R, Montgomery DM, Kurz LT. 1997 Volvo award winner in clinical studies. Degenerative lumbar spondylolisthesis with spinal stenosis: a prospective, randomized study comparing decompressive laminectomy and arthrodesis with and without spinal instrumentation. Spine (Phila Pa 1976). 1997;22(24):2807–12.
17. Kornblum MB, Fischgrund JS, Herkowitz HN, Abraham DA, Berkower DL, Ditkoff JS. Degenerative lumbar spondylolisthesis with spinal stenosis: a prospective long-term study comparing fusion and pseudarthrosis. Spine (Phila Pa 1976). 2004;29(7):726–33.
18. Song KJ, Kim GH, Choi BY. Efficacy of PEEK cages and plate augmentation in three-level anterior cervical fusion of elderly patients. Clin Orthop Surg. 2011;3(1):9–15.
19. Burwell RG. The fate of bone grafts. In: Apley AG, editor. Recent advances in orthopaedics. London: Churchill Livingstone; 1969. p. 115–207.
20. Enneking WF, Burchardt H, Puhl JJ, Piotrowski G. Physical and biological aspects of repair in dog cortical-bone transplants. J Bone Joint Surg Am. 1975;57(2):237–52.
21. Khan SN, Cammisa FP Jr, Sandhu HS, Diwan AD, Girardi FP, Lane JM. The biology of bone grafting. J Am Acad Orthop Surg. 2005;13(1):77–86.
22. Gore DR, Sepic SB. Anterior cervical fusion for degenerated or protruded discs. A review of one hundred forty-six patients. Spine (Phila Pa 1976). 1984;9(7):667–71.
23. Krag MH, Robertson PA, Johnson CC, Stein AC. Anterior cervical fusion using a modified tricortical bone graft: a radiographic analysis of outcome. J Spinal Disord. 1997;10(5):420–30.
24. Mutoh N, Shinomiya K, Furuya K, Yamaura I, Satoh H. Pseudarthrosis and delayed union after anterior cervical fusion. Int Orthop. 1993;17(5):286–9.
25. Zdeblick TA, Ducker TB. The use of freeze-dried allograft bone for anterior cervical fusions. Spine (Phila Pa 1976). 1991;16(7):726–9.
26. Wright IP, Eisenstein SM. Anterior cervical discectomy and fusion without instrumentation. Spine (Phila Pa 1976). 2007;32(7):772–4.
27. Samartzis D, Shen FH, Matthews DK, Yoon ST, Goldberg EJ, An HS. Comparison of allograft to autograft in multilevel anterior cervical discectomy and fusion with rigid plate fixation. Spine J. 2003;3(6):451–9.
28. Stevenson S, Horowitz M. The response to bone allografts. J Bone Joint Surg Am. 1992;74:939–50.
29. Hamer AJ, Strachan JR, Black MM, et al. Biomechanical properties of cortical allograft bone using a new method of bone strength measurement: a comparison of fresh, freshfrozen, and irradiated bone. J Bone Joint Surg Br. 1996;78:363–8.
30. Tomford WW. Transmission of disease through transplantation of musculoskeletal allografts. J Bone Joint Surg Am. 1995;77:1742–54.

31. Mroz TE, Joyce MJ, Lieberman IH, Steinmetz MP, Benzel EC, Wang JC. The use of allograft bone in spine surgery: is it safe? Spine J. 2009;9(4):303–8.
32. Cloward RB. The anterior approach for removal of ruptured cervical discs. J Neurosurg. 1958;15:602.
33. Brown MD, Malinin TI, Davis PB. A roentgenographic evaluation of frozen allografts versus autografts in anterior cervical spine fusions. Clin Orthop. 1976;119:231–6.
34. Jagannathan J, Shaffrey CI, Oskouian RJ, Dumont AS, Herrold C, Sansur CA, Jane JA. Radiographic and clinical outcomes following single-level anterior cervical discectomy and allograft fusion without plate placement or cervical collar. J Neurosurg Spine. 2008;8(5):420–8.
35. Young WF, Rossenwasser RH. An early comparative analysis of the use of fibular allograft versus autologous iliac crest graft for interbody fusion after anterior cervical discectomy. Spine. 1993;18:1123–4.
36. Kozak JA, Heilman AE, O'Brian JP. Anterior lumbar fusion options: techniques and graft materials. Clin Orthop. 1994;300:45–51.
37. Thalgott JS, Fogarty ME, Giuffre JM, Christenson SD, Epstein AK, Aprill C. A prospective, randomized, blinded, single-site study to evaluate the clinical and radiographic differences between frozen and freeze-dried allograft when used as part of a circumferential anterior lumbar interbody fusion procedure. Spine (Phila Pa 1976). 2009;34(12):1251–6.
38. Butterman GR, Glazer PA, Hu SS, Bradford DS. Revision of failed lumbar fusions. A comparison of anterior autograft and allograft. Spine. 1997;22:2748–55.
39. Jones KC, Andrish J, Kuivila T, Gurd A. Radiographic outcomes using freeze-dried cancellous allograft bone for posterior spinal fusion in pediatric idiopathic scoliosis. J Pediatr Orthop. 2002;22(3):285–9.
40. Knapp DR Jr, Jones ET, Blanco JS, Flynn JC, Price CT. Allograft bone in spinal fusion for adolescent idiopathic scoliosis. J Spinal Disord Tech. 2005;18(Suppl):S73–6.
41. Tay BK, Patel VV, Bradford DS. Calcium sulfate and calcium phosphate- based bone substitutes. Mimicry of the mineral phase of bone. Orthop Clin North Am. 1999;30:615–23.
42. Jarcho M. Calcium phosphate ceramics as hard tissue prosthetics. Clin Orthop. 1981;157:259–78.
43. Buser Z, Brodke DS, Youssef JA, Meisel HJ, Myhre SL, Hashimoto R, Park JB, Tim Yoon S, Wang JC. Synthetic bone graft versus autograft or allograft for spinal fusion: a systematic review. J Neurosurg Spine. 2016;27:1–8. [Epub ahead of print]
44. Lee JH, Hwang CJ, Song BW, Koo KH, Chang BS, Lee CK. A prospective consecutive study of instrumented posterolateral lumbar fusion using synthetic hydroxyapatite (BongrosHA) as a bone graft extender. J Biomed Mater Res A. 2009;90:804–10.
45. Hsu CJ, Chou WY, Teng HP, Chang WN, Chou YJ. Coralline hydroxyapatite and laminectomy-derived bone as adjuvant graft material for lumbar posterolateral fusion. J Neurosurg Spine. 2005;3:271–5.
46. Acharya NK, Kumar RJ, Varma HK, Menon VK. Hydroxyapatite-bioactive glass ceramic composite as stand-alone graft substitute for posterolateral fusion of lumbar spine: a prospective, matched, and controlled study. J Spinal Disord Tech. 2008;21:106–11.
47. Yoshii T, Yuasa M, Sotome S, Yamada T, Sakaki K, Hirai T, Taniyama T, Inose H, Kato T, Arai Y, Kawabata S, Tomizawa S, Enomoto M, Shinomiya K, Okawa A. Porous/dense composite hydroxyapatite for anterior cervical discectomy and fusion. Spine (Phila Pa 1976). 2013;38(10):833–40.
48. Dai LY, Jiang LS. Single-level instrumented posterolateral fusion of lumbar spine with beta-tricalcium phosphate versus autograft: a prospective, randomized study with 3-year follow-up. Spine (Phila Pa 1976). 2008;33:1299–304.
49. Kong S, Park JH, Roh SW. A prospective comparative study of radiological outcomes after instrumented posterolateral fusion mass using autologous local bone or a mixture of beta-tcp and autologous local bone in the same patient. Acta Neurochir (Wien). 2013;155:765–70.
50. Moro-Barrero L, Acebal-Cortina G, Suárez-Suárez M, Pérez-Redondo J, Murcia-Mazón A, López-Muñiz A. Radiographic analysis of fusion mass using fresh autologous bone marrow with ceramic composites as an alternative to autologous bone graft. J Spinal Disord Tech. 2007;20:409–15.
51. Neen D, Noyes D, Shaw M, Gwilym S, Fairlie N, Birch N. Healos and bone marrow aspirate used for lumbar spine fusion: a case controlled study comparing Healos with autograft. Spine (Phila Pa 1976). 2006;31:E636–40.
52. Cho DY, Lee WY, Sheu PC, Chen CC. Cage containing a biphasic calcium phosphate ceramic (Triosite) for the treatment of cervical spondylosis. Surg Neurol. 2005;63:497504.
53. Alexander DI, Manson NA, Mitchell MJ. Efficacy of calcium sulfate plus decompression bone in lumbar and lumbosacral spinal fusion: preliminary results in 40 patients. Can J Surg. 2001;44:262–6.
54. Chen WJ, Tsai TT, Chen LH, Niu CC, Lai PL, Fu TS, McCarthy K. The fusion rate of calcium sulfate with local autograft bone compared with autologous iliac bone graft for instrumented short-segment spinal fusion. Spine (Phila Pa 1976). 2005;30:2293–7.
55. Niu CC, Tsai TT, Fu TS, Lai PL, Chen LH, Chen WJ. A comparison of posterolateral lumbar fusion comparing autograft, autogenous laminectomy bone with bone marrow aspirate, and calcium sulphate with bone marrow aspirate: a prospective randomized study. Spine (Phila Pa 1976). 2009;34:2715–9.
56. Licina P, Coughlan M, Johnston E, Pearcy M. Comparison of silicate-substituted calcium phosphate (Actifuse) with recombinant human bone morphogenetic protein-2 (infuse) in posterolateral instrumented lumbar fusion. Global Spine J. 2015;5(6):471–8.

57. Nandyala SV, Marquez-Lara A, Fineberg SJ, Pelton M, Singh K. Prospective, randomized, controlled trial of silicate-substituted calcium phosphate versus rhBMP-2 in a minimally invasive transforaminal lumbar interbody fusion. Spine (Phila Pa 1976). 2014;39(3):185–91.
58. Salih E, Wang J, Mah J, Fluckiger R. Natural variation in the extent of phosphorylation of bone phosphoproteins as a function of in vivo new bone formation induced by demineralized bone matrix in soft tissue and bony environments. Biochem J. 2002;364(Pt 2):465–74.
59. Blum B, Moseley J, Miller L, Richelsoph K, Haggard W. Measurement of bone morphogenetic proteins and other growth factors in demineralized bone matrix. Orthopedics. 2004;27(1 Suppl):s161–5.
60. Lee YP, Jo M, Luna M, Chien B, Lieberman JR, Wang JC. The efficacy of different commercially available demineralized bone matrix substances in an athymic rat model. J Spinal Disord Tech. 2005;18:439–44.
61. Peterson B, Whang PG, Iglesias R, Wang JC, Lieberman JR. Osteoinductivity of commercially available demineralized bone matrix. Preparations in a spine fusion model. J Bone Joint Surg Am. 2004;86-A:2243–50.
62. Wang JC, Alanay A, Mark D, Kanim LE, Campbell PA, Dawson EG, Lieberman JR. A comparison of commercially available demineralized bone matrix for spinal fusion. Eur Spine J. 2007;16:1233–40.
63. Choi Y, Oldenburg FP, Sage L, Johnstone B, Yoo JU. A bridging demineralized bone implant facilitates posterolateral lumbar fusion in New Zealand white rabbits. Spine. 2007;32:36–41.
64. Louis-Ugbo J, Murakami H, Kim HS, Minamide A, Boden SD. Evidence of osteoinduction by Grafton demineralized bone matrix in nonhuman primate spinal fusion. Spine. 2004;29:360–6.
65. Martin GJ Jr, Boden SD, Titus L, Scarborough NL. New formulations of demineralized bone matrix as a more effective graft alternative in experimental posterolateral lumbar spine arthrodesis. Spine. 1999;24:637–45.
66. Girardi FP, Cammisa FP Jr. The effect of bone graft extenders to enhance the performance of iliac crest bone grafts in instrumented lumbar spine fusion. Orthopedics. 2003;26:s545–8.
67. Sassard WR, Eidman DK, Gray PM, Block JE, Russo R, Russell JL, Taboada EM. Augmenting local bone with Grafton demineralized bone matrix for posterolateral lumbar spine fusion: avoiding second site autologous bone harvest. Orthopedics. 2000;23:1059–64.
68. Cammisa FP Jr, Lowery G, Garfin SR, Geisler FH, Klara PM, McGuire RA, Sassard WR, Stubbs H, Block JE. Two-year fusion rate equivalency between Grafton DBM gel and autograft in posterolateral spine fusion: a prospective controlled trial employing a side-by-side comparison in the same patient. Spine. 2004;29:660–6.
69. Vaccaro AR, Stubbs HA, Block JE. Demineralized bone matrix composite grafting for posterolateral spinal fusion. Orthopedics. 2007;30:567–70.
70. An HS, Simpson JM, Glover JM, Stephany J. Comparison between allograft plus demineralized bone matrix versus autograft in anterior cervical fusion. A prospective multicenter study. Spine. 1995;20:2211–6.
71. Park HW, Lee JK, Moon SJ, Seo SK, Lee JH, Kim SH. The efficacy of the synthetic interbody cage and Grafton for anterior cervical fusion. Spine (Phila Pa 1976). 2009;34(17):E591–5.
72. Moon HJ, Kim JH, Kim JH, Kwon TH, Chung HS, Park YK. The effects of anterior cervical discectomy and fusion with stand-alone cages at two contiguous levels on cervical alignment and outcomes. Acta Neurochir. 2011;153(3):559e65.
73. Lu SS, Zhang X, Soo C, Hsu T, Napoli A, Aghaloo T, Wu BM, Tsou P, Ting K, Wang JC. The osteoinductive properties of Nell-1 in a rat spinal fusion model. Spine J. 2007;7:50–60.
74. Weiner BK, Walker M. Efficacy of autologous growth factors in lumbar intertransverse fusions. Spine. 2003;28:1968–70.
75. Carreon LY, Glassman SD, Anekstein Y, Puno RM. Platelet gel (AGF) fails to increase fusion rates in instrumented posterolateral fusions. Spine. 2005;30:E243–6.
76. Hee HT, Majd ME, Holt RT, Myers L. Do autologous growth factors enhance transforaminal lumbar interbody fusion? Eur Spine J. 2003;12:400–7.
77. Jenis LG, Banco RJ, Kwon B. A prospective study of autologous growth factors (AGF) in lumbar interbody fusion. Spine J. 2006;6(1):14–20.
78. Muschler GF, Nitto H, Boehm CA, Easley KA. Age- and gender-related changes in the cellularity of human bone marrow and the prevalence of osteoblastic progenitors. J Orthop Res. 2001;19(1):117–25.
79. Muschler GF, Boehm CA, Easley K. Aspiration to obtain osteoblast progenitor cells from human bone marrow: the influence of aspiration volume. J Bone Joint Surg Am. 1997;79(11):1699–709.
80. Taghavi CE, Lee KB, Keorochana G, Tzeng ST, Yoo JH, Wang JC. Bone morphogenetic protein-2 and bone marrow aspirate with allograft as alternatives to autograft in instrumented revision posterolateral lumbar spinal fusion: a minimum two-year follow-up study. Spine (Phila Pa 1976). 2010;35(11):1144–50.
81. Khashan M, Inoue S, Berven SH. Cell based therapies as compared to autologous bone grafts for spinal arthrodesis. Spine (Phila Pa 1976). 2013;38(21):1885–91.
82. Urist MR. Bone: formation by auto induction. Science. 1965;150:893–9.
83. Wozney JM. Overview of bone morphogenetic proteins. Spine (Phila Pa 1976). 2002;27:S2–8.
84. Graff JM, Bansal A, Melton DA. Xenopus MAD proteins transduce distinct subsets of signals for the TGF beta superfamily. Cell. 1996;85:479–87.

85. Boden SD, Kang J, Sandhu H, Heller JG. Use of recombinant human bone morphogenetic protein-2 to achieve posterolateral lumbar spine fusion in humans: a prospective, randomized clinical pilot trial. Spine. 2002;27:2662–73.
86. Burkus JK, Gornet MF, Dickman CA, Zdeblick TA. Anterior lumbar interbody fusion using rhBMP-2 with tapered interbody cages. J Spinal Disord Tech. 2002;15:337–49.
87. Ong KL, Villarraga ML, Lau E, et al. Off-label use of bone morphogenetic proteins in the United States using administrative data. Spine. 2010;35:1794–800.
88. Bozic K. ORS clinical research forum, AAOS meeting 2/6/12.
89. FDA Public Health Notification. Life-threatening complications associated with recombinant human bone morphogenetic protein in cervical spine fusion, issued July 1, 2008.
90. Mroz TE, Wang JC, Hashimoto R, et al. Complications related to osteobiologics use in spine surgery: a systematic review. Spine. 2010;35:S86–S104.
91. Carragee EJ, Hurwitz EL, Weiner BK. A critical review of recombinant human bone morphogenetic protein-2 trials in spinal surgery: emerging safety concerns and lessons learned. Spine J. 2011;11:471–91.
92. Fu R, Selph S, McDonagh M, et al. Effectiveness and harms of recombinant human bone morphogenetic protein-2 in spine fusion: a systematic review and meta-analysis. Ann Intern Med. 2013;158(12):890–902.
93. Simmonds MC, Brown J, Heirs MK, et al. Safety and effectiveness of recombinant human bone morphogenetic protein-2 for spinal fusion. Ann Intern Med. 2013;158(12):877–89.
94. Huang J-W, Lin S-S, Chen L-H, et al. The use of fluorescence-labeled mesenchymal stem cells in poly(lactideco-glycolide)/hydroxyapatite/collagen hybrid graft as a bone substitute for posterolateral spinal fusion. J Trauma. 2011;70(6):1495–502.
95. Abbah SA, Lam CX, Ramruttun AK, Goh JC, Wong H-K. Fusion performance of low-dose recombinant human bone morphogenetic protein 2 and bone marrow derived multipotent stromal cells in biodegradable scaffolds: a comparative study in a large animal model of anterior lumbar interbody fusion. Spine. 2011;36(21):1752–9.
96. Lopez MJ, McIntosh KR, Spencer ND, et al. Acceleration of spinal fusion using syngeneic and allogeneic adult adipose derived stem cells in a rat model. J Orthop Res. 2009;27(3):366–73.
97. Wang JC, Kanim LE, Yoo S, Campbell PA, Berk AJ, Lieberman JR. Effect of regional gene therapy with bone morphogenetic protein-2-producing bone marrow cells on spinal fusion in rats. J Bone Joint Surg Am. 2003;85-A(5):905–11.
98. Miyazaki M, Zuk PA, Zou J, Yoon SH, Wei F, Morishita Y, Sintuu C, Wang JC. Comparison of human mesenchymal stem cells derived from adipose tissue and bone marrow for ex vivo gene therapy in rat spinal fusion model. Spine (Phila Pa 1976). 2008;33(8):863–9.
99. Nakajima T, Iizuka H, Tsutsumi S, Kayakabe M, Takagishi K. Evaluation of posterolateral spinal fusion using mesenchymal stem cells: differences with or without osteogenic differentiation. Spine. 2007;32(22):2432–6.
100. Barba M, Cicione C, Bernardini C, Campana V, Pagano E, Michetti F, Logroscino G, Lattanzi W. Spinal fusion in the next generation: gene and cell therapy approaches. ScientificWorldJournal. 2014; 2014:406159. doi:10.1155/2014/406159. eCollection 2014
101. Rao PJ, Pelletier MH, Walsh WR, Mobbs RJ. Spine interbody implants: material selection and modification, functionalization and bioactivation of surfaces to improve osseointegration. Orthop Surg. 2014;6(2):81–9. doi:10.1111/os.12098.
102. Ramakrishna SMJ, Wintermantel E, Leong KW. Biomedical applications of polymer-composite materials: a review. Compos Sci Technol. 2001;61:1189–224.

Basic Science of Bone Fusion

35

Joseph A. Weiner and Wellington K. Hsu

Introduction

Bone regeneration is critical for many orthopedic procedures such as fracture repair, osteotomies, and spine fusion. Understanding the molecular and cellular mediators of bone healing is essential for the treating surgeon who must ensure that the critical components of bone repair are present during surgery. Spine arthrodesis is frequently performed in the treatment of spine trauma, deformity, and complex degenerative disorders. With an estimated 413,000 fusion procedures performed in the United States annually, the number of procedures performed has increased by 2.4-fold since 1998 [1]. The success of spine surgery in these conditions depends on the reestablishment of spinal stability. While spinal instrumentation may afford temporary support, a bony union must be formed to provide enduring stability.

Failure of fusion, or pseudarthrosis, is associated with poor long-term clinical outcomes and an increase in the 10-year reoperation rate [2, 3]. Recently, pseudarthrosis rates for lumbar spine fusions have been reported from 5% to 48% [4–6] with a higher incidence in fusions spanning three or more spinal levels [7]. The rate of nonunion following anterior cervical discectomy and fusion (ACDF) can vary depending on the number of levels fused, the allograft type used, and the surgical technique; however, it is frequently reported to be between 0% and 20% in single-level ACDF to over 60% in multilevel fusions [8]. Given the rising number of spine fusions performed, it is essential that surgeons be aware of the pathophysiologic processes that can lead to this complication. This chapter will review the basic biological and physiological principles of bone healing in an effort to assist the spine surgeon in selecting the most efficacious techniques for achieving successful arthrodesis. Furthermore, we will briefly discuss promising areas of research in the treatment and prevention of pseudarthrosis.

Basic Science of Bone

Bone Anatomy and Histology

Bone is a dynamic biological tissue comprised of metabolically active cells incorporated into a rigid mineralized matrix framework. An understanding of the relationship between the anatomic structure and histology of bone tissue is

J.A. Weiner, MD (✉) • W.K. Hsu, MD
Department of Orthopaedic Surgery, Northwestern University Feinberg School of Medicine,
676 N. St. Clair St., #1350, Chicago, IL 60611, USA
e-mail: Joseph.Weiner@northwestern.edu; Whsu@nm.org

L.T. Holly, P.A. Anderson (eds.), *Essentials of Spinal Stabilization*,
DOI 10.1007/978-3-319-59713-3_35

critical to understand the process of bone healing and fusion. On a cellular level, bone consists of four main cell types: osteogenic precursor cells (stem cells), osteoblasts, osteoclasts, and osteocytes [9–11]. Contained within the marrow space are numerous other cells types critical for hematopoiesis. Osteogenic progenitor cells, a derivative of mesenchymal stem cells, serve as the cellular reserve of bone tissue. They are present within the inner layer of the periosteum which envelops the outer surface of bone and on the endosteum that lines the medullary surface of compact bone. Similarly, these osteogenic progenitor cells are also found within the endosteum lining the surface of trabecular bone within vertebrae.

Osteoblasts, derived from osteogenic precursor cells, are mature bone-forming cells. They secrete osteoid that subsequently undergoes mineralization, providing strength and rigidity. As osteoblasts lay down osteoid, cells become incorporated into the matrix and become osteocytes, while others remain on resorptive surfaces to participate in bone turnover alongside osteoclasts. From each osteocyte a web of cytoplasmic processes extends through canaliculi to blood vessels and other osteocytes, forming a critical network that allows bone to function as a living tissue. Osteocytes are involved in the control of the extracellular concentration of calcium and phosphorus, as well as in adaptive remodeling behavior via cell-to-cell interactions in response to the local environment [12–14].

Osteoclasts, derived from macrophages, are multinucleated, bone-resorbing cells controlled by hormonal and cellular mechanisms. These cells function in cutting cones and dissolve the inorganic and organic matrices of bone and calcified cartilage via the release of catabolic enzymes. This process results in the formation of shallow erosive pits on the bone surface called Howship's lacunae. The delicate balance between osteoblast and osteoclast activity mediates the metabolic turnover of bone. When these processes are disrupted, conditions such as Paget's disease are seen.

Bone Metabolism

Bone metabolism is under continual regulation by a multitude of hormonal factors and local mediators, many of which play a critical role in bone healing during spine fusion. Three of the hormones that play a crucial role in calcium-phosphate homeostasis and bone metabolism are parathyroid hormone (PTH), vitamin D, and calcitonin. PTH increases free serum calcium and maintains the body's extracellular calcium levels at a relatively constant level [15–17]. Interestingly, while PTH is typically considered to be a bone catabolic agent, when delivered intermittently at low doses, PTH potently stimulates cortical and trabecular bone growth by increasing osteoblast proliferation and differentiation, decreasing osteoblast apoptosis and reducing the inhibitory effects of peroxisome proliferator activator (PPAR)γ receptor on osteoblast differentiation [15].

Calcitonin, a peptide hormone secreted by the parafollicular cells of the thyroid gland, serves to counteract the activities of PTH. Rising serum calcium levels cause calcitonin to be released in an attempt to return calcium levels to a homeostatic level. More specifically, calcitonin lowers blood calcium levels through four mechanisms: inhibiting calcium absorption by the intestines, inhibiting osteoclast activity, stimulating osteoblast activity, and inhibiting renal tubular cell reabsorption of calcium allowing excretion in the urine [18, 19].

With the finding of the vitamin D receptor (VDR) in nearly all tissues and the recent discovery of thousands of VDR binding sites throughout the genome, the interest in vitamin D and its impact on multiple biologic processes has accelerated tremendously [20, 21]. In the arena of bone metabolism, vitamin D's role is well established. Vitamin D stimulates intestinal and renal calcium-binding proteins and facilitates active calcium transport [22]. Vitamin D is also critical to the process of osteoid mineralization [21]. Together, the interplay between vitamin D, PTH, and calcitonin helps to maintain bone homeostasis, a process critical to osteoid mineralization and normal bone healing following surgery.

Principles of Bone Healing

While understanding bone metabolism is critical, it does not fully explain the process of bone healing after a fracture or following fusion surgery. Bone healing is dependent on four elements: an osteoinductive stimulus, an osteoconductive matrix, a source of osteogenic cells, and a viable vascular supply (Fig. 35.1). The mechanical environment is also vital, as bone is remodeled in response to load (Wolff's law). If any of these crucial factors is absent, new bone formation is significantly diminished [23, 24].

Osteoinduction is the process of recruitment of immature osteogenic precursor cells and subsequent stimulation to differentiate into osteoblasts. This process requires a stimulus to trigger differentiation of precursor cells into mature osteoblasts; often this stimulus comes in the form of local growth factors released from platelets, macrophages, and fibroblasts in response to bone injury [25, 26]. Examples of important growth factor mediators include bone morphogenetic peptides, fibroblast growth factor (FGF), insulin-like growth factor (IGF), platelet-derived growth factor (PDGF), and transforming growth factor-β (TGF-β). The most widely studied growth factors are those in the bone morphogenetic protein (BMP) family. BMPs are soluble cytokines of the transforming growth factor beta superfamily involved in the differentiation, maturation, and proliferation of mesenchymal precursor cells into osteogenic cells. To date, over 20 types have been described and are typically present in only minute quantities in the body. However, two commercial forms of recombinant BMP are available for clinical use: rhBMP-2 (INFUSE) (Medtronic – Memphis, TN) and rhBMP-7 (OP-1) (Olympus Biotech Corporation – Hopkinton, MA) [27]. BMPs act via serine-threonine kinase receptors found on the surface of target cells and transduce their signal via the SMAD pathway, leading to nuclear translocation and subsequent expression of target genes involved in osteogenesis [28, 29].

Osteoconduction is the physical property of the matrix or graft to serve as a scaffold for viable bone healing. Physiologically, osteoid deposition by osteoblasts serves as an initial osteoconductive scaffold during fracture healing. Osteoconduction allows for neovasculaturization and the infiltration of osteogenic precursor cells into the fusion or healing site. In the context of spine fusion, numerous graft materials such as cancellous autografts and allografts, demineralized bone matrix, ceramics, and collagen sponges can serve as osteoconductive scaffolds for new bone growth to occur [7, 30, 31]. Scaffold properties such as compressive strength, biocompatibility, and pore size determine its ability to successfully aid bone regeneration [31, 32].

Osteogenesis refers to the process of creating new bone and typically denotes the presence of viable mesenchymal stem cells, osteoblasts, and osteocytes in a graft material [31]. During the early stages of bone healing, these cell types are essential to new bone formation and bony union.

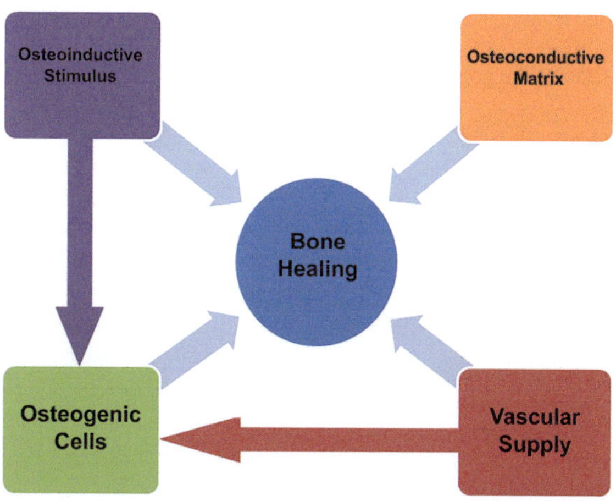

Fig. 35.1 Key elements of bone healing. Bone healing requires interplay between four factors: an osteoinductive stimulus, an osteoconductive matrix, a source of osteogenic cells, and a viable vascular supply

In spine surgery, osteogenic potential is classically provided by decortication of the fusion bed and supplementation with autogenous graft material – the most widely used being iliac crest and local bone. The process of decortication exposes underlying cancellous bone and releases growth factors critical to the recruitment and differentiation of osteogenic progenitor cells. These grafts offer a source of viable osteoblasts and stem cells that begin the process of bone healing.

Bone Healing Process

While the mechanism of bone injury in fractures is remarkably different than spine fusion, it has been established that the process of bone healing is extraordinarily similar [33]. Bone healing has been classified into three distinct yet overlapping phases: early inflammatory, repair or proliferative, and late remodeling [34]. The inflammatory phase begins immediately following a fracture with hematoma formation in the injured bone and generally lasts 1–3 days [35]. This hematoma results from bleeding vessels within the damaged periosteum and cancellous bone. The inflammatory phase is mediated via a growth factor cascade, which includes TGF-β, BMPs, FGF, PDGF, IGF-1, osteoprotegerin, and VEGF. These factors are released from platelets, macrophages, and fibroblasts within the local hematoma during the first week and serve to begin the process of osteoinduction and osteogenesis (Table 35.1) [36]. During this critical period, cells involved in the healing process receive their nutrient and oxygen supply from the exposed cancellous bone and muscle. Toward the end of the inflammatory phase, deposition of matrix results in the formation of an immature callus.

During the repair or proliferative phase, fibroplasia occurs, leading to the replacement of the crude callus by immature woven bone over the course of several weeks. More specifically, the necrotic bone at the margins of the fracture site or decorticated bone is resorbed by recruited osteoclasts [36]. A periosteal response also occurs with angiogenesis and formation of soft callus [37]. Within the fracture site or fusion bed, recruited mesenchymal stem cells differentiate into chondrocytes within the hypoxic fracture regions. Within these areas, soft callus will steadily take on the appearance of cartilage and help to stabilize

Table 35.1 Local factors involved in bone healing

Type	Source	Role
Bone morphogenetic protein	Mesenchymal stem cells Extracellular matrix Vascular endothelium	Recruitment and differentiation of mesenchymal cells Mineralization of extracellular matrix
Fibroblast growth factor	Vascular endothelium Basement membrane	Mitogen Supports vascularization and bone development
Insulin-like growth factor	Liver Paracrine signaling	Activation of osteocytes Anabolic for bone tissue
Platelet-derived growth factor	Platelets Smooth muscle cells Activated macrophages Vascular endothelium	Mitogen for mesenchymal cells Supports angiogenesis
Vascular endothelium growth factor	Vascular endothelium Smooth muscle	Angiogenesis
Osteoprotegerin (TNF-α[alpha] superfamily)	Vascular endothelium Smooth muscle cells Osteocytes	Blocks RANK ligand interaction with RANK receptor → promotes bone formation
RANK ligand	Vascular endothelium Smooth muscle Osteocytes	Osteoclastic differentiation and activation

the fracture site [36]. Chondrocyte growth and differentiation are stimulated by growth factors released during the inflammatory phase, including TGF-β, BMPs, FGF, PDGF, and IGF-1. Irregular woven bone gradually replaces this cartilage via the process of endochondral ossification [34].

During the last phase of bone repair, irregular woven bone within the callus is transformed into lamellar bone. This process occurs when osteoclasts resorb the newly woven bone and osteoblasts replace this matrix with the lamellar bone. Importantly, this remodeling phase leads to restoration of mechanical strength and stability. A critical aspect of appropriate remodeling is the biomechanical force applied to the healing site. Lamellae are aligned parallel to the axis of the greatest force, and adequate mechanical loading is required to augment osteogenesis and generate bone with the proper anatomic configuration [38].

Through the concepts of fracture fixation, it has been well established that proper biomechanical forces are necessary for bone healing [39]. When sufficient osteogenic cells and biologic factors are present, the course of bone healing is influenced mainly by the amount of strain and mechanical load across a bone defect. The forces across a fracture or bone defect, along with the fixation, determine the interfragmentary movement. A stiff fixation minimizes interfragmentary movements and results in limited stimulation of callus formation, while a flexible fixation can enhance the callus formation. However, an unstable fixation can cause the interfragmentary strain to exceed the rupture strain of bone leading to nonunion [40]. Ideally, the proliferating osteoblasts respond to the mechanical strain, and the final product of bone healing has the same biomechanical properties of the original bone it replaced.

Clinical Application of the Basic Science of Bone Healing

While the basic science of bone healing can be quite complex, it is critical that spine surgeons have a thorough understanding of how bone healing principles apply to their fusion patients. As demonstrated above, bone repair in the context of spine fusion is a multifaceted process that requires five major components: a sufficient population of osteogenic cells, an osteoconductive matrix within the region where new bone tissue is needed, osteoinductive signals within the fusion bed, a local blood supply, and desirable biomechanical forces.

	Critical components of bone healing
1	Sufficient population of osteogenic cells
2	Osteoconductive matrix
3	Osteoinductive signals
4	Local blood supply
5	Desirable biomechanical forces

A deficiency in any one of those elements can have a profoundly detrimental effect on spine fusion. To date, numerous systemic factors have been identified both in the laboratory and clinically that directly or indirectly impact bone regeneration [41–45] (Table 35.2). A working knowledge of the bony repair mechanisms can allow the surgeon to maximize chances for successful fusion.

Table 35.2 Systemic factors/conditions affecting bone healing

Positive factors	Negative factors
Adequate nutrition	Malnourishment (iron deficiency anemia, negative nitrogen balance)
Vitamin D	Vitamin D deficiency
Parathyroid hormone	Tobacco
Calcitonin	Sepsis
Insulin	Corticosteroids
Insulin-like growth factor	Calcium deficiency/osteoporosis
Testosterone	Nonsteroidal anti-inflammatory drugs
Estrogen	Adriamycin
Thyroxine	Methotrexate
Vitamin A	Rheumatoid arthritis
Growth hormone	Syndrome of inappropriate antidiuretic hormone
Anabolic steroids	Castration
Vitamin C	

Nutritional Deficiency

Nutritional status has been well established as a predictor of surgical outcomes in the general surgical literature for decades [46–48]. Nutritional deficiencies lead to increased complication rates, length of hospitalization, and mortality. The impact of poor nutrition on orthopedic procedures and bone healing has more recently become a focus of research [49]. Jensen et al. established that nearly 35% of patients undergoing elective orthopedic procedures are clinically malnourished, defined by serum albumin <3.5 g/dL [50]. This rate of malnutrition should be highly concerning for the spine surgeon because of associations with delayed wound healing, diminished immunocompetence, surgical site infection, prolonged hospitalizations, and poor bone healing [51, 52].

Identification of a nutritional deficit in preoperative spine fusion patients, especially those undergoing an elective procedure, is critical for maximizing the chances of a successful outcome. While numerous methods such as anthropomorphic measurements, skin antigen testing, and nitrogen balance studies exist for nutritional evaluation, the clinical tests most commonly used to assess the nutritional status of surgical patients are the serum albumin level and the total lymphocyte count. These tests are practical, cost-effective, widely available, and highly reproducible in the surgical patient population [53]. Serum albumin is a representative marker of visceral protein mass; decreased levels are due to both decreased synthesis and increased catabolism. The conditions leading to decreased albumin levels are often found in patients with poor functional and nutritional statuses. Furthermore, decreased albumin levels are associated with poor wound healing, postoperative infectious, complications, mortality, and immune suppression [54]. Serum albumin levels less than 3.5 g/dL are widely accepted to represent a state of malnutrition [55]. Furthermore, the severity of the deficiency is correlated with the incidence of complications. In 2016, Kamath et al. reported that joint arthroplasty patients with preoperative albumin <3.0 g/dL had a 15.4% rate of unplanned ICU admission compared to 3.8% for patients with an albumin 3.0–3.5 g/dL [56].

Similarly, poor nutritional status causes a decrease in total lymphocyte count – a marker of immune competence [57]. This decrease in immune competence is believed to underlie the increased risk for surgical site infection in this patient population. Current research indicates that protein-calorie malnutrition causes a catabolic state which limits the body's ability to undertake anabolic processes, including forming new lymphocytes. A total lymphocyte count less than 1500–2000 cells/mm^3 is considered by most authors to represent a clinical state of malnutrition [57].

When this diagnosis is made, correction of all nutritional deficiencies should be part of the preoperative optimization process. Correction for malnutrition is primarily accomplished conservatively through dietary counseling, as well as meal fortification with protein and energy-rich foods [58]. However, when patients fail conservative management, oral nutritional supplements, such as Ensure, can be effective in improving nutritional status [55, 59]. Risk factors for correction failure include complex medical comorbidities, such as gastrointestinal disease, psychiatric conditions, or cancer. These patients should be medically optimized with the aid of a comprehensive care team before undergoing surgery.

Vitamin D Deficiency

Vitamin D plays a critical role in maintaining metabolic bone homeostasis. Vitamin D deficiency, a condition present in 33% of healthy young adults and more than 50% of general medicine inpatients [60], can have serious deleterious effects on bone health. As vitamin D is depleted, absorption of calcium decreases and parathyroid hormone is upregulated. This hormonal dysregulation can cause an increase in osteoclast bone resorption and predisposes patients to osteoporosis, osteomalacia, and fractures [61].

The previously unknown prevalence of vitamin D deficiency has led to a recent awareness of this problem. In 2010, Bogunovic et al. reported that 43% of a 723-patient cohort scheduled to undergo an orthopedic procedure were deficient in vitamin D [62]. In addition to predisposing to fractures, an overabundance of osteoclastic resorption may impede bone formation needed for spinal arthrodesis [63]. Considering the financial and clinical burden of pseudarthrosis, knowledge of the prevalence, evaluation, and treatment for hypovitaminosis D is critical for all spine surgeons.

Despite the established importance of vitamin D in musculoskeletal health, most spine surgeons fail to recognize the value in testing preoperative levels. A 2009 study by Dipaola et al. revealed that only 12% of spine surgeons order metabolic tests, including serum levels of vitamin D, before fusion surgery and only 20% as part of a pseudarthrosis workup [64]. This is despite the fact that nearly 70% of patients with spine pathology are insufficient or deficient in vitamin D, those with severe pain being the most deficient [65, 66]. Numerous studies, both in animal models and humans, have established vitamin D as a critical mediator of fracture healing [67–70]. More recently, Metzger et al. demonstrated that vitamin D modulates the consolidation of bone after grafting for posterolateral spinal fusion in a rat model. Specifically, their results indicate that increased levels of dietary vitamin D correlate directly with the density of the fusion mass [71].

Given the impact of vitamin D on spine fusion and the prevalence of deficiency, it is the authors' recommendation that preoperative testing of serum vitamin D levels should be routine. Thresholds for vitamin D levels which are well established in the literature (Table 35.3) [61, 72] should be used to institute treatment. Patients deficient in vitamin D are typically prescribed 50,000 IU of oral vitamin D2 (ergocalciferol) per week for 8 weeks followed by maintenance therapy of 1500–2000 IU/day [61]. Furthermore, the relatively brief treatment duration often allows completion before surgery and provides for high patient compliance [73]. Given the high prevalence of vitamin D deficiency and low risk of treatment, it is also acceptable to consider supplementation with 2000 IU/day of oral vitamin D3.

Table 35.3 Serum 25-hydroxyvitamin D [25(OH)D] concentrations and health

nmol/L	ng/mL	Health status
<30	<12	Vitamin D deficiency, leading to rickets in infants and children and osteomalacia in adults
30 to <50	12 to <20	Vitamin D insufficiency
≥50	≥20	Generally considered adequate for bone and overall health in healthy individuals
>125	>50	Emerging evidence links potential adverse effects to such high levels, particularly >150 nmol/L (>60 ng/mL)

Cigarette Smoking

The impact of tobacco smoke on human health remains a critical problem facing the orthopedic surgeon worldwide. Cigarette smoke has a well-established role in the pathogenesis of numerous smoking-related disorders including chronic obstructive pulmonary disease (COPD), cancer, and atherosclerosis [74, 75]. More recently recognized, smoking also exacerbates musculoskeletal disease and presents serious challenges in the treatment of orthopedic conditions [76]. In addition to promoting osteoporosis, degenerative disk disease, and surgical site infections, smoking impedes osseointegration and bony union – deleterious effects associated with higher rates of revision procedures [77–79]. In spine surgery, smoking has been shown to have a negative impact on outcomes with a lumbar pseudarthrosis rate nearly double that of nonsmokers (26.5% vs. 14.2%) [80].

Defining a single mechanism by which cigarette smoke impedes bone healing is challenging, as cigarette smoke contains upward of 4000 distinct chemical components. However, several mechanisms are postulated to be involved. Carbon monoxide present in the smoke displaces oxygen from hemoglobin, significantly diminishing the capacity for blood to carry vital oxygen to proliferating osteoblasts at the site of bone healing or growth [81]. Nicotine, a potent anti-inflammatory and immunosuppressive substance, has been shown to have deleterious effects on fibroblasts, red blood cells, and macrophages [82–84], in addition to diminishing blood flow to tissues by promoting vasoconstriction [84, 85]. Numerous other studies have proposed that reactive oxygen species and other pro-inflammatory constituents are responsible for the dysregulation of bone homeostasis, reduction in bone mineral density, and inhibition of fracture healing [86–88].

More recent research has identified dioxin, a potent carcinogenic by-product of combustion, as playing a major role in the inhibition of osteogenesis [43]. In vitro and in vivo work has shown that dioxin has toxic effects on bone, adversely affecting bone growth and remodeling, matrix composition, mechanical strength, and osteoblast differentiation [89]. These effects occur independent of nicotine and have a dramatically larger impact. Although the exact mechanism of osteoblastic inhibition from smoking remains somewhat unclear, many surgeons currently associate nicotine with the negative impact of smoking on bone healing. The association of dioxin and the AhR pathway with bone healing inhibition from cigarettes offers a promising new approach to the mitigation of these effects.

With the negative effects of smoking so well established, spine surgeons must consider their options when treating patients who smoke. All patients have both modifiable and non-modifiable risk factors that can impact patient outcomes after spine procedures. Therefore, it is critical that modifiable risk factors, like smoking, are minimized before taking a patient to surgery. Many have advocated for smoking cessation programs before elective procedures [80, 90]. These programs have demonstrated that an active smoking intervention program started 6–8 weeks before surgery can halve the frequency of postoperative complications, with the greatest effect on wound-related and cardiovascular complications [90]. Furthermore, given the emerging evidence that nicotine may not be the primary culprit behind inhibition of bone healing [43], surgeons should consider nicotine replacement therapy as method for increasing patient compliance with cessation programs. Given the deleterious consequences of smoking and the large impact of cessation, preoperative counseling and enrollment in cessation programs are an essential aspect of preoperative patient care.

Bisphosphonates and Teriparatide

With an overall low bone mass prevalence of 43.9%, there are an estimated 43.4 million adults in the United States at increased risk for fracture. In 2008, 15.8% of women over the age of 55 were prescribed bisphosphonates to increase their bone mineral density and reduce their risk for fracture [91]. More recently, many patients have been prescribed anabolic agents such as teriparatide. However, due to the cost of anabolic agents, most physicians still recommend anti-catabolic drugs as the first-line treatment for osteoporosis. Bisphosphonates inhibit osteoclastic bone resorption, preventing bone loss and improving bone strength [92, 93]. However, the effect of bisphosphonates on bone healing remains controversial. As previously discussed, osteoclasts are essential for remodeling during the transformation from immature callus into mature bone. The impact on remodeling causes adverse effects such as atypical femur fractures and osteonecrosis [94]. While the association with abnormal remodeling is well defined, the overall effect of bisphosphonates on bone healing is less clear. A recent meta-analysis of eight randomized control trials revealed that bisphosphonates do not cause a clinically detectable delay to bone healing regardless of the timing of bisphosphonate delivery [95].

Teriparatide, a recombinant PTH analog, has been utilized since 2002 to increase bone mineral density in postmenopausal women suffering from osteoporosis. Unlike bisphosphonates, teriparatide is an anabolic agent that has the ability to stimulate new bone formation. There has been abundant evidence from animal studies that indicate teriparatide can improve fracture healing [96, 97]. Significant improvements in callus volume, callus mineralization, bone mineral content, strength, and rate of successful union at the fracture site have been demonstrated [98]. However, studies in humans have been relatively limited, and further research is needed to delineate the impact of anabolic agents on bone healing in humans. Currently, teriparatide is being used "off label" for the management of fractures and nonunions, as well as perioperative optimization of surgical patients.

Electrical Stimulation

The role for electrical stimulation in bone healing has been somewhat controversial. Basic science research suggests that pulsed electromagnetic field (PEMF) therapy likely enhances bone healing through stimulation of the calcium-calmodulin pathway secondary to the upregulation of bone morphogenetic proteins, transforming growth factor-β, and other cytokines [99, 100]. A recent meta-analysis of 15 trials, performed in 2016, indicated that that electrical stimulation reduced the relative risk for radiographic nonunion or persistent nonunion by 35% and the absolute risk by 15% [101]. Four trials found that stimulation produced a significant improvement in patient-reported pain scores [101]. However, functional outcome data are limited and further randomized controlled trials are needed.

Clinical Case

History

A 59-year-old male with grade I degenerative spondylolisthesis and severe spinal stenosis at L4–L5 causing neurogenic claudication, low back pain, and buttock pain. The patient previously failed conservative management for 2 years at which point he underwent open decompression and posterolateral spinal fusion at L4–L5. He was subsequently pain-free for 1 year and then developed recurrent back pain without neurologic symptoms. Standing exacerbates his symptoms; sitting or leaning forward temporarily relieves pain. The patient has a past medical history significant for hypertension. Of note, he is a current smoker with a 40 pack-year history. A complete workup was performed, including postoperative lumbar CT.

Examination

Physical examination demonstrated a positive straight-leg raising on the right at 30 degrees. The remainder of the examination was normal.

Pretreatment Images

MRI of the lumbar spine demonstrated recurrent degenerative spondylolisthesis (Fig. 35.2). CT scan of the lumbar spine demonstrated screw loosening at L4–L5 and lumbar pseudarthrosis (Fig. 35.3).

Diagnosis

L4–L5 pseudarthrosis.

Treatment

The patient was informed of the risk factors for pseudarthrosis, including smoking, malnutrition, and vitamin D deficiency. The patient elected to participate in a 6-week smoking cessation program and utilized nicotine patches during the perioperative period. The patient was subsequently revised with a lateral interbody fusion with Polyether ether ketone (PEEK) cage at the L4–L5 level (Fig. 35.4). A small kit of INFUSE and 5 cc of Mastergraft were utilized to promote successful arthrodesis.

Outcome

The patient had radiographic evidence of fusion on CT at 6 months. No clinical signs or symptoms of pseudarthrosis. Patient denied continued low back pain.

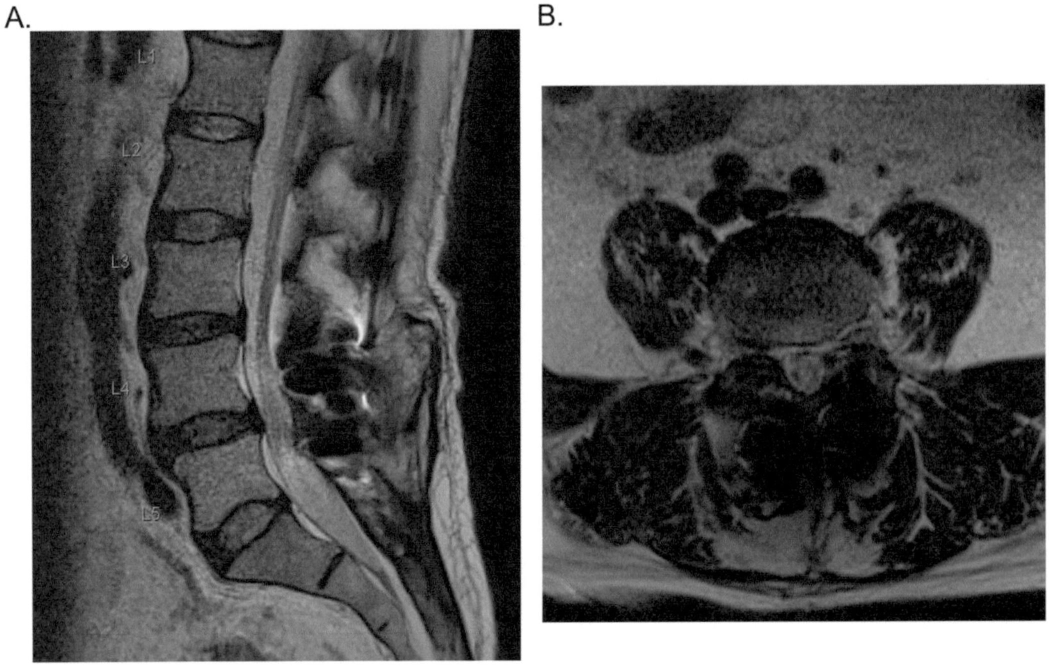

Fig. 35.2 Pre-revision (**a**) sagittal and (**b**) axial MRI of the lumbar spine demonstrating recurrence of the L4–L5 degenerative spondylolisthesis

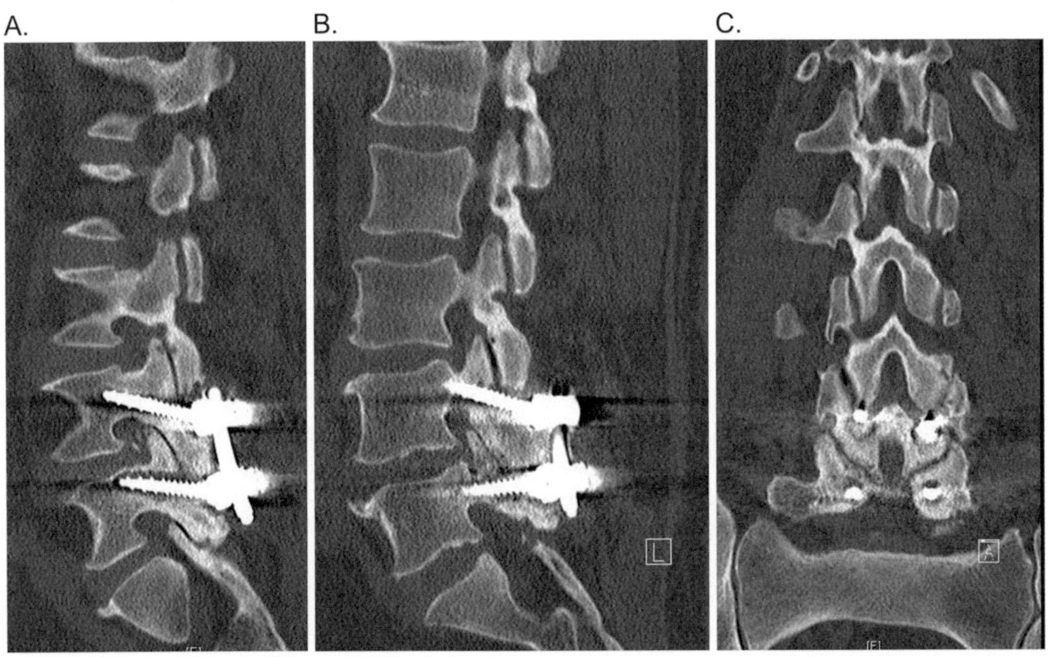

Fig. 35.3 Pre-revision (**a**, **b**) sagittal and (**c**) coronal CT scan demonstrating radiolucency surrounding the L4 and L5 pedicle screws and an L4–L5 pseudarthrosis

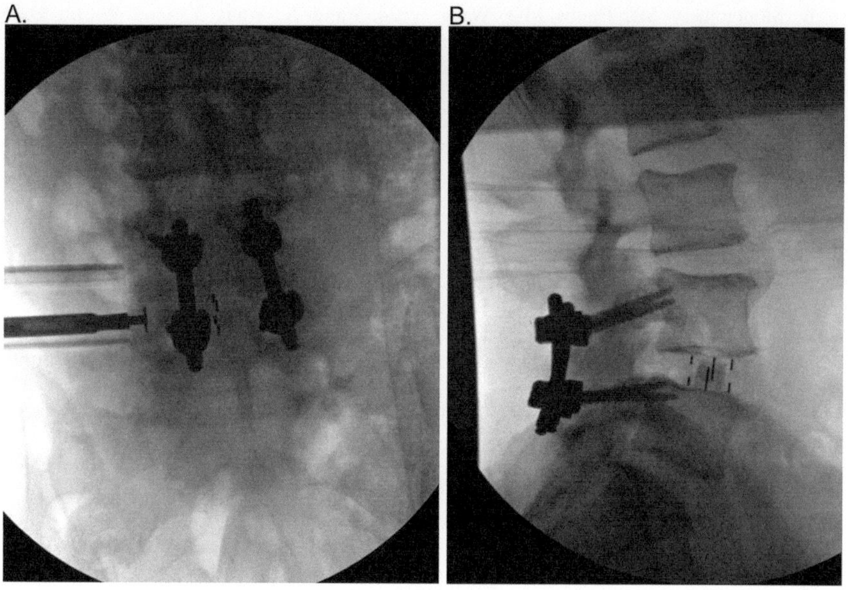

Fig. 35.4 Intraoperative (**a**) AP and (**b**) lateral fluoroscopy after placement of Polyether ether ketone (PEEK) lateral interbody cage

Conclusion

While the basic science of bone healing is complex, it is important that spine surgeons have a thorough understanding of how bone healing principles apply to their fusion patients. Bone healing requires five major components: a sufficient population of osteogenic cells, an osteoconductive matrix, osteoinductive signals, a local blood supply, and desirable biomechanical forces. Deficiency of any one component can lead to pseudarthrosis. With that knowledge, it is imperative that spine surgeons optimize their patients preoperatively by evaluating for and correcting nutritional and vitamin D deficiency, osteoporosis, and tobacco use. Surgeons must understand the importance of stress, strain, and osteogenesis to optimize their biomechanical constructs and graft choice intraoperatively. Finally, surgeons should understand the biologic mechanism, clinical role, and efficacy of adjunct therapies, such as pulsed electromagnetic field therapy and bisphosphonates, on bone healing.

References

1. Rajaee SS, Bae HW, Kanim LEA, Delamarter RB. Spinal fusion in the United States: analysis of trends from 1998 to 2008. Spine. 2012;37(1):67–76.
2. Fischgrund JS, Mackay M, Herkowitz HN, Brower R, Montgomery DM, Kurz LT. 1997 Volvo award winner in clinical studies: degenerative lumbar Spondylolisthesis with spinal stenosis: a Prospective, randomized study comparing decompressive laminectomy and arthrodesis with and without spinal instrumentation. Spine. 1997;22(24):2807–12.
3. Kornblum MB, Fischgrund JS, Herkowitz HN, Abraham DA, Berkower DL, Ditkoff JS. Degenerative lumbar spondylolisthesis with spinal stenosis: a prospective long-term study comparing fusion and pseudarthrosis. Spine. 2004;29(7):726–33.
4. Berjano P, Langella F Damilano M, Pejrona M, Buric J, Ismael M, Villafane JH, et al. Fusion rate following extreme lateral lumbar interbody fusion. Eur Spine J. 2015. (1432–0932 (Electronic)).
5. Grubb SA, Hj L, Suh PB. Results of surgical treatment of painful adult scoliosis. Spine (Phila Pa 1976). (0362–2436 (Print))
6. Herkowitz HN, Sidhu KS. Lumbar spine fusion in the treatment of degenerative conditions: current indications and recommendations. J Am Acad Orthop Surg. (1940–5480 (Electronic))

7. Aghdasi B, Montgomery SR, Daubs MD, Wang JC. A review of demineralized bone matrices for spinal fusion: the evidence for efficacy. Surgeon J R Coll Surg Edinb Irel. 2013;11(1):39–48.
8. McAnany SJ, Baird EO, Overley SC, Kim JS, Qureshi SA, Anderson PA. A meta-analysis of the clinical and fusion results following treatment of symptomatic cervical Pseudarthrosis. Global Spine J. 2015;5(2):148–55.
9. Pavelka M, Roth J. Bone. In: Functional ultrastructure. Vienna: Springer; 2015. p. 336–9.
10. Dickson GR. Bailey's textbook of histology. J Anat. 1979;129((Pt 1)):189.
11. Ross MH, Pawlina W. Histology : a text and atlas : with correlated cell and molecular biology, vol. xviii. 6th ed. Philadelphia: Wolters Kluwer/Lippincott Williams & Wilkins Health; 2011. 974p.
12. Klein-Nulend J, Nijweide PJ, Burger EH. Osteocyte and bone structure. Curr Osteoporos Rep. 2003;1(1):5–10.
13. Franz-Odendaal TA, Hall BK, Witten PE. Buried alive: how osteoblasts become osteocytes. Dev Dyn Off Publ Am Assoc Anat. 2006;235(1):176–90.
14. Aarden EM, Burger EH, Nijweide PJ. Function of osteocytes in bone. J Cell Biochem. 1994;55(3):287–99.
15. Lombardi G, Di Somma C, Rubino M, Faggiano A, Vuolo L, Guerra E, et al. The roles of parathyroid hormone in bone remodeling: prospects for novel therapeutics. J Endocrinol Investig. 2011;34(7 Suppl):18–22.
16. Morley P, Whitfield JF, Willick GE. Parathyroid hormone: an anabolic treatment for osteoporosis. Curr Pharm Des. 2001;7(8):671–87.
17. Sowa H, Kaji H, Iu MF, Tsukamoto T, Sugimoto T, Chihara K. Parathyroid hormone-Smad3 axis exerts anti-apoptotic action and augments anabolic action of transforming growth factor beta in osteoblasts. J Biol Chem. 2003;278(52):52240–52.
18. Sexton PM, Findlay DM, Martin TJ. Calcitonin. Curr Med Chem. 1999;6(11):1067–93.
19. Pondel M. Calcitonin and calcitonin receptors: bone and beyond. Int J Exp Pathol. 2000;81(6):405–22.
20. Haussler MR, Jurutka PW, Mizwicki M, Norman AW. Vitamin D receptor (VDR)-mediated actions of 1alpha,25(OH)(2)vitamin D(3): genomic and non-genomic mechanisms. Best Pract Res Clin Endocrinol Metab. 2011;25(4):543–59.
21. Bikle DD. Vitamin D metabolism, mechanism of action, and clinical applications. Chem Biol. 2014;21(3):319–29.
22. Gorter EA, Hamdy NA, Appelman-Dijkstra NM, Schipper IB. The role of vitamin D in human fracture healing: a systematic review of the literature. Bone. 2014;64:288–97.
23. Stevenson S, Emery SE, Goldberg VM. Factors affecting bone graft incorporation. Clin Orthop Relat Res. 1996;324:66–74.
24. Wang X, Wang Y, Gou W, Lu Q, Peng J, Lu S. Role of mesenchymal stem cells in bone regeneration and fracture repair: a review. Int Orthop. 2013;37(12):2491–8.
25. Wang EA, Rosen V, D'Alessandro JS, Bauduy M, Cordes P, Harada T, et al. Recombinant human bone morphogenetic protein induces bone formation. Proc Natl Acad Sci U S A. 1990;87(6):2220–4.
26. Reddi AH, Cunningham NS. Initiation and promotion of bone differentiation by bone morphogenetic proteins. J Bone Miner Res Off J Am Soc Bone Miner Res. 1993;8(Suppl 2):S499–502.
27. Rihn JA, Kirkpatrick K, Albert TJ. Graft options in posterolateral and posterior interbody lumbar fusion. Spine (Phila Pa 1976). 2010;35(17):1629–39.
28. Sykaras N, Opperman LA. Bone morphogenetic proteins (BMPs): how do they function and what can they offer the clinician? J Oral Sci. 2003;45(2):57–73.
29. Hoffmann A, Gross G. BMP signaling pathways in cartilage and bone formation. Crit Rev Eukaryot Gene Expr. 2001;11(1–3):23–45.
30. Fillingham Y, Jacobs J. Bone grafts and their substitutes. Bone Joint J. 2016;98-b(1 Suppl A):6–9.
31. Khan SN, Cammisa FP Jr, Sandhu HS, Diwan AD, Girardi FP, Lane JM. The biology of bone grafting. J Am Acad Orthop Surg. 2005;13(1):77–86.
32. McKee MD. Management of segmental bony defects: the role of osteoconductive orthobiologics. J Am Acad Orthop Surg. 2006;14(10):S163–S7.
33. Boden SD, Schimandle JH, Hutton WC. An experimental lumbar intertransverse process spinal fusion model. Radiographic, histologic, and biomechanical healing characteristics. Spine (Phila Pa 1976). 1995;20(4):412–20.
34. Oryan A, Monazzah S, Bigham-Sadegh A. Bone injury and fracture healing biology. Biomed Environ Sci. 2015;28(1):57–71.
35. Mountziaris PM, Mikos AG. Modulation of the inflammatory response for enhanced bone tissue regeneration. Tissue Eng Part B Rev. 2008;14(2):179–86.
36. Kwong FN, Harris MB. Recent developments in the biology of fracture repair. J Am Acad Orthop Surg. 2008;16(11):619–25.
37. Goldhahn J, Feron JM, Kanis J, Papapoulos S, Reginster JY, Rizzoli R, et al. Implications for fracture healing of current and new osteoporosis treatments: an ESCEO consensus paper. Calcif Tissue Int. 2012;90(5):343–53.
38. LaStayo PC, Winters KM, Hardy M. Fracture healing: bone healing, fracture management, and current concepts related to the hand. J Hand Ther.Off J Am Soc Hand Ther. 2003;16(2):81–93.
39. Claes LE, Heigele CA, Neidlinger-Wilke C, Kaspar D, Seidl W, Margevicius KJ, et al. Effects of mechanical factors on the fracture healing process. Clin Orthop Relat Res. 1998;355 Suppl S132–47.

40. Goodship AE, Kenwright J. The influence of induced micromovement upon the healing of experimental tibial fractures. J Bone Joint Surg. 1985;67(4):650–5.
41. Gaston M, Simpson A. Inhibition of fracture healing. J Bone Joint Surg Br. 2007;89(12):1553–60.
42. Pountos I, Georgouli T, Blokhuis TJ, Pape HC, Giannoudis PV. Pharmacological agents and impairment of fracture healing: what is the evidence? Injury. 2008;39(4):384–94.
43. Hsu EL, Sonn K, Kannan A, Bellary S, Yun C, Hashmi S, et al. Dioxin exposure impairs BMP-2-mediated spinal fusion in a rat arthrodesis model. J Bone Joint Surg Am. 2015;97(12):1003–10.
44. Geusens P, Emans PJ, de Jong JJ, van den Bergh J. NSAIDs and fracture healing. Curr Opin Rheumatol. 2013;25(4):524–31.
45. Einhorn TA, Boskey AL, Gundberg CM, Vigorita VJ, Devlin VJ, Beyer MM. The mineral and mechanical properties of bone in chronic experimental diabetes. J Orthop Res Off Publ Orthop ResSoc. 1988;6(3):317–23.
46. Jones CM, Eaton FB. Postoperative nutritional edema. Arch Surg. 1933;27(1):159–77.
47. Khuri SF, Daley J, Henderson W, Barbour G, Lowry P, Irvin G, et al. The National Veterans Administration Surgical Risk Study: risk adjustment for the comparative assessment of the quality of surgical care. J Am Coll Surg. 1995;180(5):519–31.
48. Mullen JL, Gertner MH, Buzby GP, Goodhart GL, Rosato EF. Implications of malnutrition in the surgical patient. Arch Surg. 1979;114(2):121–5.
49. Guo JJ, Yang H, Qian H, Huang L, Guo Z, Tang T. The effects of different nutritional measurements on delayed wound healing after hip fracture in the elderly. J Surg Res. 2010;159(1):503–8.
50. Jensen JE, Jensen TG, Smith TK, Johnston DA, Dudrick SJ. Nutrition in orthopaedic surgery. J Bone Joint Surg Am. 1982;64(9):1263–72.
51. Smith TK. Prevention of complications in orthopedic surgery secondary to nutritional depletion. Clin Orthop Relat Res. 1987;222:91–7.
52. Klein JD, Hey LA, Yu CS, Klein BB, Coufal FJ, Young EP, et al. Perioperative nutrition and postoperative complications in patients undergoing spinal surgery. Spine (Phila Pa 1976). 1996;21(22):2676–82.
53. Harris D, Haboubi N. Malnutrition screening in the elderly population. J R Soc Med. 2005;98(9):411–4.
54. Goldwasser P, Feldman J. Association of serum albumin and mortality risk. J Clin Epidemiol. 1997;50(6):693–703.
55. Adogwa O, Martin JR, Huang K, Verla T, Fatemi P, Thompson P, et al. Preoperative serum albumin level as a predictor of postoperative complication after spine fusion. Spine (Phila Pa 1976). 2014;39(18):1513–9.
56. Kamath AF, McAuliffe CL, Kosseim LM, Pio F, Hume E. Malnutrition in joint Arthroplasty: prospective study indicates risk of unplanned ICU admission. Arch Bone Jt Surg. 2016;4(2):128–31.
57. Gariballa SE, Sinclair AJ. Nutrition, ageing and ill health. Br J Nutr. 1998;80(1):7–23.
58. Nieuwenhuizen WF, Weenen H, Rigby P, Hetherington MM. Older adults and patients in need of nutritional support: review of current treatment options and factors influencing nutritional intake. Clin Nutr. 2010;29(2):160–9.
59. Norman K, Kirchner H, Freudenreich M, Ockenga J, Lochs H, Pirlich M. Three month intervention with protein and energy rich supplements improve muscle function and quality of life in malnourished patients with non-neoplastic gastrointestinal disease--a randomized controlled trial. Clin Nutr. 2008;27(1):48–56.
60. Holick MF. High prevalence of vitamin D inadequacy and implications for health. Mayo Clin Proc. 2006;81(3):353–73.
61. Holick MF. Vitamin D deficiency. N Engl J Med. 2007;357(3):266–81.
62. Bogunovic L, Kim AD, Beamer BS, Nguyen J, Lane JM. Hypovitaminosis D in patients scheduled to undergo orthopaedic surgery: a single-center analysis. J Bone Joint Surg Am. 2010;92(13):2300–4.
63. Ponnusamy KE, Iyer S, Gupta G, Khanna AJ. Instrumentation of the osteoporotic spine: biomechanical and clinical considerations. Spine J Off J N Am Spine Soc. 2011;11(1):54–63.
64. Dipaola CP, Bible JE, Biswas D, Dipaola M, Grauer JN, Rechtine GR. Survey of spine surgeons on attitudes regarding osteoporosis and osteomalacia screening and treatment for fractures, fusion surgery, and pseudoarthrosis. Spine J Off J N Am Spine Soc. 2009;9(7):537–44.
65. Kim TH, Lee BH, Lee HM, Lee SH, Park JO, Kim HS, et al. Prevalence of vitamin D deficiency in patients with lumbar spinal stenosis and its relationship with pain. Pain Physician. 2013;16(2):165–76.
66. Ravindra VM, Godzik J, Guan J, Dailey AT, Schmidt MH, Bisson EF, et al. Prevalence of vitamin D deficiency in patients undergoing elective spine surgery: a cross-sectional analysis. World Neurosurg. 2015;83(6):1114–9.
67. Erben RG, Bromm S, Stangassinger M. Therapeutic efficacy of 1alpha,25-dihydroxyvitamin D3 and calcium in osteopenic ovariectomized rats: evidence for a direct anabolic effect of 1alpha,25-dihydroxyvitamin D3 on bone. Endocrinology. 1998;139(10):4319–28.
68. Erben RG, Scutt AM, Miao D, Kollenkirchen U, Haberey M. Short-term treatment of rats with high dose 1,25-dihydroxyvitamin D3 stimulates bone formation and increases the number of osteoblast precursor cells in bone marrow. Endocrinology. 1997;138(11):4629–35.
69. Fu L, Tang T, Miao Y, Hao Y, Dai K. Effect of 1,25-dihydroxy vitamin D3 on fracture healing and bone remodeling in ovariectomized rat femora. Bone. 2009;44(5):893–8.

70. Omeroglu H, Omeroglu S, Korkusuz F, Ates Y. Effect of 25-OH-vitamin D on fracture healing in elderly rats. J Orthop Res Off Publ Orthop ResSoc. 1999;17(5):795.
71. Metzger MF, Kanim LE, Zhao L, Robinson ST, Delamarter RB. The relationship between serum vitamin D levels and spinal fusion success: a quantitative analysis. Spine (Phila Pa 1976). 2015;40(8):E458–68.
72. Rosen CJ. Clinical practice. Vitamin D insufficiency. N Engl J Med. 2011;364(3):248–54.
73. Rodriguez WJ, Gromelski J. Vitamin D status and spine surgery outcomes. ISRN Orthop. 2013;2013:12.
74. Middlekauff HR, Park J, Moheimani RS. Adverse effects of cigarette and noncigarette smoke exposure on the autonomic nervous system: mechanisms and implications for cardiovascular risk. J Am Coll Cardiol. 2014;64(16):1740–50.
75. Sasco AJ, Secretan MB, Straif K. Tobacco smoking and cancer: a brief review of recent epidemiological evidence. Lung Cancer. 2004;45(Suppl 2):S3–9.
76. Porter SE, Hanley EN Jr. The musculoskeletal effects of smoking. J Am Acad Orthop Surg. 2001;9(1):9–17.
77. Sloan A, Hussain I, Maqsood M, Eremin O, El-Sheemy M. The effects of smoking on fracture healing. Surgeon J R Coll Surg Edinb Irel. 2010;8(2):111–6.
78. Schmitz MA, Finnegan M, Natarajan R, Champine J. Effect of smoking on tibial shaft fracture healing. Clin Orthop Relat Res. 1999;365:184–200.
79. Martin CT, Gao Y, Duchman KR, Pugely AJ. The impact of current smoking and of smoking cessation on short-term morbidity risk after lumbar spine surgery. Spine. 2016;41(7):577–84.
80. Glassman SD, Anagnost SC, Parker A, Burke D, Johnson JR, Dimar JR. The effect of cigarette smoking and smoking cessation on spinal fusion. Spine (Phila Pa 1976). 2000;25(20):2608–15.
81. Castillo RC, Bosse MJ, MacKenzie EJ, Patterson BM, Group LS. Impact of smoking on fracture healing and risk of complications in limb-threatening open tibia fractures. J Orthop Trauma. 2005;19(3):151–7.
82. Zevin S, Gourlay SG, Benowitz NL. Clinical pharmacology of nicotine. Clin Dermatol. 1998;16(5):557–64.
83. Jorgensen LN, Kallehave F, Christensen E, Siana JE, Gottrup F. Less collagen production in smokers. Surgery. 1998;123(4):450–5.
84. Leow YH, Maibach HI. Cigarette smoking, cutaneous vasculature, and tissue oxygen. Clin Dermatol. 1998;16(5):579–84.
85. Bornmyr S, Svensson H. Thermography and laser-Doppler flowmetry for monitoring changes in finger skin blood flow upon cigarette smoking. Clin Physiol. 1991;11(2):135–41.
86. Syversen U, Nordsletten L, Falch JA, Madsen JE, Nilsen OG, Waldum HL. Effect of lifelong nicotine inhalation on bone mass and mechanical properties in female rat femurs. Calcif Tissue Int. 1999;65(3):246–9.
87. Rothem DE, Rothem L, Soudry M, Dahan A, Eliakim R. Nicotine modulates bone metabolism-associated gene expression in osteoblast cells. J Bone Miner Metab. 2009;27(5):555–61.
88. Holzer N, Braun KF, Ehnert S, Egana JT, Schenck TL, Buchholz A, et al. Green tea protects human osteoblasts from cigarette smoke-induced injury: possible clinical implication. Langenbeck's Arch Surg. 2012;397(3):467–74.
89. Jamsa T, Viluksela M, Tuomisto JT, Tuomisto J, Tuukkanen J. Effects of 2,3,7,8-tetrachlorodibenzo-p-dioxin on bone in two rat strains with different aryl hydrocarbon receptor structures. J Bone Miner Res. 2001;16(10):1812–20.
90. Moller AM, Villebro N, Pedersen T, Tonnesen H. Effect of preoperative smoking intervention on postoperative complications: a randomised clinical trial. Lancet. 2002;359(9301):114–7.
91. Jha S, Wang Z, Laucis N, Bhattacharyya T. Trends in media reports, oral bisphosphonate prescriptions, and hip fractures 1996-2012: an ecological analysis. J Bone Miner Res Off J Am Soc Bone Miner Res. 2015;30(12):2179–87.
92. van der Poest CE, Patka P, Vandormael K, Haarman H, Lips P. The effect of alendronate on bone mass after distal forearm fracture. J Bone Miner Res Off J Am Soc Bone Miner Res. 2000;15(3):586–93.
93. Watkins MP, Norris JY, Grimston SK, Zhang X, Phipps RJ, Ebetino FH, et al. Bisphosphonates improve trabecular bone mass and normalize cortical thickness in ovariectomized, osteoblast connexin43 deficient mice. Bone. 2012;51(4):787–94.
94. Schilcher J, Koeppen V, Aspenberg P, Michaëlsson K. Risk of atypical femoral fracture during and after bisphosphonate use. N Engl J Med. 2014;371(10):974–6.
95. Xue D, Li F, Chen G, Yan S, Pan Z. Do bisphosphonates affect bone healing? A meta-analysis of randomized controlled trials. J Orthop Surg Res. 2014;9:45.
96. Komatsubara S, Mori S, Mashiba T, Nonaka K, Seki A, Akiyama T, et al. Human parathyroid hormone (1-34) accelerates the fracture healing process of woven to lamellar bone replacement and new cortical shell formation in rat femora. Bone. 2005;36(4):678–87.
97. Andreassen TT, Willick GE, Morley P, Whitfield JF. Treatment with parathyroid hormone hPTH(1-34), hPTH(1-31), and monocyclic hPTH(1-31) enhances fracture strength and callus amount after withdrawal fracture strength and callus mechanical quality continue to increase. Calcif Tissue Int. 2004;74(4):351–6.

98. Babu S, Sandiford NA, Vrahas M. Use of Teriparatide to improve fracture healing: what is the evidence? World J Orthop. 2015;6(6):457–61.
99. Haddad JB, Obolensky AG, Shinnick P. The biologic effects and the therapeutic mechanism of action of electric and electromagnetic field stimulation on bone and cartilage: new findings and a review of earlier work. J Altern Complement Med. 2007;13(5):485–90.
100. Aaron RK, Boyan BD, Ciombor DM, Schwartz Z, Simon BJ. Stimulation of growth factor synthesis by electric and electromagnetic fields. Clin Orthop Relat Res. 2004;419:30–7.
101. Aleem IS, Aleem I, Evaniew N, Busse JW, Yaszemski M, Agarwal A, et al. Efficacy of electrical stimulators for bone healing: a meta-analysis of randomized sham-controlled trials. Sci Rep. 2016;6:31724.

Principles of Deformity Correction

36

Josiah N. Orina and Sigurd H. Berven

Introduction

Spinal deformity encompasses a broad spectrum of malalignments, including sagittal, coronal, and axial planes. Deformity of the spine may include segmental malalignments (olisthesis, lateral subluxation, and rotational subluxation), regional deformities such as scoliosis and kyphosis of the thoracic and lumbar regions, and global deformities with sagittal vertical axis malalignment and truncal shifts in the coronal plane. The impact of spinal deformity is determined most significantly by sagittal plane parameters [1]. Understanding the impact of malalignment on health status of patients is important in guiding an evidence-based approach to deformity correction. The purpose of this chapter is to describe the impact of deformity on health status and to detail principles and techniques for correction of spinal deformity.

Deformity of the spine is an important condition affecting the growing spine and a common condition in the aging spine. The burden of disease on population health is defined by consideration of the prevalence of disease within the population and the impact of the disease on health of the individual patient [2]. The Institute of Medicine has concluded that priorities for healthcare research and funding should be based upon the burden of disease. The high prevalence and impact of adult spinal deformity make an evidence-based approach to this condition an important healthcare priority. Deformity of the spine has a significant and measurable impact on health-related quality of life. Patients with symptomatic adult deformity report a health status preference for their condition that is significantly worse than other common medical conditions [3, 4]. With an aging population, spinal deformity presents a considerable health and financial challenge to our healthcare economy [5]. Appropriate management of the condition may encompass a spectrum of options including nonoperative care, limited decompression surgeries, limited fusion, and complex realignment of the spine [6]. The treatment strategy that is most appropriate for the individual patient requires consideration of symptoms, pathoanatomy, comorbidities, and patient preference. Appropriate care strategies maximize the expected benefits of care while limiting the risks and costs of care [7].

Patients seeking care for spinal deformity characteristically present with symptoms that may include back pain, radicular symptoms such as dermatomal pain, neurogenic claudication, weakness or numbness, functional decline, concern about appearance, and disability. Treatment is multidisciplinary and comprises nonoperative

J.N. Orina, MD • S.H. Berven, MD (✉)
Department of Orthopaedic Surgery,
University of California, San Francisco,
500 Parnassus Avenue, MU320W, San Francisco,
CA 94143-0728, USA
e-mail: josiah.orina@ucsf.edu; sigurd.berven@ucsf.edu

L.T. Holly, P.A. Anderson (eds.), *Essentials of Spinal Stabilization*,
DOI 10.1007/978-3-319-59713-3_36

and operative management strategies [8]. Nonoperative care utilizes analgesics, physical therapy, and injections to improve patient pain and function. Surgical treatment aims to improve health status by decompressing the neural elements, correcting the deformity, and stabilizing the spine. The last decade (2000–2010) has seen a rapid increase in the operative management of spinal deformity with a twofold increase in the number of surgeries performed for this condition [9]. The rate of rise of surgery in elderly patients is greater than the rate of rise in younger populations [10, 11]. Understanding the principles of deformity correction is important to guide an evidence-based approach to care that applies across the broad spectrum of clinical presentations, pathoanatomies, and demographics of patients with spinal deformity.

Goals of Deformity Correction

A fundamental principle in deformity correction is establishing appropriate goals of care. Goals of surgical correction of deformity include improvement of pain, function, appearance, and health status of the patient. Improvement in patient-reported health status (pain, function, self-esteem) is an important benchmark in assessing the effectiveness of surgical management [12–14]. Patient improvement can be quantified using a number of health-related quality of life metrics such as the Oswestry Disability Index (ODI), EuroQol five dimensions questionnaire (EQ-5D), and Short Form (36) Health Survey (SF-36) [15–17]. There is a moderate correlation between radiographic measures of deformity and health status. Specifically, Glassman et al. identified global sagittal alignment – the distance of the C7 plumb line from the posterior margin of the sacrum – to be the radiographic parameter most highly correlated with clinical health status in adult deformity [1]. Sagittal plane deformity is more strongly associated with impaired clinical health status than coronal plane deformity, but there are weak to moderate correlations of clinical health status with coronal plane malalignment. Subsequent research extended analysis to the lumbopelvic region, and Schwab et al. identified the mismatch of lumbar lordosis and pelvic incidence and pelvic retroversion as significant radiographic correlates with pain and disability [18, 19]. The correlation between radiographic measures of deformity and health status defines specific goals for surgical correction of deformity. In the young adult, the goal of surgical reconstruction of the spine is to correct global balance so that the C7 sagittal vertical axis (SVA) falls within 4 cm of the posterior aspect of the sacrum, the lumbar lordosis is within 10° of the pelvic incidence, and the pelvic tilt is less than 20° [18]. Figure 36.1 demonstrates the method for calculating SVA, lumbar lordosis, pelvic incidence, and pelvic tilt.

Indications and Patient Selection

The decision to perform surgical reconstruction on the patient with spinal deformity is based upon informed discussion between the patient and the spine surgeon. Understanding the expected benefits of surgery, with knowledge of potential risks and costs, is the basis of informed choice and appropriate care [20]. Indications for surgical correction of spinal deformity include pain and functional limitations that are unresponsive to nonoperative care, progression of deformity, neural deficits, and impairment of health status related to deformity. In the absence of progressive deformity or neural deficit, a nonoperative approach focused on improving pain and functionality may be an appropriate initial approach to care. Nonoperative approaches to deformity may encompass analgesics, exercise and physical therapy, physiatry, spinal epidural or facet injections, and orthotics. Unfortunately, despite the significant costs of nonoperative care, there is indeterminate evidence (levels 3 and 4) to support the efficacy of any specific form of nonoperative care [21, 22]. Studies have shown poorer outcomes in symptomatic deformity patients treated conservatively compared to patients treated surgically [23–25]. While bracing is an effective treatment in preventing progression in the skeletally immature spine [26],

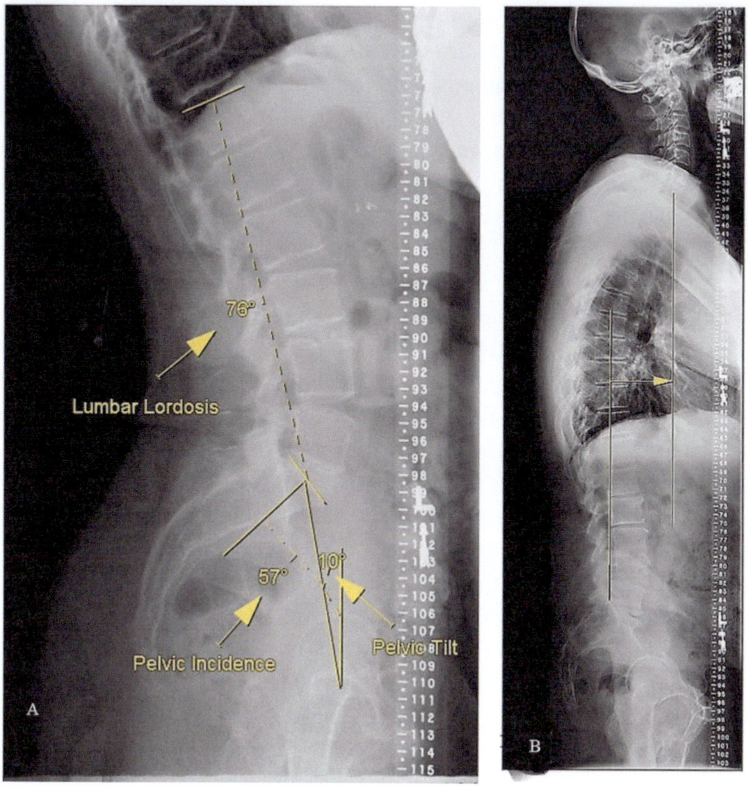

Fig. 36.1 Radiographic parameters important in treatment decisions for adult spinal deformity. (**a**) Lumbar lordosis is measured from the superior endplate of T12 to the superior endplate of S1. Pelvic incidence is the angle subtended by a line perpendicular to the midpoint of the superior endplate of S1 and a line from this midpoint to the center of the femoral heads. Pelvic tilt is the angle between a line from the midpoint of the superior endplate of S1 to the center of the femoral heads and a vertical line passing through the center of the femoral heads. (**b**) Sagittal vertical axis (SVA) is the distance between a plumb line from the center of C7 and the posterior-superior margin of the sacrum

bracing has not been shown to successfully slow progression of spinal deformity in the mature adult skeleton [27], and the authors do not recommend orthotics for this purpose. Orthotics in the adult with spinal deformity may be useful intermittently for pain relief and to enable function in patients with limitations related to pain with movement.

Patients with progressive deformity, symptomatic neural compromise, and pain and functional limitations that are unresponsive to nonoperative care are most appropriate for surgical treatment. The operative management of deformity in the adult with spinal deformity is characterized by significant variability. An appropriate approach to care requires a multidisciplinary team skilled in preoperative optimization of the patient's health status, intraoperative strategies to decompress the neural elements and restore alignment of the spine, and postoperative rehabilitation with a focus on early mobilization and function. Essential members of the team during preoperative optimization may include primary care providers, cardiologists, pulmonologists, endocrinologists, physiatrists, and social workers depending on the patient's comorbidities, disability, and social issues. Reversible comorbidities such as poor nutritional status, poor pulmonary and cardiac function, osteoporosis, obesity, and nicotine use should be addressed and treated prior to elective surgery [28–30]. Patients with osteoporosis (T-score of −2.5 or less) must undergo medical treatment to improve their bone quality prior to undergoing elective deformity surgery as this can reduce the risk of postoperative pseudarthrosis and instrumentation failure. These patients should be referred to an endocrinologist to consider initiation of teriparatide, an anabolic agent that stimulates osteoblastic activity and significantly improves bone mineral density [31]. While bisphosphonates could be considered, these are less efficacious than teriparatide in improving bone mineral density [32]. Additionally, animal studies have suggested that bisphosphonates may delay bone remodeling after fusion. The impact they have on fusion rates when used in the perioperative period in humans is unknown [33]. Those patients with low bone mass or osteopenia (T-score between −1.0 and −2.5) can be considered for nutritional supplementation with calcium and vitamin D. Preoperative optimization of the patient's health status with treatment of reversible medical comorbidities such as osteoporosis may limit complications of care.

Intraoperative Strategies

Surgical Techniques for Deformity Correction

Surgical techniques for deformity correction can be grouped into anterior, posterior, and combined approaches. The choice of surgical technique is influenced by the goals of surgery, patient comorbidities, and patient and surgeon preference. The observed variability in surgical approaches to deformity correction is a reflection of the broad spectrum of goals and preferences that guide care as well as the heterogeneity in patient presentation.

Anterior Surgery

Indications for Anterior Spine Surgery

The anterior approach to the spine is a powerful technique for mobilization of the spinal column and for correction of spinal deformity. Removal of the intervertebral disc, annulus, and anterior longitudinal ligament permits excellent mobilization of the motion segment in lateral bending and rotation. Complete discectomy including endplate preparation creates an excellent environment for bone healing. The advantages of the anterior approach include mobilization of deformity and interbody healing. Anterior surgery has several applications in spinal deformity.

Anterior instrumented surgery for treatment of spinal deformity was first described by Hodgson and Stock for the management of kyphosis in Pott's disease and paraplegia. Allen Dwyer introduced the anterior approach to the spine for the management of scoliosis in 1964 and published his experience in 1969 [34]. The original technique involved a two-stage operation. The first stage consisted of a posterior release with resection of ligaments and facet capsules along the concavity of the deformity. This was followed by an anterior operation as a second stage in which discectomies were performed along the deformity followed by placement of screws into the lateral vertebral bodies along the convexity. The screws were then compressed using cables along the convexity to correct the curve [35, 36]. While arthrodesis rates were high, the Dwyer approach was associated with late curve progression, increased thoracic kyphosis, and inadequate vertebral body derotation [36]. More rigid anterior fixation systems and the use of interbody implants have improved the ability to preserve sagittal alignment and maintenance of correction in anterior spine approaches.

In deformity correction surgery, the anterior approach to the spine can be useful in the thoracic and thoracolumbar spine. Anterior surgery may permit minimization of the number of levels fused, allowing shorter constructs with preservation of motion segments [37, 38]. Limitations can include pseudarthrosis in the thoracic spine and kyphotic decompensation in the lumbar spine. Deviren and colleagues reviewed outcomes in 15 adult and 15 adolescent patients with scoliosis treated with anterior instrumentation and reported 67% curve correction in adults and 80% curve correction in adolescents. All patients achieved solid fusion, and there were no cases of kyphotic decompensation or

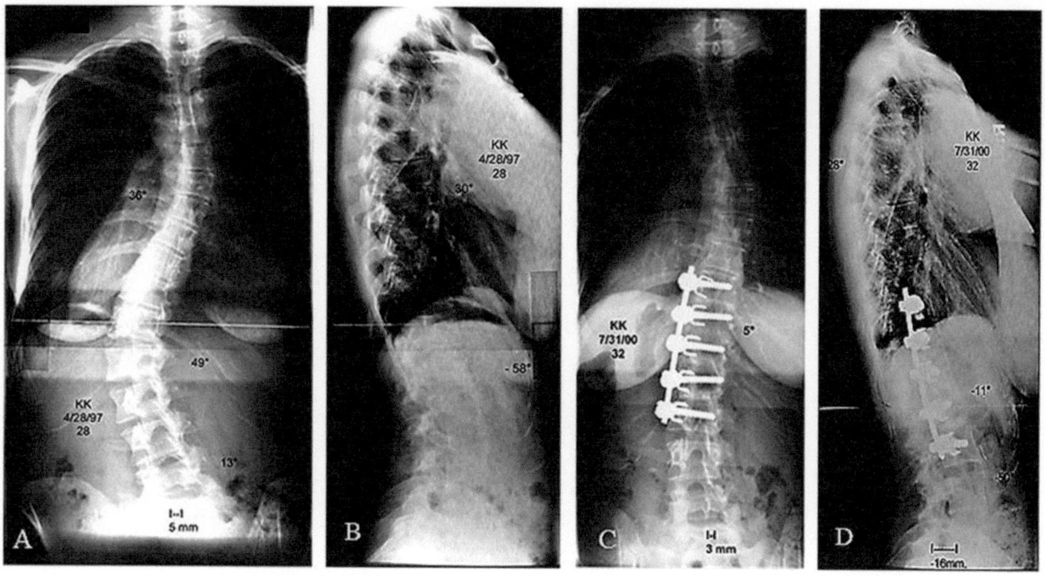

Fig. 36.2 A 32-year-old female with Lenke 5C deformity and progressive thoracolumbar curvature associated with pain. Patient underwent T10–L2 single rod anterior fusion. (**a**) Preoperative anteroposterior (AP) scoliosis X-rays. (**b**) Preoperative lateral scoliosis X-rays. (**c**) Postoperative AP scoliosis X-rays. (**d**) Postoperative lateral scoliosis X-rays

loss of lumbar lordosis [38]. Figure 36.2 is a single rod anterior fusion for a Lenke 5C deformity.

Anterior surgery can also be useful in fixed multiplanar adult deformity for release and mobilization of rigid spinal deformity and improvement of sagittal and coronal balance. The anterior approach can improve the efficacy of arthrodesis by involving the large surface of the interbody space in the fusion area and by capitalizing on a biomechanical environment of compression which promotes bone fusion. Indications for combined anterior and posterior surgery include planned fusion across the lumbosacral junction (L5–S1), post-laminectomy deformity, osteoporosis, lumbar pseudarthrosis, and large coronal deformities/imbalance (structural curves greater than 60° and coronal imbalance greater than 5 cm). Long posterior-only fusions across the lumbosacral junction have a high rate of pseudarthrosis, and the addition of anterior supplementation has been shown to improve fusion rates [39, 40]. Figure 36.3 is an example of a patient with osteoporosis and progressive post-laminectomy deformity. A posterior-only revision approach would have been compromised in healing due to absent posterior elements for interlaminar fusion.

Anterior surgery is a powerful tool for increasing segmental lumbar lordosis, particularly in patients with lumbar hypolordosis and a high pelvic incidence – lumbar lordosis mismatch. Studies demonstrate that approximately 70% of the total segmental lumbar lordosis comes from L4 to S1 vertebral segments, and nearly 50% of total segmental lumbar lordosis comes from the L5 to S1 segment [41, 42]. Total segmental lumbar lordosis also correlates strongly with spinal sagittal balance [41]. In patients with hypolordotic deformity and significant sagittal plane imbalance, sagittal alignment can be improved by restoring lumbar lordosis via L4–S1 anterior lumbar interbody fusion (ALIF). Hsieh and colleagues reviewed a series of 32 patients treated with ALIF and 26 patients treated with transforaminal lumbar interbody fusion (TLIF) and found that ALIF was superior to TLIF in improving lumbar lordosis [43]. ALIF resulted in a 6° improvement in lumbar lordosis whereas TLIF actually led to a 2° decrease in lumbar lordosis.

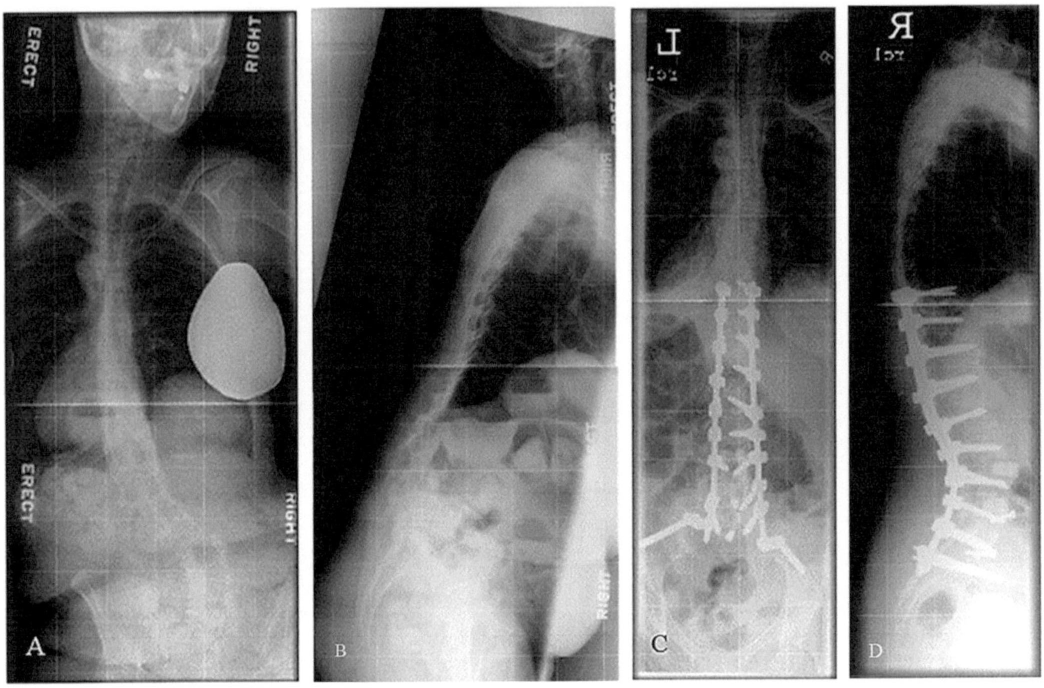

Fig. 36.3 A 68-year-old female with osteoporosis (T-score = −2.8) and three prior laminectomies for neurogenic claudication. Patient developed post-laminectomy deformity with progressive sagittal and coronal plane malalignment. The surgical approach was a combined anterior fusion with structural allograft at L3–S1 and a posterior instrumented fusion at T10–S1. A posterior-only revision approach would have been compromised in bony healing due to absent posterior elements for interlaminar fusion. (**a**) Preoperative AP scoliosis X-rays. (**b**) Preoperative lateral scoliosis X-rays. (**c**) Postoperative AP scoliosis X-rays. (**d**) Postoperative lateral scoliosis X-rays

Patients with major thoracolumbar or lumbar coronal curves often have a compensatory fractional curve at the lumbosacral junction. This compensatory curve can be quite rigid in the region of L4–5 and L5–S1 and may have a significant impact on coronal and sagittal alignment of the spine. Additionally, the proximal end vertebra of this lumbosacral fractional curve can be significantly tilted. Attempting to correct the major thoracolumbar/lumbar scoliotic curve without also addressing the fractional curve can result in suboptimal coronal correction or even worsening of coronal balance postoperatively. A balanced correction of the major thoracolumbar deformity and the fractional curve is an important goal in adult deformity correction. Correcting the stiff fractional curve can be accomplished by horizontalizing the tilted proximal end vertebra via ALIFs at L4–S1. Because the ALIF procedure involves removing the anterior longitudinal ligament and the concave annulus, the surgeon may apply distractive forces across the disc space to horizontalize and derotate the tilted proximal end vertebrate. In contrast, TLIFs do not involve sectioning of the anterior longitudinal ligament which can result in less correction of a stiff fractional curve than can be achieved with the ALIF. Figure 36.4 is an example of a 52-year-old female with progressive lumbar kyphosis and severe lumbosacral pain. Her trunk shift is ipsilateral to the concavity of the fractional lumbosacral curve. Inadequate correction of L4–S1 compared with the major curve from T11 to L4 may have resulted in exacerbation of coronal plane deformity. An anterior approach to the spine at L3–S1 facilitated correction of lumbar lordosis and permitted correction of the deformity from T11 to L4 from a posterior approach.

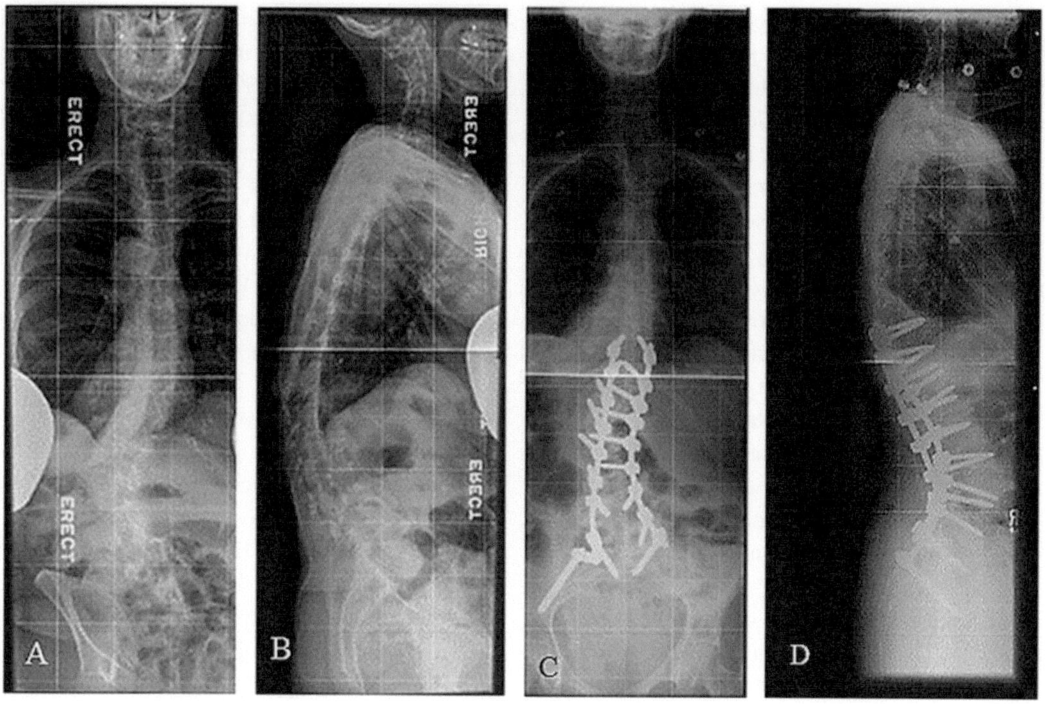

Fig. 36.4 52-year-old female with lumbar hypolordosis and a T11–L4 levoscoliotic major curve. She presented with progressive deformity and a rigid fractional lumbosacral compensatory curve from L4 to S1. Her trunk shift is ipsilateral to the concavity of the fractional curve. Correction of the major curve from T11 to L4 without adequate correction of the fractional curve from L4 to S1 may have resulted in exacerbation of the coronal plane deformity. An anterior approach to the spine at L3–S1 facilitated both restoration of the lumbar lordosis and reduction of the fractional curve. This permitted correction of the deformity from T11 to L4 from a posterior approach without precipitating further coronal imbalance. (**a**) Preoperative AP scoliosis X-rays. (**b**) Preoperative lateral scoliosis X-rays. (**c**) Postoperative AP scoliosis X-rays. Patient underwent L3–S1 anterior lumbar interbody fusion followed by T10 to pelvis posterior instrumented fusion. (**d**) Postoperative lateral scoliosis X-rays

Limitations of Anterior Surgery

While anterior surgery – especially when combined with posterior surgery – has been shown to have good clinical outcomes in spinal deformity cases, it has been associated with significant perioperative morbidity. Any anterior approach through the chest wall and into the pleural space can lead to decline in pulmonary function. Graham and colleagues reported the pulmonary function tests of 51 patients with scoliosis treated with an anterior procedure (thoracotomy, thoracoplasty, and minimally invasive thoracoplasty). The authors found a significant decline in postoperative pulmonary function test values at the 3-month mark compared to preoperative values [44]. Vascular complications can also occur, and control of the great vessels, segmental vessels, and recurrent iliolumbar vein is vital to the safety of the anterior approach. Avulsions of great vessels or venous injury can be life threatening.

Neural injury can result from compromise of the segmental vascular supply to the spinal cord secondary to vessel ligation. Direct nerve trauma can also result from retraction and cauterization at the neural foramen and within the psoas muscle. The surgeon should be keenly aware of risk factors for neural injury and paraplegia during the anterior approach for spinal deformity correction such as intraoperative hypotension, kyphosis, preoperative neural deficits, prior ligation of contralateral vessels, and congenital deformity.

Intraoperative neuromonitoring is a valuable adjunct as motor evoked potentials and somatosensory evoked potentials can signal early changes in spinal cord function. Electromyography and motor evoked potentials are also useful in detecting injury to peripheral nerves.

Anterior surgery may also result in complications related to genitourinary injury. Identification of the ureter and retraction of the ureter with the peritoneum can minimize risk of ureteral injury during anterior approach to the lumbar spine. Preoperative ureteral stent placement may be useful in revision surgery. Retrograde ejaculation is a well-reported complication of anterior lumbar surgery in men and is due to thermal injury or direct injury to the autonomic fibers of the superior hypogastric plexus supplying the internal vesicular sphincter [45].

In addition to the complications of the approach, anterior surgery often requires staged procedures. This increases the cost of care, recovery time, and length of hospitalization, all of which consume more healthcare resources. Therefore, the use of anterior surgery should offer an incremental benefit over a posterior-only approach to add value as a strategy for care.

Specific Surgical Approaches to the Anterior Spine

The anterior spine can be accessed via different approaches depending on the location of the spinal pathology. The transthoracic approach provides an anterolateral corridor that allows spine access from T5 to L2. Access above T5 is limited by the scapula and is more effective using a transsternal approach. Access between T12 and L2 requires a thoracolumbar approach with release of the diaphragm from the chest wall. The patient is placed in the lateral position, and careful attention is given to protecting the axillary region, eyes, and arms. The incision is made along the axis of a rib 1–2 segments above the level of the uppermost disc to be excised. In kyphosis, the incision may be placed at the level of the upper disc to be excised. In the setting of coronal deformity, access to the spine is more direct when approaching from the convex side of the deformity. Ligation of segmental vessels may compromise segmental vascular supply to the spinal cord. This is an important consideration in the setting of kyphotic deformity, previous anterior surgery, and at the watershed levels (T8–L1).

The thoracoabdominal approach permits access to the spine from T8 to the sacrum. The thoracolumbar approach requires release of the diaphragm from the chest wall and permits continuity in the exposure of the thoracic and lumbar spine. The incision of the diaphragm may begin at the costochondral junction anteriorly or from the costovertebral junction posteriorly. Instrumentation using vertebral body screws is difficult below the level of L4 due to the position of the iliac crest. However, interbody instrumentation can be extended to the pelvis. It is important to identify and mobilize the ipsilateral ureter during this approach. Placement of a ureteral stent preoperatively may be useful in revision surgeries. Vascular considerations include identification and control of the recurrent iliolumbar vein and the L5 segmental vessel. Preoperative assessment of aortic calcification is also useful to avoid plaque rupture and embolization. Abdominal wall pseudohernia after surgery is common and can be minimized by direct visualization of abdominal muscle innervation during exposure. A direct hernia is prevented by meticulous closure of the transversus abdominis and internal oblique, followed by separate closure of the external oblique layer and by limiting the distal extent of the incision.

The paramedian approach gives the spine surgeon access from the L2–3 interspace to S1. A transverse incision permits access to one or two motion segments, whereas a longitudinal incision may be used for access from L2 to the sacrum. The patient is positioned supine, and a lumbosacral roll is useful in increasing lordosis. The L5–S1 level is accessed between the common iliac arteries as they bifurcate from the aorta. L4–5 is commonly exposed lateral to the common iliac vessels.

The direct lateral approach to the anterior column permits access to all disc spaces above L5–S1. In the lumbar spine, the approach may be transpsoas or antepsoas. The direct lateral approach significantly reduces the length of the incision and muscle dissection compared to a traditional thoracoabdominal exposure. The anatomy of the transpsoas exposure is variable, and the position of the lumbar plexus may preclude access to the disc spaces, especially at L4–L5. Spinal deformity significantly reduces the safe zone for a direct lateral approach to the lumbar spine [46]. Intraoperative nerve monitoring is useful in identifying motor nerves, but direct visualization is important to minimize risk to sensory nerves including the ilioinguinal and the genitofemoral nerves. Nerve injury may be due to direct injury or to retraction against a fixed transverse process.

Posterior-Based Osteotomies

Posterior-based osteotomies encompass a spectrum of techniques that enable effective correction of mobile and rigid spinal deformities. Posterior-based osteotomies may be used in combination with an anterior approach in severe sagittal or coronal deformities. The spectrum of posterior-based osteotomies can be divided into six different grades, as described by Schwab and colleagues [47], or six different types as described by Berven and Bradford [48]. The six types are a continuum with each type building upon the bony removal performed in its predecessor. Because the bone resection is sequential, from facet resection to transpedicular resections and corpectomies, the surgeon may often find that facet resections alone yield adequate correction or progress to a three-column osteotomy if the spine is more rigid. Figure 36.5 illustrates the spectrum of osteotomies from posterior-based facet resections to vertebral column resection.

Types 1 and 2 (Complete Facet Resection)

Type 1 and 2 osteotomies both involve a complete facetectomy bilaterally at a given level. They involve resection of the posterior elements from the mid pars above to the pedicle below, including removal of the interspinous ligaments and ligamentum flavum. The osteotomy is then closed by compressing posteriorly. Ponte (type 1) and Smith-Petersen (type 2) osteotomies are commonly used terms that fall under this category. There are important distinctions between the two. The Ponte osteotomy as originally described is characterized by deformity correction through a non-fused disc space anteriorly. The osteotomy uses an axis of rotation at the center of the vertebra, with distraction of the anterior longitudinal ligament and posterior compression to realign a mobile spine [49]. The elasticity of the anterior longitudinal ligament determines the amount of correction that may be achieved at a single segment. In contrast, Smith-Petersen osteotomy is performed at a level with a fused disc space, and correction is gained by osteoclasis of the anterior column with a center axis of rotation at the posterior longitudinal ligament and anterior column opening [50]. Type 1 osteotomies can achieve on average 5–10° of correction per level in a mobile disc level; type 2 osteotomies may yield up to 30° in patients with a Smith-Peterson approach [49, 51].

Types 3 and 4 (Pedicle Subtraction Osteotomies)

Type 3 and 4 osteotomies build upon the posterior element resection performed in type 2 to include resection of the pedicles bilaterally at a given level with an intraosseous partial resection of the vertebral body. Heinig described the eggshell osteotomy in which the surgeon decancellates the vertebral body from a transpedicular approach and then achieves correction of the spine with a controlled fracture of the decancellated vertebral body [52]. Thomasen described the transpedicular wedge resection osteotomy in which correction of deformity is gained through resection of a wedge of pedicle and vertebral body, followed by closure of the wedge. The posterior and middle portions of the index vertebral body are resected while the anterior vertebral cortex is left intact. The fulcrum for closure of the osteotomy is the superior one-third of the vertebral body. This results in shortening of the posterior column without lengthening of the anterior column [53]. Type 3 and 4 osteotomies are best applied in the lumbar spine for rigid deformities with fused disc

Fig. 36.5 Spectrum of posterior-based osteotomies. Reprinted with permission from Berven S, Mummaneni P. Lumbar pedicle subtraction osteotomy. In: Zdeblick T, Albert T, editors. The Spine. Master Techniques in Orthopaedic Surgery. Third ed. Philadelphia: Lippincott Williams & Wilkins; 2014. p. 258

TABLE 20-1 Spectrum of Posterior-Based Osteotomies

Type	Description	Diagram	Reference
1	Resection of posterior elements from mid-pars above to pedicle below with realignment of the spine through hinging through a mobile disc anteriorly	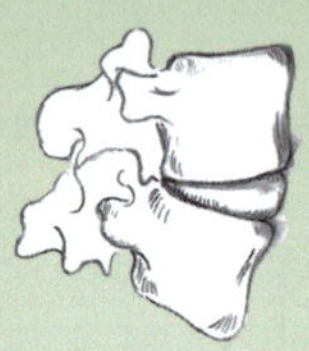	Ponte
2	Resection of posterior elements from mid-pars above to pedicle below with realignment of the spine through hinging hinging through the anterior column of the spine which is ankylosed. The opening involves osteoclasis rather than movement through a mobile intervertebral disc	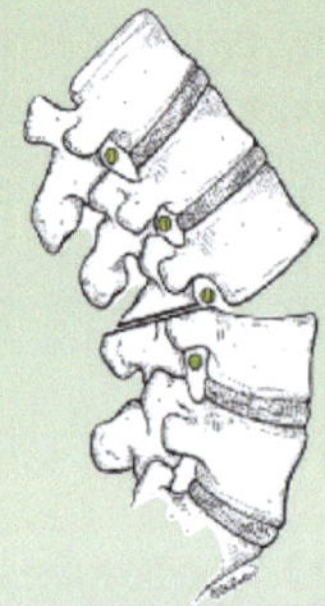	Smith-Peterson
3	Posterior-based transpedicular decancellation of the vertebral body with realignment through controlled fracture of the anterior column	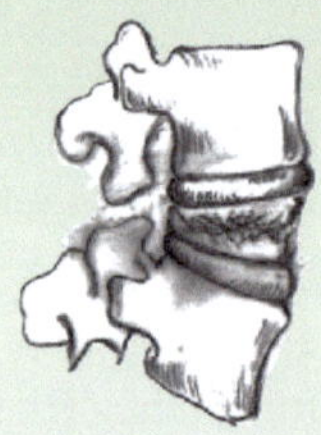	Heinig
4	Posterior-based intraosseous wedge resection of the vertebral body with realignment through osteoclasis of the proximal third of the anterior vertebral body	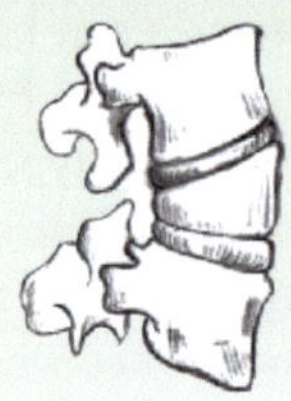	Thomasen
5	Posterior-based wedge resection with extension of the osteotomy into the supraadjacent disc and realignment hinging on the anterior column at the intervertebral space	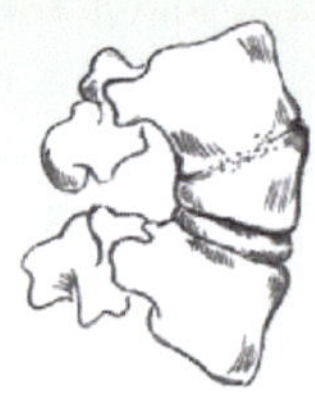	Modified Thomasen
6	Posterior-based vertebral column resection including one or more vertebra with adjacent discs	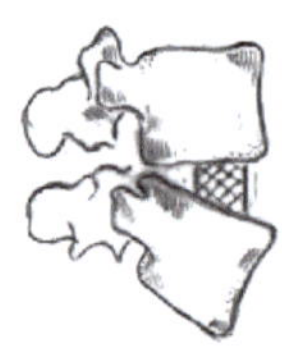	Suk

spaces. Although it can also be performed in the cervical or thoracic spine, the amount of sagittal correction achieved from this technique is greatest the more distally in the spine it is done based upon the distance of the osteotomy from C7 (i.e., an L4 pedicle subtraction osteotomy leads to greater sagittal correction than an L1 pedicle subtraction osteotomy). Pedicle subtraction osteotomy can achieve between 25 and 35° of correction depending on the location in the spine at which it is performed [54].

Type 5 (Extended Pedicle Subtraction Osteotomy)

Type 5 involves a pedicle subtraction osteotomy with wider wedge resection of the vertebral body, its superior endplate, and resection of the supra-adjacent disc. An interbody spacer can be placed into the supra-adjacent disc space to facilitate arthrodesis and prevent shortening of the anterior and posterior spinal column. The extended pedicle subtraction osteotomy is useful to gain a circumferential fusion at the level of a three-column osteotomy with an open disc above the osteotomy. Figure 36.6 demonstrates the stages of an extended PSO. The patient is a 62-year-old male with flatback deformity and sagittal plane malalignment following a prior L2-5 posterior instrumented fusion with TLIFs. Symptoms consisted of lower back pain and inability to stand upright. An L5-S1 ALIF followed by an extended PSO at L2 resulted in excellent correction of his sagittal plane deformity.

Type 6 (Vertebral Column Resection)

The type 6 osteotomy involves complete resection of one or more vertebral bodies and the adjacent superior and inferior intervertebral discs. Bradford described the vertebral column resection from a combined anterior and posterior approach [55], and Suk described the posterior-based vertebral column resection [56]. This is a complex osteotomy that is reserved for rigid multiplanar deformities and deformities involving translation of the trunk. In the thoracic spine, the osteotomy requires the surgeon to perform rib resection with a lateral extracavitary exposure of the vertebral body, often with sacrifice of exiting thoracic nerve roots and segmental vessels. The vertebral column resection results in circumferential disconnection of the spine, leading to shortening of the anterior and posterior columns. An anterior cage may be placed to prevent severe shortening of the anterior column and to serve as a fulcrum for osteotomy closure.

Figure 36.7 demonstrates a type 6 vertebral column resection. The patient is a 62-year-old female with severe trunk translation above a prior fusion from L3 to S1. Traditional techniques of angular correction with segmental compression and distraction would be ineffective in correcting the deformity because compression of the convexity of the thoracolumbar curve would lead to increased trunk shift and compression of the convexity of the lumbosacral curve would increase shoulder asymmetry [54]. In cases with severe kyphosis and trunk shift, a vertebral column resection is most appropriate to facilitate translation of the trunk relative to the pelvis.

Limited Versus Extensive Surgery

The surgical approach to spinal deformity is characterized by significant variability between providers. Surgical correction of spinal deformity may involve extensive surgeries with combined anterior and posterior approaches to the spine and complex osteotomies or more limited approaches to the deformity including decompression alone or decompression with a limited fusion. The appropriate approach to spinal deformity is the approach which maximizes benefit while limiting risk and costs of care [7]. Informed choice regarding an appropriate surgical approach requires consideration of the goals of care, patient preference, and surgeon preference [6]. A decompression alone may be appropriate in patients with primarily radicular pain and stable deformity, without progression of curvature and absent global sagittal or coronal malalignment [20]. A decompression with a limited fusion may be appropriate for patients with focal pain or neural compression that may require realignment of limited segments of the spine. Figure 36.8 illustrates a case of a 32-year-old female with adult idiopathic scoliosis. Her deformity has not progressed in the past 8 years, and she is well aligned in her global sagittal and coronal measures. She presents with limited left L4 and L5 radicular pain and significant lumbosacral pain. A limited decompression and fusion permit maintenance of mobility of the thoracolumbar spine and limited morbidity of the surgical approach. More extensive approaches to deformity including combined anterior and posterior approaches and multilevel

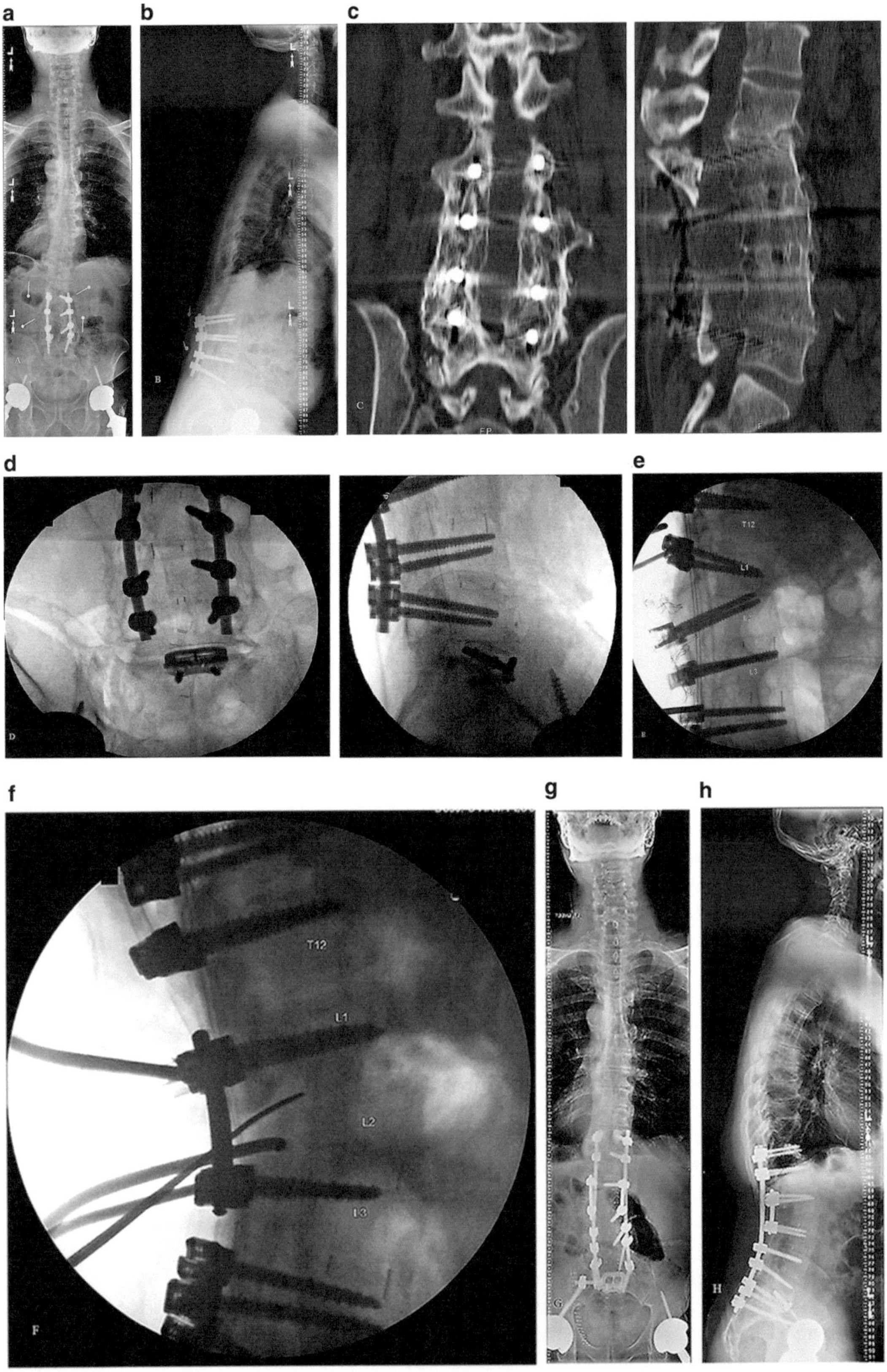

Fig. 36.6 62-year-old male with flatback deformity and sagittal malalignment following prior L2-5 posterior fusion with transforaminal lumbar interbody fusion and inferior L2 to superior L5 laminectomies. (**a**) Preoperative AP

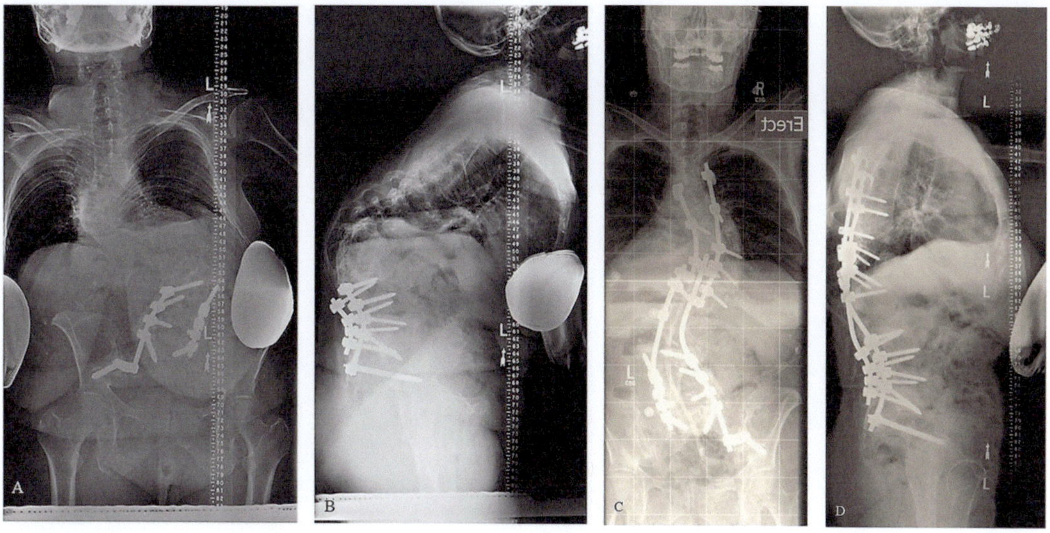

Fig. 36.7 A 62-year-old female with rightward trunk shift and progressive kyphosis above a prior limited L3–S1 spine fusion. A type 6 osteotomy with vertebral column resection at L1 and L2 faciliated translation of the trunk (without the loss of shoulder balance that may have occurred from an angular correction) and significant sagittal plane correction. (**a**) Preoperative AP scoliosis X-rays. (**b**) Preoperative lateral scoliosis X-rays. (**c**) Postoperative AP scoliosis X-rays. (**d**) Postoperative lateral scoliosis X-rays

fusions may be most appropriate for patients in good health with severe symptomatic deformity that is progressive and involves global sagittal or coronal malalignment [20].

Technical Pearls

- Establishing the goals of surgery is a foundational principle in deformity correction. There is a correlation between radiographic measures of deformity and health-related quality of life that can define specific goals for surgical reconstruction of the spine: SVA less than 4 cm, lumbar lordosis within 10° of the pelvic incidence, and pelvic tilt less than 20°.
- Ensure each patient has undergone careful preoperative optimization with a multidisciplinary team prior to elective deformity surgery. Identify and treat reversible medical comorbidities, consider physiatry for deconditioning and obesity, address nicotine cessation, and

Fig. 36.6 (continued) scoliosis X-rays. (**b**) Preoperative lateral scoliosis X-rays. He has an SVA of + 20 cm. Pelvic incidence is 80 degrees and lumbar lordosis is 30 degrees, with a mismatch of 50 degrees between the two parameters. Pelvic tilt is 39 degrees indicating significant pelvic retroversion to compensate for the sagittal plane deformity. (**c**) Preoperative CT lumbar spine. He has a solid arthrodesis from L2 to L5. (**d**) Stage 1. AP and lateral intraoperative fluoroscopy. He was treated in a staged fashion with an L5-S1 ALIF to increase segmental lumbar lordosis and improve efficacy of arthrodesis across the lumbosacral junction. (**e**) Stage 2. Lateral intraoperative fluoroscopy prior to the L2 extended PSO. Notice the kyphosis between the L1 and L3 pedicle screws. (**f**) Stage 2. Lateral intraoperative fluoroscopy during the L2 extended PSO. The posterior elements were resected from the mid-pars of L1 to the top of the pedicle of L3, thus isolating the L2 pedicles bilaterally. The L2 pedicles were subsequently removed. A wedge of the L2 vertebral body was resected with extension into the L1-2 disk space. The osteotomy was then closed. Notice the orientation between the L1 and L3 pedicles is now lordotic and that a wedge of bone has been resected from the L2 vertebral body. The Penfield No. 2 indicates bone-on-bone contact between the inferior endplate of L1 and the wedged L2 vertebral body. (**g**) Postoperative AP scoliosis X-rays. (**h**) Postoperative lateral scoliosis X-rays. SVA and lumbar lordosis are much improved

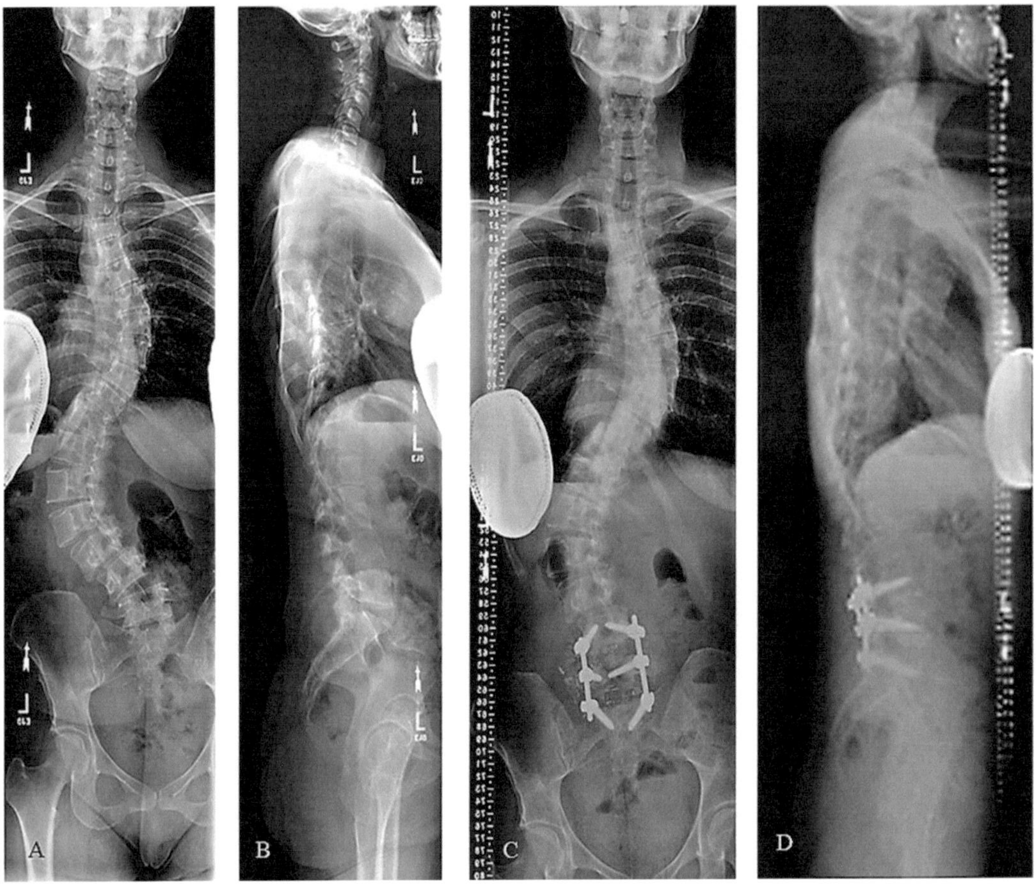

Fig. 36.8 A 32-year-old female with adult idiopathic scoliosis. She presents with limited L4 and L5 radicular pain and significant lumbosacral pain. (**a**) Preoperative AP scoliosis X-rays. Her deformity has not progressed in the past 8 years. She is well aligned globally in the coronal plane. (**b**) Preoperative lateral scoliosis X-rays. She is also well aligned globally in the sagittal plane. (**c**) Postoperative AP scoliosis X-rays. She was treated with a limited fusion from L4 to S1 with the goal of alleviating her radicular pain. (**d**) Postoperative lateral scoliosis X-rays

optimize bone mineral density to minimize the risks of complications of care.

- Anterior surgery is a powerful tool to restore lumbar lordosis in patients with flat back deformity and significant pelvic incidence – lumbar lordosis mismatch. Anterior surgery is also an effective approach to correct a rigid fractional lumbosacral compensatory curve and increase arthrodesis rates in patients at risk for pseudarthrosis.
- Posterior-based osteotomies may be used in combination with an anterior approach in severe sagittal or coronal deformities. Type 5 and 6 osteotomies may lead to severe shortening of the anterior and posterior spinal columns. Place an anterior cage to mitigate shortening and serve as a fulcrum for osteotomy closure.
- Perform less extensive surgery in patients with stable spinal deformity, normal global balance, and symptoms primarily consisting of radiculopathy. Less extensive surgery may include decompression alone or limited decompression and fusion.

Complications and Strategies for Avoidance

Surgical correction of adult spinal deformity is associated with a high risk of perioperative and postoperative complications [14, 57, 58]. A key principle in deformity correction is ensuring that both the surgeon and the patient have a thorough understanding of potential complications so an informed decision can be made by both parties regarding surgical intervention and strategy. Recognition of potential complications encourages the surgeon to anticipate adverse events and exercise prudence in selecting the techniques, tools, and implants that best achieve the goals of deformity correction while minimizing the risk of harm to the patient. In addition to the complications specific to anterior surgery discussed previously, perioperative complications may include neurological injury and causes of revision surgery such as pseudarthrosis and proximal junctional kyphosis (PJK).

Neurological injury can occur intraoperatively from direct trauma to the neural elements by instrumentation or surrounding bony and soft tissue structures during deformity correction. Deformity correction can also lead to neural injury from elongation of the spinal cord or a compromise of its vascular supply. The incidence of neurological injury depends on many factors including surgical approach, use of osteotomies, presence of kyphosis, and revision surgery [59]. Sansur et al. reviewed the Scoliosis Research Society Morbidity and Mortality Database and identified 4980 cases of patients with adult scoliosis treated between 2004 and 2007. Ninety patients experienced a neurological complication (1.8%). Of these 90 patients, 71 (78.9%) patients experienced a nerve root injury, 11 (12.2%) patients had an incomplete spinal cord injury, 1 (1.1%) patient had a complete spinal cord injury, and 5 (5.6%) patients had cauda equina syndrome [60]. Lenke et al. reported a much higher rate of motor deficits in patients with complex three-column osteotomies, with measurable deficits in lower extremity motor scores in 22.2% of patients after surgery [61].

Intraoperative spinal cord and nerve root monitoring is appropriate for use in complex spinal realignment surgery. Somatosensory evoked potentials, motor evoked potentials, and electromyography are valuable adjuncts for early detection of neurological injury and rapid treatment of reversible causes. Motor evoked potentials provide direct monitoring of the corticospinal tracts and are the most sensitive neuromonitoring modality for detecting spinal cord injury. If any changes in neuromonitoring occur, the intraoperative Stagnara wake-up test can be performed to directly examine the patient's neurological function.

Pseudarthrosis and proximal junctional kyphosis are complications that are common sources of revision surgery. Kim et al. retrospectively reviewed 144 patients with adult spinal deformity undergoing long fusions to the sacrum and reported a pseudarthrosis rate of 24% [62]. Similarly, Dickson et al. retrospectively reviewed 171 patients undergoing lumbar pedicle subtraction osteotomy and found a pseudarthrosis rate of 10.5% [63]. In the authors' practice, strategies to avoid pseudarthrosis in adult spinal deformity include consideration and modification of patient factors (obesity, nicotine use, osteoporosis), meticulous preparation of the fusion surface, and use of recombinant human bone morphogenetic protein (rhBMP) for bone grafting. Studies have shown the use of rhBMP to be associated with significantly lower rates of pseudarthrosis compared to use of iliac crest bone graft [64]. Complications reported in the literature to be associated with rhBMP use include radiculopathy, seroma, and heterotopic ossification as well as possible tumorigenicity [64]. Thus, the surgeon should carefully balance these risks and benefits when considering its use.

Proximal junctional kyphosis is defined as a postoperative proximal junctional Cobb angle greater than or equal to 10° between the inferior endplate of the uppermost instrumented vertebra and the superior endplate of the two vertebrae supra-adjacent and an increase in the proximal junctional Cobb angle greater than or equal to 10° from preoperatively. The reported incidence varies widely, from 10 to 40% [65, 66]. Risk factors include the proximal instrumented level selected, combined anterior-posterior surgeries, correction of SVA greater than 5 cm, and osteoporosis [67, 68]. Strategies to prevent PJK include avoiding terminating a construct at a level that has 10 or greater degrees of proximal junctional kyphosis preoperatively. Additionally, the surgeon should avoid overcorrecting patients with significant sagittal plane deformity given the risk of PJK developing in patients with a change in SVA from preoperatively to postoperatively of greater than 5 cm. Future research may be aimed at designing techniques to reconstruct the posterior tension band at the proximal levels.

Conclusion

Spinal deformity has a significant and measurable impact on health-related quality of life. The principles of deformity correction are based upon defining appropriate goals of care including presenting symptoms, radiographic alignment goals, patient safety, and patient and physician preference. There is a broad spectrum of surgical options for deformity correction, and the presence of variability in surgical approaches is a clear indication of the absence of a uniform consensus regarding an evidence-based approach to care. Informed choice regarding a surgical approach to deformity in the adolescent and the adult requires information on the natural history of deformity progression, symptoms, patient comorbidities, and patient and surgeon preference. A dogmatic or monolithic approach to deformity correction is not appropriate, and the most appropriate approach to care is the one that maximizes patient benefit while minimizing the risks and costs of care.

References

1. Glassman SD, Berven S, Bridwell K, Horton W, Dimar JR. Correlation of radiographic parameters and clinical symptoms in adult scoliosis. Spine (Phila Pa 1976). 2005;30(6):682–8.
2. Institute of Medicine. Scientific opportunities and public needs: improving priority setting and public input at the NIH, National Institutes of Health priority steering committee. Washington, DC: National Academy Press; 1998. Available from: http://www.nap.edu. Accessed November 11, 2016.
3. Pellise F, Vila-Casademunt A, Ferrer M, Domingo-Sabat M, Bago J, Perez-Grueso FJ, et al. Impact on health related quality of life of adult spinal deformity (ASD) compared with other chronic conditions. Eur Spine J. 2015;24(1):3–11.
4. Schwab F, Dubey A, Gamez L, El Fegoun AB, Hwang K, Pagala M, et al. Adult scoliosis: prevalence, SF-36, and nutritional parameters in an elderly volunteer population. Spine (Phila Pa 1976). 2005;30(9):1082–5.
5. Waldrop R, Cheng J, Devin C, McGirt M, Fehlings M, Berven S. The burden of spinal disorders in the elderly. Neurosurgery. 2015;77(Suppl 4):S46–50.
6. Gussous Y, Than K, Mummaneni P, Smith J, Steinmetz M, Ohya J, et al. Appropriate use of limited interventions vs extensive surgery in the elderly patient with spinal disorders. Neurosurgery. 2015;77(Suppl 4):S142–63.
7. Fitch K. The RAND/UCLA appropriateness method user's manual. Santa Monica: RAND Corporation; 2001.
8. Berven S, Jain D, O'Neill C, Selinger A, Mummaneni P. Team approach: degenerative spinal deformity. J Bone Joint Surg Rev. 2017. [Epub ahead of print].
9. McCarthy I, O'Brien M, Ames C, Robinson C, Errico T, Polly DW Jr, et al. Incremental cost-effectiveness of adult spinal deformity surgery: observed quality-adjusted life years with surgery compared with predicted quality-adjusted life years without surgery. Neurosurg Focus. 2014;36(5):E3.
10. Sing D, Khanna R, Shaw J, Metz L, Burch S, Berven S. Increasing rates of surgical management of multilevel spinal curvature in elderly patients. Spine Deformity. 2016;4:365–72.
11. Rajaee SS, Bae HW, Kanim LE, Delamarter RB. Spinal fusion in the United States: analysis of trends from 1998 to 2008. Spine (Phila Pa 1976). 2012;37(1):67–76.
12. Li G, Passias P, Kozanek M, Fu E, Wang S, Xia Q, et al. Adult scoliosis in patients over sixty-five years of age: outcomes of operative versus nonoperative treatment at a minimum two-year follow-up. Spine (Phila Pa 1976). 2009;34(20):2165–70.
13. Smith JS, Shaffrey CI, Glassman SD, Berven SH, Schwab FJ, Hamill CL, et al. Risk-benefit assessment of surgery for adult scoliosis: an analysis based on patient age. Spine (Phila Pa 1976). 2011;36(10):817–24.
14. Bridwell KH, Glassman S, Horton W, Shaffrey C, Schwab F, Zebala LP, et al. Does treatment (nonoperative and operative) improve the two-year quality of life in patients with adult symptomatic lumbar scoliosis: a prospective multicenter evidence-based medicine study. Spine (Phila Pa 1976). 2009;34(20):2171–8.
15. Fairbank JC, Pynsent PB. The Oswestry disability index. Spine (Phila Pa 1976). 2000;25(22):2940–52. Discussion 52
16. EuroQol G. EuroQol – a new facility for the measurement of health-related quality of life. Health Policy. 1990;16(3):199–208.
17. Ware JE Jr, Sherbourne CD. The MOS 36-item short-form health survey (SF-36). I. Conceptual framework and item selection. Med Care. 1992;30(6):473–83.
18. Schwab F, Ungar B, Blondel B, Buchowski J, Coe J, Deinlein D, et al. Scoliosis Research Society-Schwab adult spinal deformity classification: a validation study. Spine (Phila Pa 1976). 2012;37(12):1077–82.

19. Lafage V, Schwab F, Patel A, Hawkinson N, Farcy JP. Pelvic tilt and truncal inclination: two key radiographic parameters in the setting of adults with spinal deformity. Spine (Phila Pa 1976). 2009;34(17):E599–606.
20. Chen PG, Daubs MD, Berven S, Raaen LB, Anderson AT, Asch SM, et al. Surgery for degenerative lumbar scoliosis: the development of appropriateness criteria. Spine (Phila Pa 1976). 2016;41(10):910–8.
21. Glassman SD, Carreon LY, Shaffrey CI, Polly DW, Ondra SL, Berven SH, et al. The costs and benefits of nonoperative management for adult scoliosis. Spine (Phila Pa 1976). 2010;35(5):578–82.
22. Everett CR, Patel RK. A systematic literature review of nonsurgical treatment in adult scoliosis. Spine (Phila Pa 1976). 2007;32(19 Suppl):S130–4.
23. Farcy JP, Schwab FJ. Management of flatback and related kyphotic decompensation syndromes. Spine (Phila Pa 1976). 1997;22(20):2452–7.
24. Scheer JK, Hostin R, Robinson C, Schwab F, Lafage V, Burton DC, et al. Operative management of adult spinal deformity results in significant increases in QALYs gained compared to non-operative management: analysis of 479 patients with minimum 2-year follow-up. Spine (Phila Pa 1976). 2016. [Epub ahead of print].
25. Smith JS, Lafage V, Shaffrey CI, Schwab F, Lafage R, Hostin R, et al. Outcomes of operative and non-operative treatment for adult spinal deformity: a prospective, multicenter, propensity-matched cohort assessment with minimum 2-year follow-up. Neurosurgery. 2016;78(6):851–61.
26. Weinstein SL, Dolan LA, Wright JG, Dobbs MB. Effects of bracing in adolescents with idiopathic scoliosis. N Engl J Med. 2013;369(16):1512–21.
27. Heary RF, Bono CM, Kumar S. Bracing for scoliosis. Neurosurgery. 2008;63(3 Suppl):125–30.
28. Hu SS, Berven SH. Preparing the adult deformity patient for spinal surgery. Spine (Phila Pa 1976). 2006;31(19 Suppl):S126–31.
29. Soroceanu A, Burton DC, Diebo BG, Smith JS, Hostin R, Shaffrey CI, et al. Impact of obesity on complications, infection, and patient-reported outcomes in adult spinal deformity surgery. J Neurosurg Spine. 2015:1–9.
30. Glassman SD, Anagnost SC, Parker A, Burke D, Johnson JR, Dimar JR. The effect of cigarette smoking and smoking cessation on spinal fusion. Spine (Phila Pa 1976). 2000;25(20):2608–15.
31. Neer RM, Arnaud CD, Zanchetta JR, Prince R, Gaich GA, Reginster JY, et al. Effect of parathyroid hormone (1-34) on fractures and bone mineral density in postmenopausal women with osteoporosis. N Engl J Med. 2001;344(19):1434–41.
32. Black DM, Delmas PD, Eastell R, Reid IR, Boonen S, Cauley JA, et al. Once-yearly zoledronic acid for treatment of postmenopausal osteoporosis. N Engl J Med. 2007;356(18):1809–22.
33. Hirsch BP, Unnanuntana A, Cunningham ME, Lane JM. The effect of therapies for osteoporosis on spine fusion: a systematic review. Spine J. 2013;13(2):190–9.
34. Dwyer AF, Newton NC, Sherwood AA. An anterior approach to scoliosis. A preliminary report. Clin Orthop Relat Res. 1969;62:192–202.
35. Dwyer AF, Schafer MF. Anterior approach to scoliosis. Results of treatment in fifty-one cases. J Bone Joint Surg Br. 1974;56(2):218–24.
36. Heary RF, Madhavan K. The history of spinal deformity. Neurosurgery. 2008;63(3 Suppl):5–15.
37. Lowe TG, Betz R, Lenke L, Clements D, Harms J, Newton P, et al. Anterior single-rod instrumentation of the thoracic and lumbar spine: saving levels. Spine (Phila Pa 1976). 2003;28(20):S208–16.
38. Deviren V, Patel VV, Metz LN, Berven SH, Hu SH, Bradford DS. Anterior arthrodesis with instrumentation for thoracolumbar scoliosis: comparison of efficacy in adults and adolescents. Spine (Phila Pa 1976). 2008;33(11):1219–23.
39. Saer EH 3rd, Winter RB, Lonstein JE. Long scoliosis fusion to the sacrum in adults with nonparalytic scoliosis. An improved method. Spine (Phila Pa 1976). 1990;15(7):650–3.
40. Balderston RA, Winter RB, Moe JH, Bradford DS, Lonstein JE. Fusion to the sacrum for nonparalytic scoliosis in the adult. Spine (Phila Pa 1976). 1986;11(8):824–9.
41. Gardocki RJ, Watkins RG, Williams LA. Measurements of lumbopelvic lordosis using the pelvic radius technique as it correlates with sagittal spinal balance and sacral translation. Spine J. 2002;2(6):421–9.
42. Bernhardt M, Bridwell KH. Segmental analysis of the sagittal plane alignment of the normal thoracic and lumbar spines and thoracolumbar junction. Spine (Phila Pa 1976). 1989;14(7):717–21.
43. Hsieh PC, Koski TR, O'Shaughnessy BA, Sugrue P, Salehi S, Ondra S, et al. Anterior lumbar interbody fusion in comparison with transforaminal lumbar interbody fusion: implications for the restoration of foraminal height, local disc angle, lumbar lordosis, and sagittal balance. J Neurosurg Spine. 2007;7(4):379–86.
44. Graham EJ, Lenke LG, Lowe TG, Betz RR, Bridwell KH, Kong Y, et al. Prospective pulmonary function evaluation following open thoracotomy for anterior spinal fusion in adolescent idiopathic scoliosis. Spine (Phila Pa 1976). 2000;25(18):2319–25.
45. Christensen FB, Bunger CE. Retrograde ejaculation after retroperitoneal lower lumbar interbody fusion. Int Orthop. 1997;21(3):176–80.
46. Regev GJ, Chen L, Dhawan M, Lee YP, Garfin SR, Kim CW. Morphometric analysis of the ventral nerve roots and retroperitoneal vessels with respect to the minimally invasive lateral approach in normal and deformed spines. Spine (Phila Pa 1976). 2009;34(12):1330–5.

47. Schwab F, Blondel B, Chay E, Demakakos J, Lenke L, Tropiano P, et al. The comprehensive anatomical spinal osteotomy classification. Neurosurgery. 2015;76(Suppl 1):S33–41. Discussion S
48. Berven S, Mummaneni P. Lumbar pedicle subtraction osteotomy. In: Zdeblick T, Albert T, editors. The spine. Master techniques in orthopaedic surgery. 3rd ed. Philadelphia: Lippincott Williams & Wilkins; 2014. p. 257–67.
49. Geck MJ, Macagno A, Ponte A, Shufflebarger HL. The Ponte procedure: posterior only treatment of Scheuermann's kyphosis using segmental posterior shortening and pedicle screw instrumentation. J Spinal Disord Tech. 2007;20(8):586–93.
50. Smith-Petersen MN, Larson CB, Aufranc OE. Osteotomy of the spine for correction of flexion deformity in rheumatoid arthritis. Clin Orthop Relat Res. 1969;66:6–9.
51. La Marca F, Brumblay H. Smith-Petersen osteotomy in thoracolumbar deformity surgery. Neurosurgery. 2008;63(3 Suppl):163–70.
52. Heinig C. Eggshell procedure. In: Luque E, editor. Segmental spinal instrumentation. Thorofare: Slack; 1984. p. 221–30.
53. Thomasen E. Vertebral osteotomy for correction of kyphosis in ankylosing spondylitis. Clin Orthop Relat Res. 1985;194:142–52.
54. Bridwell KH. Decision making regarding Smith-Petersen vs. pedicle subtraction osteotomy vs. vertebral column resection for spinal deformity. Spine (Phila Pa 1976). 2006;31(19 Suppl):S171–8.
55. Boachie-Adjei O, Bradford DS. Vertebral column resection and arthrodesis for complex spinal deformities. J Spinal Disord. 1991;4(2):193–202.
56. Suk SI, Kim JH, Kim WJ, Lee SM, Chung ER, Nah KH. Posterior vertebral column resection for severe spinal deformities. Spine (Phila Pa 1976). 2002;27(21):2374–82.
57. Emami A, Deviren V, Berven S, Smith JA, Hu SS, Bradford DS. Outcome and complications of long fusions to the sacrum in adult spine deformity: luque-galveston, combined iliac and sacral screws, and sacral fixation. Spine (Phila Pa 1976). 2002;27(7):776–86.
58. Smith JS, Klineberg E, Lafage V, Shaffrey CI, Schwab F, Lafage R, et al. Prospective multicenter assessment of perioperative and minimum 2-year postoperative complication rates associated with adult spinal deformity surgery. J Neurosurg Spine. 2016;25(1):1–14.
59. Iorio JA, Reid P, Kim HJ. Neurological complications in adult spinal deformity surgery. Curr Rev Musculoskelet Med. 2016;9(3):290–8.
60. Sansur CA, Smith JS, Coe JD, Glassman SD, Berven SH, Polly DW Jr, et al. Scoliosis research society morbidity and mortality of adult scoliosis surgery. Spine (Phila Pa 1976). 2011;36(9):E593–7.
61. Lenke LG, Fehlings MG, Shaffrey CI, Cheung KM, Carreon L, Dekutoski MB, et al. Neurologic outcomes of complex adult spinal deformity surgery: results of the prospective, multicenter Scoli-RISK-1 study. Spine (Phila Pa 1976). 2016;41(3):204–12.
62. Kim YJ, Bridwell KH, Lenke LG, Rhim S, Cheh G. Pseudarthrosis in long adult spinal deformity instrumentation and fusion to the sacrum: prevalence and risk factor analysis of 144 cases. Spine (Phila Pa 1976). 2006;31(20):2329–36.
63. Dickson DD, Lenke LG, Bridwell KH, Koester LA. Risk factors for and assessment of symptomatic pseudarthrosis after lumbar pedicle subtraction osteotomy in adult spinal deformity. Spine (Phila Pa 1976). 2014;39(15):1190–5.
64. Kim HJ, Buchowski JM, Zebala LP, Dickson DD, Koester L, Bridwell KH. RhBMP-2 is superior to iliac crest bone graft for long fusions to the sacrum in adult spinal deformity: 4- to 14-year follow-up. Spine (Phila Pa 1976). 2013;38(14):1209–15.
65. Glattes RC, Bridwell KH, Lenke LG, Kim YJ, Rinella A, Edwards C 2nd. Proximal junctional kyphosis in adult spinal deformity following long instrumented posterior spinal fusion: incidence, outcomes, and risk factor analysis. Spine (Phila Pa 1976). 2005;30(14):1643–9.
66. Liu FY, Wang T, Yang SD, Wang H, Yang DL, Ding WY. Incidence and risk factors for proximal junctional kyphosis: a meta-analysis. Eur Spine J. 2016;25(8):2376–83.
67. Yagi M, Akilah KB, Boachie-Adjei O. Incidence, risk factors and classification of proximal junctional kyphosis: surgical outcomes review of adult idiopathic scoliosis. Spine (Phila Pa 1976). 2011;36(1):E60–8.
68. Kim HJ, Lenke LG, Shaffrey CI, Van Alstyne EM, Skelly AC. Proximal junctional kyphosis as a distinct form of adjacent segment pathology after spinal deformity surgery: a systematic review. Spine (Phila Pa 1976). 2012;37(22 Suppl):S144–64.

Image-Guided Spinal Stabilization

37

Jang W. Yoon and Eric W. Nottmeier

Introduction

Since its introduction in the mid-1990s, image guidance has been gaining popularity among spine surgeons [1–4]. Image guidance technology allows the surgeon to navigate the patient's anatomy on preoperative or intraoperative images by tracking surgical instruments in three-dimensional (3D) space using infrared light. With standard pedicle screw insertion techniques, misplacement rates of up to 29% [5–8] and neurologic injury rates of up to 7% [9] have been reported [10] in the literature. With widespread utilization of 3D image guidance for pedicle screw placement, the malposition rates have been significantly decreased [11, 12]. With continual technological advancement, 3D image guidance technique has become even more user-friendly and efficient for spine surgeons.

A significant step forward in this process was the introduction of cone-beam computed tomography (cbCT) registration for spinal image guidance. During cbCT acquisition, multiple fluoroscopic images are obtained while the device rotates around the patient. These images are then reconstructed into a 3D data set, essentially a CT scan, which can then be navigated after the data is transferred to the image-guided system. Advantages of 3D cbCT image guidance include the ability to register multiple vertebral segments at once without the need to expose the bony dorsal elements, and, therefore, it is now being utilized in minimally invasive spinal surgery procedures.

This chapter will review the key concepts that are critical in completing a successful image-guided spinal surgery. Though the use of image guidance is increasing in spinal surgery, this technology is still not used by a majority of spine surgeons. A large part of the literature concerning spinal image guidance describes its use in open procedures, with a smaller part of the literature reporting on minimally invasive procedures. Spinal image guidance has been used as an adjunct for instrumentation placement from the ilium to the occiput [13–21].

J.W. Yoon, MD, MS (✉)
Department of Neurosurgery, Mayo Clinic,
4500 San Pablo Road, Jacksonville, FL 32224, USA
e-mail: yoon.jang@mayo.edu

E.W. Nottmeier, MD
Department of Neurosurgery, St. Vincent's Spine and Brain Institute, Jacksonville, FL, USA
e-mail: Enottmeier@me.com

Indications and Patient Selection

Patient Factors

Obese patients pose a challenge to the spine surgeon for multiple reasons. Placement of instrumentation in obese patients can be quite challenging

L.T. Holly, P.A. Anderson (eds.), *Essentials of Spinal Stabilization*,
DOI 10.1007/978-3-319-59713-3_37

due to the lack of fluoroscopic visualization of the anatomy. Image guidance can be particularly useful in these patients for visualizing the anatomy when used in conjunction with cbCT. Though cbCT image quality can be degraded in obese patients, the images are typically adequate enough to allow visualization of the essential anatomy by the surgeon.

Image guidance also proves useful in patients undergoing revision spinal surgery. When exposing the spine in these patients, image guidance can help the surgeon avoid dural penetration through previous laminectomy defects while at the same time allow for maximum exposure of the remaining bony elements. Additionally, in patients with previous fusion mass and obscuration of anatomical landmarks, image guidance allows for 3D visualization of the spine for instrumentation placement.

In minimally invasive cases, the location of the skin incisions can be ascertained with image guidance to allow the best trajectory to the underlying spinal anatomy. Additionally, percutaneous non-cannulated pedicle screws can be placed without the use of K-wires, thereby decreasing instrumentation costs for the hospital since non-cannulated screws typically cost less than cannulated screws [22].

In trauma cases, careful attention needs to be directed toward navigation accuracy given the instability of the spine. To minimize inaccuracy, the surgeon can place one screw on each side of the fracture and then use a temporary rod in these screws to help minimize the motion across the fracture while placing the remaining screws. In the upper cervical spine, drilling the holes for all the screws to be placed should be accomplished prior to tapping and placing screws. This is because drilling typically results in less movement of the spine and the subsequent navigation inaccuracy that can occur as a result.

Regional Consideration

Cervical Spine

To easily maintain line of site between the navigated instruments and the tracking camera, the reference arc should be located between the camera and the region of the spine that is to be navigated. In our experience, the Mayfield head holder allows a stable and rigid fixation point for the reference arc during posterior cervical spine surgery and is preferred over placing the reference arc on a cervical spinous process [16]. This way, the reference arc does not get in the way of instrumentation placement. Additionally, with the tracking camera located at the head of the bed, the instruments can be easily tracked as the line of sight is maintained. It is also possible to place the arc at the most distally exposed spinous process; however, due to the flexibility of cervical spine, the position of the arc can be moved during spine instrumentation and introduces errors in the accuracy. Also, if the reference arc is placed on the most distal spinous process, then the camera should be located at the foot of the bed so as to keep the reference arc between the tracking camera and the navigated instruments. In addition, acquisition of images should be performed following dissection to expose bone anatomy and also after the placement of retractors. After image acquisition with the retractors in place, the table position and the retractors should not be moved. Such movement can cause inaccuracy of navigation due to mobility of the cervical spine in relation to the reference arc, which is attached to the skull via the Mayfield head holder. Especially, Trendelenburg or reverse Trendelenburg movement of the table can cause dramatic shift of the patient's weight in either direction and change the position of the cervical spine. The shift can also occur when the retractors are repositioned in the cervical spine.

Thoracic

For posterior approaches to the thoracic spine, the reference arc should be placed on the most superiorly exposed spinous process, and the image acquisition should take place after the bony anatomy is exposed as to minimize errors in accuracy. For anterior and lateral approaches to the thoracic spine, the use of cbCT 3D navigation system is challenging due to the difficulty of placing the reference arc. The size and depth of the bore, patient positioning, and orientation make the use of 3D navigation difficult in these cases. In the author's experience, utilizing surgical landmarks and fluoroscopy-based imaging as guides for the procedure is preferable in these cases. Alternatively, percutaneous placement of reference arc in the iliac crest can be done; however, the access surgeon may find the arc to be impedance during the exposure. The spine surgeon should keep in mind that navigation is useful for bone anatomy and not typically useful in delineating the adjacent vascular anatomy or soft-tissue structures.

Lumbar

Spinal navigation systems have been adapted to lateral approaches to the lumbar spine for interbody fusions in patients with spinal deformity, spondylosis adjacent to a previous fusion, or degenerative disc disease. The dissection, discectomy, and implant tools can be paired to navigation. Use of navigation can simplify patient positioning and eliminate the need to spend OR time to perfectly align the pedicle and disc space with anteroposterior and lateral fluoroscopy. In lateral lumbar cases, preoperative planning with proper placement of the reference arc is crucial. We have found that placing a percutaneous reference arc into the posterior iliac crest serves better than placing into the lateral iliac crest. This allows the reference arc to be seen by the camera while still being close enough to the operative field to maintain accuracy and stays out of the line of sight to the operative tools. Once the navigation accuracy is confirmed and the patient positioning is finalized, the navigated discectomy and interbody implant can be performed safely and efficiently. If a navigated interbody placement tool is not available to the surgeon, then the image-guided probe can be inserted into the disc space to ascertain the trajectory and depth that the cage should be inserted.

In large deformity cases requiring iliac instrumentation, the reference arc can still be placed on the most superiorly exposed spinous process. In degenerative scoliosis patients, the spine is typically stiff enough that, in our experience, navigation has been accurate for placement of iliac and sacral fixation, even when the reference arc is placed on a spinous process in the upper thoracic spine. In pediatric and adolescent scoliosis cases, the spine is more flexible and the reference arc may have to be placed at shorter distances to the instrumented levels to maintain navigation accuracy. In these instances, multiple registration spins with the cbCT device may have to be accomplished as the reference arc is moved.

Preoperative Considerations

There are many factors that a surgeon must consider before starting image-guided spinal fusion. In some institutions, spinal image guidance is accomplished by point-matching registration from a preoperative CT scan. An advantage of this is that a preoperative CT scan is usually of higher quality than an intraoperative cbCT scan. However, a preoperative CT scan is performed when the patient is in a supine position. Because of this, single-segment registration is typically needed because of intersegmental shifts in the patient's spine that occur in the prone position. Additionally, a thorough dissection of the dorsal spinal bony elements is needed with this technique to be able to match points to the preoperative CT scan. This can be tedious and add OR time. It is also more difficult to perform point-matching registration in a patient who has had a previous laminectomy. The Fluoromerge technique allows for the surgeon to acquire an anteroposterior and lateral fluoroscopic image of the spinal anatomy of which the navigation system will use to perform the registration to a preoperative CT scan. This technique is advantageous over the point-matching technique in that a tedious dissection of the spine is not needed and it can be performed in patients who have had previous laminectomy. This technique can also be used for minimally invasive cases. Because this technique navigates from a preoperative CT scan, the same disadvantage exists with intersegmental motion that can occur between the supine position of the spine during the preoperative CT scan and the prone position of the spine at surgery, which can result in navigation inaccuracy when instrumenting multiple segments.

Other preoperative considerations include patient factors, positioning, neuromonitoring, and different surgical tools depending on the type of spinal fusion. At our institution, the surgeon, the residents, and the operating room staff meet on the morning of the surgery to review the surgeries for the day and discuss all necessary setups in the operating room to decrease potential disruption in the workflow during the cases. For all image-guided spine surgeries, a surgeon must be aware of key steps for completing a successful surgery. The typical operating room must be set up in a manner that allows for efficient surgical workflow. Our operating room setup is demonstrated in Fig. 37.1. This setup allows for easy maneuvering of O-arm in and out of the surgical field with the navigation camera pointed toward the reference arc. As stated earlier, the line of sight between the camera and navigated instruments is best maintained when the reference arc is located in between the tracking camera and the navigated instruments [23]. Details of important preoperative considerations are described below.

Surgical Table Selection

Surgical table selection is critical for the success of image-guided spine surgery. An ideal surgical table should allow for easy patient positioning, exposure, and intraoperative imaging. Many operating room tables can be used for 2D fluoroscopy as long as the patient is positioned appropriately. For 3D image guidance using the O-arm, the apparatus should be able to fit around the patient on the table and move up and down without any obstruction from the base of the surgical table. Standard operating room tables may hinder one's ability to perform imaging with cone-beam CT-based imaging systems such as the O-arm. The dimensions and designs of the Jackson table allow the maintenance of the patient's lumbar lordosis in the prone position [24]. In addition, it does not have a base obstructing movement along the long axis of the patient and table. The Jackson table enables the O-arm to be positioned along any level of the spinal axis. The table is well designed for imaging purposes, with its core structure such that the table has minimal radiodense metal resulting in minimal radiographic artifact.

Sterile Draping

Sterile draping can be a source of frustration and delays if not done properly. Draping the entire O-arm is quite cumbersome, and the device can be contaminated during image acquisition. In addition, the sterile cover can become loose and can get caught when the O-arm is being closed. If this occurs, the O-arm has to be manually opened to remove the jammed drape. To circumvent this frequently encountered problem, covering of the patient in a 360° circumferential manner with sterile drapes is a much more efficient way to maintain sterility of the field (Fig. 37.2). However, the reference arc on the patient cannot be covered by the sterile drape and has to be visible to the camera on the navigation system.

Registration Process

The registration process is a critical step in determining the accuracy of image acquisition and subsequent navigation information. There are multiple sources of error during this critical step; thus, the surgeon must validate and assess accuracy of navigation on a continuous basis. The size of the pedicle, size of the screw, and distance to the isthmus or narrowest point on the pedicle determine the margin of error in screw placement. In the midcervical spine, the mid-thoracic spine, and the thoracolumbar junction, there is a maximum permissible translational error of less than 1 mm and rotational error of less than 5° [25]. This leaves little room for any error in pedicle screw placement. Intraoperative image acquisition and registration should therefore be performed after surgical access is completed to avoid angular and translational movements that may occur with exposing the spine and subsequently alter the image registration. With open midline access, image acquisition and registration should

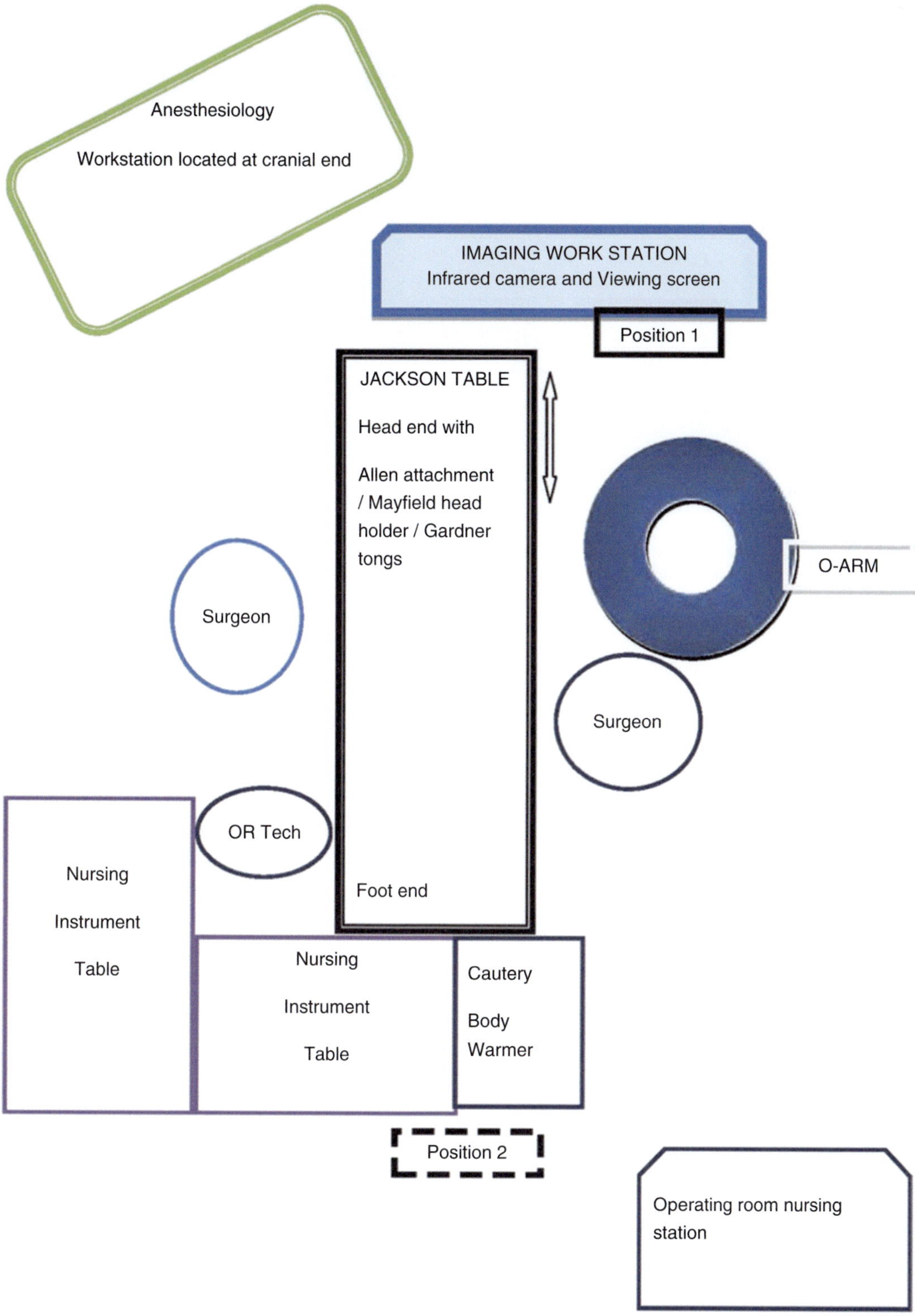

Fig. 37.1 Outline of OR setup for a spinal fusion case with the image guidance camera and viewing screen placed cranially (*Position 1*). The O-arm can be moved in and out of position depending on the case and location of imaging required. The camera and screen can be moved to the foot end of the table (*Position 2*) for certain cases to obtain a clear line of sight and images for navigation

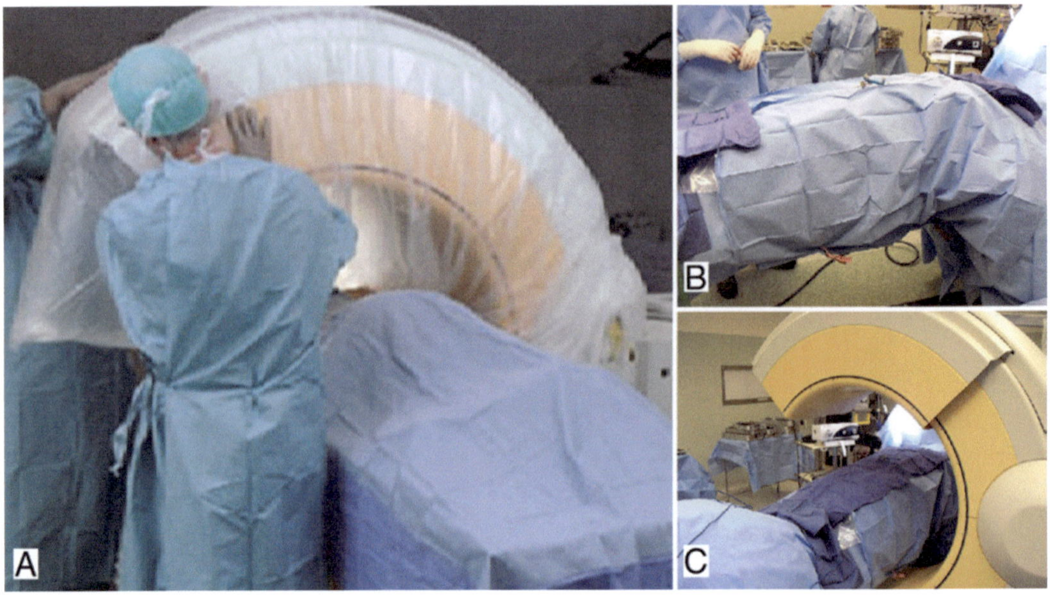

Fig. 37.2 Intraoperative photographs demonstrating our draping technique. (**b**) Sterile tube drape is designed with a great deal of redundancy to accommodate the O-arm; therefore, it can easily get stuck while the gantry tries to close and open. (**b**) Our sterile draping technique requires filling the surgical wound with antibiotic irrigation solution and using surgical split-sheet drapes to circumferentially enclose the patient while keeping the reference arc just above the drapes. (**c**) With gantry closure there is no contact between the patient, the reference arc, and the tube. Following image acquisition, these drapes are removed and procedure is continued

be performed after completing exposure necessary to perform instrumentation in order to eliminate motion-related inaccuracy. The deep retractors should also be left in situ, especially for mobile cervical spine segments. In contrast, percutaneous minimally invasive instrumentation may begin immediately after the intraoperative registration procedure without prior anatomical landmark dissection, as significant manipulation of the surgical field and landmarks do not occur in these procedures [26]. If body warmers are used intraoperatively, they should be temporarily turned off to maintain visibility of the reference arc during registration. Additionally, movements during respiration and image acquisition can cause significant changes and inaccuracies with registration so respirations are temporarily held during the registration process to minimize errors secondary to motion artifact.

The surgeon should avoid changing the position of the table and attempt to avoid any potential movements with instruments that may cause distortion of the anatomy. Excessive force on the spine during screw placement should be avoided. In areas of excessive mobility, such as traumatic injury to the spine or when navigating cervical segments, all holes for the screws should be drilled first under navigation as this maneuver results in the least force being applied to the spine. Tapping and screw placement should occur after all the holes are drilled as these maneuvers can result in movement of the spine relative to the reference arc and subsequent navigation inaccuracy. Navigation accuracy should be continuously checked, and if inaccuracy exists, then the surgeon at least has the holes for the instrumentation drilled and can freehand place the screws into the already drilled holes. Navigation is beneficial in identifying complex bone anatomy, maintaining midline orientation in rotary scoliosis, and identifying important anatomic structures during complex tumor cases where they may be involved or displaced. Key landmarks need to be marked out prior to bone removal as navigation may become inaccurate the more the spine is manipulated.

Radiation Exposure to the OR Staff and the Patient

With minimally invasive spinal instrumentation using active fluoroscopy, radiation exposure to the surgeon and the OR staff has been an increasing concern. In a prospective study, Bindal et al. reported a mean fluoroscopy time of 1.69 min per case, with a mean radiation exposure of 27 mRem to the surgeon's torso (under a lead apron), 76 mRem to the surgeon's dominant hand, and 32 mRem to an unprotected thyroid during transforaminal lumbar interbody fusion procedures [27]. With cbCT-based 3D image guidance techniques, radiation exposure to OR staff and the surgeon can be minimized. Nottmeier et al. report no radiation exposure when standing 10 feet behind the lead shield during O-arm image acquisition [28]. Radiation scatter from the O-arm was not a concern when this simple precaution was undertaken. Radiation exposure to the patient during cbCT-based image acquisition is approximately half the radiation dose of a 64-slice CT scanner [29], which is well below the recommended annual limit of 5 Rem to the torso as set forth by the National Council on Radiation Protection and Measurements [28]. Thus, utilization of cbCT registration techniques eliminates the risk of radiation exposure to the surgeon and OR staff while at the same time resulting in less radiation exposure to the patient as compared with registration techniques that utilize preoperative CT scans.

Surgical Technique

General Principles

Surgeons must remember that 3D navigation images are generated at the time of image acquisition, which means images are not in real time when surgeons are instrumenting the spine. The surgeon must use the navigation system as an adjunct and cannot be used to replace thorough knowledge of spinal anatomy. The surgeon must verify navigation accuracy on continuous basis and be cognizant of inaccuracy when the anatomic landmark does not correlate with navigation.

Verification and Sequence of Instrumentation

Before placing any instrumentation into the spine, the surgeon must verify the accuracy of the registration by correlating anatomic landmarks to what is shown on the navigation screen. This can be accomplished by placing a navigation wand on exposed lamina, spinous processes, or transverse process to verify navigation accuracy. It is known that increased distance from the reference arc and longer duration of surgery are two main factors that will negatively affect accuracy. Based on previous investigation, there is an average of 3 mm inaccuracy in 7% of the patients when surgery is three levels away from the reference arc and inaccuracy of 3 mm in 17% about 1 hour into surgery in the lumbar region [30]. Therefore, the registration is most accurate immediately after image acquisition and registration and before the interbody or decompression tasks of the procedure are performed. In patients with degenerative spines, we have accurately placed instrumentation in the sacrum with the reference arc placed on an upper thoracic spinous process. However, in more flexible spines such as adolescent scoliosis or trauma, navigation inaccuracy is more likely at distances further away from the reference arc. To maximize navigation accuracy and efficiency, pedicle screw placement should be the initial step of the procedure. In our experience, it is beneficial to begin with the pedicle screw insertion at the level that is furthest away from the reference arc and then proceed proximally toward the level closer to the reference arc. The rationale for this sequence of instrumentation is that the accuracy of navigation will remain more accurate closer to the reference arc, while the accuracy at the most distal segment will degrade as the time goes on. In addition, the accuracy of navigation can also be affected by pedicle screw placement itself. In our practice, we revalidate and recheck the accuracy of navigation after completing pedicle screw placement at each level with known anatomic landmark (e.g., spinous process, lamina, or other bony landmarks). If inaccuracy is detected, then we will obtain a new intraoperative scan to update the navigation images. As a principle, when using the pedicle probe, extreme downward pressure should be avoided to prevent pedicle breaches. It can also cause shift in bony anatomy and degrade navigation accuracy.

Pedicle Screw Insertion Technique

A starting point is chosen based on anatomic landmark in an open case and verified with the navigation screen. In minimally invasive cases, the pedicle screw starting point is chosen based on the navigation. After a satisfactory starting point is chosen, a plan is created in the navigation computer system. This plan must be meticulously created along the long axis of the pedicle without bony breaches. The size and trajectory of the screws can be chosen, and this plan can be locked in, which will overlay this information over the navigation images. Then, a pilot hole is created at the starting point with the high-speed burr. The initial passage through the pedicle tract is made with either a handheld power drill with an image-guided drill guide or a sharp image-guided pedicle probe. A ball-tipped sounder is used to confirm that there are no bony breaches, and the image-guided pointer is passed down the tract to confirm the proper trajectory. Then, image-guided undertapping further develops the tract, followed again by sounding. An image-guided screwdriver is then utilized to deliver the screw in the path. If there is concern about pedicle breach, the screw is immediately removed. The proper trajectory can be accomplished by passing the navigated pointer down the intended path, placing a Kirschner wire (K-wire) along that path, and placing a cannulated screw with the navigated screwdriver over the K-wire. However, as illustrated in the case below, even percutaneous screws can be placed without a K-wire when navigation is used. After all instrumentation has been placed, we obtain new images using O-arm to confirm proper placement of hardware. If pedicle screw malposition is noted during this step, then we can revise the screw using an updated scan.

Minimally Invasive Percutaneous Pedicle Screw Insertion

Image guidance can be used to place percutaneous cannulated pedicle screws using a K-wire. In this technique, an image-guided Jamshidi needle is used to place the wire using guidance. Image-guided taps and screwdrivers are then used to tap the pedicle and place the screw over the K-wire. An advantage of this technique is that the surgeon can easily locate the pedicle entry point as the instruments follow the K-wire. However, live fluoroscopy is typically not used with this technique so inadvertent advancement of the K-wire may go unnoticed. Additionally, K-wires can fracture with the tip remaining in the vertebral body. With image guidance, K-wires do not have to be used as the surgeon can use a sharp image-guided awl to enter the pedicle. An image-guided tap is then used to tap the hole in which a non-cannulated screw can be placed [22].

Image-Guided Implant Placement

Three-dimensional image guidance technique can be helpful in the placement of interbody grafts and cages. In author's experience, this technique can be applied when performing direct lateral interbody fusion (DLIF) or extreme lateral interbody fusion (XLIF) procedures. Patient positioning is crucial in these surgeries to open up the space between the top of iliac crest and the bottom of the rib cage. The patient is positioned in lateral decubitus position on Wilson frame and secured with strong adhesive tapes and straps (Fig. 37.3). A Jackson table is recommended since this allows easy access for O-arms to move in and out. The navigation arc can either be taped onto the patient's body (Fig. 37.4a) or it can be securely tapped into iliac crest (Fig. 37.4b). It is important to ensure that the arc is not taped on top of the Bair Hugger or loose drapes: if so, the position of the arc can move rendering image guidance unreliable. In addition, position of the arc has to be cleared from the trajectory of your image-guided tools; therefore, this has to be

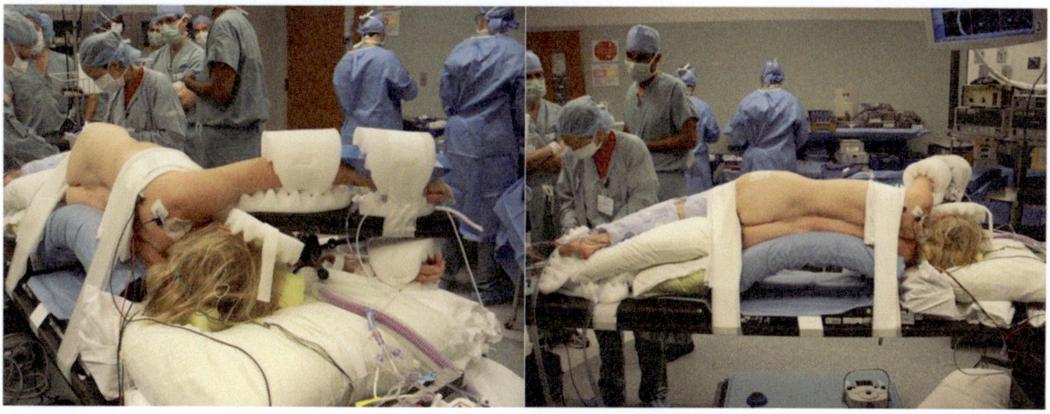

Fig. 37.3 Patient positioning in DLIF or XLIF procedure. Wilson frame on top of Jackson table is our preferred setup for this procedure. The patient is positioned in lateral decubitus position, so that the space between the bottom of rib cage and the top of iliac crest is at the apex of Wilson frame, allowing maximal access to this region. Jackson table allows easy access for O-arm to move in and out

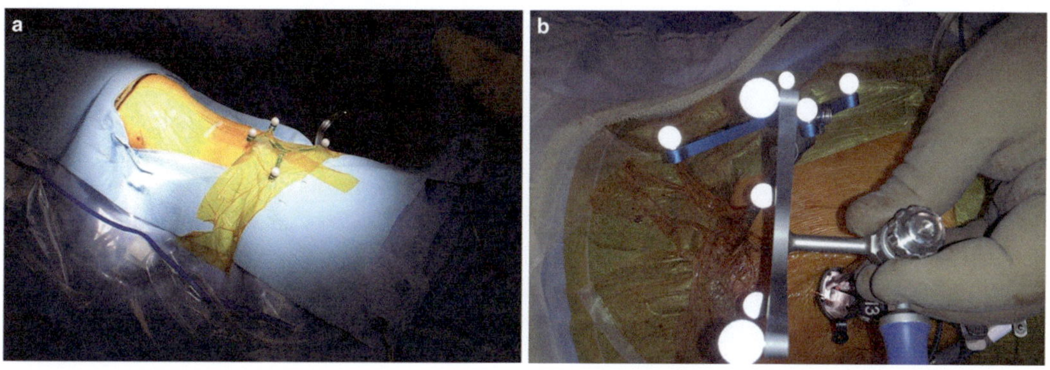

Fig. 37.4 (**a**) The navigation arc can either be taped or (**b**) securely tapped into patient's iliac crest. It is important to ensure that the arc is not on top of Bair Hugger or loose draping when it is taped. The most important step when securing the navigation arc is to ensure the position of navigation arc does not interfere with the trajectory of navigation tools; therefore, situation like this does not happen

checked prior to the beginning of the case (Fig. 37.4b). After patient positioning and the navigation arc are secured using either method described above, the case can begin. In our experience, the navigation wand can be used periodically throughout the case to determine the extent of the diskectomy, implant location, and trajectory of implant (Fig. 37.5). It should be noted that spinal image guidance is FDA approved in cases in which the reference arc is attached to the bone. Taping the reference arc to the skin is an off-label use of the technology and does have a higher incidence of navigation inaccuracy.

Illustrative Case

This 39-year-old male presented with symptomatic L5–S1 degenerative disc disease (DDD) confirmed by discography (Fig. 37.6). Surgical intervention was an image-guided, minimally invasive L5–S1 transforaminal lumbar interbody fusion (TLIF).

A Jackson table was used with the patient in the prone position. A percutaneous reference arc was used in this case and placed on the right iliac crest. Following patient registration with the O-arm, the location of the paraspinal incision was

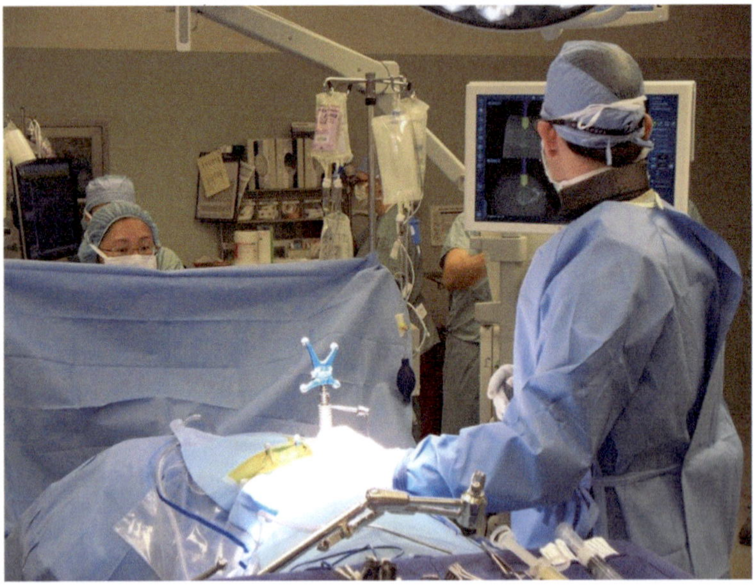

Fig. 37.5 Navigation information can be useful in determining the level of discectomy and extent of discectomy and estimating the size of the interbody graft as well as the location and depth of the implant

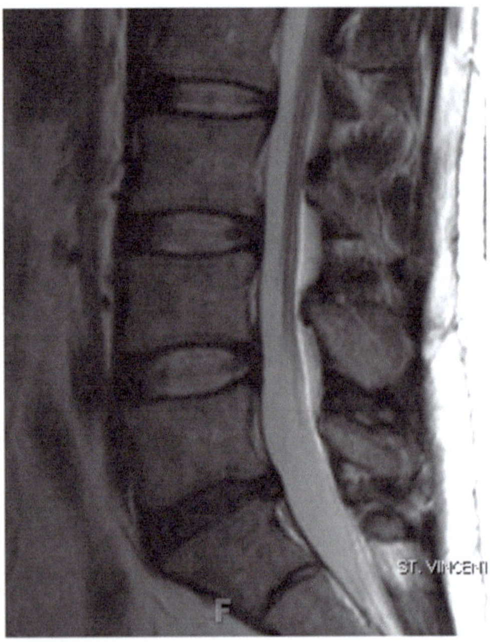

Fig. 37.6 Sagittal T2-weighted MRI showing L5–S1 degenerative disc disease

ascertained on the skin so as to give appropriate trajectory to the pedicles and interbody space. After the incision was made and extended through the fascia, the probe was then placed down onto the facet joint, and the navigation accuracy was checked (Fig. 37.7). Once adequate navigation accuracy was confirmed, the navigated awl was placed down onto the pedicle entry point, and a virtual plan was sized to the pedicle. This plan was then locked, and the awl was tamped into the pedicle prior to removing it, which created a pilot hole (Fig. 37.8). The navigated awl was then inserted into the pilot hole, and the pedicle was tapped. The pilot hole was at the base of the plan and was easily found with the navigated tap. Although an option, K-wires were not used during this case. After the pedicle was tapped, a probe was inserted to palpate the pedicle walls (Fig. 37.9). The screw was then placed with the navigated screwdriver, and the process was repeated for each pedicle (Fig. 37.10). Prior to wound closure, the O-arm was used to check instrumentation placement, and the patient was followed as an outpatient in clinic with serial radiographs (Fig. 37.11).

Technical Pearls

- In-line force is essential when placing instrumentation with image guidance. If a pedicle is significantly angled medially, then the surgeon will have a tendency to push the instruments against the paraspinal muscles to obtain

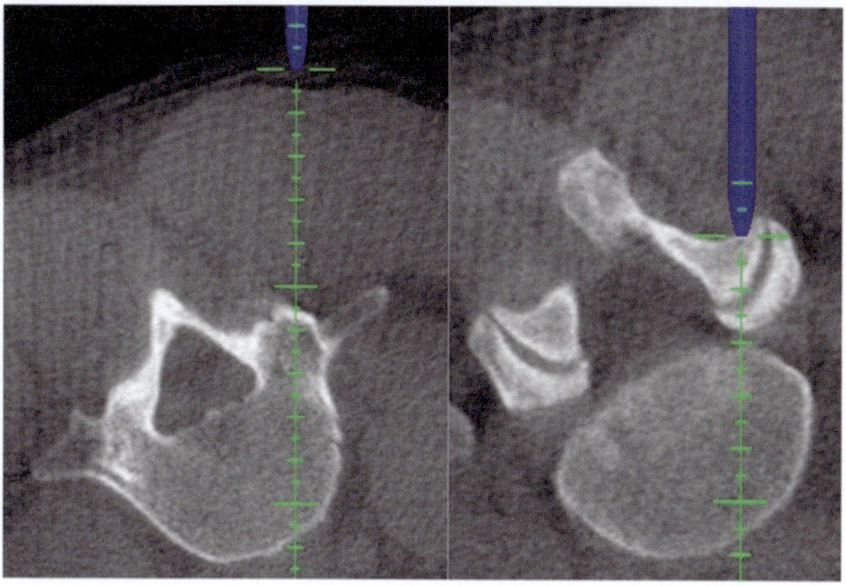

Fig. 37.7 (**a**) The navigated probe is used to mark the location of the skin incision. (**b**) The navigated probe placed down on the facet joint to check navigation accuracy

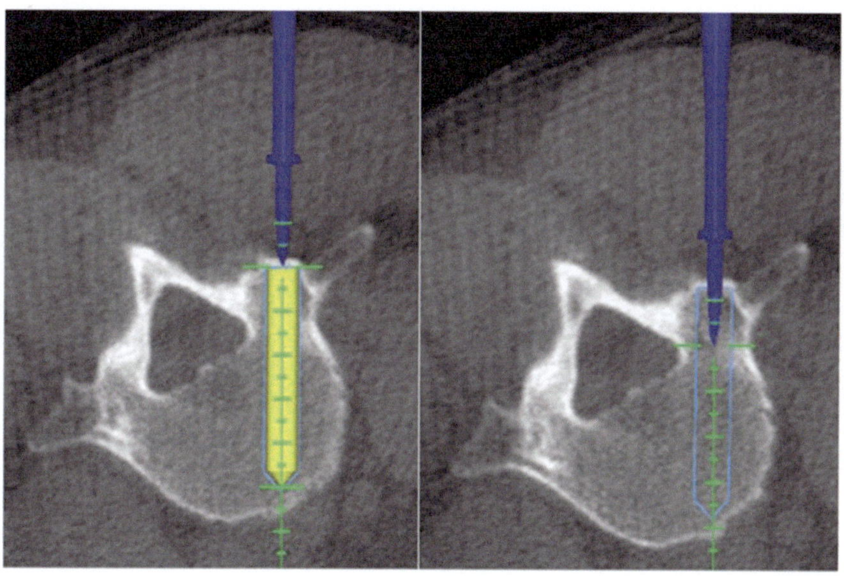

Fig. 37.8 (**a**) The navigated awl is placed on the pedicle entry point, and a virtual plan is positioned and sized. (**b**) After the plan is locked into place, the awl is tamped down the pedicle thereby creating a pilot hole

adequate medial trajectory of the instrument down the pedicle. In these cases, the image-guided instrument shafts can bend, which results in the instrument tip appearing to be in the pedicle when actually it is lateral to the pedicle.

- If there is any question as to the location of the instrument tip in the pedicle, then the surgeon should relax the grip and pressure on the instrument so as to return the instrument to its true trajectory. The actual position of the instrument can then be determined on the

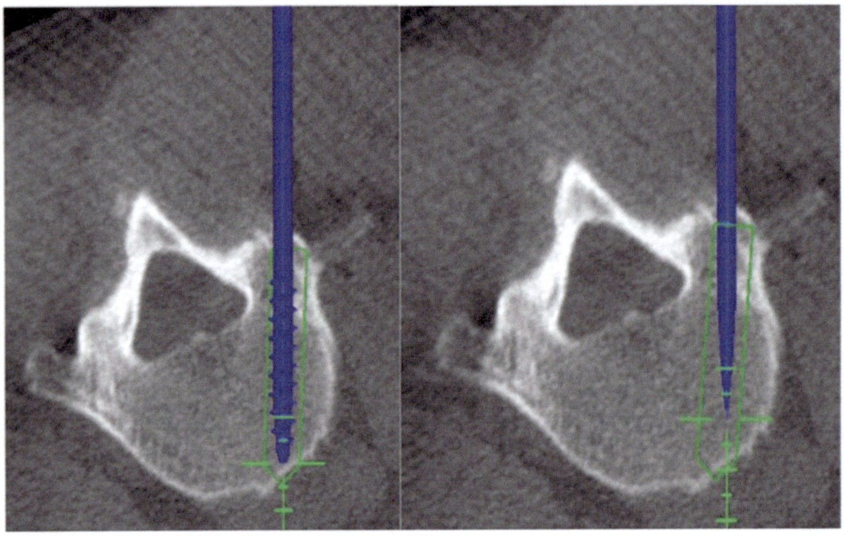

Fig. 37.9 (**a**) The pedicle is tapped with the navigated tap. (**b**) The pedicle is probed with the navigated probe to check for pedicle breach

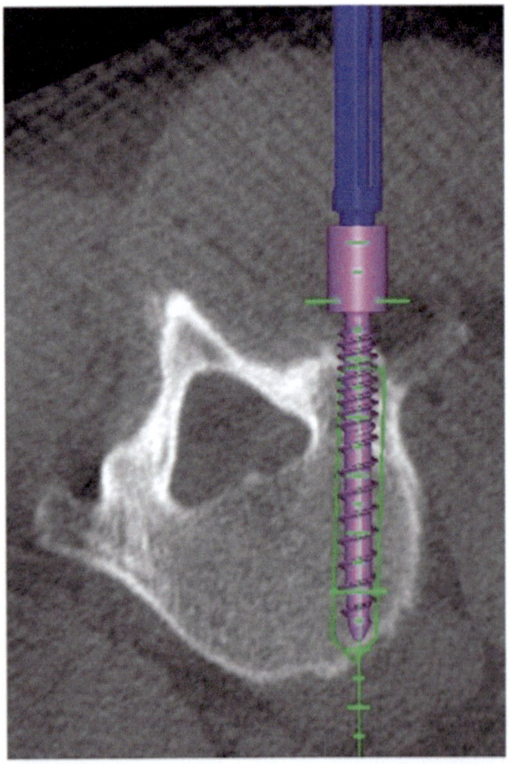

Fig. 37.10 Placement of the pedicle screw with the navigated screwdriver

navigation screen, and corrective action can be taken if necessary.

- Transfascial screw placement may be required in patients with a low-set lumbosacral junction in which trajectory down the pedicle is impeded by the paraspinal muscles that cannot be adequately retracted secondary to the iliac crest. In these instances, placing the screw transfascially through the muscle allows for appropriate trajectory without being impeded by the need to retract or push against the paraspinal muscles (Fig. 37.12).
- The pedicle can be sized via an intraoperative plan. If the pedicle is being tapped and the surgeon desires a larger screw, then the projected tap size can be adjusted on the navigation system to ascertain the largest diameter screw that the pedicle can accommodate (Fig. 37.13). The advantage of this technique is that the screw should lie in the same exact position as the tap as it appears on the navigation screen, thereby allowing the largest diameter screw to be placed without a pedicle breach.
- In the navigation window, the surgeons should periodically check all views (axial,

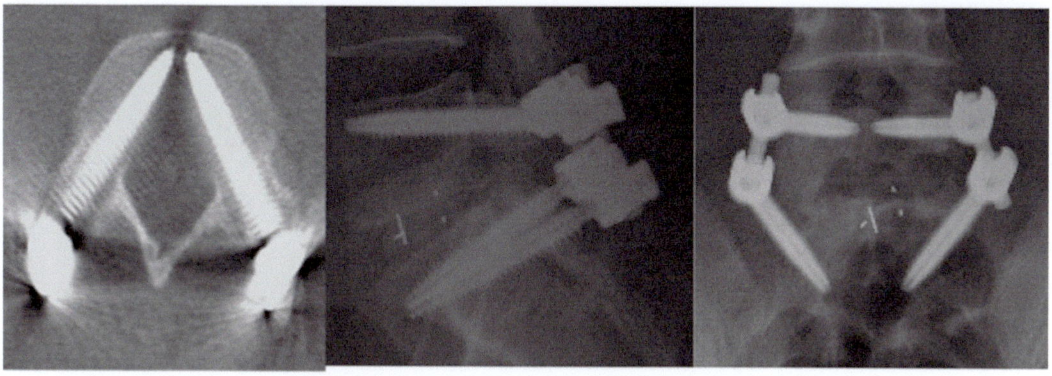

Fig. 37.11 (**a**) Intraoperative cbCT scan. (**b**) Postoperative X-rays showing adequate instrumentation placement

Fig. 37.12 Placement of a transfascial screw to allow for in-line force to be applied to the instrument without the need for pushing the instrument against the paraspinal muscles

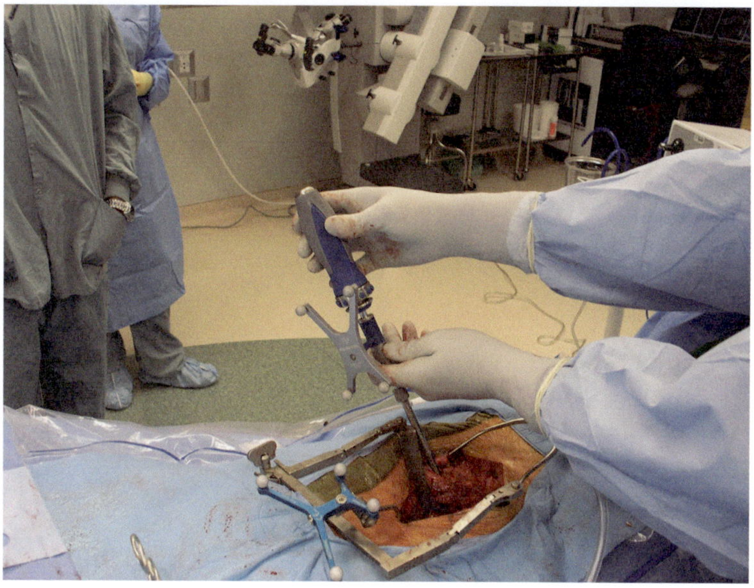

sagittal, coronal, trajectories 1 and 2) to ensure that the pedicle screw is following the saved plan. If there is deviation from the saved plan, the surgeon should stop advancing the screw and relax all pressure on the screw. If there are any concerns of breach based on tactile feedback or navigation images, then the screw should be revised. The authors prefer the trajectory 1 and trajectory 2 views on the Medtronic navigation system and the inline 1 and inline 2 views on the BrainLab navigation system.

- We recommend using a pedicle probe in thoracic and lumbar spine since probes are safer than high-speed drill. We use high-speed drill for lateral mass screws in cervical spine and pedicle screw at C2. With high-speed drill, you do not have the tactile feedback when probing into the pedicle; thus, we prefer using the probe whenever possible. In cervical spine where ventral pressure can cause a large shift in bony anatomy, a high-speed drill can be an effective tool to probe into the pedicle/lateral masses.

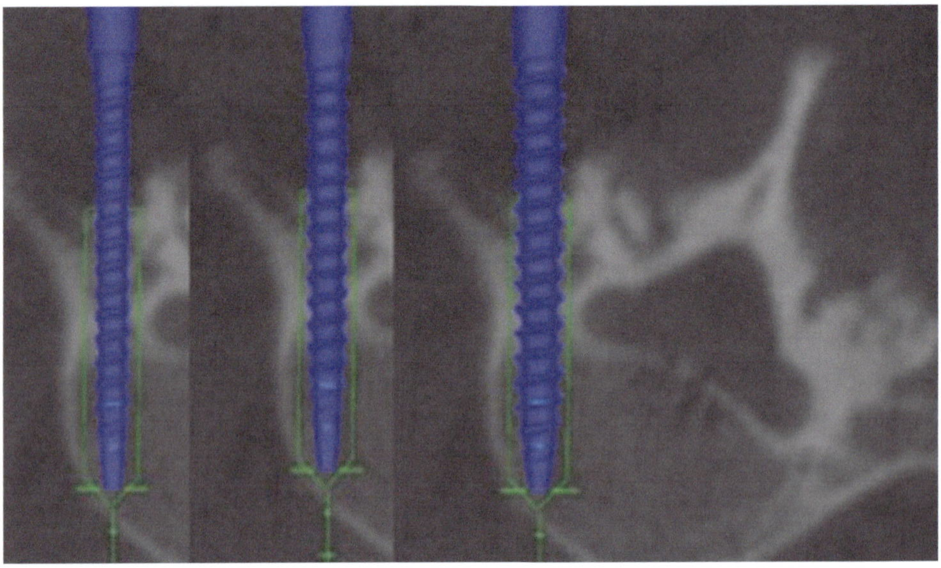

Fig. 37.13 The image-guided tap size can be adjusted on the navigation system while the tap is in the pedicle to allow for proper sizing of the screw to the pedicle

Complications and Strategies for Avoidance

Wrong-Level Surgery

Wrong-level surgery is a potential pitfall. The lack of visual anatomical landmarks, a steep learning curve, and tactile feedback readily available in open surgery make the risks of wrong-level screw insertion higher with minimally invasive techniques [31]. To ensure the correct level, the lumbosacral junction should be used as a point of reference in cases involving lumbar and lower thoracic spine. It is extremely important to thoroughly review preoperative imaging prior to surgery to identify anatomic variations such as sixth lumbar vertebra, which can result in counting errors intraoperatively. For mid-thoracic spine, the reference arc placed on the spinous process serves as a marker, and its location should be confirmed by counting levels from the lumbosacral junction using the fluoroscopy function on the cbCT device prior to implementing the scan for registration. In general, the reference arc should always be included in the cbCT scan in these cases to always serve as a point of reference for confirmation of appropriate levels. During navigation, the image-guided platform will allow the field of view to be expanded for visualization of the lumbosacral junction and/or reference arc to confirm appropriate levels. Once appropriate levels are confirmed, the field of view can be zoomed in to allow better visualization of the spinal anatomy for instrumentation placement.

Pedicle Breach and Redirection Technique

If pedicle breach is suspected after screw placement, then the screw can be redirected with guidance of navigation. Adequate redirection of previously misplaced pedicle screws can be challenging secondary to the tendency of the redirected screw to follow the tract of previously misplaced screw. After removing the previously misplaced pedicle screw, a new starting point can be selected using the navigated pointer tool and residual bony anatomy. Occasionally, the same starting point with a new screw trajectory has to be utilized because of lack of residual anatomy. A new screw plan must avoid bony breaches and communication with the previous screw tract. To confirm the proper redirection of pedicle screw, the image-guided pointer can be placed in the new tract before the final screw placement. In addition, a ball-tipped sounder can provide tactile feedback to confirm the breaches. If there is still a concern of breach, then a cannulated screw with the navigated screwdriver over the K-wire can be used to redirect the pedicle screw. Yoon et al. reported successful redirection of 50 pedicle screws in 30 patients with 0% breach rate using cbCT-based 3D image guidance [32]. Although there are many strategies available to redirect pedicle screws after pedicle breach, the redirection of pedicle screws using 3D image guidance can be safe and effective.

Conclusion

Image guidance technology can be a useful adjunct tool for spine surgeons for both open and minimally invasive spine surgeries. With technological advancement, integration of image guidance technology into the surgical workflow is becoming more seamless and efficient. It must be remembered that this technology cannot replace a surgeon's working knowledge of surgical anatomy, and the surgeon should not rely on image guidance alone for placement of spine instrumentation. In this chapter, we summarized and presented our surgical techniques and strategies that were formulated through experience. The authors hope that the readers find this chapter helpful in identifying and avoiding potential pitfalls with utilization of image guidance technology. This chapter can serve as a guide to close a gap in the learning curve associated with image-guided spinal surgery.

References

1. Nolte LP, Visarius H, Arm E, Langlotz F, Schwarzenbach O, Zamorano L. Computer-aided fixation of spinal implants. J Image Guid Surg. 1995;1(2):88–93.
2. Merloz P, Tonetti J, Eid A, Faure C, Lavallee S, Troccaz J, et al. Computer assisted spine surgery. Clin Orthop. 1997;337:86–96.
3. Lavallee S, Sautot P, Troccaz J, Cinquin P, Merloz P. Computer-assisted spine surgery: a technique for accurate transpedicular screw fixation using CT data and a 3-D optical localizer. J Image Guid Surg. 1995;1(1):65–73.
4. Kalfas IH, Kormos DW, Murphy MA, McKenzie RL, Barnett GH, Bell GR, et al. Application of frameless stereotaxy to pedicle screw fixation of the spine. J Neurosurg. 1995;83(4):641–7.
5. Bolger C, Carozzo C, Roger T, McEvoy L, Nagaria J, Vanacker G, et al. A preliminary study of reliability of impedance measurement to detect iatrogenic initial pedicle perforation (in the porcine model). Eur Spine J. 2006;15:316–20.
6. Laine T, Schlenzka D, Makitalo K, Tallroth K, Nolte LP, Visarius H. Improved accuracy of pedicle screw insertion with computer-assisted surgery. A prospective clinical trial of 30 patients. Spine. 1997;22(11):1254–8.
7. Vaccaro AR, Rizzolo SJ, Balderston RA, Allardyce TJ, Garfin SR, Dolinskas C, et al. Placement of pedicle screws in the thoracic spine. Part II: an anatomical and radiographic assessment. J Bone Joint Surg (Am Vol). 1995;77(8):1200–6.
8. Xu R, Ebraheim NA, Ou Y, Yeasting RA. Anatomic considerations of pedicle screw placement in the thoracic spine. Roy-Camille technique versus open-lamina technique. Spine. 1998;23(9):1065–8.
9. Amiot LP, Lang K, Putzier M, Zippel H, Labelle H. Comparative results between conventional and computer-assisted pedicle screw installation in the thoracic, lumbar, and sacral spine. Spine. 2000;25(5):606–14.
10. Santos ER, Sembrano JN, Yson SC, Polly DW Jr. Comparison of open and percutaneous lumbar pedicle screw revision rate using 3-D image guidance and intraoperative CT. Orthopedics. 2015;38(2):e129–34.
11. Kosmopoulos V, Schizas C. Pedicle screw placement accuracy: a meta-analysis. Spine. 2007;32(3):E111–20.
12. Bourgeois AC, Faulkner AR, Pasciak AS, Bradley YC. The evolution of image-guided lumbosacral spine surgery. Ann Transl Med. 2015;3(5):69.
13. Garrido BJ, Wood KE. Navigated placement of iliac bolts: description of a new technique. Spine J. 2011;11(4):331–5.
14. Nottmeier EW, Foy AB. Placement of C2 laminar screws using three-dimensional fluoroscopy-based image guidance. Eur Spine J. 2008;17(4):610–5.
15. Nottmeier EW, Seemer W, Young PM. Placement of thoracolumbar pedicle screws using three-dimensional image guidance: experience in a large patient cohort. J Neurosurg Spine. 2009;10(1):33–9.
16. Nottmeier EW, Young PM. Image-guided placement of occipitocervical instrumentation using a reference arc attached to the headholder. Neurosurgery. 2010;66(3 Suppl Operative):138–42.
17. Bledsoe JM, Fenton D, Fogelson JL, Nottmeier EW. Accuracy of upper thoracic pedicle screw placement using three-dimensional image guidance. Spine J. 2009;9(10):817–21.

18. Holly LT, Foley KT. Percutaneous placement of posterior cervical screws using three-dimensional fluoroscopy. Spine. 2006;31(5):536–40. Discussion 41
19. Welch WC, Subach BR, Pollack IF, Jacobs GB. Frameless stereotactic guidance for surgery of the upper cervical spine. Neurosurgery. 1997;40(5):958–63. Discussion 63-4
20. Nottmeier EW, Pirris SM, Balseiro S, Fenton D. Three-dimensional image-guided placement of S2 alar screws to adjunct or salvage lumbosacral fixation. Spine J. 2010;10(7):595–601.
21. Lekovic GP, Potts EA, Karahalios DG, Hall G. A comparison of two techniques in image-guided thoracic pedicle screw placement: a retrospective study of 37 patients and 277 pedicle screws. J Neurosurg Spine. 2007;7(4):393–8.
22. Nottmeier EW, Fenton D. Three-dimensional image-guided placement of percutaneous pedicle screws without the use of biplanar fluoroscopy or Kirschner wires: technical note. Int J Med Robot. 2010;6(4):483–8.
23. Rahmathulla G, Nottmeier EW, Pirris SM, Deen HG, Pichelmann MA. Intraoperative image-guided spinal navigation: technical pitfalls and their avoidance. Neurosurg Focus. 2014;36(3):E3.
24. Peterson MD, Nelson LM, McManus AC, Jackson RP. The effect of operative position on lumbar lordosis. A radiographic study of patients under anesthesia in the prone and 90-90 positions. Spine. 1995;20(12):1419–24.
25. Rampersaud YR, Simon DA, Foley KT. Accuracy requirements for image-guided spinal pedicle screw placement. Spine. 2001;26(4):352–9.
26. Scheufler KM, Franke J, Eckardt A, Dohmen H. Accuracy of image-guided pedicle screw placement using intraoperative computed tomography-based navigation with automated referencing. Part II: thoracolumbar spine. Neurosurgery. 2011;69(6):1307–16.
27. Bindal RK, Glaze S, Ognoskie M, Tunner V, Malone R, Ghosh S. Surgeon and patient radiation exposure in minimally invasive transforaminal lumbar interbody fusion. J Neurosurg Spine. 2008;9(6):570–3.
28. Nottmeier EW, Pirris SM, Edwards S, Kimes S, Bowman C, Nelson KL. Operating room radiation exposure in cone beam computed tomography-based, image-guided spinal surgery: clinical article. J Neurosurg Spine. 2013;19(2):226–31.
29. Zhang J, Weir V, Fajardo L, Lin J, Hsiung H, Ritenour ER. Dosimetric characterization of a cone-beam O-arm imaging system. J Xray Sci Technol. 2009;17(4):305–17.
30. Quinones-Hinojosa A, Robert Kolen E, Jun P, Rosenberg WS, Weinstein PR. Accuracy over space and time of computer-assisted fluoroscopic navigation in the lumbar spine in vivo. J Spinal Disord Tech. 2006;19(2):109–13.
31. Ravi B, Zahrai A, Rampersaud R. Clinical accuracy of computer-assisted two-dimensional fluoroscopy for the percutaneous placement of lumbosacral pedicle screws. Spine. 2011;36(1):84–91.
32. Yoon JW, Nottmeier EW, Rahmathulla G, Fenton DS, Pirris SM. Redirecting pedicle screws: a revision spinal fusion strategy using three-dimensional image guidance. Int J Med Robot. 2016;12(4):758–64.

Neurophysiological Monitoring During Placement of Spinal Instrumentation

38

Marc R. Nuwer

Introduction

Neurophysiologic intraoperative monitoring (NIOM) tests spinal cord integrity classically by monitoring nervous system conduction between the limbs and head. Intact conduction confirms intact spinal tracts. Multiple modalities can be examined which test different components of the neurologic function. Somatosensory evoked potentials (SEPs) test dorsal column function and can be tested more or less continuously. If SEP findings deteriorate, the neurophysiology team alerts the surgeon to changes. These changes may potentially forewarn of imminent complications and can do so in time for interventions to reverse or halt complications. Motor evoked potentials (MEPs) usually are tested periodically. While MEPs are more specific for identifying potential motor complications, they are not performed continuously. Electromyography (EMG) monitoring often accompanies SEP and MEP. It is used most often to screen for root compression, e.g., with pedicle screw implantation. Multiple modalities can be monitored simultaneously (Fig. 38.1).

The neurophysiology team establishes baseline values early in a procedure. These values may be obtained prior to positioning or after the patient has been positioned, depending on surgeon preference. The baseline findings are compared to current status of amplitude, latencies, or presence of discharges during the remainder of the procedure. Changes from baseline are the basis for alerts. The thresholds for alerts typically are predetermined, such as a 50% amplitude drop in the SEP cortical peak amplitude.

Preoperative assessment can refine monitoring tactics. Preexisting conditions that influence monitoring techniques include diabetes, older age, and peripheral neuropathy, which can alter tactics for lower extremity SEPs. Myelopathy resets expectations for ease of finding baseline signals and heightens desire for obtaining baselines before positioning.

Somatosensory Evoked Potentials

Somatosensory evoked potentials typically are recorded from the median or ulnar nerve of the upper extremities and peroneal or posterior tibial nerves in the lower extremities. They are used for a variety of NIOM purposes, most often for spinal cord monitoring.

M.R. Nuwer, MD, PhD (✉)
Department of Neurology, David Geffen School of Medicine at UCLA, Reed Bldg, room 1190, 710 Westwood Plaza, Los Angeles, CA 90095, USA

Clinical Neurophysiology, Ronald Reagan UCLA Medical Center, Los Angeles, CA, USA
e-mail: mnuwer@mednet.ucla.edu

L.T. Holly, P.A. Anderson (eds.), *Essentials of Spinal Stabilization*,
DOI 10.1007/978-3-319-59713-3_38

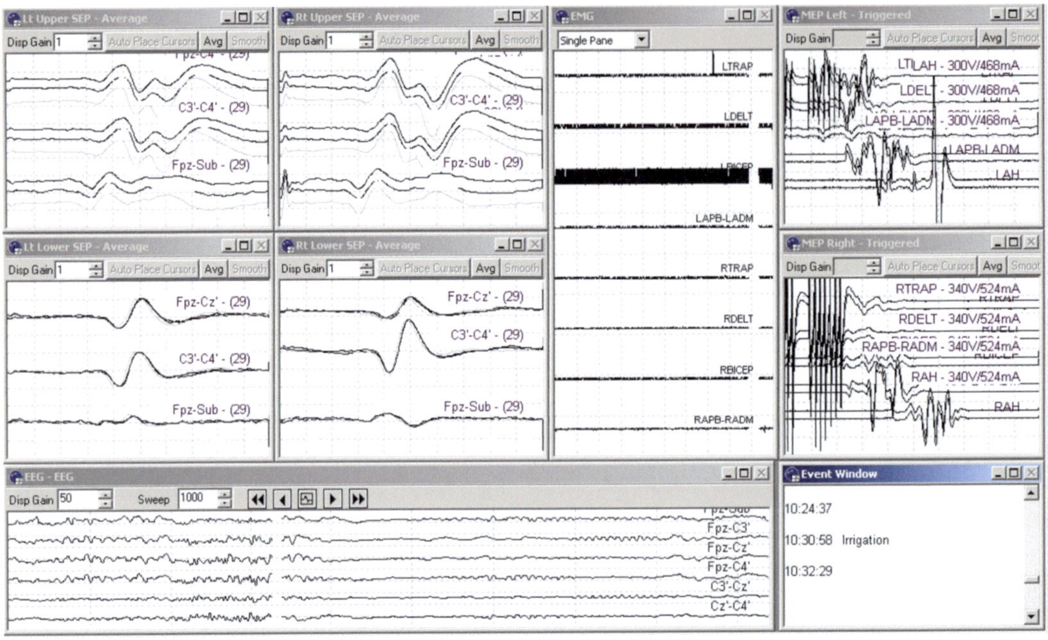

Fig. 38.1 Multimodality monitoring simultaneously assesses four-limb somatosensory evoked potentials, four-limb motor evoked potentials, the multichannel ongoing electromyogram, and several channels of ongoing electroencephalogram. A chat dialog box communicates notes to the remote supervising neurophysiologist. This typical spinal surgery page allows the monitoring team to overview many modalities. Other available screen pages focus on specific modalities in greater detail

Stimulation

Ulnar nerve pathway testing begins with stimulation applied at the wrist. Stimulus intensity of 20–40 mA is above the motor threshold to produce fifth finger abduction. The ulnar nerve is used rather than the median nerve for cervical cases. That is because the ulnar pathway gives more complete cervical spinal cord coverage. Ulnar monitoring can be used in lumbar cases because of the risk of ulnar palsy due to arm positioning [1].

Posterior tibial nerve stimulation is used for lower extremities in many cases. Stimulation is delivered posterior to the medial malleolus. The peroneal nerve also is set up for monitoring patients who have a peripheral neuropathy and diabetes or whose age is greater than 65 years. The peroneal nerve is stimulated where it crosses the fibular head just below the knee. By preparing both nerves, the team can choose which produces the better results. Posterior tibial nerve stimulation produces plantar foot bending. Peroneal nerve stimulation produces foot dorsiflexion. Without the use of neuromuscular junction blockade, these movements can become disruptive during surgery and can limit the stimulus intensity used.

Nerves are stimulated at rates of several per second. Stimulation in older patients often is around 2.5 per second, whereas twice as fast can be used in young patients. Faster rates result in smaller amplitude peaks [2]. Faster stimulation rates produce SEP tracings more quickly. The monitoring team adjusts the rate to find the best "rate vs. amplitude" trade-off. For example, for low amplitude baseline potentials, a typical strategy is slowing the stimulation rate to improve peak amplitudes.

Commonly 300 stimulation repetitions are needed to obtain each evoked potential trial. In some cases, background noise and low amplitude peaks require larger sample sizes, e.g., 500–1000 repetitions. Two minutes is needed to acquire 300 repetitions at a 2.5 stimulation rate producing a new SEP tracing. Electrocautery and other problems can prevent recording and slow this ideal rate of acquiring new tracings.

Recordings

The main recording electrodes are placed at the scalp and neck. Scalp site named locations use the modified 10% extension of the 10/20 system [3]. Extra scalp recording channels are helpful in finding the highest amplitude cortical peaks. Flexibility in scalp recording channels is desirable as opposed to always using a preset recording montage. Individual patients' peaks are seen at different scalp locations because the generator dipoles vary among patients in their geometric orientation on gyri and in sulci. Scouting for best sites early in the case can locate optimal or adequate monitoring channels for an individual patient. The monitoring team should not feel constrained to use a simple cookbook formula to always monitor every patient using the identical simple techniques. An example of monitoring over half an hour is illustrated in Fig. 38.2a.

A cervical recording electrode is placed over the fifth cervical spinous process for thoracolumbar spinal cases. During cervical surgery, a substitute site is the mastoid or ear. A peripheral recording channel may be used over the shoulder, lumbar spine, or popliteal fossa.

The recording low filter usually is set to 30 Hz. The high filter is set between 500 Hz and 1500 Hz. A higher setting records more background noise, whereas a lower setting attenuates the cortical peak amplitude. The notch filter removes the 50 or 60 Hz line noise commonly encountered in the operating room. Unfortunately, SEPs themselves have a 50–60 Hz basic frequency so the notch filter can attenuate the desired SEP peaks. The notch filter also can produce artifact that can mimic SEP peaks. The best tactic to eliminate electrical environmental noise is turning off responsible equipment rather than turning on the notch filter.

Interpreting Changes

Ulnar nerve pathway measurements are the cortical N20 (from the primary somatosensory cortex), the subcortical N18 (midbrain-thalamus), and the cervical N13 (mid-cervical spinal cord) peaks [4]. See Fig. 38.3b. Both latency and amplitude are measured. For posterior tibial or peroneal SEPs, measurement is to the P37 (primary somatosensory cortex) amplitude and latency (Fig. 38.3b). A subcortical P30 (cervicomedullary) peak also may be found in a cervical channel. Classically, a 50% drop in amplitude is considered the criterion for raising an alarm. A 10% increase in latency is a secondary criterion for alarm (Table 38.1).

Amplitude is reduced by anesthesia. Inhalation anesthetics attenuate cortical peak amplitudes. Inhalation agents affect subcortical N18 and P30 peak amplitudes less. Bolus medications transiently affect cortical peak amplitudes, e.g., after a propofol bolus (see Fig. 38.4). Anesthetic fade is the gradual cumulative effect of anesthesia reducing cortical peak amplitudes. For SEPs, fade is more noticeable in the first 40 min after induction.

The monitoring team quickly must decide whether technical problems, surgical problems, or anesthesia or systemic issues caused the observed change. Technical problems include loose electrodes or equipment malfunction. Systemic problems include hypothermia, hypotension, and hypoxia. Anesthesia effects are considered. If no obvious causes are identified, the surgeon and anesthesiologist are alerted.

In response to an alert, the surgeon reviews steps undertaken in the past 20 min. Some surgical maneuvers or actions may take 20 min to alert SEPs. The delay between surgical action and SEP alert may be because of the gradual accumulating physiologic effect of some compression or stretching or more marginal degrees of ischemia or secondary autonomic vasospasm. Many alert responses are available to the surgeon, anesthesiologist, and monitoring team [5]. See Table 38.2 for a summary of certain responses to monitoring alerts.

Clinical Risk of Change

SEP amplitude decreases do not always predict an adverse neurologic outcome. A several minute 50–80% decrease in SEP amplitude poses only a

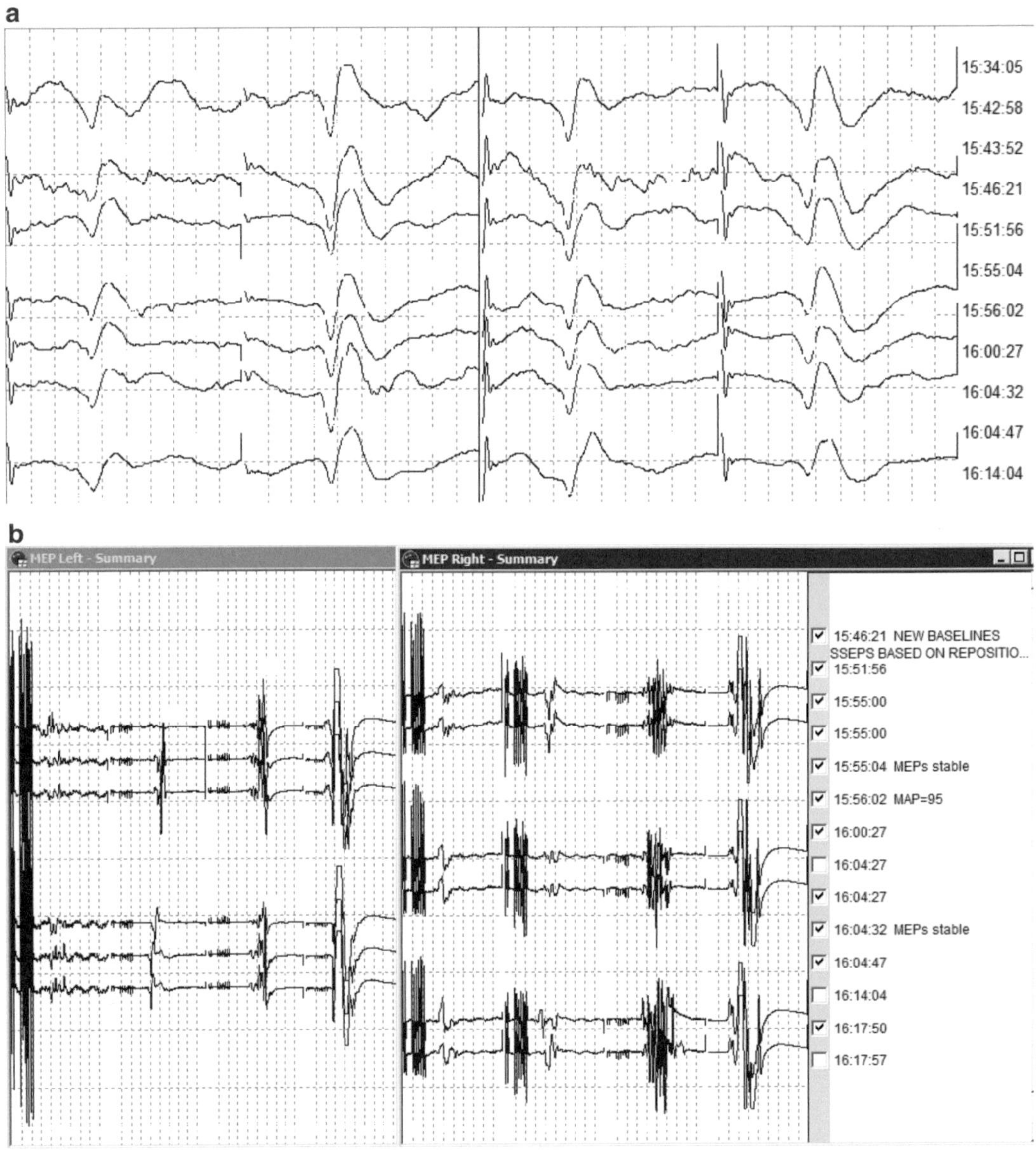

Fig. 38.2 Typical routine reproducible SEPs and MEPs in waterfall displays. (**a**) Posterior tibial nerve SEPs shown with a moderate amount of background variability, 10 ms/div, 0.5 uV/div. (**b**) MEP muscles are abductor halluces (AH), medial gastroc (MG), tibialis anterior (TA), and abductor pollicis brevis (APB), 10 ms/div, 100–1000 uV/div. A stimulus artifact is seen at the beginning of each MEP recording column. The double pulse technique shows in the artifact as the brief first artifact followed by the longer second stimulus artifact

small to modest risk of postoperative deficit. See Fig. 38.5 for an example of tracings. That is true especially if the SEP amplitude subsequently returns to baseline. If SEPs are abruptly completely lost and remain absent for the remainder of the case, the risk of adverse outcome is 50–75%.

Motor Evoked Potentials

Motor evoked potentials (MEPs) monitor corticospinal tracts. This is a particularly important modality because of the importance of preserving

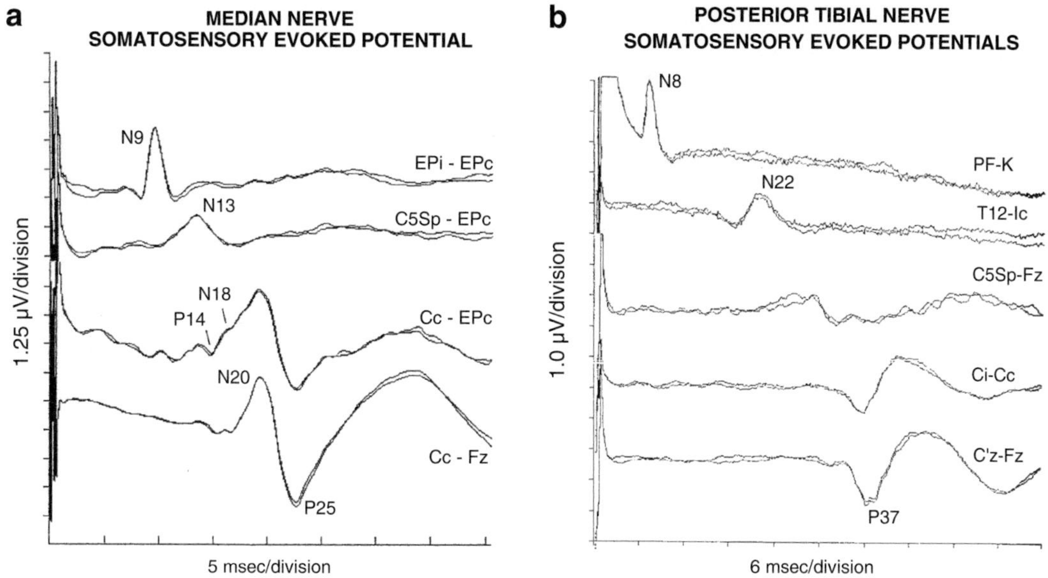

Fig. 38.3 Examples of the peaks seen in normal short latency (**a**) median nerve and (**b**) posterior tibial nerve SEP testing. Negative potentials are upward deflections here. Recording sites EPi and EPc are at shoulders ipsilateral and contralateral to the side stimulated; C5Sp and T12 over the 5th cervical and 12th thoracic spine; PF, K, and IC at the popliteal fossa, knee, and iliac crest; and Ci, Cc, C'z, and Fz on central and frontal scalp. The several standard peaks are identified here From [4]

motor function. MEPs use transcranial electrical (tce) stimulation.

Stimulation

tceMEP electrodes are secured at the scalp near the motor cortex over each hemisphere. An anode electrode is placed 2 cm anterior to C3 or C4 scalp sites, and a cathode electrode is at Cz or CPz, with sites named according to the 10% extension of the 10–20 electrode systems [3]. Sometimes alternate scalp sites obtain better responses.

Stimulus intensity of 200–400 mA usually is adequate. Stronger stimulation sometimes is used as high as 600 mA, which may correspond to 1000–1200 mV. The stimulus pulse width is set to 0.05 ms, with a longer pulse width used if responses are difficult to find.

Single MEP pulses usually fail to produce adequate responses. A brief stimulus train is effective in many patients. Simple pulse trains are five to seven stimuli each separated by a 1.0–3.0 ms interpulse interval. This train builds up excitatory postsynaptic potentials at spinal anterior horn cells. It results in the cell firing an action volley and in recordable tceMEP muscle activity.

Double pulse trains are more effective than simple pulse trains. An initial priming of two to three pulses is followed by an inter-train interval of approximately 10 ms. The second train is like a regular simple pulse train of five to seven pulses. The first train primes anterior horn cells; the second train more effectively discharges the anterior horn cells.

Each tceMEP pulse discharges corticospinal axons in the cerebral hemispheres. Stronger intensities discharge axons in deeper white matter. Strong stimuli can shorten muscle response latencies by discharging corticospinal axons at deeper anatomical levels.

Table 38.1 Intraoperative neuromonitoring alert criteria

Somatosensory evoked potentials			
Stimulation site or type of test	Criteria for change	Which recordings are affected	Common kinds of change
Median or ulnar	50% decrease in amplitude	N20 cortical peak N13, P14 cervical peak	Abrupt, bilateral, peripheral, or anesthesia-related
	10% increase in latency	N20 cortical peak N13, P14 cervical peak	Could be temperature-related
	Completely absent signal	N20 cortical peak N13, P14 cervical peak	Abrupt, bilateral, peripheral, or technical
Posterior tibial or peroneal	50% decrease in amplitude	P37 cortical peak N30 cervical peak	Abrupt, bilateral, peripheral, or anesthesia-related
	10% increase in latency	P37 cortical peak N30 cervical peak	Could be temperature-related
	Completely absent signal	P37 cortical peak N30 cervical peak	Abrupt, bilateral, peripheral, or technical
Motor evoked potentials			
Spinal cord monitoring	Complete loss of MEP	At all or most muscles, two to four in each limb	Lowers only or uppers + lowers
	80% amplitude loss	Excludes peaks small at baseline	
	Polyphasic loss of phases	Measures turns or complexity in recordings	
	Increase of stimulation current >100 V	Subject to anesthetic fade in long cases	
D-waves	50% decrease in amplitude	Loss seen distally, preserved rostrally	Avoid inadvertent movement of electrodes
Electromyography			
Spontaneous	Neurotonic discharge	Muscle recordings associated with a root	Mechanical, thermal, ischemic
	Irritability	Muscle recordings associated with a root	Baseline disorder, mechanical, thermal, ischemic
Triggered EMG	Threshold response in milliamperes	Muscle recordings associated with a root	Assesses medial wall breach or proximity to nerve

Recording

Electrodes in arm and leg muscles record tce-MEP responses. Both proximal and distal limb muscles are often chosen. Distal sites are often more responsive to MEP because of their greater representation of those muscles in the motor cortex. Recording from several sites in each limb is appropriate because good results may appear in one muscle group, whereas only marginally recordable or absent results appear in other muscles. Figure 38.2b illustrates MEPs. At baseline, tce stimulation intensity is gradually increased until adequate muscle recordings are found.

The tceMEP muscle responses are polyphasic complex compound muscle action potentials (CMAPs) at each site. Primary measurement is the CMAP amplitude. Secondary criterion is the complexity of the response in terms of the number of polyphasic turns in the response.

MEPs also can be recorded from the epidural space. These recordings measure axon volleys from the corticospinal cord. This technique, known as *D-wave*, detects direct conduction of the corticospinal track. D-waves are recorded

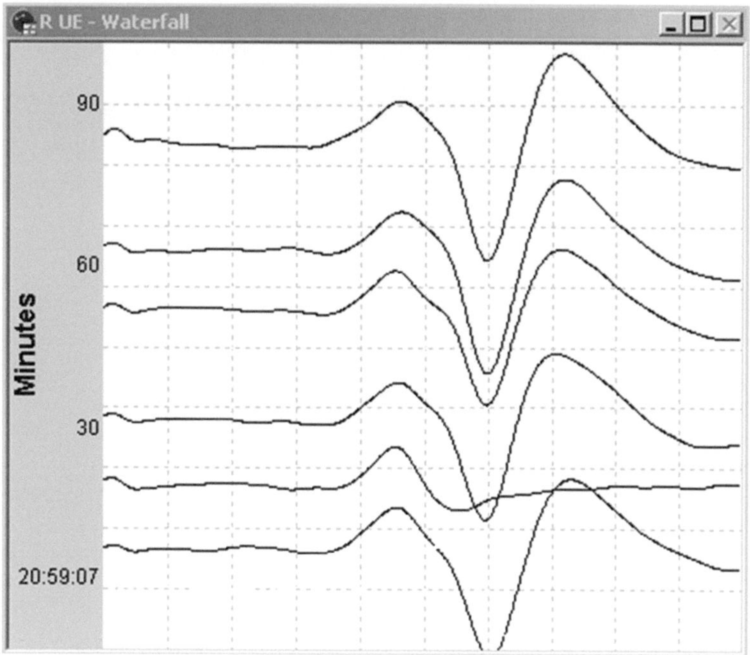

Fig. 38.4 Anesthesia effect: SEP ulnar nerve N20 cortical peaks in a waterfall display. Six tracings are displayed over 75 min. At 20 min before the present time (second trace from the bottom), a tracing shows a sudden drop in N20 cortical peak amplitude. A propofol bolus caused this change

using epidural electrodes either bipolar or with a nearby reference. Since the very small amplitude of D-waves decreases more caudally, they are more easily recorded at cervical and upper thoracic levels.

Safety

MacDonald [6] found few adverse events associated with tceMEP stimulation. Tongue and lip lacerations are occasionally reported. The stimulation activates not only cerebral hemisphere axons but also muscles on the skull surface, resulting in a brisk jaw muscle contraction. A mouth guard is placed as a precaution prior to surgery and checked again after turning the patient prone for spine surgery. Seizures are rare; many teams monitor EEG during tceMEP as a precaution just to check for any adverse EEG discharges associated with stimulation. One should consider monitoring EEG in the case of patients with epilepsy. The electrical field during stimulation fills a small area in the head. It does not spread significantly to the thorax so that metal placed in the neck or thorax is generally considered relatively safe. That includes a cardiac pacemaker, although in that case anesthesiologist should monitor the EKG when MEP stimulation is used. Cardiac arrhythmia is not likely due to tce stimulation which does not significantly travel beyond the head. Minor scalp burns are rare. No spinal epidural recording electrode complications were found for the D-wave technique. Relative contraindications include epilepsy, cortical lesions, convexity skull defects, raised intracranial pressure, cardiac disease, proconvulsant medications or anesthetics, and cardiac pacemakers. Absolute contraindications include intracranial electrodes (e.g., Parkinson's deep brain stimulators) and vascular aneurysm clips. One report suggests that implant devices are not adversely affected by MEP [7]. Unexplained intraoperative seizures and cardiac arrhythmias are relative indications to avoid MEP stimulation. With appropriate precautions, the benefits of MEP monitoring outweigh the associated risks.

Interpretation

Many monitoring teams use all-or-none criteria for MEP alerts due to a tendency for potentials to vary. If the potential is present and then

Table 38.2 Responses to intraoperative monitoring alert

Anesthesia team	Maintain or achieve mean arterial pressure (MAP) above 70 mmHg	Higher MAP if cord already is compressed
	Review anesthesia changes in the past 20 min	
	Review any boluses given	For all drugs administered
	Assess depth of anesthesia	Is EEG burst suppression? Is BIS <45? Consider lightening
	Replace gas agents with TIVA	
	Check hemoglobin/hematocrit	Is Hgb >10 g/dl? Replace if questionable
	Check I/O status	Replace if questionable
	Check blood pressure cuff	If one arm SEP lost
	Check arm position, reposition arm	If one arm SEP lost
	Check train of four	For remaining blockade effects
	Prepare for possible wake-up test	
Monitoring team	Repeat trials of MEPs, SEPs	Rule out false alarms
	Check electrodes, impedances, connections, settings	Evaluate for technical failures
	Check technical settings	Did screen display sensitivities reset? Did stimulus setting reset to *off*?
	Check stimulus artifacts	As same as before the change
	Consider rebooting	If questioning software error
	Increase stimulation intensities, change recording parameters	To reestablish signals, many technical changes may help
	Evaluate the potential effect of anesthesia changes, boluses, MAP, other systemic factors	As clues toward an anesthesia cause
	Review recent subalert SEP and MEP changes	Clues are anesthetic vs. technical vs. clinical-surgical
Surgeon	Stop current manipulation	
	Search for mechanical compression or ischemia	Retractor, hematoma, osteophyte, bone fragment, hardware
	Consider further decompression of spinal cord	If preexisting cord compression
	Reduce spinal column distraction	Especially if recently distracted
	Consider hardware removal	For example, pedicle screws
	Consider imaging	X-ray, CT or MRI
Further action	Increase MAP further	
	Consider wake-up test	Takes time to awaken, especially with propofol
	Pause surgery, await return of signals	Consider abort surgery
	Administer steroids	
	Consider calcium channel blockers	

disappears, that is possibly an alarm. The monitoring team takes into account that muscle response's baseline amplitude because low amplitude, simple responses may disappear just due to anesthesia fade. The monitoring team also takes into account the responses from other muscles in the same limb. If a limb has several muscles with good well-defined MEP responses, the loss of just one may not be of clinical significance. Some variable amplitude changes are common. A small potential may disappear upon anesthesia fade or for no

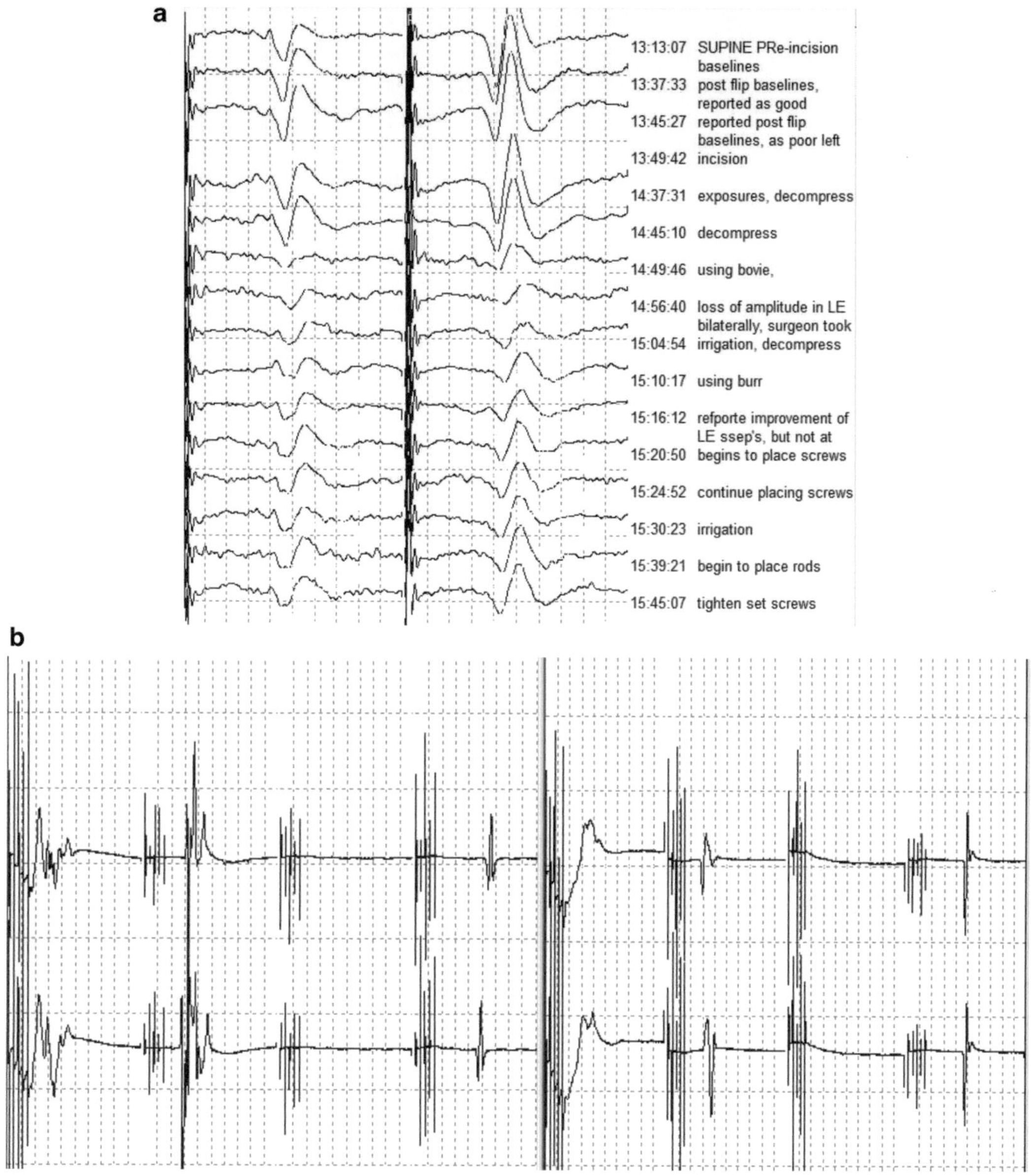

Fig. 38.5 Amplitude loss during a cervical case. The surgeon reported that he bumped the cervical spinal cord. (**a**) Left and right leg SEP cortical peaks decreased abruptly and then partially improved and remained stable. 100 ms/div, 0.5 uV/div. (**b**) Two repetitions of MEP testing just after the event. Prominent stimulus artifacts are present at the start of each recording column. Left and right sided recordings from deltoid, abductor pollicis brevis, and abductor hallucis channels show good, brief responses

particular reason. A sudden loss of all MEPs from several muscles in one limb is a reason for an alert. Sudden loss of all MEPs from both lower extremities is a clear reason for an alert, especially in the absence of an anesthetic reason for the loss.

Other monitoring teams apply a more graded method to assess an alert [8]. In this alternative system, an 80% amplitude loss is considered sufficient to raise an MEP alarm [9, 10]. In another alternative scoring system, the degree of polyphasic turns in the MEP tracing is counted.

For example, an alert may be raised if a polyphasic response becomes simplified to just two phases. See Fig. 38.8 for an example of a case in which an 80% loss of MEPs guided clinical decision-making. Some teams increase the transcranial current until a motor response is found. An increase more than 100 mA from the baseline threshold is the criterion to raise an alarm [11]. When monitoring D-waves along with tceMEPs in intramedullary tumor resection, relatively stable D-waves predict good motor outcome even if MEPs are lost [12, 13]. A formula combining loss of phases, loss of amplitude, delayed latency, and other parameters may be more stable and more predictable than any one parameter alone [14], although this formula is not yet available on most commercial equipment.

Anesthesia plays a significant role in the ability to obtain MEPs. Classically, total intravenous anesthesia (TIVA) was required, and neuromuscular blockade must be avoided. Neither of those ideal requirements is completely true. Some inhalation anesthesia can be tolerated, especially in younger patients with robust baseline MEPs and no preexisting neurologic conditions. Inhalation anesthesia may be poorly tolerated among older patients with preexisting neurologic conditions, e.g., elderly patients with cervical myelopathy. A continuous low-dose drip of neuromuscular blockade, one that still allows three of four responses on the train of four test, can temper the excess MEP body movement.

D-waves persist despite neuromuscular junction blockade, since they are direct recordings of spinal axon volleys. Recording electrode movement during surgery can attenuate them. They can be used along with tceMEPs. When neuromuscular blockade is required, they offer a possible method for following motor pathways.

Anesthetic fade, as was mentioned for SEP, is the gradual cumulative effect of anesthesia reducing peak amplitudes. For MEPs, anesthetic fade is more noticeable as the case proceeds over hours. Peaks that start as low amplitude, simple MEP muscle responses may be expected to disappear over hours due to anesthetic fade.

The clinical decision to raise a tceMEP alert can be complex. The decision integrates which muscles changed, how many muscles changed, the loss of phases or degree of amplitude change (80% loss vs. total loss), how robust were baseline recordings in those muscles, whether anesthesia fade is occurring, whether inhalation anesthesia has increased, and whether a bolus of centrally active medication recently was given.

Electromyography

EMG can monitor peripheral motor pathways from the limbs or trunk during surgery. EMG monitoring can check for neurotonic discharges, or A-trains, which are signs of nerve injury [6]. Lesser degrees of nerve irritation produce motor unit CMAP discharges seen in the EMG recordings. EMG is also used to assess placement of pedicle screws or passage of a dilator through psoas muscle. EMG monitoring is conducted in the absence of neuromuscular blockade or with minimal continuous drip blockade with three of four responses in train of four testing. EMG monitoring tests motor pathways, but not sensory or autonomic function.

Recordings

Needle electrodes are inserted into muscles innervated by roots, nerves, or spinal levels at risk during surgery. Electrodes are uninsulated over an extended portion of the needle shaft, unlike traditional needle electrodes used in outpatient EMG diagnostic testing. Recordings are monitored in real time. High-frequency filters are set to 3 k–10 kHz.

Many channels are used, one for each muscle recorded. Often ten or more muscles are monitored, e.g., five from each limb on the left and right side at the level of surgery. Proximal and distal muscles are chosen, and muscles should represent the regions at risk in the particular surgery. In the cervical region, EMG is covered through muscles across the relevant root levels which often include recording sites chosen from among trapezius, deltoid, biceps, triceps, brachioradialis, flexor carpi ulnaris, flexor carpi radialis, abductor pollicis, and abductor digiti minimi. It is more difficult to monitor the upper thoracic region with EMG, but electrodes carefully inserted in intercostal muscles or placed in paraspinal muscles are sometimes used. For monitoring for the T6 through L1 levels, the rectus abdominal muscles are monitored typically with electrodes placed at upper, middle, and lower abdominal levels. In the lumbosacral region, EMG is covered through muscles across the relevant root levels which often include recording sites chosen from among iliopsoas, quadriceps, adductor magnus, biceps femoris, tibialis anterior, medial gastroc, extensor digitorum brevis, and flexor hallucis. Needle electrodes in the anal sphincter sometimes are added when the conus or cauda equina region is included in the surgical region. Vocal cords are monitored with surface electrodes, instead of needle electrodes, which are attached to the sides of the endotracheal tube when the recurrent laryngeal nerve is at risk in cervical surgery.

Triggered EMG

Pedicle screw testing is performed to assess if the screw is placed correctly. If the medial wall is breached, the screw can injure a nerve or the spinal cord. To use EMG as a placement aid, the walls of the guide hole and the screw itself can be stimulated electrically. If the guide hole wall is breached or the screw breaches the medial pedicle wall, low-intensity electrical stimulation will stimulate a nearby nerve or the spinal cord. Nerve stimulation results in EMG discharges from muscles in that dermatome. Pedicle screws are stimulated at constant current up to 20–25 mA in lumbar levels. Stimulation at upper thoracic levels may be conducted up to 15 mA, a lower intensity because the tested bone is thinner. Triggered EMG for cervical instrumentation may be used at lower intensity levels still.

Stimulation of pedicle screw may fail in several circumstances. The screw itself may be unsuitable for stimulation studies. Some screws are coated with hydroxyapatite to help bone ingrowth and osseointegration into the screw. The hydroxyapatite coating is an electrical insulator. Other screws are titanium and have been anodized which produces an electrically insulating titanium oxide coating. Both hydroxyapatite and titanium oxide impede adequate electrical conduction from the screw during stimulation studies. A polyaxial screw construct, i.e., when the mobile head is not firmly connected to the shank, causes a gap where electrical conduction may not bridge the gap. Testing electrical stimulation at the head will not necessarily give correct results about a wall breach.

Pedicle screw stimulation is about 85% accurate at generating an EMG response when a medial wall breach occurs [15]. That is well below the ideal 100% sensitivity. Some failures are due to screw deficiencies. Chronically injured nerves are more difficult to make respond to electrical stimulation, and some are silent despite a breach. Sometimes the NIOM team does not monitor the correct muscles, or suitable muscles are not readily available, e.g., around L1 or at upper thoracic.

Stimulation also can be delivered through a dilator as it is passed through the psoas muscle during a lateral transpsoas approach to the lumbar spine in minimally invasive procedures. The goal is to identify nerves adjacent to the dilator tip and to avoid damage to the nerve if the dilator were to be advanced.

Interpretation

EMG recordings are monitored continuously in real time. During the baseline portion of the procedure, any ongoing irregular background CMAP activity is observed. Baseline ongoing activity may result from the pathophysiology that is the reason for the surgery, e.g., radiculopathy. EMG channels usually are silent during the baseline recording. When a surgeon causes mechanical compression or stretches a nerve or root, such as placing a retractor too close to a nerve, a series of CMAPs may be seen. A greater degree of compression or stretching can result in a continuous

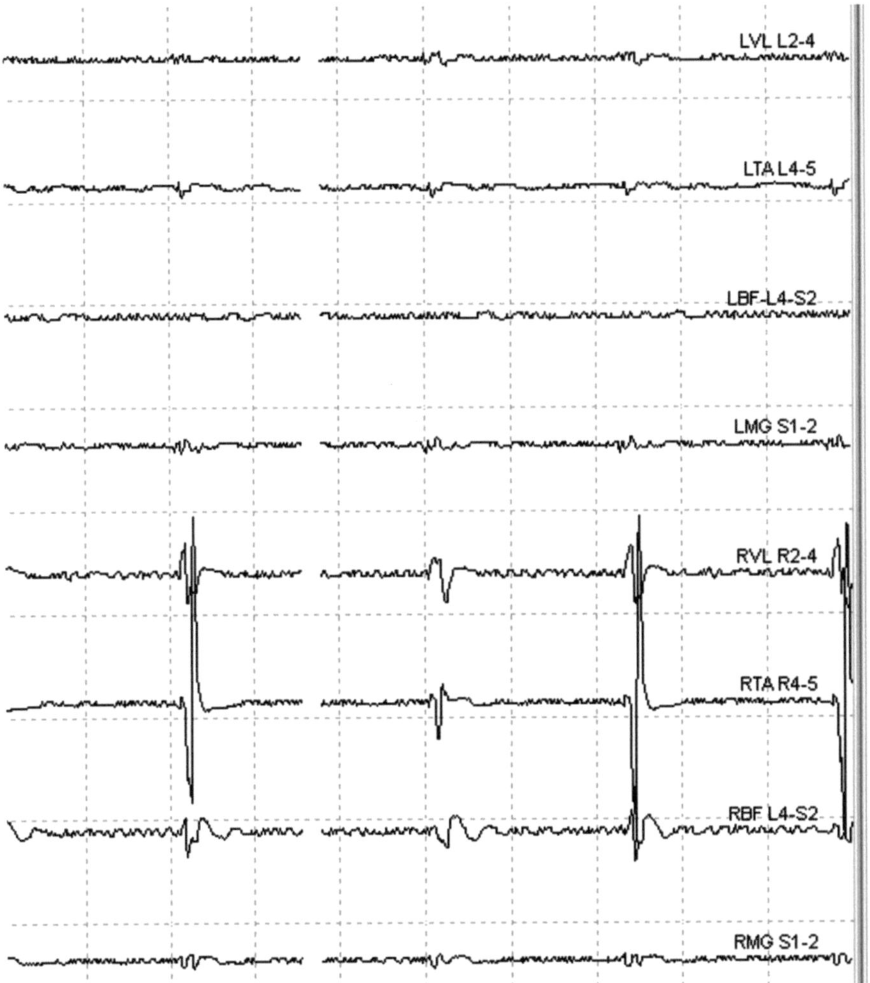

Fig. 38.6 Electrical stimulations were applied to the right L4 pedicle screw at 8 mA. Responses are seen at the right vastus lateralis, tibialis anterior, and biceps femoris muscles. This 68-year-old woman had a left L3–L4 lateral transpsoas approach for lumbar stenosis followed by posterior spinal fusion with instrumentation. This suggested a medial pedicle wall breach. 150 ms/div, 200 uV/div

EMG interference pattern. A classical sign of more acute irritation or injury is a neurotonic discharge, or A-train, a dense high-frequency EMG discharge often lasting 30–45 s [16].

Pedicle screws are stimulated at constant current of up to 20 mA for lumbar and lower intensities at more rostral levels. Figure 38.6 illustrates an example of a recording during pedicle screw testing. In clinical settings a stimulus intensity threshold is checked. At lumbar and lower thoracic spinal levels, a threshold 10 mA is generally considered adequate. A threshold of 5 mA or lower is considered a sign of a wall breach. Values for thresholds are lower for higher spinal levels, i.e., cervical spine. Osteoporosis also produces lower thresholds through poorly mineralized bone. If a testing suggests that a screw is malpositioned, then the surgeon can reposition it. Checking the guide hole before screw placement is often undertaken as a safety precaution at the surgeon's option.

EMG monitoring detects most, but not all, nerve injuries. Signs of nerve injury can appear transiently. If not watched consistently, a neurotonic

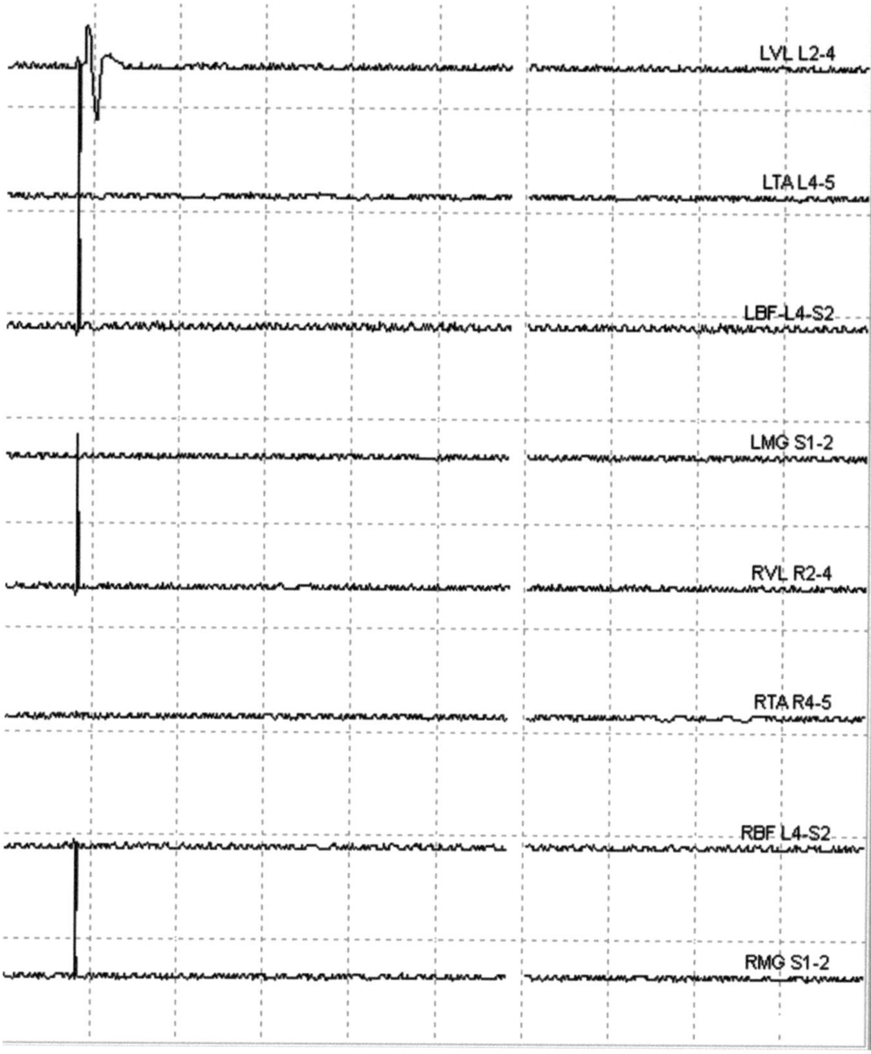

Fig. 38.7 Stimulation is delivered through a lateral transpsoas dilator at 7 mA intensity. This 68-year-old woman had a left L3–L4 lateral transpsoas procedure for lumbar stenosis. Muscles tested are vastus lateralis, tibialis anterior, biceps femoris, and medial gastroc. The stimulus artifact is seen in several channels, followed by an EMG discharge in the left vastus lateralis channel. A small response also had been seen in the left tibialis anterior channel. This showed proximity to an L4 nerve root. 500 ms/div, 200 uV/div

discharge can appear briefly, disappear, and be overlooked by the monitoring technologist and physician. Not all nerve injuries produce an EMG discharge. A nerve might be cleanly cut but generate no discharges [17]. A chronically compressed nerve is not so sensitive for generating discharges. Since compressed or chronically injured nerves are the ones for which surgery most often is undertaken, EMG monitoring fails to detect some compressive, mechanical, or ischemic nerve injuries. EMG monitoring is useful because it detects most nerve injuries, even though it fails to detect about 15%.

For lateral transpsoas dilator stimulation, stimulations should not produce muscle responses except for the local direct response of psoas itself. Figure 38.7 illustrates muscle responses recorded during dilator stimulation. A sufficient group of muscles should be monitored relevant to the level through which the dilator is passed, recognizing that nerves from higher lumbar level also may be encountered. Monitoring from too few muscles may miss relevant responses. This technique assesses monitored motor pathways only, but not sensory or autonomic nerves. The dilator is stimulated and responses sought repeatedly as the instrument tip is advanced in small increments. The less current needed to trigger a muscle response, the closer the dilator is to the motor nerve in question.

Spinal Cord Monitoring

SEP and MEP techniques monitor the spinal cord. SEP and MEP often are used together. SEP monitors continuously, whereas MEP is tested intermittently as needed. MEP carries disadvantages such as stimulation-related movement and restrictions on inhalation agents. For reasons such as those, some cases are monitored with SEP alone.

False alerts are false-positive monitoring events, i.e., alerts without postoperative neurological deficits. Many may be true detections of neurologic risk which averted a postoperative deficit because the surgeon responded. Those could be called true save events. Methodologically one cannot differentiate between false alerts and true saves. Investigations in animal models show that failure to respond to SEP alerts carries a high risk of an adverse postoperative deficit [18–23]. Similarly, in those studies, responding to alerts prevents postoperative deficits. Such literature supports strongly the conclusion that NIOM alerts are effective in reducing adverse postoperative outcomes.

False-negative monitoring is the highly undesirable outcome when the patient awakens with a new neurologic deficit despite no NIOM alert. NIOM false-negative events are very rare during spinal cord monitoring [24] (Table 38.3).

Table 38.3 Neurologic outcome prediction rates for SEP monitoring in spinal surgery

Total procedures monitored	51,263	(100%)
False-negative (FN) rate: neurologic postoperative deficits despite stable SEPs		
Definite	34	(0.063%)
Equivocal	13	(0.025%)
Delayed onset	18	(0.035%)
Total	65	(0.127%)
False-positive rate: no neurologic deficits despite SEP changes		
Definite	504	(0.983%)
Equivocal	270	(0.527%)
Total	774	(1.510%)
True-positive (TP) rate: neurologic deficits predicted by SEP changes		
Definite	150	(0.293%)
Equivocal	67	(0.131%)
Total	217	(0.423%)
Neurologic deficits (FN plus TP)		
Definite	184	(0.356%)
Equivocal	80	(0.156%)
Delayed onset	18	(0.035%)
Total	282	(0.550%)
True-negative rate: no neurologic deficit and stable SEPs		
Total	50,207	(97.94%)

These data are from the multicenter outcome study of SEP spinal cord monitoring by 153 US surgeons [11]. Note the very low rate of definite false-negative cases (0.063%). Equivocal cases were transient or minor degrees of impairment. Delayed onset cases awoke from surgery intact but developed impairment within the first day postoperatively

SEPs and MEPs in clinical practice detect spinal cord impairment relatively early in the course of complications. The clinical alerts occur early enough to avert many deficits. The American Academy of Neurology and American Clinical Neurophysiology Society published an evidence-based assessment of NIOM spinal cord monitoring [25]. That assessment included Class 1 and 2 studies of MEP and SEP alerts [26–37]. The joint assessment concluded, based on the published evidence, that NIOM is established as effective to predict an increased risk of the adverse outcomes of paraparesis, paraplegia, and quadriplegia in spinal surgery. The assessment went on to recommend interventions to attempt to reduce the risk of adverse neurologic outcomes when alerts occur.

A large multicenter study [24] evaluated more than 100,000 spinal surgery cases. Surgical outcomes over 7 years for a cohort of 184 surgeons were tracked, among which half the cases were monitored. Outcomes compared cases with and without monitoring and compared monitored cases against historical controls for the same cohort. Monitoring was associated with a 60% reduction in paraparesis and paraplegia. False-negative cases were very rare, less than 0.1%.

More recent evidence-based outcome studies continue to find similar diagnostic and prognostic reliability for SEP and tceMEP spinal cord monitoring. Kobayashi [10] found two false-negative SEP and tceMEP monitoring cases during surgery for intramedullary spinal cord tumors. He found a high sensitivity (95%) and specificity (91%) for intraoperative spinal cord monitoring and favorable accuracy especially for spinal cord tumor, spinal deformity, and ossification of the posterior longitudinal ligament (OPLL). Pastorelli [38] found 100% sensitivity and 98% specificity for spinal deformity surgery. Lee and colleagues [39] found excellent sensitivity and specificity and yet noted C5 palsy cases with weakness onset hours after surgery. Monitoring cannot accurately predict impairment with a future onset.

Sala [13] used historical controls and assessed motor exam changes with McCormick grading. The aggregate motor ability grade improved +0.28 in monitored patients, whereas without monitoring it deteriorated to –0.16 ($p < 0.002$).

Studies have assessed both SEP and MEP, but no definitive comparison has been done. Each monitors a different spinal pathway. SEP can be performed continuously, whereas MEPs are intermittent. MEP produces movements, so some surgeons use them sparingly. Some reports show MEP changing a few minutes before SEPs during alerts, if the MEPs were done at just the right time.

Staffing

NIOM requires a knowledgeable, experienced team both for the technical skills and for the clinical interpretations. Staffing NIOM services includes three individuals with different kinds of skills, knowledge, ability, training, and experience: (a) In the operating room, a technologist runs the equipment and applies the electrodes. If the monitoring professional is remote, the technologist arranges for Internet connectivity and assists with communication. A trained, certified EEG technologist usually fills this role. The recognized US national technologist's certificate is *Certified in Neurophysiologic Intraoperative Monitoring* (CNIM). (b) A professional with substantial knowledge, training, and experience in intraoperative monitoring assists the technologist in decision-making and problem solving and helps train technologists to perform their jobs well. (c) A licensed physician, knowledgeable about both neurophysiology and medicine, continuously monitors the findings, makes determinations about alerts, and discusses the meaning of the changes. The physician is in the best position to recommend changes in anesthesia, surgery, wake-up testing, or medical interventions. The physician integrates NIOM findings with the patient's medical history. The physician provides medical quality assurance. Among these three positions described above, one person may fill more than one role. For example, some physicians serve both the second and third roles when they are sufficiently expert in NIOM. Sometimes a highly skilled nonphysician PhD neurophysiologist fills the second role, while a physician fills the third role.

In general, neither the operating surgeon nor the anesthesiologist is charged with interpreting and problem solving the neurophysiologic monitoring. Rather, a third physician neurophysiologist carries out that service, one who is able to devote full attention to problems that require detailed time and effort. Many cases involve such decision-making to judge whether developing changes require an alert to the surgeon, modify tactics to meet the individual patient's clinical circumstances, integrate findings with anesthetic and surgical events, improve quality of recordings, eliminate artifacts, or overcome technical problems. The physician neurophysiologist has extended special training in clinical neurophysiology and intraoperative monitoring. That brings to the case the knowledge about the monitoring literature and lore, ability to communicate effectively, skills at technological tricks to improve recordings, and experience with many events as they may occur during cases.

The monitoring neurophysiology physician may be outside the operating room supervising remotely [40]. Continuous communication with the operating room is needed. The simple remote monitoring method screen displays only what the technologist selects on the operating room equipment screen. Advanced remote monitoring method allows the neurophysiologist to change among various screens and to manipulate the data. This advanced method allows the monitoring physician to monitor at his or her discretion all aspects of the case rather than being simply dependent on the technologist to display one aspect. The advanced method is desirable because it allows for an independent assessment of multiple aspects of data and different views of an evolving clinical situation.

Alternative models to traditional monitoring include (a) automated monitoring, (b) surgeon-directed monitoring, (c) technologist-directed monitoring, and (d) proctored monitoring. Automated monitoring deploys a computer algorithm to search recorded signals, score peaks for desired criteria, and identify if alert criteria are met. No person checks the computer's answer, and the data itself may not be readily accessible for an expert's review. Surgeon-directed monitoring has the disadvantage that the surgeon is generally not trained in the technical details, problem solving, artifact elimination, tactics for improving recording quality, or the monitoring literature and lore. The surgeon is too busy to pay ongoing attention to the tracings. Technologist-directed monitoring without a neurophysiologist supervisor has the disadvantage that many technologists are not familiar with the literature in the monitoring field, not in a position to answer questions about why signals changed, and often monitor in a simple cookbook fashion. Unsupervised technologists do mistake real clinical changes for technical problems and may fail to raise timely alerts.

Proctoring differs from traditional active monitoring by the dilution effect of divided attention. The proctoring physician may supervise many online cases simultaneously, e.g., up to six or ten at a time. Attention is divided among all those cases. The proctoring physician relies on the technologist to screen for significant events and to bring them to the physician's attention. When events or problems occur, the technologist asks for the physician's advice or intervention. In contrast, the traditional active monitoring neurophysiology physician supervises few cases, e.g., one to three at a time [41]. In the traditional monitoring model, the neurophysiology physician gives substantial attention to each case. The monitoring physician is actively involved with each case and identifies changes that the technologist may have missed. This brings to the case a professional level of attention and decision-making. Whenever a physician is supervising remotely more than one case, he or she must be able to turn over the additional cases to a colleague when one case requires individual attention.

In one study of common practices [40], physicians who monitored at their local hospitals typically supervised one case and one-quarter of the time supervised two or three simultaneous cases. For monitoring remotely at multiple distant hospitals, one-quarter of the time physicians supervised four or more simultaneous cases. During busier portions of the workday, that remote distant caseload could exceed six simultaneous cases.

An unfortunate example of surgeon-directed monitoring was published. The case claimed to show a failure of MEP spinal cord monitoring [42]. The authors reported a thoracic case in which upper extremity MEPs disappeared, whereas lower extremity MEPs were preserved. The patient awoke paraplegic. The authors reported this as a false-negative MEP monitoring. Figures showed that the authors were unaware that they had mixed up the arms and the legs in their technical setup. The case actually was a true-positive MEP alert, not a false-negative lack of change. No neurophysiology team was used to assist the surgeon for reviewing the setup and data. An important lesson is that neurophysiology teams are needed, ones with the substantial skills, knowledge, ability, training, and experience in monitoring to set up, recognize, and correctly interpret monitoring tracings.

Multiple spinal pathways and tests can be monitored at the same time. The monitoring team displays ongoing status for multiple monitored tests on a single screen simultaneously. Figure 38.1 shows a combined display of somatosensory, motor, EMG, and EEG channels. The monitoring physician can also change the view to other screens as desired to view detailed trends for individual modalities which display data over hours on particular channels.

Illustrative Case

A 30 M was admitted with traumatic cervical fractures, subluxation, and cord compression. He had trauma also to his head, chest, and abdomen. He arrived at the emergency department on a backboard. On exam he was alert, his power was 5/5 in all extremities, sensation was intact C5-T1 and L2-S1, and DTRs were normal with downgoing toes. Imaging showed left C5 facet fracture, subluxed right C5 facet, kyphotic deformity, anterolisthesis of C5 on C6, and mild cord compression.

After initial treatment with cervical traction, he was brought to the operating room for instrumented fusion. At the time of positioning on the table, baseline MEPs and SEPs were robust. Upon prone positioning, SEPs and MEPs lost 80–90% amplitudes. See Fig. 38.8. The surgeon was alerted, and the patient was returned to the supine position. Upon returning to supine position, the MEPs and SEPs returned to baseline. After 10–15 min of normal SEPs and MEPs, prone positioning again was attempted with the same extensive signal attenuation. The patient again was returned to the supine position. A wake-up test showed that the patient was able to move all extremities. The surgery was postponed. Patient was taken to the ICU in a halo brace. Imaging revealed good spinal alignment. The patient was brought back to the OR 2 days later for spinal fusion. On that second date, the monitoring showed no significant events and remained at the normal baseline. The surgery proceeded without incident, and he was discharged neurologically intact.

Technical Pearls

- Set up both peroneal and posterior tibial nerves for lower extremity SEPs in patients who:
  - Are older than 65 years
  - Have diabetes
  - Have a peripheral neuropathy
- Use alternate scalp recording sites if scalp signals are small.
- Set up foot and leg MEP channels in cervical cases along with arm and hand channels.
- Set up for EMG at least five muscles in arms for cervical and at least five muscles in legs for lumbar cases.
- For upper lumbar cases, consider including iliopsoas muscle for MEPs.
- Slow the SEP stimulus repetition rate to improve amplitude in small signals.
- Increase the SEP stimulus repetition rate to obtain results faster when signals are high amplitude.
- Avoid using the notch filter with SEP and MEP because it can produce ringing artifacts and reduce SEP amplitudes.
- Expect anesthetic fade over long cases, and avoid false alarm alerts based on this attenuation.

Complications and Strategies for Avoidance

- Tongue and lip bites are avoided with well-placed MEP bite blocks; check they don't dislodge with prone positioning.
- To avoid burns, use ground plates instead of needle ground leads.
- Secure leads well to avoid dislodging electrodes, e.g., during position changes and table movement.
- Take care to avoid needle sticks when turning patients; consider placing some needle electrodes after positioning.
- Record some EEG channels along with MEPs to identify any nonconvulsive seizures resulting from stimulation.
- Avoid MEP stimulation adjacent to deep brain stimulation electrode implantation sites or

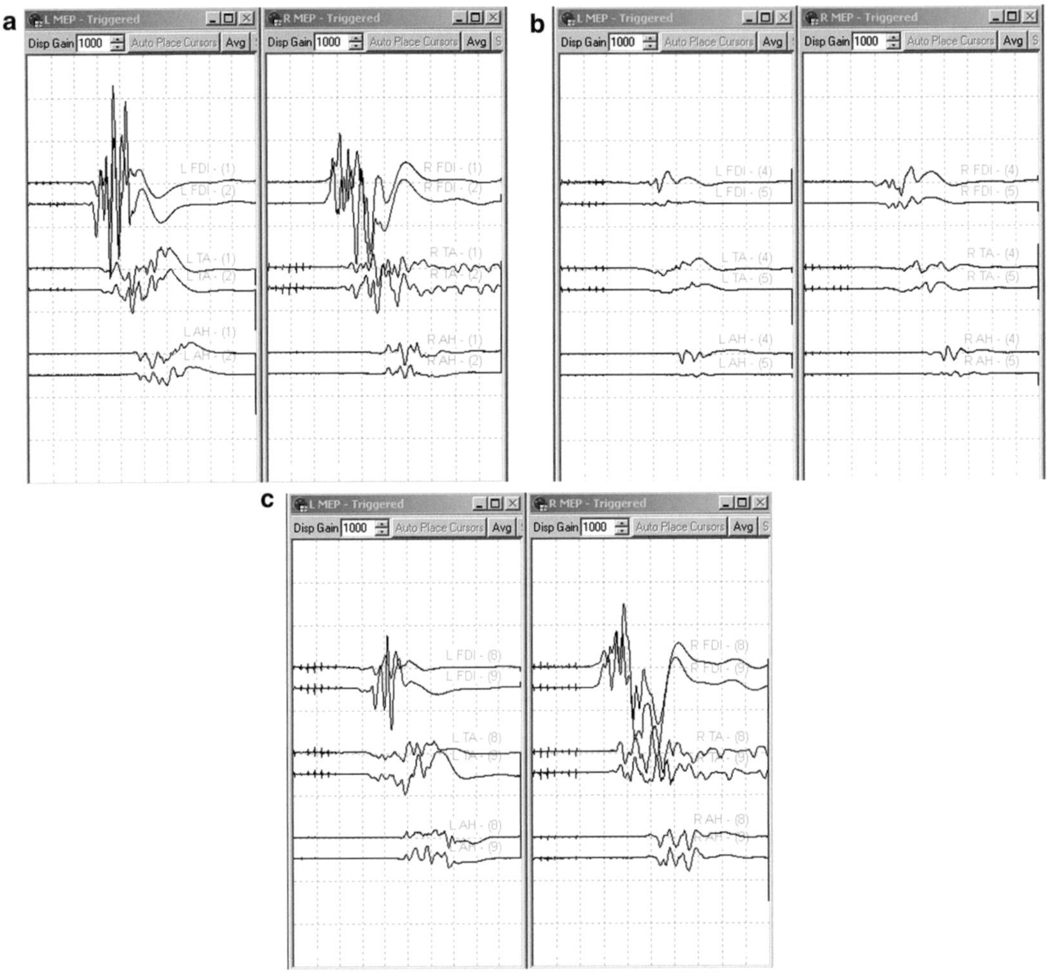

Fig. 38.8 (**a**) Baseline supine, left on left, right on right, pairs of MEP stimulations at flexor digiti minimi, tibialis anterior, and abductor hallucis muscles. (**b**) Upon prone positioning, MEPs lost 80% amplitudes. The SEPs also lost >75% amplitudes (not shown). (**c**) Upon returning to the supine position, the potentials returned to close to baseline, no longer in an alert status

other brain electrode implantation sites. Cochlear implants have been shown to be safe for MEPs.

- Avoid pedicle screws with hydroxyapatite or anodized coating or a polyaxial screw construct, because they may conduct electrical testing poorly and give false results in triggered EMG testing.
- Use ulnar SEPs in lumbar cases to check for impending nerve palsy from arm and shoulder position problems. When a unilateral peripheral ulnar SEP is lost, reposition the arm and shoulder, adjust taping, deflate the BP cuff, and check stimulating electrodes.
- Avoid "automated" SEP and MEP interpretation software, which are subject to "interpretation" errors.
- Monitoring technologist should remain in the room attending to your case, screening the data for technical and clinical changes. The technologist should not cover multiple cases simultaneously. Absence of a technologist can miss critical changes and leave no one to respond to technical problems.

- Monitoring neurophysiology physician may be remote. The physician should avoid simultaneously supervising too many cases. Divided attention causes lack of attention to detail, which can result in delay identifying critical changes. Attention to detail for an individual case drops off when simultaneously monitoring. Surgeons should ask that their monitoring physicians limit the number of simultaneous cases or at least be aware of how many other cases are being monitored.

Conclusion

Intraoperative neurophysiologic monitoring involves SEP, MEP, and EMG. In experienced hands, monitoring reduces the risk of postoperative adverse neurologic outcomes, e.g., reducing by 60% the risk of paraplegia and paraparesis. SEP is continuous, whereas MEP is performed intermittently. Both constrain the choice of anesthesia, MEP more than SEP. Pedicle screw testing with EMG is moderately successful in detecting medial wall breach, but occasional breach or nerve impingement can be undetected for a variety of reasons described here. The monitoring team requires a technologist in the room and a neurophysiology physician supervisor who can be remote. A variety of tactics are now well known for obtaining good recordings in a surgical setting. Limits of normal variability have been established as alarm levels for alerting the surgeon.

References

1. Schwartz DM, Sestokas AK, Hilibrand AS, Vaccaro AR, Bose B, Li M, Albert TJ. Neurophysiological identification of position-induced neurologic injury during anterior cervical spine surgery. J Clin Monit Comput. 2006;20(6):437–44.
2. Nuwer MR, Dawson EG. Intraoperative evoked potential monitoring of the spinal cord: enhanced stability of cortical recordings. Electroencephalogr Clin Neurophysiol. 1984;59:318–27.
3. Nuwer MR, Comi G, Emerson R, Fuglsang-Frederiksen A, Guérit JM, Hinrichs H, Ikeda A, Luccas FJC, Rappelsberger PIFCN. Standards for digital recording of clinical EEG. Electroencephalogr Clin Neurophysiol. 1998;106:259–61.
4. Nuwer MR, Aminoff M, Desmedt J, et al. IFCN recommended standards for short latency somatosensory evoked potentials. Electroencephalogr Clin Neurophysiol. 1994;91:6–11.
5. Ziewacz JE, Berven SH, Mummaneni VP, Tu T-H, Akinbo OC, Lyon R, Mummaneni PV. The design, development, and implementation of a checklist for intraoperative neuromonitoring changes. Neurosurg Focus. 2012;33:1–10.
6. MacDonald DB. Safety of intraoperative transcranial electrical stimulation motor evoked potential monitoring. J Clin Neurophysiol. 2002;19:416–29.
7. Yellin JL, Wiggins CR, Franco AJ, Sankar WN. Safe transcranial electric stimulation motor evoked potential monitoring during posterior spinal fusion in two patients with cochlear implants. J Clin Monit Comput. 2016;30:503–6.
8. MacDonald DB. Overview on criteria for MEP monitoring. J Clin Neurophysiol. 2017;34:4–11.
9. Journée HL, Berends HI, Kruyt MC. The percentage of amplitude decrease warning criteria for transcranial MEP monitoring. J Clin Neurophysiol. 2017;34:22–31.
10. Kobayashi S, Matsuyama Y, Shinomiya K, et al. A new alarm point of transcranial electrical stimulation motor evoked potentials for intraoperative spinal cord monitoring: a prospective multicenter study from the spinal cord monitoring working Group of the Japanese Society for spine surgery and related research. J Neurosurg Spine. 2014;20:102–7.
11. Calancie B. Intraoperative neuromonitoring and alarm criteria for judging MEP responses to transcranial electric stimulation: the threshold-level method. J Clin Neurophsiol. 2017;34:12–21.
12. Kothbauer KF. The interpretation of muscle motor evoked potentials for spinal cord monitoring. J Clin Neurophysiol. 2017;34:32–7.
13. Sala F, Palandri G, Basso E, et al. Motor evoked potential monitoring improves outcome after surgery for intramedullary spinal cord tumors: a historical control study. Neurosurgery. 2006;58:1129–43.
14. Segura MJ, Talarico ME, Noel MA. A multiparametric alarm criterion for motor evoked potential monitoring during spine deformity surgery. J Clin Neurophysiol. 2017;34:38–48.
15. Mikula AL, Williams SK, Anderson PA. The use of intraoperative triggered electromyography to detect misplaced pedicle screws: a systematic review and meta-analysis. J Neurosurg Spine. 2016;24:624–38.
16. Daube JR, Harper CM. Surgical monitoring of cranial and peripheral nerves. In: Desmedt JE, editor. Neuromonitoring in surgery. Amsterdam: Elsevier; 1989. p. 115–38.
17. Crum BA, Strommen JA. Peripheral nerve stimulation and monitoring during operative procedures. Muscle Nerve. 2007;35:159–70.
18. Coles JG, Wilson GJ, Sima AF, Klement P, Tait GA. Intraoperative detection of spinal cord ischemia using somatosensory cortical evoked potentials during thoracic aortic occlusion. Ann Thorac Surg. 1982;34:299–306.

19. Kojima Y, Yamamoto T, Ogino H, Okada K, Ono K. Evoked spinal potentials as a monitor of spinal cord viability. Spine. 1979;4:471–7.
20. Laschinger JC, Cunningham JN Jr, Catinella FP, Nathan IM, Knopp EA, Spencer FC. Detection and prevention of intraoperative spinal cord ischemia after cross-clamping of the thoracic aorta: use of somatosensory evoked potentials. Surgery. 1982;92:1109–17.
21. Cheng MK, Robertson C, Grossman RG, Foltz R, Williams V. Neurological outcome correlated with spinal evoked potentials in a spinal cord ischemia model. J Neurosurg. 1984;60:786–95.
22. Nordwall A, Axelgaard J, Harada Y, Valencia P, McNeal DR, Brown JC. Spinal cord monitoring using evoked potentials recorded from feline vertebral bone. Spine. 1979;4:486–94.
23. Bennett MH. Effects of compression and ischemia on spinal cord evoked potentials. Exp Neurol. 1983;80:508–19.
24. Nuwer MR, Dawson EG, Carlson LG, Kanim LEA, Sherman JE. Somatosensory evoked potential spinal cord monitoring reduces neurologic deficits after scoliosis surgery: results of a large multicenter survey. Electroencephalogr Clin Neurophysiol. 1995;96:6–11.
25. Nuwer MR, Emerson RG, Galloway G, Legatt AD, Lopez J, Minahan R, Yamada T, Goodin DS, Armon C, Chaudhry V, Gronseth GS, Harden CL. Evidence-based guideline update: intraoperative spinal monitoring with somatosensory and transcranial electrical motor evoked potentials. J Clin Neurophysiol. 2012;29:101–8.
26. Cunningham JN Jr, Laschinger JC, Spencer FC. Monitoring of somatosensory evoked potentials during surgical procedures on the thoracoabdominal aorta. IV: clinical observations and results. J Thorac Cardiovasc Surg. 1987;94:275–85.
27. Sutter M, Eggspuehler A, Grob D, et al. The validity of multimodal intraoperative monitoring (MIOM) in surgery of 109 spine and spinal cord tumors. Eur Spine J. 2007;16:S197–208.
28. Costa P, Bruno A, Bonzanino M, et al. Somatosensory- and motor-evoked potential monitoring during spine and spinal cord surgery. Spinal Cord. 2007;45:86–91.
29. Weinzierl MR, Reinacher P, Gilsbach JM, Rohde V. Combined motor and somatosensory evoked potentials for intraoperative monitoring: intra- and postoperative data in a series of 69 operations. Neurosurg Rev. 2007;30:109–16.
30. Etz CD, Halstead JC, Spielvogel D, et al. Thoracic and thoracoabdominal aneurysm repair: is reimplantation of spinal cord arteries a waste of time? Ann Thorac Surg. 2006;82:1670–8.
31. May DM, Jones SJ, Crockard HA. Somatosensory evoked potential monitoring in cervical surgery: identification of pre- and post-operative risk factors associated with neurological deterioration. J Neurosurg. 1996;85:566–73.
32. Lee JY, Hilibrand AS, Lim MR, et al. Characterization of neurophysiologic alerts during anterior cervical spine surgery. Spine. 2006;31:1916–22.
33. Pelosi L, Lamb J, Grevitt M, Mehdian SMH, Webb JK, Blumhardt LD. Combined monitoring of motor and somatosensory evoked potentials in orthopaedic spinal surgery. Clin Neurophysiol. 2002;113:1082–91.
34. Hilibrand AS, Schwartz DM, Sethuraman V, Vaccaro AR, Albert TJ. Comparison of transcranial electrical motor and somatosensory evoked potential monitoring during cervical spine surgery. J Bone Joint Surg. 2004;86A:1248–53.
35. Jacobs MJ, Elenbass TW, Schurink GWH, Mess WH, Mochtar B. Assessment of spinal cord integrity during thoracoabdominal aortic aneurysm repair. Ann Thorac Surg. 2000;74:S1864–6.
36. Langeloo DD, Lelivelt A, Journee L, Slappendel R, de Kleuver M. Transcranial electrical motor-evoked potential monitoring during surgery for spinal deformity: a study of 145 patients. Spine. 2003;28:1043–50.
37. Khan MH, Smith PN, Balzer JB, et al. Intraoperative somatosensory evoked potential monitoring during cervical spine corpectomy surgery: experience with 508 cases. Spine. 2006;31:E105–13.
38. Pastorelli F, Di Silvestre M, Plasmati R, et al. The prevention of neural complications in the surgical treatment of scoliosis: the role of the neurophysiological intraoperative monitoring. Eur Spine J. 2011; 20:S105–14.
39. Lee HJ, Kim IS, Sung JH, Lee SW, Hong JT. Significance of multimodal intraoperative monitoring for the posterior cervical spine surgery. Clin Neurol Neurosurg. 2016;143:9–14.
40. Nuwer MR, Cohen BH, Shepard KM. Practice patterns for intraoperative neurophysiologic monitoring. Neurology. 2013;80:1156–60.
41. American Clinical Neurophysiology Society. Guideline 11A: recommended standards for neurophysiologic intraoperative monitoring – principles. 1994. Available from: http://www.acns.org/pdf/guidelines/Guideline-11A.pdf
42. Modi HN, Suh SW, Yang JH, Yoon JY. False-negative transcranial motor evoked potentials during scoliosis surgery causing paralysis. Spine. 2009;34:E896–900.

Index

L.T. Holly, P.A. Anderson (eds.), *Essentials of Spinal Stabilization*,
DOI 10.1007/978-3-319-59713-3

B

U

V

W

X

Y

MIX
Papier aus verantwortungsvollen Quellen
Paper from responsible sources
FSC® C105338

If you have any concerns about our products,
you can contact us on
ProductSafety@springernature.com

In case Publisher is established outside the EU,
the EU authorized representative is:
Springer Nature Customer Service Center GmbH
Europaplatz 3, 69115 Heidelberg, Germany

Printed by Libri Plureos GmbH
in Hamburg, Germany